AF734457

Medical Radiology

Diagnostic Imaging

Series editors
Hans-Ulrich Kauczor
Hedvig Hricak
Marco Essig

Editorial Board
Andy Adam, London
Fred Avni, Brussels
Richard L. Baron, Chicago
Carlo Bartolozzi, Pisa
George S. Bisset, Durham
A.Mark Davies, Birmingham
William P. Dillon, San Francisco
D. David Dershaw, New York
Sam Sanjiv Gambhir, Stanford
Nicolas Grenier, Bordeaux
Gertraud Heinz-Peer, Vienna
Robert Hermans, Leuven
Theresa McLoud, Boston
Konstantin Nikolaou, Munich
Caroline Reinhold, Montreal
Donald Resnick, San Diego
Rüdiger Schulz-Wendtland, Erlangen
Stephen Solomon, New York
Richard D. White, Columbus

For further volumes:
http://www.springer.com/series/4354

Mariano Scaglione • Ulrich Linsenmaier
Gerd Schueller • Ferco Berger
Stefan Wirth
Editors

Emergency Radiology of the Chest and Cardiovascular System

ESER
European Society of
Emergency Radiology

Springer

Editors
Mariano Scaglione
Department of Radiology
Pineta Grande Hospital
Castel Volturno
Italy

Royal Stoke University Hospital
University Hospitals of North Midlands
NHS Trust
UK

Ulrich Linsenmaier
Ludwig-Maximilians-Universität
München
München
Germany

Gerd Schueller
Vienna
Austria

Ferco Berger
VU University Medical Center
Amsterdam
The Netherlands

Stefan Wirth
University Hospital Munich
Munich
Germany

On behalf of the European Society of Emergency Radiology.

ISSN 0942-5373 ISSN 2197-4187 (electronic)
Medical Radiology
ISBN 978-3-319-42582-5 ISBN 978-3-319-42584-9 (eBook)
DOI 10.1007/978-3-319-42584-9

Library of Congress Control Number: 2016956625

© Springer International Publishing Switzerland 2017
This work is subject to copyright. All rights are reserved by the Publisher, whether the whole or part of the material is concerned, specifically the rights of translation, reprinting, reuse of illustrations, recitation, broadcasting, reproduction on microfilms or in any other physical way, and transmission or information storage and retrieval, electronic adaptation, computer software, or by similar or dissimilar methodology now known or hereafter developed.
The use of general descriptive names, registered names, trademarks, service marks, etc. in this publication does not imply, even in the absence of a specific statement, that such names are exempt from the relevant protective laws and regulations and therefore free for general use.
The publisher, the authors and the editors are safe to assume that the advice and information in this book are believed to be true and accurate at the date of publication. Neither the publisher nor the authors or the editors give a warranty, express or implied, with respect to the material contained herein or for any errors or omissions that may have been made.

Printed on acid-free paper

This Springer imprint is published by Springer Nature
The registered company is Springer International Publishing AG
The registered company address is Gewerbestrasse 11, 6330 Cham, Switzerland

To ESER members, supporters, contributors and friends who are making the ESER Society bigger and bigger! To the ESER founding members who shared with me the dream of setting up a Society of Emergency Radiologists in Europe.

To my parents, Pietro and Ida, and my sons, Pietro and Ruben, with all my love…

Mariano Scaglione

I thank my family and my friends for encouraging and supporting me to work in academic emergency radiology, which is the music of life.

I dedicate this book to my family and my beloved great children, Lukas and Laura, being so nice and understanding to me.

Uli Linsenmaier

This one is for my beloved daughters Nadja, Mona, and Linda. Perhaps one day, you will consider it as helpful in your life.

Gerd Schueller

To my parents and family for their everlasting support.

Ferco Berger

I would like to thank all the active ESER members, the Emergency Radiology community, the other editors, the various authors and the whole Springer Lecture team and editorial staff for making this book possible.

My dedication goes to my family for always having ears for me, supporting me, supplying me with tips and altogether for just being there for me.

Stefan Wirth

Preface

It was only in early January 2011 that a couple of European radiologists sat in Munich, Germany, and aimed to propagate an international platform for a comprehensive academic, scientific, methodologic interdisciplinary communication in emergency radiology. Eventually, the European Society of Emergency Radiology (ESER) was founded under the umbrella of the European Society of Radiology (ESR). From the beginning, this society's aim has on the one hand been transformed and highlighted by annual scientific meetings throughout Europe, serving the needs for a stringent, continuous education and communication regarding our discipline.

On the other hand, it came into light already at an early stage, that annual meetings, as a matter of fact, do not entirely cover intrinsic education in all fields of traumatic as well as nontraumatic emergencies. However, since we face potentially life threatening conditions, imaging the emergencies is a critical issue. Consequently, radiologists must be aware of the great variability of trauma and internal diseases and their adequate characterization in the light of clinical information. In order to share the knowledge in emergency radiology, we initiated a series of dedicated textbooks in 2012 with a publication about abdominal emergencies. We were more than happy having brought together many experts in the field, and up to now the book succeeds in both to immediately resolve diagnostic uncertainties and as a reference source for radiologists interested in the broad field of emergency imaging. In addition, we just started to offer an ongoing series of webinars and began to develop a dedicated European Emergency Radiology training with the aim of offering an European Diploma in Emergency Radiology (EDER).

We are now ready for the next step. It is our pleasure to introduce this new book in your hands about emergent thoracic and cardiovascular disorders to an international readership. Once again it is our true belief that this book will continue to help organize this distinctive body of knowledge in emergency radiology. As compared to its predecessor, this one has an unchanged comprehensively structured outline. The book is divided in three parts: blunt chest trauma, nontraumatic, nonvascular chest emergencies, and vascular chest emergencies which is completed by an emphasis of pulmonary embolism. We aimed to bring as many illustrations as feasible to the reader. Moreover, all chapters provide reflections of the authors' personal insights and opinions about complex and sometimes controversially discussed issues.

In our opinion, it is not by fortune that in this book most disorders introduced are described and discussed on the basis of computed tomography (CT) images. CT has actually changed our insights into emergency-related disorders not later as by the advent of multidetector machines. Indeed, this book provides latest state-of-the art knowledge of a mindset that is considered as the result of a shift of paradigm from modality-based approaches to process-specific practices. In this regard, this book is dedicated to all radiologists who understand emergency imaging as a continuous training as well as an integral part of their highly sophisticated and specialized profession.

We truly believe that this new book continues to help fulfilling the unique demands of modern emergency radiology and thus bringing the European Community of Emergency Radiology both together and forward.

Castel Volturno, Caserta, Italy	Mariano Scaglione, MD
Munich, Germany	Ulrich Linsenmaier, MD
München, Austria	Gerd Schueller, MD, MBA
Amsterdam, The Netherlands	Ferco Berger, MD
Munich, Germany	Stefan Wirth, MD, MBA

Contents

Contributors

P. Agarwal Department of Biomedical Imaging and Image-guided Therapy, Vienna General Hospital, Medical University of Vienna, Vienna, Austria

Ali Alsafi Departments of Radiology, Imperial College London, London, UK

Chiara Andreoli Radiology, Emergency Department, La Sapienza University of Rome, Rome, Italy

Raffaella Basilico Department of Imaging, University of Chieti, Chieti, Italy

Selen Bayraktaroglu Department of Radiology, Ege University Hospital, Izmir, Turkey

Ferco H. Berger Department of Radiology and Nuclear Medicine, VU University Medical Centre, Amsterdam, HZ, Netherlands

Pietro Raimondo Biondetti Fondazione IRCCS Ca' Granda, Ospedale Maggiore Policlinico, Milan, Italy

Luca Brunese Department of Medicine and Health Sciences, Università del Molise, Campobasso, Italy

Grazia Loretta Buquicchio Department of Emergency Radiology, S. Camillo Hospital, Rome, Italy

Teresa Cinque Department of Radiology, Cardarelli Hospital, Naples, Italy

Antonio R. Cotroneo Department of Imaging, University of Chieti, Chieti, Italy

John M. Curtis Aintree University Hospital, Liverpool, UK

Francesco D'Alessandro Department of Imaging, University of Chieti, Chieti, Italy

G. Dalpiaz Radiologia Ospedale Bellaria, AUSL Bologna, Bologna, Italy

Diederick W. De Boo Department of Radiology, Amsterdam Medical Center – University of Amsterdam, Amsterdam, AZ, Netherlands

Elizabeth A. Dick Departments of Radiology, Imperial College London, London, UK

Maurizio Domanin Fondazione IRCCS Ca' Granda, Ospedale Maggiore Policlinico, Milan, Italy

Maureen Dumba Departments of Radiology, Imperial College London, London, UK

Maria Cristina Firetto Fondazione IRCCS Ca' Granda, Ospedale Maggiore Policlinico, Milan, Italy

Paola Franchi Department of Radiological Sciences, Fondazione Policlinico A. Gemelli, Catholic University, Roma, Italy

Nicola Gagliardi Department of Radiology, Cardarelli Hospital, Naples, Italy

Michele Galluzzo Department of Emergency Radiology, S. Camillo Hospital, Rome, Italy

Lucas L. Geyer Institute for Clinical Radiology, LMU Ludwig-Maximilians-University Hospital Munich, Munich, Germany

Roberto Grassi Department of Radiology, Second University of Naples, Naples, Italy

Department of Imaging, Castel Volturno, Italy

Stefania Ianniello Department of Emergency Radiology, S. Camillo Hospital, Rome, Italy

Stephan Jansen Ludwig-Maximilians-University, Munich, Germany

Elika Kashef Departments of Radiology, Imperial College London, London, UK

Francesca Lacobellis Department of Radiology, Second University of Naples, Naples, Italy

Department of Imaging, Castel Volturno, Italy

Anna Rita Larici Department of Radiological Sciences, Fondazione Policlinico A. Gemelli, Catholic University, Roma, Italy

Carlo Liguori Department of Radiology, Cardarelli Hospital, Naples, Italy

Ulrich Linsenmaier Institute for Diagnostic and Interventional Radiology, HELIOS Kliniken München West, Ludwig-Maximilians-University Munich (LMU), ESER – European Society of Emergency Radiology, Munich, Germany

Maria Teresa Martino Department of Radiology, Second University of Naples, Naples, Italy

Department of Imaging, Castel Volturno, Italy

Manuela Mereu Department of Imaging, University of Chieti, Chieti, Italy

Vittorio Miele Department of Emergency Radiology, S. Camillo Hospital, Rome, Italy

R. Nicola Department of Imaging Science, Division of Emergency Imaging, University of Rochester, Rochester, NY, USA

A. Olsen Department of Imaging Science, Division of Emergency Imaging, University of Rochester, Rochester, NY, USA

Rosa Lucia Patea Department of Imaging, University of Chieti, Chieti, Italy

M. Patlas Division of Emergency/Trauma Radiology, Department of Radiology, McMaster University, Hamilton, ON, Canada

Marcello Petrini Università degli Studi di Milano, Postgraduation School in Radiodiagnostics, Milan, Italy

Claudia Lucia Piccolo Department of Emergency Radiology, S. Camillo Hospital, Rome, Italy

Department of Medicine and Health Sciences, Università del Molise, Campobasso, Italy

Antonio Pinto Department of Radiology, Cardarelli Hospital, Naples, Italy

M. Piolanti Radiologia Ospedale Maggiore, AUSL Bologna, Bologna, Italy

H. Prosch Department of Biomedical Imaging and Image-guided Therapy, Vienna General Hospital, Medical University of Vienna, Vienna, Austria

C. Raptis Mallinckrodt Institute of Radiology, Washington University School of Medicine, St Louis, MO, USA

Luigia Romano Department of Radiology, Cardarelli Hospital, Naples, Italy

Department of Emergency Radiology, Cardarelli Hospital, Naples, Italy

Roberto Ronza Department of Radiology, Second University of Naples, Naples, Italy

Department of Imaging, Castel Volturno, Italy

Claudia Rossi Department of Radiology, Second University of Naples, Naples, Italy

Department of Imaging, Castel Volturno, Italy

Francesco Sala Department of Radiology, A.O. Papa Giovanni XXIII, Bergamo, Italy

Mariano Scaglione Department of Imaging, Pineta Grande Medical Center, Castel Volturno, Italy

G. Schueller Academic Health, Opfikon, Switzerland

Florian Schwarz Institut für Klinische Radiologie, Klinikum der Universität München (LMU), München, Germany

Alessandro Stasolla Department of Emergency Radiology, S. Camillo Hospital, Rome, Italy

Giovanni Terribile Fondazione IRCCS Ca' Granda, Ospedale Maggiore Policlinico, Milan, Italy

Sujit Vaidya Department of Radiology, The Royal London Hospital, Barts and the London NHS Trust, London, UK

Tullio Valente Department of Imaging, Section of Radiology, Azienda Ospedali dei Colli, Naples, Italy

Stefan Wirth Institute for Clinical Radiology, Hospital of the Ludwig-Maximilians-University, Munich, Germany

Part I

Blunt Chest Trauma

Lung Injury

Vittorio Miele, Grazia Loretta Buquicchio, Claudia Lucia Piccolo, Alessandro Stasolla, and Michele Galluzzo

Contents

Abstract

Thoracic trauma is the most common injury in polytrauma patients, with an incidence rate of 45–65%, and the most common cause of trauma deaths (about 20 % of all deaths), second only to head injuries.

In the time-sensitive acute care setting, efficiency and rapidity are basic. The Chest-X-Ray (CXR) may be considered as an adjunct to the initial assessment or primary survey of unstable traumatic patients. It helps to identify a tension pneumothorax (PNX) and pleural effusions that may suggest a hemothorax, until further evidence.

MultiSlice Computed Tomography (MSCT) is always the last step of the diagnostic procedures for stable patients, regardless of the positive or negative results on CXR, being the gold standard for the radiologic evaluation of the chest in traumatic patients.

This chapter will review the wide spectrum of radiographic and MSCT findings in patients undergoing a thoracic trauma, both blunt and penetrating, with a particular focus on the role of the radiologist in the management of major trauma, together with the "trauma team".

V. Miele (✉) • G.L. Buquicchio • C.L. Piccolo
A. Stasolla • M. Galluzzo
Department of Emergency Radiology,
S. Camillo Hospital, Circonvallazione
Gianicolense, 87, Rome 00152, Italy
e-mail: vmiele@sirm.org

Med Radiol Diagn Imaging (2016)
DOI 10.1007/174_2016_51,

© Springer International Publishing Switzerland

1 Introduction

1.1 Epidemiology and Mechanism of Injury

Thoracic trauma is the most frequent injury in polytrauma patients, with an incidence rate of 45–65 %, second only to head injuries. Even though some mechanisms of injury may result in thoracic penetrating trauma from sharp objects, thoracic trauma is more often due to high-energy blunt trauma, with a mortality rate approaching 60 %. According to some statistics, thoracic trauma represents the most common cause of trauma deaths (about 20 % of all deaths), next to head trauma (Gaillard M 1990).

Among the causes of a high-energy blunt trauma (high-height falls, workplace accidents, etc.), traffic accidents account for 70–80 % of the patients; moreover, one-third of hospitalized patients following a traffic accident may present signs of major thoracic trauma.

Several studies have shown that, when a car crash occurs, passengers wearing a seat belt may sustain significant thoracic injuries at a speed of at least 48 km/h, whereas unrestrained passengers may suffer severe injuries even at an impact speed of 16 km/h. Therefore, a lot of authors recommend the use of multi-slice computed tomography (MSCT), irrespective of the findings of the chest X-ray (CXR), supine anterior-posterior projection (AP view) of the thorax, to avoid ignoring potentially fatal chest injuries (Traub M et al 2007; Van Hise ML et al. 1998).

However, other authors have highlighted the importance of not underestimating falls from low heights, particularly in the aging population, to whom even minor trauma may be fatal. The mechanisms of injury of pleuro-parenchymal traumas will be treated in the sections concerning the different types of injuries: here, it is only pointed out that the elastic characteristics of the chest wall, particularly in infants and young children, can frequently result in the presence of significant pleuro-parenchymal injuries (e.g., hemopneumothorax) associated with an intact rib cage (about ¼ of cases).

As regards lungs and abdominal organs, it is available a scientific and clinical classification, an injury grading system from the American Association for the Surgery of Trauma (AAST). However, this injury scale will not be reported in this study, because there is not much literature available.

1.2 The Role of the Radiologist

The radiologist should always play a central role in the management of major traumas (Injury Severity Score >15), together with the "trauma team" (surgeon, anesthetist, nursing staff, and radiographers). Moreover, the radiologist should be familiar with the general principles of the state-of-the-art clinical polytrauma management that in many institutions is based on the Advanced Trauma Life Support (ATLS) protocols (periodically updated) from the American College of Surgeons Committee on Trauma. Nevertheless, it is not stated that the role of the radiologist involved in the polytrauma management is unquestionably that provided by the ATLS protocols, but that a sound knowledge of the general ATLS principles is essential to have full awareness of his clinical role: only such "self-awareness" will allow him to express himself to the best as well as to defend himself from undue and unfounded demands.

For the radiologist, the key principles of ATLS are probably two: "treat first that kills first" and "imaging should not intervene with or postpone treatment." Ultimately, this means that any condition that threatens airway, breathing, circulation, and disability (ABCD) is to be treated according to priorities for the immediate patient survival, using diagnostic imaging if and when very appropriate, however, never before the stabilization of the patient's vital signs, knowing that "the lack of a definitive diagnosis should never delay an indicated treatment." (Mayberry JC et al. 2000)

In the following chapter, only limited to consider lungs and pleura, it is suggested that, when an appropriate radiological assessment is obtained, the radiologist has to evaluate the findings according to the well-known priorities ABC: airway, breathing, and circulation. Regarding the pleura and lung parenchyma, there are two diagnostic high priorities: tension pneumothorax and bleeding, particularly active bleeding within the parenchyma and the pleural space (pulmonary hematoma and hemothorax).

In brief: obtaining diagnostic assessments according to ABCD priorities and evaluating images according to the same ABCD priorities.

1.3 Diagnostic Imaging

In the emergency setting, the CXR, anteroposterior radiogram of the thorax, acquired with the patient in clinostasis, may be considered as an adjunct to the initial assessment or primary survey of trauma patients. An appropriate diagnostic imaging cannot interfere with the resuscitation process and, if necessary, can and has to be postponed until the secondary survey.

According to some authors, in the initial assessment of trauma patients, CXR should be done together with the cervical rachis and pelvis X-ray: it should be performed only on unstable patients as well as on patients with abnormal findings on chest examination.

Regarding the pleura and lung assessment, the first aim of a radiologist performing a CXR is to inspect for evidence of a tension pneumothorax (PNX) and pleural effusions that may suggest a hemothorax, until further evidence (Ianniello S et al. 2014). The diagnosis of hematoma is difficult, and the differential diagnosis for parenchymal contusion essentially remains a prerogative of MSCT. (Peters S et al. 2010; Rivas LA et al 2003)

MSCT is always performed in the secondary survey of the trauma patients; it is only addressed to hemodynamically stable patients or to patients already stabilized by the trauma team.

An unstable patient should not be moved in an MSCT suite in life-threatening conditions. Diagnostic assessment should be obtained simultaneously with the appropriate therapeutic procedures during the exploratory laparotomy and/or thoracotomy. When the patient's clinical conditions require an immediate surgical intervention, CXR closes the chest preoperative diagnostic procedures (further assessments are postponed to potential postoperative MSCT follow-up), remaining, moreover, the imaging modality of choice for subsequent assessments. (Roy-Choudhury SH et al. 2007; Ryan MF et al. 2004).

On the contrary, after the trauma team has obtained the patient's stabilization, it is necessary to continue with a second, more accurate diagnostic assessment (secondary survey) to be performed on MSCT (Miele V et al. 2015).

Stabilized patients, with normal physical examination for thoracic injury, should undergo a MSCT scan, regardless the findings on CXR. It has been proved that 39–50 % of trauma patients with unremarkable CXR may present multiple lesions on CT scan, leading to a change in the therapeutic management in 5 % of cases; on the other hand, trauma patients with remarkable CXR present further lesions on CT in the 66 % of cases, resulting in a treatment change in 20 % of cases.

In a recent population-based survey of patients admitted to ED following a high-energy trauma (such as falls from a height exceeding 3 m; traffic accidents at a speed higher than 50 km/h; ejections from the vehicle; vehicle rollovers; severe deformity of the passenger compartment; pedestrian accidents >10 km/h; bicycle collisions at a speed higher than 30 km/h; crush injury), the findings on a routine chest MSCT (even with unremarkable chest X-ray as well as normal physical examination) have allowed to diagnose additional findings in 43 % of the patients, compared with the conventional chest radiography, and have required a change in the management in 17 % of all patients.

Finally, some authors suggest to directly perform MSCT, which is by far more accurate in the detection of silent but potentially life-threatening clinical findings on stable patients with normal chest examination (such as small flaps of pneumothoraces, which in case of following intubation can lead to tension PNX).

With regard to the penetrating trauma, the previously stated principles are valid, but with a distinction: even if pneumothorax and hemothorax may be diagnosed on CXR, the MSCT screening is strictly recommended even in patients with an unremarkable CXR, in order to rule them out. Furthermore, patients with penetrating thoracic injuries may be likely to suffer abdominal injuries, until further evidence (Scaglione M et al. 2008; Scott et al. 2015; Sivit CJ et al. 1989).

In brief: the diagnostic procedures of the thorax for unstable patients finish with the execution of CXR, as part of the primary survey; the execution of MSCT is always the last step of the diagnostic procedures for stable patients, regardless of the positive or negative results on CXR. Some authors suggest the immediate execution of MSCT scan in stable patients presenting normal thoracic examination; but, according to the standard practice of many institutions, the CXR comes before MSCT anyway.

2 Pulmonary Contusion

Pulmonary contusion is the most common parenchymal lung injury seen in blunt thoracic trauma, with a prevalence of 30–75 % of cases. Pulmonary contusion is a hemorrhagic-edematous focal deposit, suggestive of a damage to the capillary-alveolar membrane, in the alveolar and interstitial space. The parenchymal architecture remains overall intact, even if associated parenchymal lacerations can be sometimes detected within the areas of contusion (Cohn SM 1997; Shanmuganathan K et al. 1999; Wagner 1988).

The mechanism of injury of pulmonary contusion is represented by a direct trauma (contusion on the lung immediately adjacent to the area of impact) or by a contrecoup trauma (contusion at the site opposite the impact). In the setting of high-energy deceleration trauma (i.e., motor-vehicle accidents), alveoli are subjected to sudden frictional forces (shear stress) from the bronchovascular peduncles; direct trauma may disrupt pulmonary alveoli (pulmonary contusions associated with lacerations, as in the case of a fractured rib); and the transmitted kinetic energy may deposit locally at a liquid-gas interface such as air-blood relationship in pulmonary alveoli.

Clinical symptoms, which about 50 % of patients present, include hemoptysis (transudation of blood within the alveolar spaces and the airways), mild fever, tachypnea, hypoxia, bronchorrhea, and acute respiratory failure.

Reduced lung compliance, reduced ventilation per unit volume, and increased shunt fraction are typical signs of contused pulmonary areas; the thickening of the alveolar septa reduces the locoregional gas diffusion in the contused lung.

In severe pulmonary contusion, the local response to the injury has systemic consequences, being related to a rise of the bronchoalveolar lavage (BAL) protein as well as an increase in capillary permeability: macroscopic and microscopic alterations, increased polymorphonuclear cells (neutrophils) even within the uninjured lung tissue, as well as increased local and systemic complement levels.

Most severe contusions requiring mechanical ventilation are associated with severe rib cage injury, although they are not necessarily associated with rib or sternal fracture. In particular, flail chest, the most severe form of blunt chest wall injury with mortality rates of 10–20 %, is typically associated with significant pulmonary contusion. The diagnosis of contusion is associated with the deterioration in the prognosis, above all, in the pediatric population (Trindade LM et al. 2009).

A strong correlation exists between the size of the pulmonary contusions and the mortality rate as well as the comorbidities for ARDS or pneumonia. Mortality rate for lung contusion varies from 14 to 40 %, depending on the severity of the extension. It is important to underline that the actual extension of a contusion cannot be detected at the initial radiologic work-up but it may be evident by 72 h following injury.

2.1 Diagnostic Imaging

Parenchymal contusion is the most common cause of pulmonary opacity on CXR after blunt chest trauma, occurring in 30–75 % of patients.

Radiographically, pulmonary contusion presents as focal or multifocal areas of confluent "ground-glass" opacity (Figs. 1 and 2) or consolidation (Fig. 3). Contusions are not limited by segmental boundaries and are usually visible in the lung periphery adjacent to the area of direct trauma. If contusion does not reveal perifocal injury site associated with parenchymal laceration, its pattern appears homogeneous, without any cavitation. Contusions may not be radiographically visible within 6 h after the

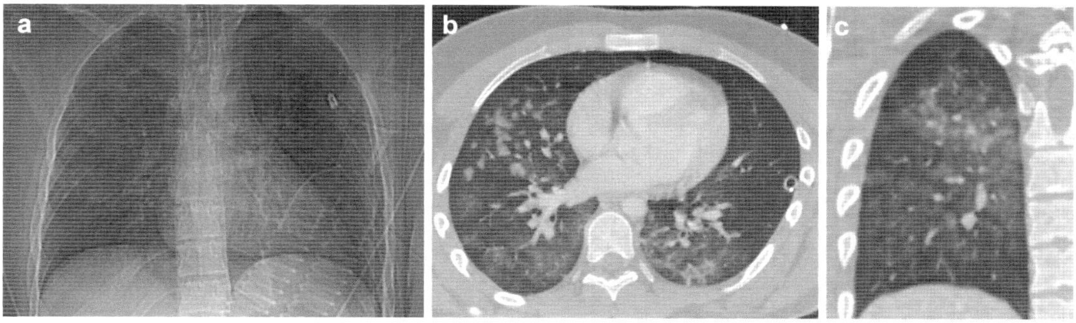

Fig. 1 (**a**) CXR: pulmonary contusions may appear as single or multifocal "ground-glass" area. The ground-glass pattern is indicative of an interstitial damage with partial alveolar filling. (**b**) Axial CT scan and (**c**) coronal reconstruction well depict the ground glass

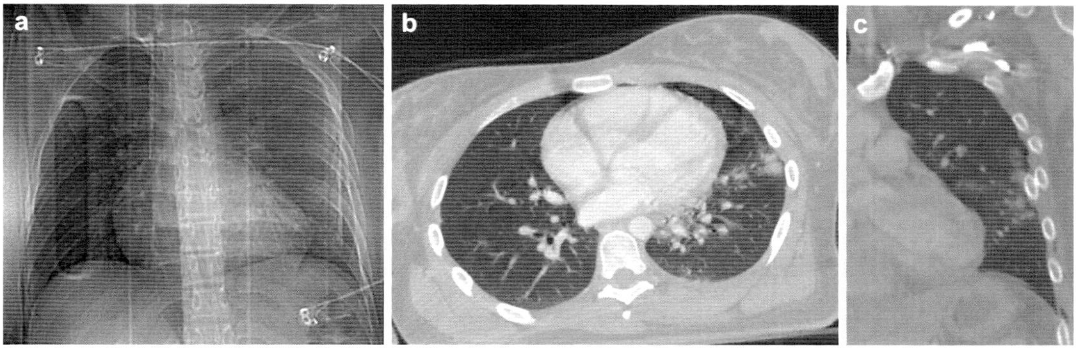

Fig. 2 (**a**) CXR, (**b**) axial CT scan, and (**c**) coronal reconstruction demonstrate the presence of contemporary ground-glass and parenchymal consolidation pattern

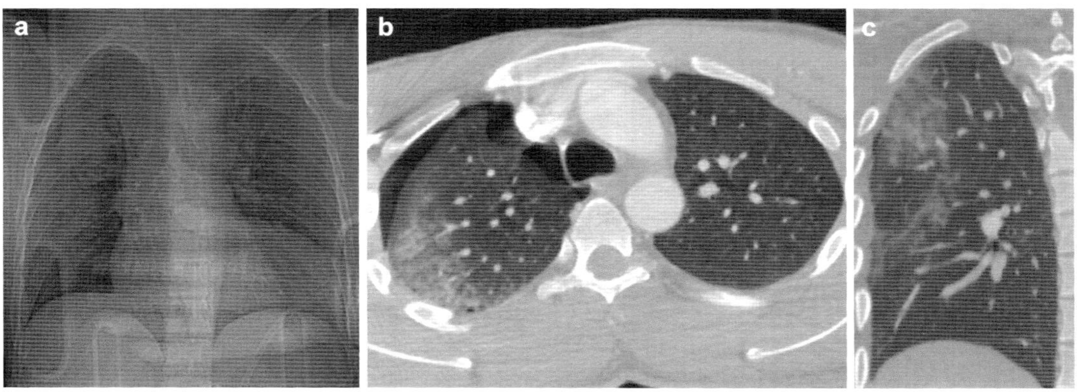

Fig. 3 (**a**) CXR, (**b**) axial CT scan, and (**c**) coronal reconstruction show severe contusion, which can appear as a parenchymal consolidation. The consolidation pattern is indicative of severe alveolar damage. In this patient it is associated with a wide apical ipsilateral pneumothorax

trauma; they may develop progressively within 24–72 h, when maximum conspicuity is reached. Finally, uncomplicated contusions may resolve gradually after 3–10 days: pulmonary opacities, which do not clear or increase within such a period, raise the suspicion of developing secondary infection or acute respiratory distress syndrome (ARDS).

CT is highly sensitive in detecting pulmonary contusions: in experimental models, CT can detect pulmonary contusion in 100 % of cases compared with 37.5 % by chest radiographs, and it provides an accurate detection of the extent of the injury. However, there is a possibility that pulmonary contusions only visible on CT are not clinically significant. The feature on CT is dependent on the injury severity: "ground-glass opacity" is indicative of a mainly interstitial damage with partial alveolar filling, whereas consolidation is indicative of a severe alveolar damage, often associated with lacerations.

2.2 Differential Diagnosis

It may manifest as pathology of the airspaces, and differential diagnosis considers aspiration, atelectasis, and pneumonia. They all may have identical radiographic findings. Radiographic features of atelectasis include triangular shape and signs associated with volume loss; those of laceration the cavitating pattern within the radiopaque area. Lack of contusion clearance within 7–8 days should raise the suspicion of either associated laceration, pneumonia, or ARDS.

Air bronchogram sign is rare because distal airways are usually filled with blood or edema.

3 Pulmonary Laceration

Pulmonary lacerations are evident tears in the lung parenchyma, usually resulting either from shearing stress forces, secondary to high-energy trauma, or from direct puncture, i.e., due to fractured rib fragments. They may be associated with contusions that should represent a minor parenchymal damage. Clinically, pulmonary lacerations may manifest as hemoptysis.

Multiple types of lacerations can be seen in the same injured parenchyma simultaneously. They are usually benign lesions, although some complications may arise: infection, bronchopleural fistula, enlargement and subsequent compression of the surrounding parenchyma, and hemorrhage.

3.1 Diagnostic Imaging

The radiographic findings are variable and can change after admission to ED in subsequent examinations. The elastic recoil properties of the surrounding lung parenchyma give a round shape to the lacerations that are often difficult to identify on CXR. The space created by the tissue disruption may be filled with air, blood (hematoma), or more often both air and blood, creating air-fluid levels. In the acute stage, the blood, collected in the laceration, shows up a well-defined homogenous opacity, with density of soft tissue. Lacerations, sometimes masked by associated pulmonary contusions, become clearly detectable on serial follow-up examination, thanks to the clearance of the contusions. Lacerations, in fact, become more visible days after the trauma, with the shrinking of the edema and the hemorrhage, both associated with contusion. On occasion, small and multiple lacerative lesions are visible within areas of parenchymal contusion, in the form of focal uniform density, with a "Swiss cheese appearance." Within areas of contusion, the detection of round, homogeneously dense focuses, indicative of multiple hematomas, is not rare.

With time, the hematoma within the laceration resolves, and it is replaced with a round or oval air cavity, referred to as posttraumatic pneumatocele. The posttraumatic pneumatocele appears within few days from trauma, but, in some cases, it can be evident after months; its size is usually 2–5 cm.

The detection of pulmonary lacerations is highly sensitive on MSCT, and, consequently, a classification into four types is possible:

Type 1: it is the most common type, centrally located; it results from shearing stress forces, developed between the lung parenchyma and the tracheobronchial tree (Fig. 4).

Type 2: often seen as a tubular lesion in the lower lobes, resulting from a compression force of the parenchyma across the vertebral body (the spine) (Fig. 5).

Type 3: it is small, rounded, peripherally located, associated with rib fractures and a PNX (Fig. 6).

Type 4: it is a tear in the preexisting pleuropulmonary adhesions; it is usually diagnosed only at surgery or autopsy.

Pulmonary lacerations usually resolve over a period of 3 weeks to a year; although uncommon, they may indefinitely persist as pulmonary nodular opacity; years later, when blood is expectorated, they may appear as pulmonary cysts (Ulutas H, et al. 2015).

More rarely, due to the reduced pulmonary compliance, the laceration is visible as evident gas-filled scarring and extrabronchial development.

Within particularly large lesions, the hematoma may have expanding force and may be associated with hemodynamically significant hemorrhage.

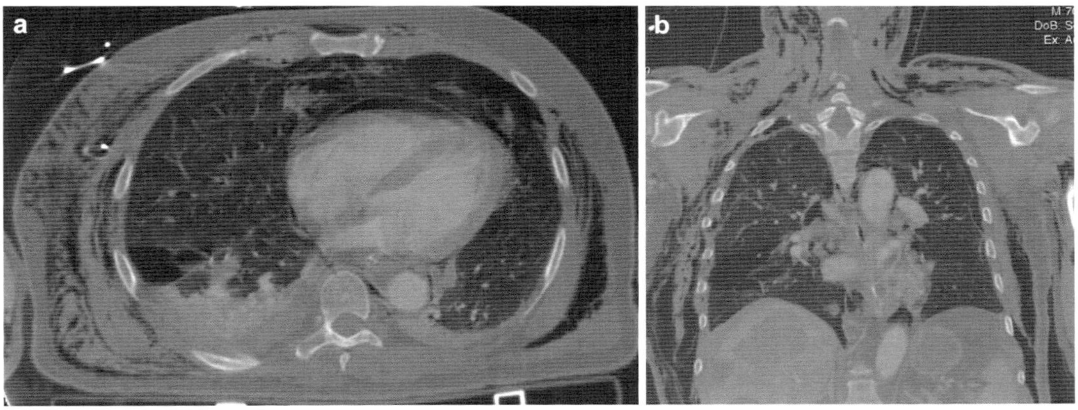

Fig. 4 (**a**) Axial CT scan, (**b**) coronal reconstruction: pulmonary laceration, type 1. Large parenchymal lacerations, peripherally located. In this patient, associated are pneumopericardium and extensive subcutaneous emphysema of the chest wall

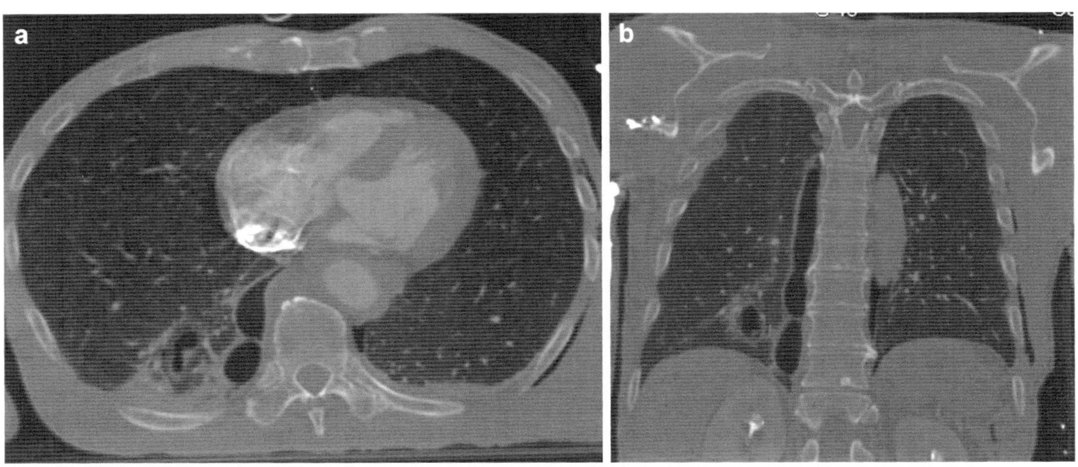

Fig. 5 (**a**) Axial CT scan and (**b**) coronal reconstruction: pulmonary lacerations, type 2. They appear as tubular lesions, more frequent in lower lobes, near the spine. They are the result of a compression force of the parenchyma across the spine

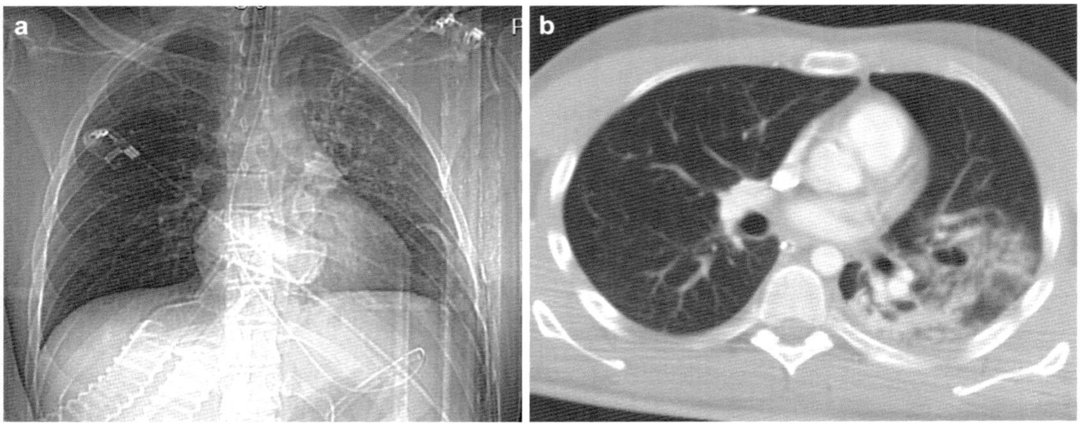

Fig. 6 (**a**) CXR, (**b**) axial CT: lacerations, type 3. This is the most common type. These lacerations are located centrally, usually in the context of a large contusion area ("Swiss cheese appearance")

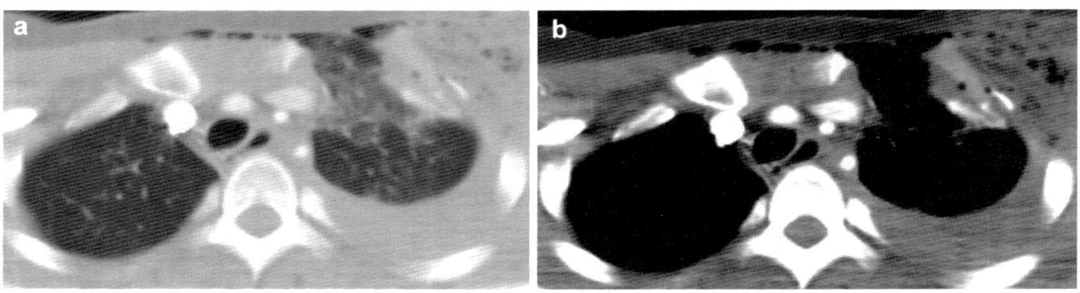

Fig. 7 (**a**, **b**) Axial CT scan. Traumatic hernia of the left lung. The anterolateral wall of the chest is thinner and more exposed to traumatic lung herniation. It often results from rib fractures, as appreciable in this case

4 Pulmonary Hernia

Lung herniation is an uncommon complication of blunt chest trauma, whereas it is more common with penetrating trauma.

It may occur through either a congenital or an acquired parietal opening, resulting from rib fractures or costochondral or sternoclavicular dislocations.

The anterolateral chest wall is more susceptible to traumatic lung herniation (Fig. 7), because of the minimal muscle thickness (intercostal muscles), compared to the posterior wall, reinforced by strong muscle planes (trapezius, latissimus dorsi, rhomboid).

The intercostal hernias may be associated with a hemothorax or a pneumothorax, secondary to strangulation or incarceration of the lung parenchyma. In symptomatic cases, a rarely necessary surgical reduction is indicated.

5 Atelectasis

Following a blunt chest trauma, large or small parts of the lung parenchyma may present atelectasis, correlated with the following pathogenic mechanisms: obstructive, compressive, passive, and adhesive atelectasis.

The obstructive atelectasis is a consequence of either mucous plugging, foreign bodies (i.e., dentures), endobronchial blood clot, bronchorrhea, or airway rupture. Large lacerated and/or contused areas may cause compressive atelectasis, as a result of passive atelectasis, eliminating contact between the parietal and visceral pleurae, thereby preventing the natural lung expansion.

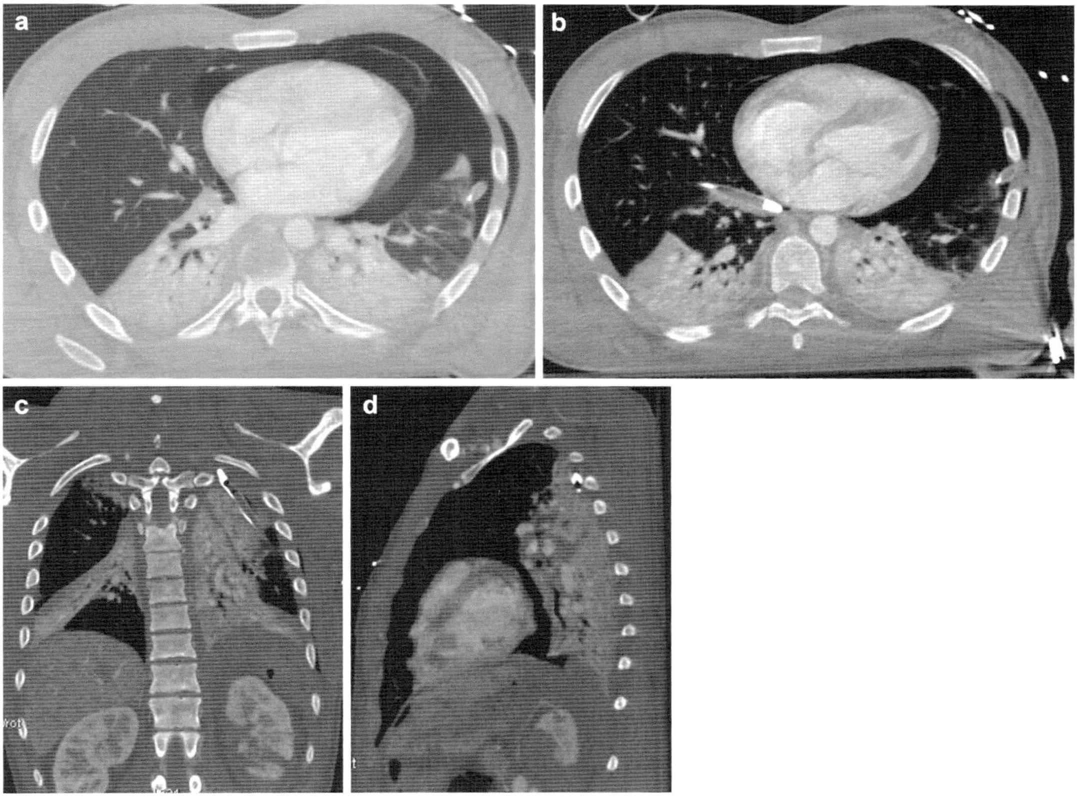

Fig. 8 (**a**, **b**) Axial CT scans: wide bilateral atelectasis of lower lobes. The greater enhancement of atelectasis is due to the associated crowding of pulmonary vessels; (**c**) coronal and (**d**) sagittal reconstructions clearly demonstrate the pulmonary volume loss. In this patient, associated is an anterobasal bilateral pneumothorax.

Finally, the so-called adhesive atelectasis is a condition of primitive alveoli collapse in association with surfactant deficiency, generally caused by concurrent contused phenomena. In the past, atelectasis was associated with dyspnea and fever, but recent studies have not suggested that fever should be considered a sign of some underlying disorder.

5.1 Diagnostic Imaging

Diagnosis of obstructive atelectasis is based on the located reduction of parenchymal volume and air: radiological signs include lobar, segmental, or subsegmental opacity, without the presence of air bronchograms, associated with displacement of fissures, hilum, mediastinum, and ipsilateral hemidiaphragm (Wanek S, Mayberry JC 2004).

In compressive atelectasis, the atelectatic lung becomes visible as radiopaque edge adjacent to the contused/lacerated area. In passive atelectasis, the parenchymal opacity may essentially remain normal, due to the consensual local-regional reduction of air and blood; air bronchogram is frequently visible if bronchial vessels are not filled with secretion or blood, as is the case in adhesive atelectasis.

It must be pointed out that the different types of atelectasis are variously associated in the traumatized. The dense, *homogeneous* appearance, associated with fissure deviation, allows a differential diagnosis between contusion and pulmonary aspiration.

On MSCT, atelectasis usually demonstrates a greater enhancement after contrast medium, compared to the consolidative lung in contusion, due to the associated crowding of pulmonary vessels. Secondary signs of volume loss are clearly visible, thanks to the MPR reconstructions (Fig. 8).

References

Cohn SM (1997) Pulmonary contusion: review of the clinical entity. J Trauma 42:973–979

Gaillard M, Hervé C, Mandin L, Raynaud P (1990) Mortality prognostic factors in chest injury. J Trauma 30:93–96

Ianniello S, Di Giacomo V, Sessa B, Miele V (2014) First-line sonographic diagnosis of pneumothorax in major trauma: accuracy of e-FAST and comparison with multidetector computed tomography. Radiol Med 119: 674–680.

Mayberry JC (2000) Imaging in thoracic trauma: the trauma surgeon's perspective. J Thorac Imaging 15:76–86

Miele V, Di Giampietro I, Ianniello S, Pinto F, Trinci M (2014) Diagnostic imaging in pediatric polytrauma management. Radiol Med 120:33–49

Peters S, Nicolas V, Heyer CM (2010) Multidetector computed tomography-spectrum of blunt chest wall and lung injuries in polytraumatized patients. Clin Radiol 65:333–338

Rivas LA, Fishman JE, Munera F et al (2003) Multislice CT in thoracic trauma. Radiol Clin North Am 41: 599–616

Roy-Choudhury SH, Gallacher DJ, Pilmer J et al (2007) Relative threshold of detection of active arterial bleeding: In vitro comparison of MDCT and digital subtraction angiography. AJR Am J Roentgenol 189:W238–W246

Ryan MF, Hamilton PA, Chu P et al (2004) Active extravasation of arterial contrast agent on post-traumatic abdominal computed tomography. Can Assoc Radiol J 55:160–169

Scaglione M, Pinto A, Pedrosa I et al (2008) Multidetector row computed tomography and blunt chest trauma. Eur J Radiol 65:377–388

Scott MF, Khodaverdian RA, Shaheen JL et al (2015) Predictors of retained hemothorax after trauma and impact on patient outcomes. Eur J Trauma Emerg Surg. Epub ahead of print

Shanmuganathan K, Mirvis SE (1999) Imaging diagnosis of nonaortic thoracic injury. Radiol Clin North Am 37:533–551

Sivit CJ, Peclet MH, Taylor GA (1989) Life-threatening intraperitoneal bleeding: demonstration with CT. Radiology 71:430

Traub M, Stevenson M, McEvoy S et al (2007) The use of chest computed tomography versus chest X-ray in patients with major blunt trauma. Injury 38:43–47

Trindade LM, Lopes LC, Cipriano GF et al (2009) Alveolar recruitment in pulmonary contusion: case report and literature review. Rev Bras Ter Intens 21:104–108

Ulutas H, Celik MR, Ozgel M et al (2015) Pulmonary pseudocyst secondary to blunt or penetrating chest trauma: clinical course and diagnostic issues. Eur J Trauma Emerg Surg 41:181–188

Van Hise ML, Primack SL, Israel RS et al (1998) CT in blunt chest trauma: indications and limitations. Radiographics 18:1071–1084

Wagner RB, Crawford WO Jr, Schimpf PP (1988) Classification of parenchymal injuries of the lung. Radiology 167:77–82

Wanek S, Mayberry JC (2004) Blunt thoracic trauma: flail chest, pulmonary contusion, and blast injury. Crit Care Clin 20:71–81

Injuries of the Pleural Spaces

Vittorio Miele, Grazia Loretta Buquicchio, Claudia Lucia Piccolo, Alessandro Stasolla, Stefania Ianniello, and Luca Brunese

Contents

V. Miele (✉) • G.L. Buquicchio • A. Stasolla
S. Ianniello
Department of Emergency Radiology,
S. Camillo Hospital, Circonvallazione Gianicolense, 87,
Rome 00152, Italy
e-mail: vmiele@sirm.org

C.L. Piccolo • L. Brunese
Department of Medicine and Health Sciences,
Università del Molise, Contrada Tappino,
Campobasso, Italy

Abstract

The presence of thoracic injuries in a multisystemic trauma can highly increase patient mortality; furthermore, injuries such as "flail chest," lung contusion, hemothorax, and pneumothorax can complicate overall case management.

Chest-X-Ray (CXR) is the first imaging step to perform in a thoracic trauma, to highlight a possible pneumothorax, hemothorax, and other life-threatening conditions. MultiSlice Computed Tomography (MDCT) is more accurate than CXR for the evaluation of pleural injuries, although it is to be performed in stable patients only.

In this chapter, pleural abnormalities following blunt thoracic trauma and the role of CXR and MSCT will be discussed (pneumothorax, hemothorax), with a small digression about pleural drainages and the importance to recognize a possible dislocation to prevent severe complications.

1 Introduction

Thoracic injuries are the third most common injuries in polytrauma patients, next to head and extremities' injuries (Ahmad et al. 2013); they have an overall fatality rate of 10.1 %, highest in patients with cardiac or tracheobronchial-esophageal injuries (Ahmad et al. 2013). Furthermore, the presence of thoracic injuries in a multisystemic trauma can highly increase patient mortality. Injuries such

Med Radiol Diagn Imaging (2016)
DOI 10.1007/174_2016_29, © Springer International Publishing Switzerland

as "flail chest," lung contusion, hemothorax, and pneumothorax can complicate overall case management (Tocino et al. 1985). More than two-thirds of cases of blunt thoracic trauma are caused by motor vehicle collisions in developed countries. The remaining cases are due to falls or of blows from blunt objects (Ahmad et al. 2013; Cothren et al. 2007; Miele et al. 2015). Imaging plays a key role in the diagnosis of blunt thoracic trauma.

Conventional radiography is typically performed as the first imaging investigation, even if computed tomography (CT) is to be performed. Chest-X-Rays (CXR), when correctly performed, may show a tension pneumothorax, a large hemothorax, a tube and line malpositioning, and other conditions that require immediate treatment. Concerning the development of CT in this setting, several studies have shown that it may demonstrate a life-threatening disease (e.g., thoracic aortic injury) in patients with normal radiographs at the beginning (Alkadhi et al. 2004). Moreover, CT has been demonstrated to change the management in up to 20% of chest trauma patients with abnormal initial radiographs (Błasińska-Przerwa et al. 2013). CT is more accurate than radiography for the evaluation of pulmonary contusion, and it is also valuable in the diagnosis of fractures of the thoracic spine, especially at the cervicothoracic junction, which is difficult to evaluate with conventional radiography (Brink et al. 2008, 2010; Detorakis and Androulidakis 2014).

In this chapter, pleural abnormalities following blunt thoracic trauma and the role of CXR and multi-slice-computed tomography (MSCT) will be discussed (pneumothorax, hemothorax), with a small digression about pleural drainages and the importance to recognize a possible dislocation to prevent severe complications.

2 Pneumothorax

The term pneumothorax (PNX) refers to the presence of air in the pleural space: it affects 60% of patients with severe thoracic trauma, and it can be rapidly fatal even in the absence of other injuries. PNX is open when it communicates with the atmosphere through an open wound; otherwise it is a closed PNX, and it may occur due to different mechanisms of injuries: fragments of fractured rib arches may lacerate the parietal pleura layer; even in the absence of rib cage fractures, the intra-alveolar pressure, following a thoracic compression, may exceed the intrapleural pressure; hence, the passage of air into the pleural space may lacerate the visceral pleura. Finally, another possible mechanism of injury is the laceration of proximal airways. The leading causes of iatrogenic pneumothorax include central venous catheter insertion, thoracentesis, and barotrauma as a result of mechanical ventilator.

Simple PNX occurs when the pressure of the air in the pleural space does not exceed that of the atmosphere; the air pressure increases (tension PNX) when a pleural-parenchymal or bronchial injury acts as a one-way valve, namely, allowing air inflow into the pleural space on inspiration but prohibiting air outflow. Tension PNX is the most severe form of PNX, which may result in a fatal cardiopulmonary failure, and it is a common cause of death for thoracic trauma.

PNX clinical relevance depends not only on its dimensions but also on the hemodynamic conditions of patients; in fact, also a small pneumothorax can become hemodynamically significant on patients under mechanical ventilation. Massive PNX and tension PNX are life-threatening conditions and should be recognized and treated before performing any radiological evaluation. In this study, it is pointed out that the detection of a PNX requires the radiologist to give an immediate communication to the trauma leader; this communication must be written in the clinical report, as well.

Considering the numerous clinical and radiological modalities for the detection of PNX as well as the availability of treatment procedures that can be adjusted to the context and the health-care providers' experience (such as needle decompression at the trauma setting, decompression with small-caliber drains, drainage tube placement, decompressive minithoracotomy), death due to PNX can be regarded as preventable; in trauma patients, death is caused by inadequate care and treatment rather than by the severity of the injuries sustained.

2.1 Diagnostic Imaging

Many authors have given evidence of the superiority of MSCT for the diagnosis of PNX and have recommended its employment. In most cases, the diagnosis of PNX on MSCT is easily successful, whereas the diagnosis is considered difficult on CXR (radiogram on anterior-posterior view with patient in supine position): it has been often proved that many cases of undetected PNX have been only diagnosed on MSCT (Gavelli et al. 2007). Occult pneumothorax is a pneumothorax that is only evident on MSCT (also in MSCT abdomen that in trauma patients should be always evaluated using the pulmonary window, with the scans covering the lung bases): occult PNX is recognizable in 40 % of trauma patients.

Autopsy experimental studies have highlighted that the lateral decubitus projection is the most sensitive in the detection of a PNX (88 % of all cases) in comparison with those obtained in upright position (59 %) or in clinostasis (38 %); nevertheless, they cannot be employed for polytrauma patients.

Furthermore, it must be taken into account that, while the minimum volume of air detected in the pleural space is about 50 ml in orthostasis (appreciable in lateral-apical site), at least 500 ml of air are needed for the detection of PNX in clinostasis, usually seen in an anteromedial and subpulmonary location.

The diagnostic difficulties in recognizing PNX are due to the not always excellent technical qualities of CXR and pertain to the specific semeiological characteristics that PNX takes on CXR. In orthostasis, the diagnosis of a PNX is based on the identification of the visceral pleura seen tangentially from the radiant beam (pleural line) better remarkable in the external apical/subclavian regions and on the complete absence of pulmonary pattern laterally to the "pleural line." In clinostasis, the semeiotics of PNX is completely different (Ianniello et al. 2014).

The lateral-costal placement of PNX is, in fact, quite uncommon, as well as the indication of the "pleural line." In fact, PNX preferably collects in the lower-anterior portion of the chest and, above all, in the anteromedial and subpulmonary site, where the flap, interposed between the base of the lung and the diaphragm, can locate both at the front and posteriorly. In cases (not uncommon) where PNX is located only in the anteromedial and subpulmonary site, the radiant beam does not tangentially detect any visceral pleural border, and the sign of the "visceral line" is not appreciable (Fig. 1).

The lung presents compliance alterations (contusion, edema) that may prevent a harmonic collapse toward the ilium; the presence of lung pattern external to the supposed "pleural line" does not rule out the diagnosis of PNX.

The radiological signs to detect a PNX in clinostasis are:

- Hyperlucency of the lower part of the chest and the upper quadrants of the abdomen (Fig. 2)
- Deep sign of the lateral pleural sinus (the deep sulcus sign) (Fig. 3)
- Double-diaphragm appearance
- Sharp appearance of the diaphragmatic outline (Fig. 4)

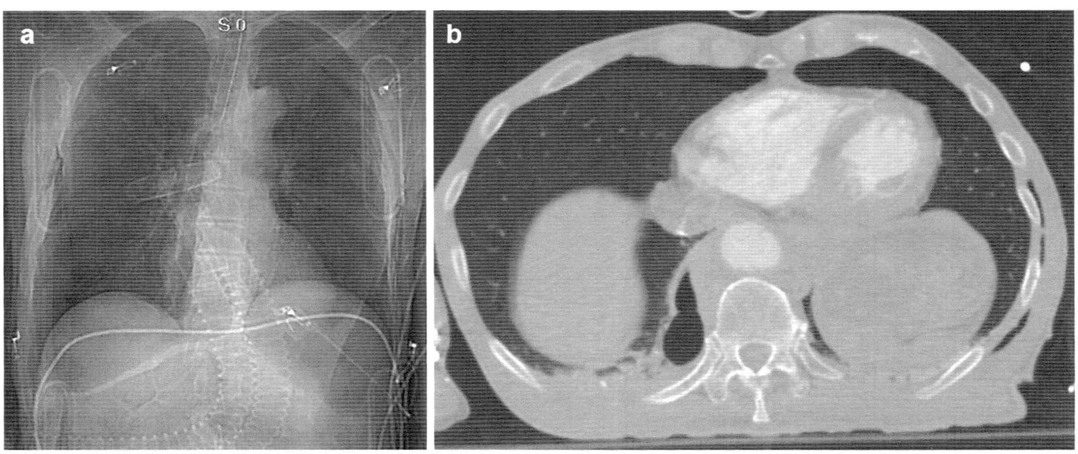

Fig. 1 (**a**) CXR: pneumothorax is located only in the anteromedial and subpulmonary site. The radiant beam does not tangentially detect any visceral pleural border, and the sign of the "visceral line" is not appreciable; (**b**) axial CT image shows very clearly the PNX located in the bilateral anterior-basal site

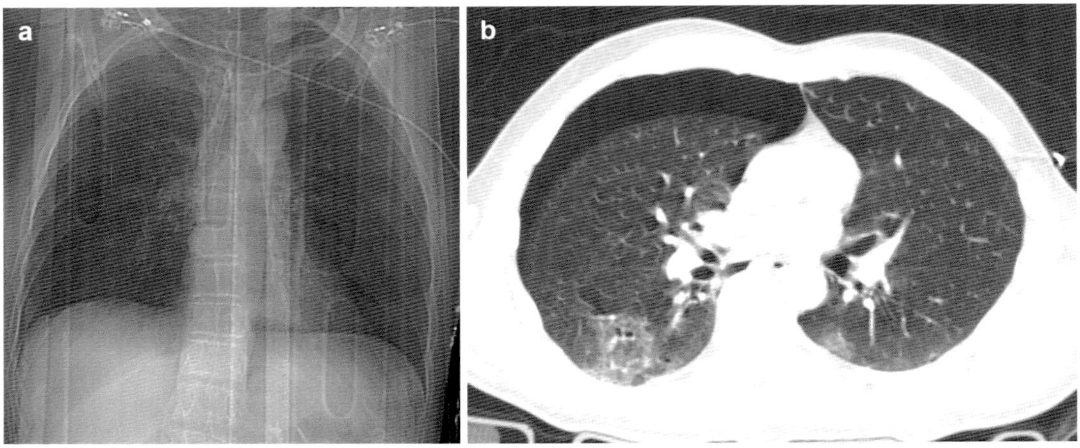

Fig. 2 (**a**) CXR image shows the hyperlucency of the right basis; (**b**) axial CT scan confirms the PNX placed in the anterior-basal site

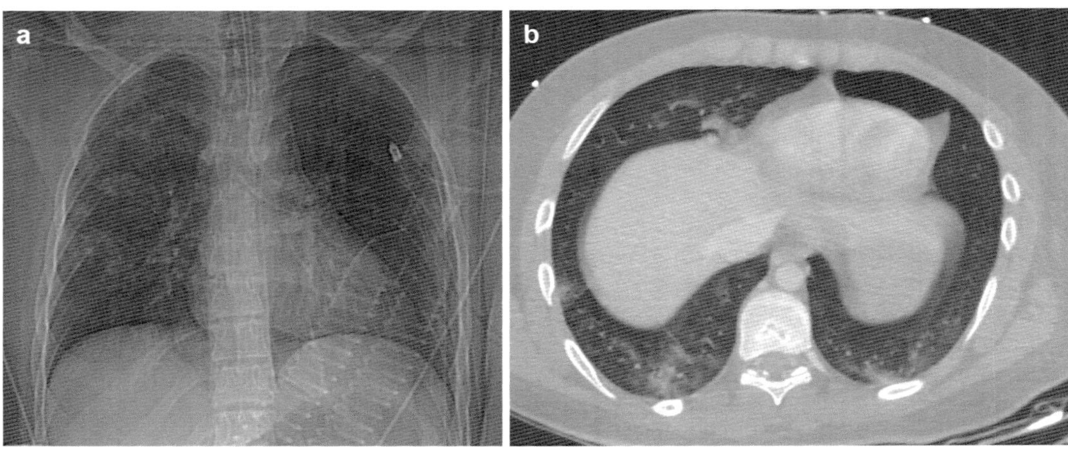

Fig. 3 (**a**) CXR image: mild deepening of the lateral pleural sinus that allows to suspect the presence of PNX in the lower left part of the chest (deep sulcus sign). (**b**) Axial CT image clearly shows the PNX located in anterobasal left site

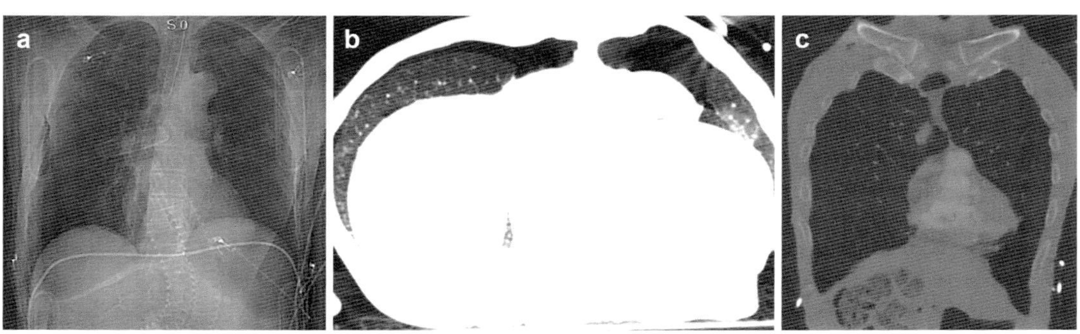

Fig. 4 (**a**) CXR image: bilaterally appreciable is the sharp appearance of the diaphragmatic outline; also evident is a clear demarcation of the profile of the aortic arch and the cardiac silhouette. (**b**) Axial CT scan and (**c**) coronal reconstruction demonstrate the presence of PNX localized in the bilateral anteromedial site

- Sharpness of the cardiophrenic fat pad
- Sharpness of the inferior surface of the lung
- High visibility of the pleural surface of the lung (more frequent in apical position)

Air can, also, separate the edges of the heart, aorta, and vena cava that take an unusual sharp appearance. The air, collected in the posteromedial pleural recess, can be recognized as radiotransparent paraspinal line, alongside the descending aorta and in the posterior costophrenic sulcus. It is essential to carefully inspect the lower lobes of the lung and the upper abdomen to avoid missing such signs. In general, if small flaps of PNX, unrecognized on AP view, have no clinical relevance, they may rapidly expand in intubated patients on positive-pressure ventilation, putting the patient's life at risk. In such a scenario, the radiographic evidence of rib fractures and homolateral subcutaneous emphysema are considered a sign of PNX even in the absence of sharp intrapleural gas folds.

3 Tension PNX

Tension PNX is an emergency clinical condition that requires an immediate treatment, being associated with a reduction of cardiac filling and compression of the homolateral lung. About one-third of the patients with unrecognized PNX progress into a tension PNX.

If the diagnostic evidence of a simple PNX must be communicated to the trauma leader in real time (and written in the report), the same is even true for the diagnosis of tension PNX (Mirvis et al. 2004, 2005).

3.1 Diagnostic Imaging

The radiological diagnosis of PNX can be guided through the following signs:

- Contralateral dislocation of the mediastinum (Figs. 5 and 6)
- Flattening/inversion of the diaphragm (Fig. 7)

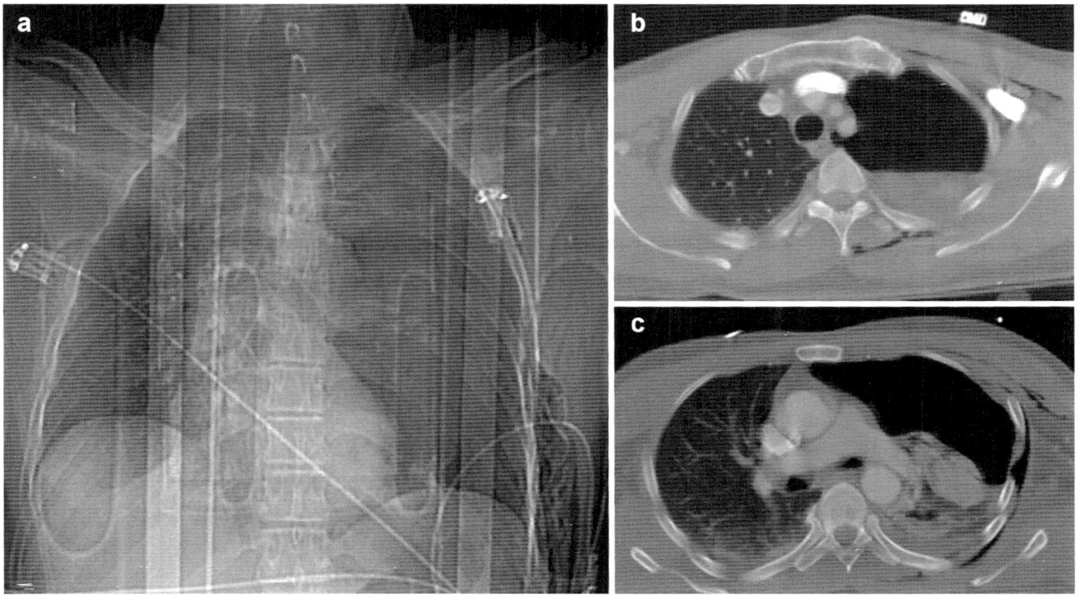

Fig. 5 (**a**) CXR and (**b**, **c**) axial CT images show the presence of large hydro-PNX on the left site caused by multiple rib fractures, resulting contralateral dislocation of the mediastinum. In CXR image, it is also visible the extension of the intercostal spaces

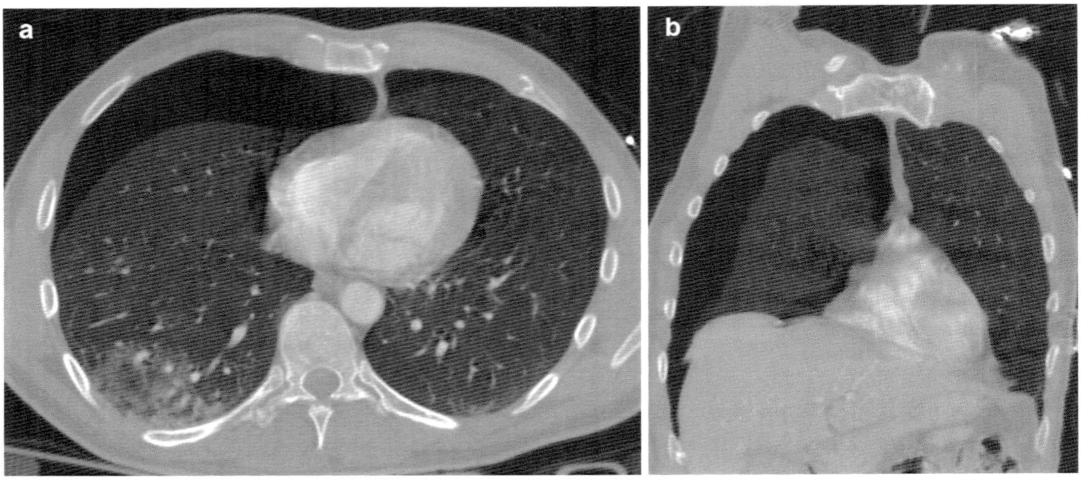

Fig. 6 (**a**) Axial and (**b**) coronal CT images demonstrate the presence of large PNX on the right site that causes contralateral displacement of the mediastinum. It is also visible the presence of a pulmonary contusion in the postero-basal right site

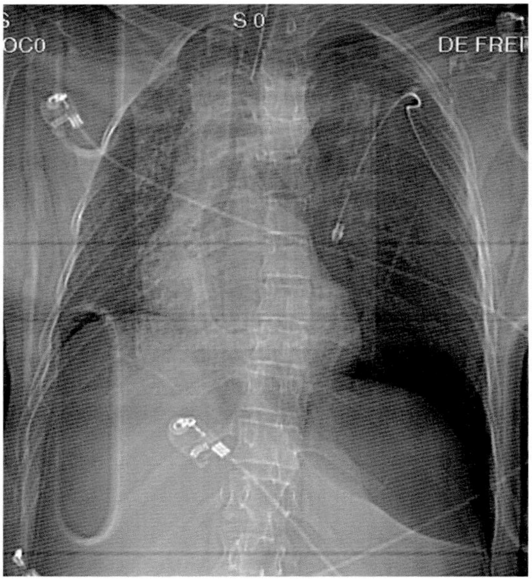

Fig. 7 CXR: Tension PNX, double-diaphragm sign. Contralateral dislocation of the mediastinum; flattening and inversion of the diaphragm and extension of the intercostal spaces

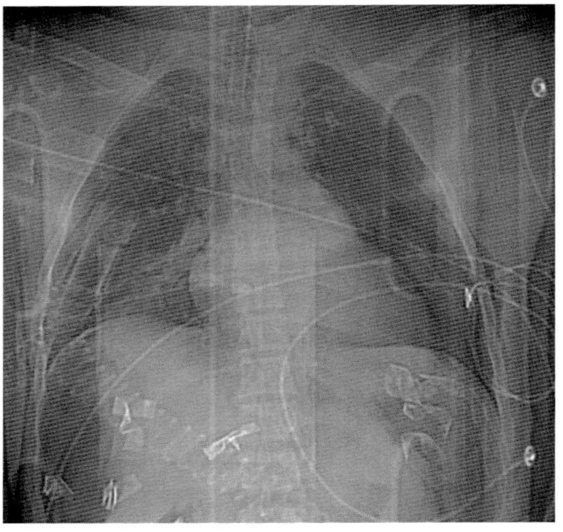

Fig. 8 CXR: Tension PNX. The image shows the flattening of the cardiac profile; this sign is related to the cardiovascular and respiratory distress

- Extension of the intercostal spaces (Fig. 7)
- Flattening of the cardiac profile (Fig. 8)

The mediastinal shift is not a specific sign of tension PNX because it may be visible, to some extent, also in simple PNX; on the other hand, the flattening of the cardiac profile may be the sign better related to the cardiovascular and respiratory distress that markedly characterizes the tension PNX. If tension PNX is persistent despite the correct functioning of the drainage, it is essential to rule out any injury of the main airways.

4 Hemothorax

In polytraumatized patients with blunt chest trauma, pleural effusion is present in approximately 30–50 % of cases, and it is usually hematic in nature (hemothorax) (Brooks et al. 2004).

However, in the acute stage, it is also possible to detect simple serous effusions (due to a reduction of the respiratory mechanics and pleural reabsorption) often associated with atelectasis or homolateral chest wall injuries that reduce the respiratory excursion. On the other hand, it is quite occasional the detection of chylous effusion, due to the rupture of either the thoracic lymphatic ducts (thoracic duct) or of the bile duct, as a result of biliopleural fistula formation that is more common in penetrating trauma.

Bleeding in the pleural cavity often occurs some hours after the trauma; it is sometimes bilateral, and it is often associated with a PNX. The causes responsible for a hemothorax include lacerations of the intercostal vessels, pulmonary contusions, pleural and pulmonary lacerations, and injuries to the diaphragm; iatrogenic lesions, for example, those following a central venous catheter, are also possible causes.

The management of hemothorax depends on its initial quantity, on the amount of blood flow, and on the health condition of the patient.

The initial, usually decisive treatment is the placement of a tube thoracostomy. Patients, who, as soon as the drainage is inserted, evacuate more than 1500 cc, need a surgical or endovascular control of the bleeding.

A hemothorax associated with contusion is usually self-limiting, whereas it may be massive and protracted, when it is associated with pulmonary lacerations or mediastinal lesions.

Venous hemorrhages are self-limited and without mass effect, whereas arterial hemorrhages are under pressure, and they may trigger a significant compression of the pulmonary parenchyma, mediastinum, and heart.

The initial recesses of the pleural cavity filled with blood effusion are declivitous; they can vary according to the decubitus, whereas, with the progressive filling of the pleural cavity, blood is invariably collected in the lateral pleural spaces over the apex of the lung (apical cap): they are very large pleural effusions, in the order of about 800–1200 cc.

4.1 Diagnostic Imaging

In orthostatic position, the most declivitous part of the pleural space is the subpulmonary space; the radiological sign is an apparent elevation of the diaphragm which appears flattened at its medial margins. When at least 200 cc of effusion are collected, the fluid, visible tangentially to the X-ray beam, has a meniscus shape and obliterates the lateral costophrenic sulcus.

On the contrary, in supine patient, the blood collects posteriorly and along the posterior pleural space; on CXR, it is acquired "face to face" (on the frontal view), not tangentially to the radiant beam. For this reason, the "formation" of meniscus sign is not usually visible, and the radiological sign is often only a homogeneous increased density in the basal medial hemithorax with visualization of the parenchymal markings associated with the obliteration of the lateral costophrenic recess. In clinostatic position, neither pleural effusions below 200–300 cc nor massive effusions collected posteriorly can usually be detected. The contralateral mediastinal shift indicates a hemithorax under pressure, probably due to an arterial bleeding (Fig. 9). Atypical radiological appearances include loculated collections that may mimic a mass in the interlobar fissures or in the mediastinal pleura and lobulated margins of the effusion which is collected along the pleural surface, due to the advanced coagulation process, however rather rare in the acute stage.

The identification of pleural effusion as well as its diversification from abdominal effusion is quite easy to acquire on MSCT, thanks to the use of multiplanar reconstruction (MPR). The density of a hemothorax generally varies from 35 to 70 HU, depending on the hematocrit, the mixture of other fluids (serous) in the pleural space, and the potential clot formation.

The presence of a liquid-liquid level may further enforce the diagnosis for a blood effusion: the

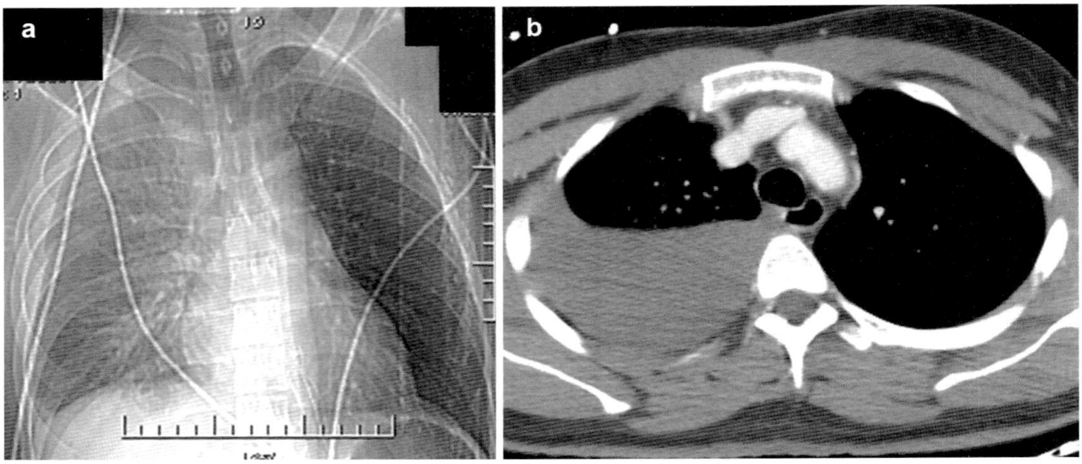

Fig. 9 (**a**) CXR demonstrates homogeneous increased density in the right hemithorax with visualization of the parenchymal markings and elevation of the diaphragmatic dome. (**b**) Axial CT scan confirms a huge hemothorax on the right side, with fluid collecting over the pulmonary apex

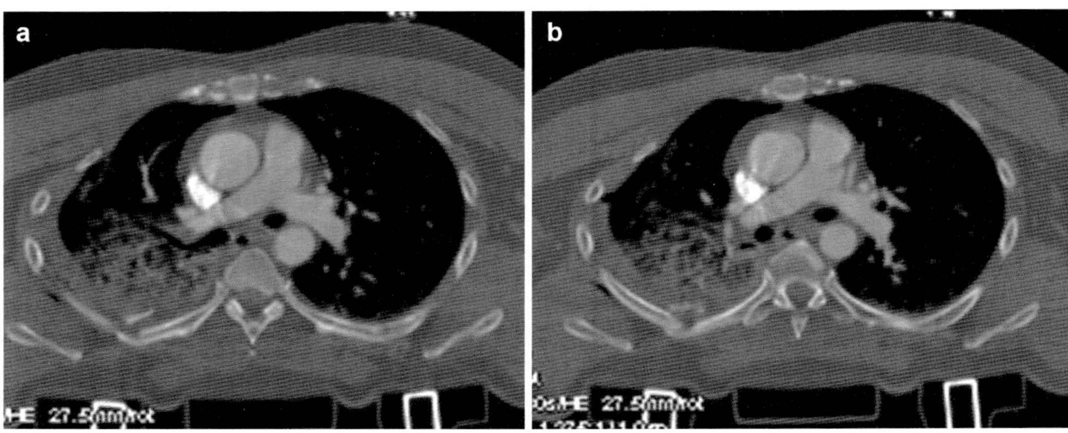

Fig. 10 (**a**, **b**) Axial CT scans demonstrate active extravasation in the context of the lung parenchyma. The pattern of extravasation is a focal area of hyperattenuation within a hematoma

blood, in fact, has a layered appearance according to its degree of coagulation ("hematocrit sign").

Occasionally, an active extravasation can be visible and it should be carefully observed, suggesting urgent hemostasis through surgical or endovascular intervention (Fig. 10).

Generally, active extravasation refers to any passage of contrast medium out of the arteries, veins, bowel, and urinary tract. Active extravasation is seen in a minority of trauma patients, in whom MSCT shows a hemothorax, whose detection is more accurate with a dual-phase protocol (Fig. 11). The classic pattern of active extravasation at dual phase is a "jet" or focal area of hyperattenuation within a hematoma that, between the initial and the delayed images acquisition, shows a visible enlargement (Fig. 12).

This finding is indicative of significant bleeding and must be quickly communicated to the clinician, since it is an indicator of the need for surgical or endovascular intervention (Hamilton 2008; Kaewlai et al. 2008; Kalsow et al. 2013).

The active extravasation may be recognized when the attenuation is greater than clotted blood

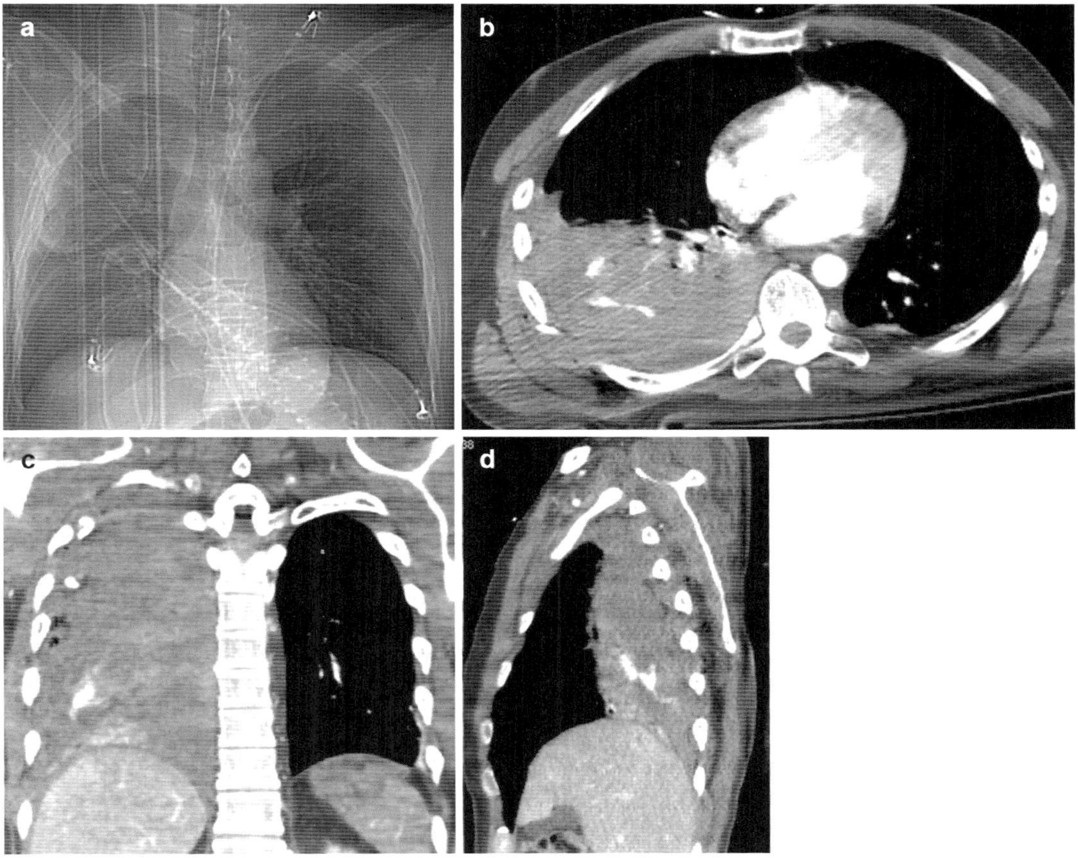

Fig. 11 (**a**) CXR: homogeneous increased density in the right parenchyma. (**b**) Axial CT scan and (**c**, **d**) multiplanar reconstructions show massive right hemothorax; active bleeding is well appreciable within the hemothorax as a focal hyperdensity

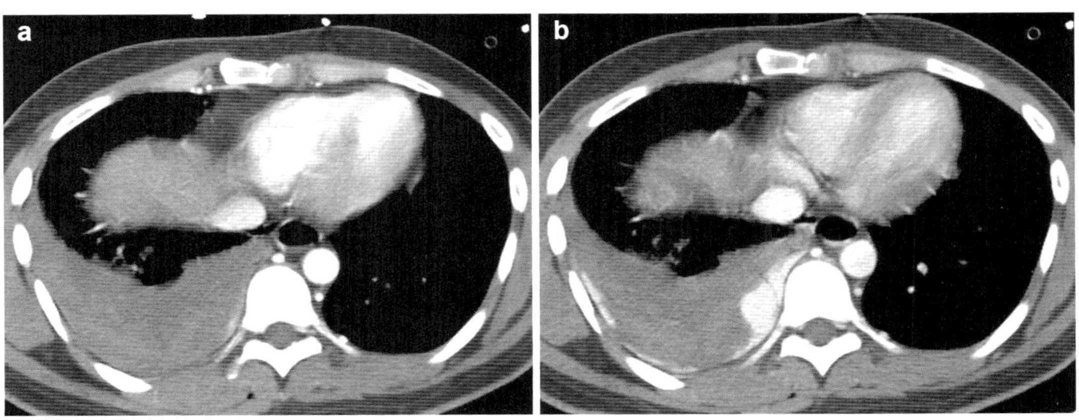

Fig. 12 (**a**) Axial CT scan in arterial phase shows the presence of an active extravasation on the right site. (**b**) Axial CT scan in late phase shows the increase in size of the hyperdensity area. The hemothorax can sometimes be better visible with a dual phase CT protocol

presenting a density of about 70–90 HU: most active extravasations present an attenuation greater than 100 HU. To obtain an optimal scanning of the active extravasation in polytrauma patients, it is suggested the use of 150 mL of contrast medium 300 mgI/l, administered at a rate of 3.5 ml/s with the beginning of the acquisition about 1 min after the start of the bolus; the delay time is slightly longer than that used in standard arterial acquisition and its purpose is to assure an optimum enhancement of the parenchymal organs. Furthermore, a delayed acquisition (for example, at a rate of 5 min) can be performed with a low-flow technique to complete the semeiotic evaluation of the findings (Lomoschitz et al. 2003, Mayberry 2000; O'Connor et al. 2009).

5 Appendix: Pleural Drainages

The placement of one or more thoracostomy tubes represents the standard procedure for treating PNX and hemothorax. The tube bore size varies from 10 to 40 F, depending on the thickness of the fluid to be drained and the physician's preference; the course's tube, inserted in the midaxillary line, is anterosuperior for the PNX drainage and posteroinferior for the evacuation of the hemothorax (McDermott et al. 2012). The chest tube is appropriately placed when its apex is within the pleural space, namely, between the parietal and visceral pleurae. The positioning procedure can be frequently considered rather safe; however, the critical conditions of polytraumatized patients are often associated with the malfunctioning of the drainage system: the chest tube does not drain air or fluid if connected to an aspiration device, or the radiological follow-up shows the persistence of a PNX or hemothorax. Causes of malfunctioning include kinking, blocked drain due to clot formation, and tube malposition (MP). Malposition of the drain is the most common complication in an emergency; it is placed in intrafissural and intraparenchymal apices, in the mediastinum, or in abdominal (through a diaphragmatic tear) and extrapulmonary subcutaneous tissues. The MP of the chest tube results in a longer length of hospital stay and risk of infectious complications. Moreover, the intraparenchymal drains may result in pulmonary abscess or may cause parenchymal hemorrhage; besides, the delay in the evacuation of hemothorax can lead to empyema (Pastore Neto et al. 2015).

The clinical recognition of MP is difficult. The CXR is usually performed as a follow-up examination, following the insertion of the drainage system, to assess the parenchymal expansion and the reduction of PNX/hemithorax flap as well as to identify the apex of the drainage tube; however, the reliability of MP detection may be considered poor and limited to ordinary cases (25 % of all cases). The identification of MP is easy on CT, with an incidence between 15 and 26 % (Corcoran et al. 2015).

A PNX is persistent when it is visible despite the drainage placement: a persistent PNX may be hypertensive, and its presence must be communicated to the team leader immediately.

References

Ahmad T, Ahmed SW, Soomro NH et al (2013) Thoracoscopic evacuation of retained post-traumatic hemothorax. J Coll Physicians Surg Pak 23: 234–236

Alkadhi H, Wildermuth S, Desbiolles L et al (2004) Vascular emergencies of the Thorax after Blunt and Iatrogenic trauma: multi-detector row CT and three-dimensional imaging. Radiographics 24:1239–1255

Błasińska-Przerwa K, Pacho R, Bestry I (2013) The application of MDCT in the diagnosis of chest trauma. Pneumonol Alergol Pol 81:518–526

Brink M, Deunk J, Dekker HM et al (2008) Added value of routine chest MDCT after blunt trauma: evaluation of additional findings and Impact on patient management. AJR Am J Roentgenol 190:1591–1598

Brink M, Deunk J, Dekker HM et al (2010) Criteria for the selective use of chest computed tomography in blunt trauma patients. Eur Radiol 20:818–828

Brooks A, Davies B, Smethhurts M et al (2004) Emergency ultrasound in the acute assessment of haemothorax. Emerg Med J 21:44–46

Corcoran JP, Acton L, Ahmed A et al (2015) Diagnostic value of radiological imaging pre- and post-drainage of pleural effusions. Respirology. doi:10.1111/resp.12675

Cothren CC, Moore EE, Hedegaard HB et al (2007) Epidemiology of urban trauma deaths: a comprehensive reassessment 10 years later. World J Surg 31:1507–1511

Detorakis EE, Androulidakis E (2014) Intercostal lung herniation- the role of imaging. J Radiol Case Rep 8:16–24

Gavelli G, Napoli G, Bertaccini P et al (2007) Imaging of thoracic injuries. In: Marincek B, Dondelinger RF (eds) Emergency radiology – imaging and intervention. Springer, Berlin Heidelberg, pp 155–178

Hamilton JD, Kumaravel M, Censullo ML et al (2008) Multidetector CT evaluation of active extravasation in blunt abdominal and pelvic trauma patients. Radiographics 28:1603–1616

Ianniello S, Di Giacomo V, Sessa B, Miele V (2014) First-line sonographic diagnosis of pneumothorax in major trauma: accuracy of e-FAST and comparison with multidetector computed tomography. Radiol Med 119: 674–680

Kaewlai R, Avery LL, Asrani AV et al (2008) Multidetector CT of blunt thoracic trauma. Radiographics 28: 1555–1570

Kalsow S, Wigle R, Johnson LW et al (2013) Delayed traumatic lung herniation. J La State Med Soc 165:163–165

Lomoschitz FM, Eisenhuber E, Linnau KF et al (2003) Imaging of chest trauma: radiological patterns of injuries and diagnostic algorithms. Eur J Radiol 48:61–70

Mayberry JC (2000) Imaging in thoracic trauma: the trauma surgeon's perspective. J Thorac Imaging 15:76–86

McDermott S, Levis DA, Arellano RS (2012) Chest drainage. Semin Intervent Radiol 29:247–255

Miele V, Di Giampietro I, Ianniello S, Pinto F, Trinci M (2014) Diagnostic imaging in pediatric polytrauma management. Radiol Med 120:33–49

Mirvis SE (2004) Diagnostic imaging of acute thoracic injury. Semin Ultrasound CT MR 25:156–179

Mirvis SE (2005) Imaging of acute thoracic injury: the advent of MDCT screening. Semin Ultrasound CT MR 26:305–331

O'Connor JV, Byrne C, Scalea TM et al (2009) Vascular injuries after blunt chest trauma: diagnosis and management. Scand J Trauma Resusc Emerg Med 17:42

Pastore Neto M, Resende V, Machado CJ et al (2015) Associated factors to empyema in post-traumatic hemotorax. Rev Col Bras Cir 42:224–230

Tocino IM, Miller MH, Fairfax WR (1985) Distribution of pneumothorax in the supine and semirecumbent critically ill adult. AJR Am J Roentgenol 144:901–905

Bony and Thoracic Chest Wall Injuries

Stefan Wirth and Stephan Jansen

Contents

S. Wirth, MD, PhD (✉)
Insitute for Clinical Radiology, Hospital of the Ludwig-Maximilians-University, Nussbaumstr. 20, Munich 80336, Germany
e-mail: Stefan.Wirth@med.uni-muenchen.de

S. Jansen
Ludwig-Maximilians-University, Geschwister-Scholl-Platz 1, Munich 80539, Germany
e-mail: Stephan.Jansen@campus.lmu.de

Abstract

Trauma is very common and has a major impact on both mortality and morbidity worldwide. More than 100,000 people die annually from the consequences of trauma in the United States. Thoracic trauma occurs in 12 persons per 1 million population daily, of which one-third require hospital admission (Mancini et al. 2014). Injuries are complexly associated with each other in up to 90 % of the cases (Traub et al. 2007) and their occurrence is regularly predictable. The following section deals with trauma mechanisms of bony and

Med Radiol Diagn Imaging (2016)
DOI 10.1007/174_2016_54, © Springer International Publishing Switzerland

thoracic chest wall injuries, as well as their significance for diagnostic workup, treatment options and outcome.

Trauma is very common and has a major impact on both mortality and morbidity worldwide. More than 100,000 people die annually from the consequences of trauma in the United States. Thoracic trauma occurs in 12 persons per 1 million population daily, of which one-third require hospital admission (Mancini et al. 2014). Injuries are complexly associated with each other in up to 90 % of the cases (Traub et al. 2007) and their occurrence is regularly predictable. The following section deals with trauma mechanisms of bony and thoracic chest wall injuries, as well as their significance for diagnostic workup, treatment options and outcome.

1 Epidemiology and Aetiology

Approximately one out of four trauma fatalities is directly caused by thoracic injuries (Calhoon and Trinkle 1997; Clark et al. 1988; Veysi et al. 2009). Up to 66 % and more of thoracic trauma cases may be blunt (Demirhan et al. 2009; Shanmuganathan and Matsumoto 2006) or penetrating. Blunt chest trauma is a potential threat to airway, breathing, as well as to circulation, and mortality rates can be as high as 60 % in the United States and Europe (Clark et al. 1988; Veysi et al. 2009; Calhoon and Trinkle 1997). As by far the most important cause, road traffic accidents account for 70–80 % of all significant blunt chest trauma cases. Falls, acts of violence and blasts are also relevant causes (Mancini et al. 2014). Particularly at risk are young adults (15–44 years) constituting 59 % of road traffic fatalities (World Health Organization 2015a). While pedestrians have a greater chance to survive a car crash at 30 km/h or less, a decrease of speed in general reduces both the likelihood of a crash as well as the severity of injuries.

Furthermore, 'drinking and driving' has a major impact on road safety. A blood alcohol concentration (BAC) above 0.4 g/l (i.e. 0.32‰) significantly boosts the risk of being involved in a car crash (World Health Organization 2015a). These facts and numbers illustrate that profound knowledge of diagnostics and treatment of patients with chest trauma is indispensable to guarantee the best possible outcome.

Secondary complications arise from blunt thoracic trauma, such as atelectasis, pneumonia, pulmonary effusion, cardiovascular and wound problems, and less frequently airway problems, emphysema, ARDS, pulmonary embolus, pneumothorax and massive subcutaneous emphysema (Clark et al. 1988). It is important to stress that significant thoracic injuries can be present even in the absence of bony fractures in up to 24.7 % of blunt chest trauma patients. Among these are haemothoraces or pneumothoraces (62.2 %), cardiac contusions (15.7 %), ruptured diaphragms (7.9 %) or aortas (7 %) and other injuries (Shorr et al. 1987).

The Injury Severity Score (ISS) is an indicator of trauma severity and correlates with mortality in patients with blunt chest trauma (Clark et al. 1988). Nevertheless, the ISS is not absolutely reliable and therefore has to be interpreted in relation to other clinical information and findings. Even worse, a correct ISS value can only be assessed with known diagnoses and thus is of limited use for both the pre-diagnostic phase and especially for the diagnostic protocol decisions. However, ISS plays a key role in databases for retrospective case group evaluation. Paffrath et al. found an increasing ISS in combination with the prevalence of risk factors, such as high age, acidosis, unconsciousness, hypotension and coagulopathy, to be associated with an increasing mortality. In this study, patients with a median ISS of 24.2 and none of these risk factors had an associated mortality of 3.1 %, while 16.0 % of patients with a median ISS of 27.8 and one risk factor died. A median ISS of 35.5 and two risk factors correlated with a mortality rate of 46.7 % (Paffrath et al. 2014). According to a study of Emircan et al. including 371 patients with thoracic trauma, an ISS over 22 is one of the most important factors affecting mortality (odds ratio (OR) = 6.27; 95 % confidence interval (CI) = 2.48–15.88; $p < 0.0001$) (Emircan et al. 2011). Patients with an ISS over 16 may have an 8.1-fold increased risk of an occult pneumothorax compared to patients with an ISS under 16 ($p < 0.0001$) (Kirkpatrick et al. 2004).

Most patients have an excellent outcome and prognosis after blunt chest trauma, and more than 80 % do not require invasive therapy or, at most, tube thoracostomy (Mancini et al. 2014). However, even if many blunt chest trauma patients do not necessarily require surgical treatment, they need accurate surveillance to identify the ones who do require operative or other intervention (LoCicero and Mattox 1989).

2 Legal Aspects

As in every medical discipline, a wrong diagnosis in radiology can be of legal medical relevance. Even an extremely precautious radiologist may overlook an injury or a disease at one point of their career. But it is possible to rule out some evitable errors. Generally, there are four reasons for lawsuits against radiologists:

- Errors in *perception*
- Errors in *interpretation*
- Failure in *communication* of findings in a clinically and timely correct manner
- Failure in *management recommendation* for the next appropriate step(s)/procedure(s)

Among these, perception errors account for the highest number of lawsuits against radiologists. Whether the error had a harmful effect on the patient or not is an important factor when the case comes before the court. The legal importance of communication failures is increasing, and it is in no way sufficient for the radiologic evaluator to solely provide a report. Additionally, important findings have to be directly communicated to the referring physician (in person or by telephone), and this *oral report* should be documented.

Moreover, prior radiology reports may influence radiologists.

If a finding was overseen in an old report, the next evaluator may miss it as well. Thus, radiologists should have a look at the films before reading prior reports (Raskin 2001).

The Institute of Forensic Medicine of the Ludwig Maximilian University in Munich, Germany, have conducted 2086 post-mortem examinations on patients who died from pneumothorax or chest trauma from 1991 until the beginning of 2016. In 4.6 % (96) of these cases, the cause of death was at least related to medical procedures or diagnostics (data with kind assistance of Dr. F. Fischer and kind permission of Prof. Dr. M. Graw, Director of the Institute of Forensic Medicine, University of Munich).

Depending on national law, in case of medical malpractice, the burden of proof is usually on the patient. They have to not only prove (e.g. with the help of a medical expert witness) that malpractice was carried out, but also that this malpractice has led to the damage of the patient's health (condicio-sine-qua-non-formula or principle of causation). If – during the course of the investigation – medical documents are found to be missing and were manipulated or necessary diagnostic was not properly performed, the burden of proof may shift onto the physician (Hager 2009). Lawsuits may be brought against physicians even if there was no medical malpractice involved. These stem from at least three problem areas:

1. The patient or their family is dissatisfied with a result, even though it is acceptable to the medical community, and the outcome was even expected.
2. Medical records are incomplete, inappropriate, inaccurate or delayed, even if the patient's care and outcome were excellent.
3. Problems regarding execution and documentation of the informed consent.

In the process of the investigation of causes and effects of chest injuries involving third parties or work-related injuries, a radiologist may be asked to write a report or statement (Vevaina et al. 2012).

3 Osteoporosis

Osteoporosis affects over 65 million people in Europe, Japan and the United States. As the societies in these countries age, osteoporosis is a growing concern. Worldwide, osteoporosis causes over 8.9 million fractures annually,

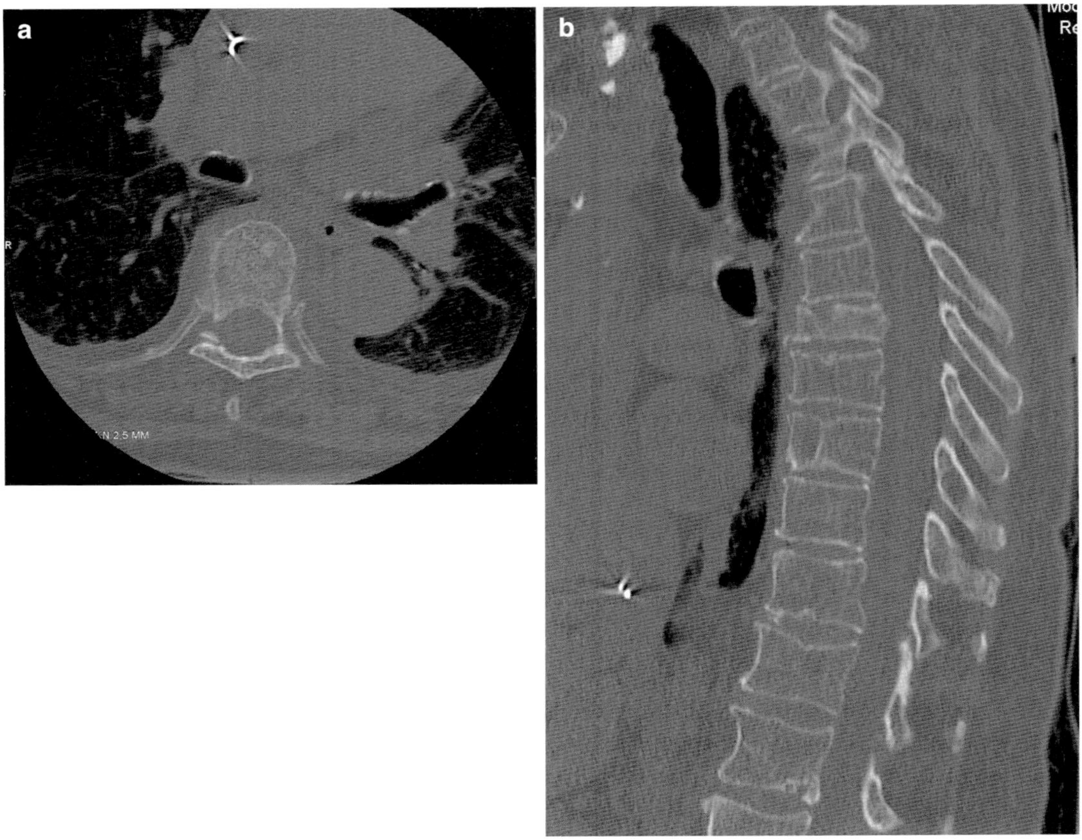

Fig. 1 Osteoporotic thoracic spine fractures in an 86-year-old female. Unenhanced CT in (**a**) axial and (**b**) sagittal plane

which makes it a major cause of bedriddenness with serious complications. With 30–40 %, the lifetime risk for an osteoporotic vertebral fracture (Fig. 1) ranges close to the risk of coronary heart disease (World Health Organization 1994, 2004). Bony thoracic fractures may be a marker for osteoporosis in men and especially in postmenopausal women, which is why a short excursion is made in order to link it with chest wall injuries.

In a study including 155,031 women in the United States, aged between 50 and 99 years, a reported rib fracture was related to a 5.4-fold raised risk of a future rib fracture, while the risk of any future clinical fracture was 2.4-fold increased (Sajjan et al. 2012).

In patients with osteoporosis or those receiving a high-dose steroid therapy, even severe cough can result in rib fractures (Katrancioglu et al. 2015). According to the findings of Pluskiewicz et al., a prior osteoporotic fracture may be the main prognostic factor for the incidence of future fractures (Pluskiewicz et al. 2011). According to Neuerburg et al., osteoporosis is evident in most men over 60 (59 %) and women over 50 (56.2 %), who present to hospital with an osseous fracture. As a consequence, osteoporosis should generally be evaluated in the management of trauma patients with the diagnosis of a fracture over 60, respectively, 50 years of age and treated if necessary to prevent future fractures (Neuerburg et al. 2015). Furthermore, the consideration whether the trauma mechanism was adequately to result in the fracture the patient presents could be a sign for a possibly impaired bone density (Sajjan et al. 2012; Wuermser et al. 2011; Palvanen et al. 2004; Barrett-Connor et al. 2010; Watts et al. 2008; Mirvis et al. 2014, p. 163).

4 Radiologic Equipment and Techniques

4.1 Ultrasound

Portable, non-invasive ultrasound (US) diagnostic can be performed at any time, in any place and on any patient and is thus very suitable for emergency situations (Reissig et al. 2011). The focused assessment with sonography for trauma (FAST), a scan for free abdominal fluid, is most widely accepted (Fleming et al. 2012; Rothlin et al. 1993; Chung et al. 2014) and was extended (EFAST) to detect pleural pathologies (Fig. 2) (Kirkpatrick et al. 2004; Matsushima and Frankel 2011).

Although some of these conditions are beyond the scope of EFAST, multiple thoracic medical conditions, such as pulmonary embolism, pneumothorax, haemothorax, pleural effusion, cardiac injuries and rib fractures, and sometimes even pneumonia can be detected with the help of US (Reissig et al. 2011). It may be surprising that US has proven to be even superior to supine chest radiography in ruling out suspected pneumothorax (sensitivity 48.8 % vs. 20.9 %; specificity 99.6 % vs. 98.7 %) (Kirkpatrick et al. 2004). This was confirmed for sensitivity in a meta-analysis from 2010 (86–98 % vs. 28–75 %), while both modalities where comparably specific (97–100 % vs. 100 %) (Wilkerson and Stone 2010). US may even be superior to chest radiography in the detection of rib fractures, but so far clear evidence is missing and further studies with a well-established gold standard have yet to be executed (Lalande and Wylie 2014).

4.2 Chest Radiography

Chest radiography is often a common part of the standard trauma workup, even if computed tomography (CT) is to be performed later on. Even mobile C-arm fluoroscopy or radiography can verify tube and line positioning (Fig. 3). In many cases pneumothorax, tension pneumothorax, haemothorax, extrapleural haematoma and injuries of the aorta (Fig. 4), heart, trachea, oesophagus, great thoracic vessels, bony chest wall and lungs can be detected, helping with patient triage without losing much time during initial emergency room care. However, in a trauma setting, patients are seldom able to stand and perform a full inspiration resulting in both limitation of chest radiographs to AP direction and impaired significance to additional motion artefacts and overlying materials (Chung et al. 2014; Kaewlai et al. 2008, pp. 1556–1557). Therefore, it is not surprising that about half of the pneumothoraces and rib fractures detected by CT are occult on AP chest radiography. Consequently, experts advise against over-reliance on chest radiography in patients with high-energy blunt thorax trauma (Ball et al. 2005; Barrios et al. 2010; Chung et al. 2014). In summary it can be stated that, although chest radiography is less accurate in case of blunt chest trauma than CT, it can still provide important information and is often faster available in the trauma bay. Thus, it can be concluded that the utilisation of chest radiography is justified in case of minor trauma or in case of high-energy trauma if CT is not available in time.

If CT is available for high-risk patients, the CT scout (i.e. topogram or scanogram) (Fig. 5) provides relevant information (about conditions that require intervention before CT) comparable to radiography but with less total time consumption (Wirth et al. 2009). However, the appropriate modality to exclude or diagnose relevant findings like pneumothorax may depend on various circumstances, such as urgency, patient condition, local conditions and others (Ball et al. 2005; Barrios et al. 2010; Chung et al. 2014; Kaewlai et al. 2008, pp. 1556–1557; Henry et al. 2014; Traub et al. 2007).

4.3 Computed Tomography

The invention of CT and CT angiography has revolutionised the blunt trauma management, allowing rapid diagnosis of complex injuries and consequently early therapeutic management like embolisation of arterial bleeding and utilisation of stents in case of vascular dissection or transection (Tillou et al. 2009). In trauma centres CT is usually 24/7 available and able to provide fast and high-quality whole body 3D cross-sectional

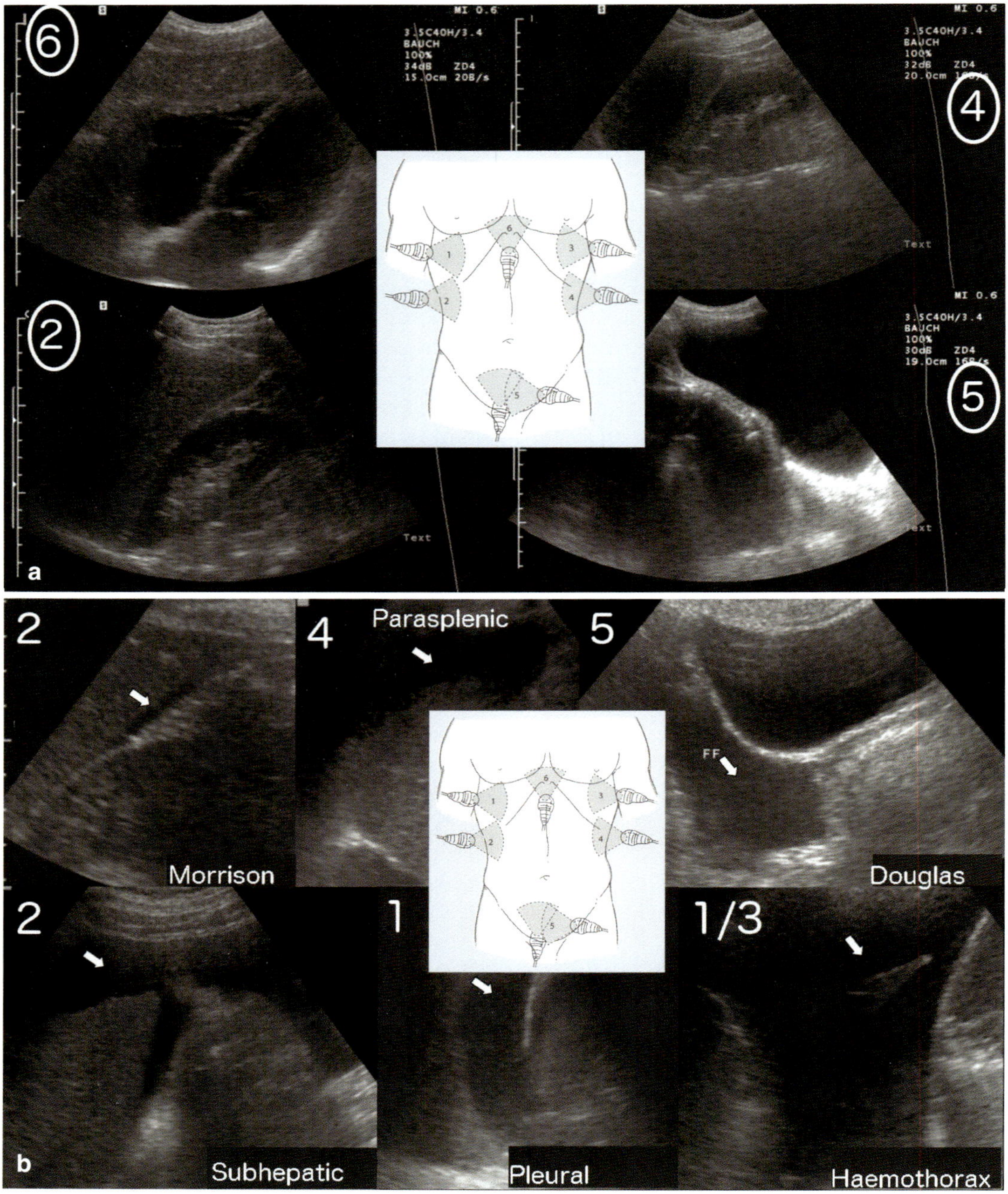

Fig. 2 EFAST: rapid ultrasound scan for free intra-abdominal and intrapleural fluids. The numbers on the left side of the top of the US pictures correspond to the positions of the Ultrasound Transducer as depicted in the central illustration. (**a**) Normal findings of the heart (*6*), the Morrison (*2*) pouch, the Koller (*4*) pouch and the Douglas space (*5*), here in sagittal orientation. (**b**) Corresponding labelling of examples with findings of free abdominal fluid as marked by *arrows* (central illustration from springer, der anaesthesist)

imaging (WB-CT). This results in the highest sensitivity (80–100 %) (Magu et al. 2009; Bier et al. 2015) among the techniques for imaging of rib fractures. Furthermore, it provides information of associated injuries. According to Traub et al., CT can reveal significant injury in about 38 % of patients with bland initial radiographs (including fractures of ribs (14.9 %, $p<0.001$),

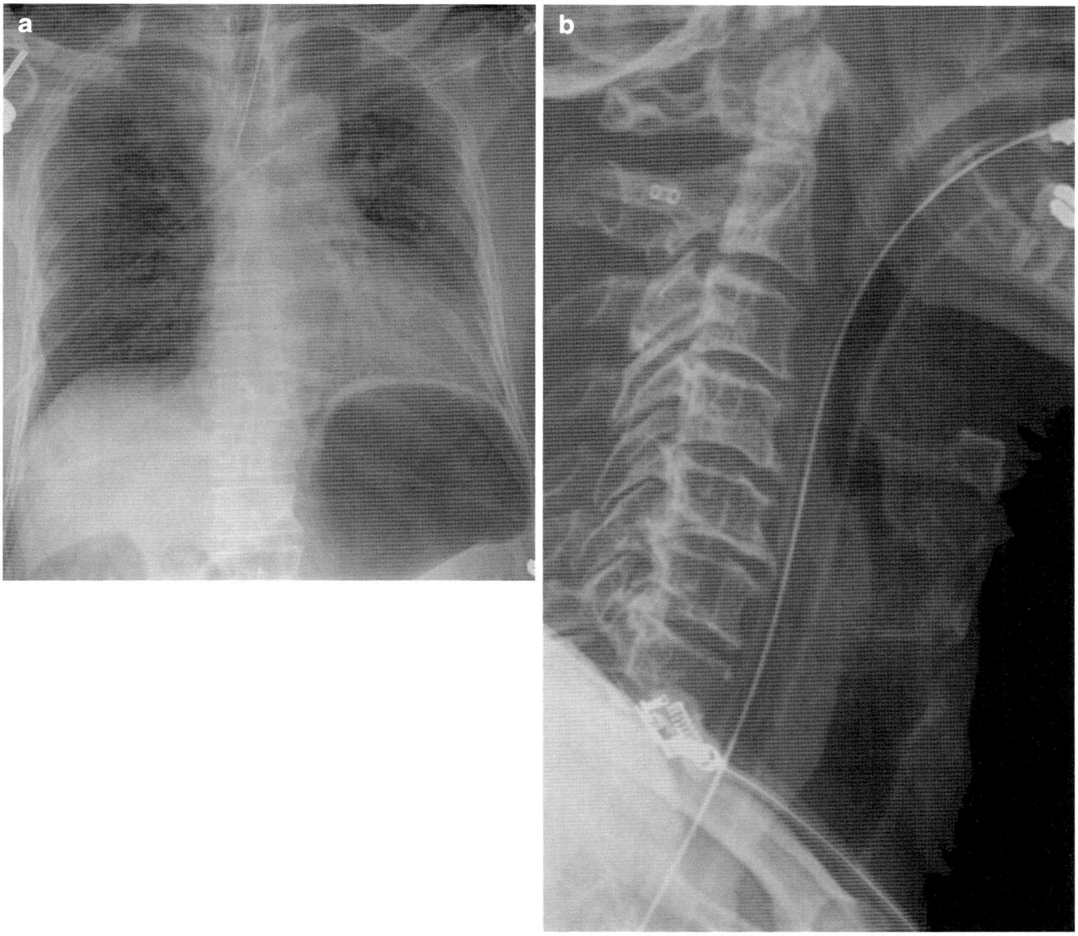

Fig. 3 Misplaced endotracheal tube. Notice huge amount of air in projection of the stomach as well as the endotracheal tube crossing the left tracheal border in AP chest projection (**a**) and the sagittal neck view (**b**) proofing the malpositioning

sternums (7.1 %, $p<0.001$), scapulae (4.9 %, $p=0.016$) and vertebrae (15.5 %, $p<0.001$)) or can possibly exclude suspected injury in patients allowing an earlier discharge (Traub et al. 2007). CT can even be performed during cardiopulmonary resuscitation (Fig. 6) (Wirth et al. 2009). Counterarguments for the utilisation of CT may be, depending on the particular setting, higher time consumption compared to radiography, higher radiation exposure (chest: average effective CT dose = 2.86–7.4 mSv vs. 0.1 mSv) and higher costs (Mettler et al. 2008; Tonkopi and Ross 2016).

As specified in the section "Epidemiology and Aetiology", a major part of trauma victims are of a young age, where the discussion about potentially harmful radiation effects is particularly relevant. This discussion should consider that it is known that we are able to save one-fourth of polytrauma patient's lives with the utilisation of whole body CT when comparing with 'dose saving' organ-based CT imaging (Huber-Wagner et al. 2009). Thus, it is of outmost importance to decide very quickly whether acute life-threatening conditions are given in a patient or not. In cases where this is given, the risk of harmful application of radiation can be expected to be far beyond the possible benefit. In addition, a polytrauma is a once in a lifetime experience for most patients – a situation that decides about living or dying. However, for children and young women, it should remain a very carefully taken case-to-case

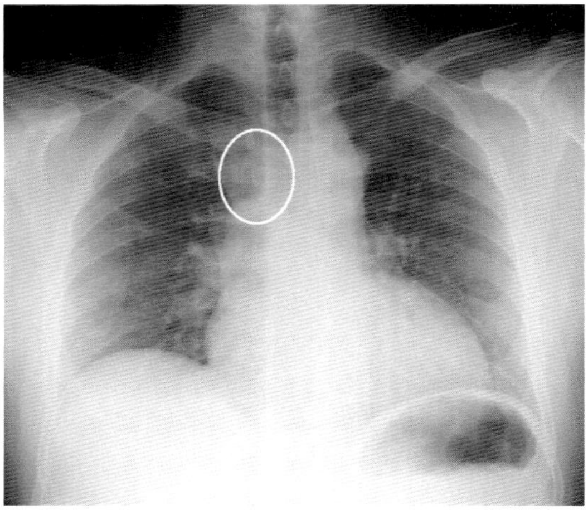

Fig. 4 Unrecognised Stanford A dissection of the aorta with secondary fatal haemopericardium. Chest radiography (p.a.) of a 46-year-old patient with mild pain after weight lifting 4 h ago. The thickening and hampered transmission of the anterior mediastinum as well as the buckling in projection of the border of the aortic root (*white circle*) was missed. As no apical cap sign was visible and there was only mild pain, the patient went home, where he died another 4 h later. CT was not performed. Autopsy revealed a massive aortic dissection

decision, depending on the very individual constellation (Mueck et al. 2016).

CT characterises pleural fluids with determination of their attenuation values, where fresh haemorrhage may have an attenuation as low as 20/30–45 Hounsfield units (HU) (Mirvis et al. 2014, p. 178; Feeman 2010). During the clotting process, the density of blood increases to up to 50–90 HU (Mirvis et al. 2014, p. 178). To distinguish blood from other fluids, the reader should routinely perform a measurement of pleural fluid attenuation in chest trauma patients (Kaewlai et al. 2008, p. 1558; Feeman 2010; Chung et al. 2014; Brink et al. 2008; Traub et al. 2007; Tillou et al. 2009; Mirvis et al. 2014, p. 178).

While the utilisation of CT is discussed contentiously in the literature, many authors consider high-energy mechanisms, chest wall tenderness, reduced air entry, abnormal respiratory effort, abnormal chest radiographs, reduced consciousness and being intubated criteria for a selective computed tomography scan (Traub et al. 2007; Tillou et al. 2009; Brink et al. 2008; Kaewlai et al. 2008, pp. 1556–1569; Feeman 2010; Chung et al. 2014; Henry et al. 2014). In a well-structured department, a standard whole body reconstruction set of CT images can be provided in about 20 min, including an in-room time for the patient of less than 10 min. Thus, up to six patients may be served per CT scanner and per hour in a mass casualty incident (Mueck et al. 2016; Wirth 2014).

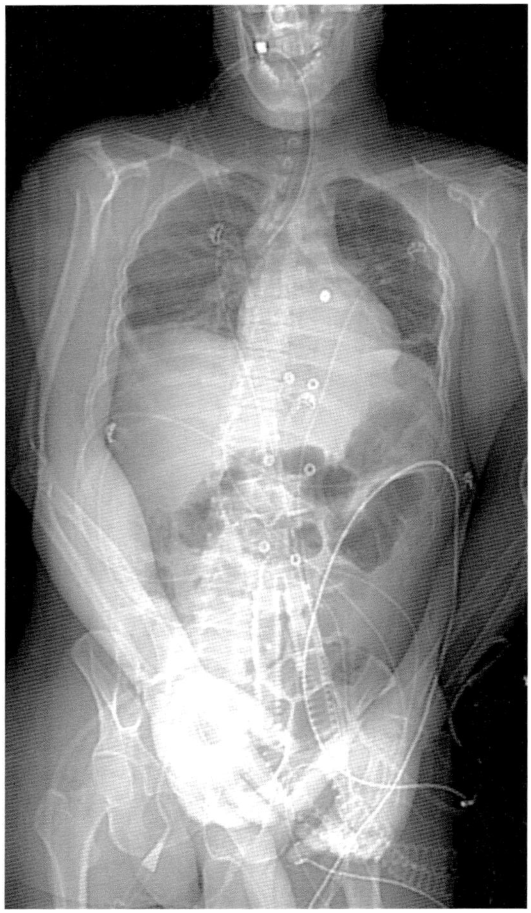

Fig. 5 Topogram of a polytrauma patient for planning the exact positioning of CT scanning. Additionally, it holds relevant information about serious patient conditions and may give hints for extension of scan regions

4.4 Magnetic Resonance Imaging

In contrast to ultrasound, computed tomography and radiography, magnetic resonance imaging (MRI) is highly time consuming (studies may take up to 1 h).

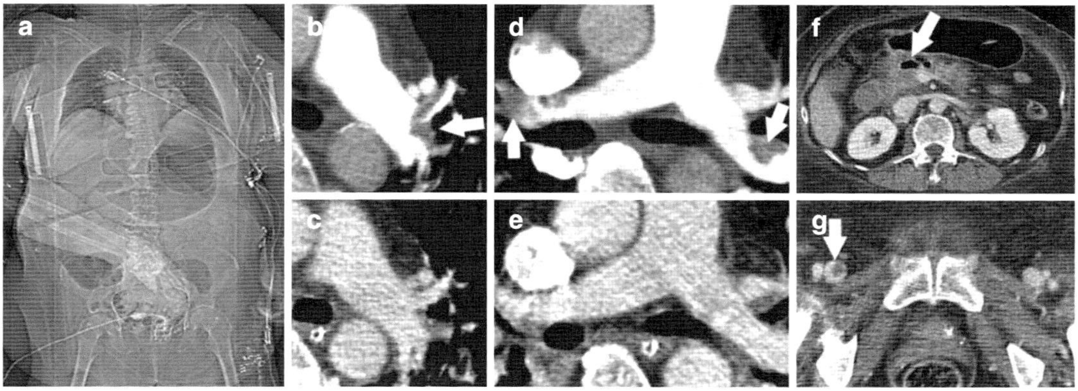

Fig. 6 CT images of a 62-year-old obese female patient with LUCAS baseplate. The patient was admitted under mechanical CPR with LUCAS. Because she did not fit into the bore of the CT gantry with the whole LUCAS system, the compression unit was lifted off for each CT data acquisition. (**a**) Planning scout for chest/abdomen and pelvis. (**b**, **d**) Thorax: CT revealed PE obstructing lobar arteries on both sides (*arrows*, 50 s delay). (**f**, **g**) Abdomen/pelvis: Because images of the abdomen/pelvis with a delay of 120 s had insufficient venous contrast enhancement (not shown), the CT acquisition was repeated with a delay of 210 s. Images depicted free peripancreatical air surrounded by small areas of contrast media (*arrow* in **f**) as well as thrombosis of the right deep femoral vein (*arrow* in **g**). (**c**, **e**) Control study of the thorax after return of spontaneous circulation confirmed successful fibrinolysis. Note the differing distribution of contrast media even though all scan parameters were identical to those of the first study shown in **b** and **d**

Patients have to remain motionless and treatment options are limited during that period. Thus, the significance of MRI in the emergency workup of severely injured trauma patients is very questionable. Nevertheless, it can be used as a problem-solving tool in case of suspected heart, pericardial and spinal injuries/acute neurologic deficit or other situations especially in pregnant women and paediatric patients (Chung et al. 2014).

For the decision for or against MRI in an emergency situation, it may be helpful to think about the following aspects:

1. Is MRI the only available modality to confirm or rule out the suspected injury, or in case of approximately equal indication, may MRI be favourable due to other reasons (e.g. radiation exposure to paediatric patients)?
2. Would the expected findings lead to alternation of patient management?
3. Would one possible finding alter the patient management to an immediate procedure that is necessary to prevent irreversible harm (e.g. refixation of damaged articular cartilage)?

If all these questions can be answered with 'yes' and thus the decision is made to execute an MRI scan, the sequences should be reduced to what is necessary to help solve the clinical problem in order to save time (Wirth 2016, pp. 54–55). Conclusively, it must be said that especially chest trauma patients have a tendency to move (e.g. due to pain) and thus have to be highly compliant in addition to the aspects above to make an MRI feasible.

5 Soft Tissue Contusion and Subcutaneous Emphysema

5.1 Epidemiology of Soft Tissue Contusion and Subcutaneous Emphysema

Blunt chest trauma may result in soft tissue injuries, such as muscle tears, haematoma, cutaneous abrasions, burns, ecchymosis or lacerations (Schnyder and Wintermark 2000, p. 9). These soft tissue injuries may be markers for more severe associated injuries. Lung contusion (Fig. 7) is a frequent injury among blunt chest trauma patients (17–70 %) and serves as a predictor of occult pneumothorax (OR = 3.25; 95 % CI = 1.62–6.54; $p = 0.001$) (Ball et al. 2005; Skinner et al. 2015; Mirvis et al. 2014, pp. 172–177; Kaewlai et al. 2008, p. 1558). Subcutaneous emphysema in patients after blunt chest trauma (approximately in

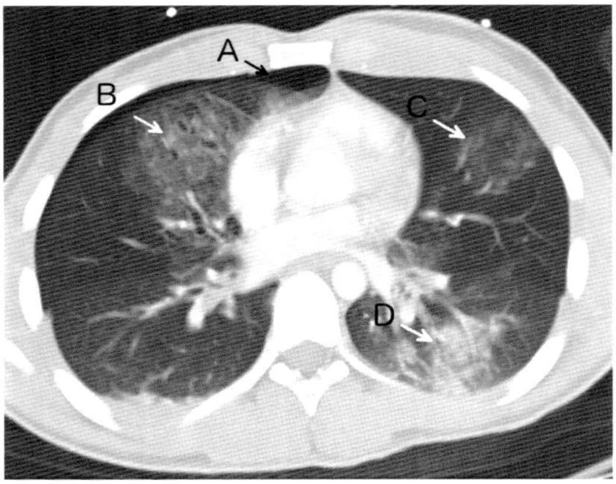

Fig. 7 Pneumothorax (*A*), pulmonary laceration (*B*), pulmonary contusion (*C*) and aspiration (*D*). Axial image of a contrast-enhanced CT of the chest, lung window settings

15 % of cases) also serves as a marker of occult pneumothorax with a crude risk ratio of 6.78 (95 % CI 2.46–18.66; $p<0.001$) and a specificity of 98 % (Ball et al. 2005; Schnyder and Wintermark 2000, pp. 9–10). Ball et al. found subcutaneous emphysema to be present in 7 % of a population of 338 trauma patients with an ISS ≥12 (Ball et al. 2005). Turkalj et al. detected subcutaneous emphysema in 34.4 % out of 61 blunt chest trauma patients (2014).

The presence of subcutaneous emphysema should also raise concern about osseous injuries. From 18.4 % to over 75 % of patients with subcutaneous emphysema have at least one associated rib fracture (Turkalj et al. 2014). The mortality rates of patients with soft tissue injuries mainly depend on associated injuries. For example, the simultaneous incidence of lung contusion and flail chest more than doubles the mortality from 16 to 42 % (Clark et al. 1988). Flail chest is a clinical finding based on osseous fractures and the breathing mechanism. If three or more contiguous ribs are broken in at least two places, they create a flail segment that moves paradoxically to the remainder of the chest wall while the patient is breathing. Flail chest usually occurs in the anterior and anterolateral regions of the middle and lower ribs, which are less protected by musculature and surrounding tissue. Compliance of the ribs is equally important in the incurrence of flail chest as the force of impact. Severe pain and respiratory insufficiency, due to a decreased vital capacity and ineffective ventilation, may possibly be the consequences. While fractures can be detected by imaging, the paradoxical motion is usually proven by clinical examination (Kaewlai et al. 2008, p. 1567; Bier et al. 2015; Sirmali et al. 2003).

5.2 Biomechanics of Soft Tissue Contusion and Subcutaneous Emphysema

Soft tissue contusion may lead to emphysema, swelling, pain and hematoma from arterial or venous vessels. While arterial hematoma can enlarge rapidly, venous haematoma is often self-limiting and enlarges rather slowly. In this context, patients under anticoagulation therapy are more likely to develop complications (75 % vs. 41 %) (Ball et al. 2005) with a complication OR of 2.3 (95 % CI 1.1–4.8; $p<0.05$) calculated for the pre-injury use of anticoagulants (Mirvis et al. 2014, p. 179; Battle et al. 2013). Fractured ribs may possibly lead to subcutaneous emphysema and pneumothorax due to air leakage by tearing the pleura and pulmonary parenchyma. Tracheobronchial injuries can induce pneumomediastinum and subcutaneous emphysema as well. According to the fact that adipose tissue is not compartmentalised, subcutaneous emphysema of thoracic origin can possibly extend to the abdomen, scrotum, limbs, mediastinum, retroperitoneum or face/skull (Fig. 8) (Schnyder and Wintermark 2000, p. 10).

Fig. 8 Tension pneumothorax with air distribution through the abdomen extension to subcutaneous spaces. Bronchial carinoma restricting the left main bronchus (*arrow*) of a 65-year-old female patient in CE axial CT (**a**) and FDG-PET-CT (**b**). One week later the same patient presents with complete atelectasis of the left lung (secondary to complete restriction of the left main bronchus by bronchial carcinoma) and tension pneumothorax on the right side (**c**, *arrows*), air distribution to the abdomen (**d**, *arrows*) and pelvis (**e**, *right arrow*). The sagittal view (**f**) demonstrates the whole extension of the abdominal emphysema portion feeding subcutaneous compartment through inguinal pathways (**e**, *left arrow*)

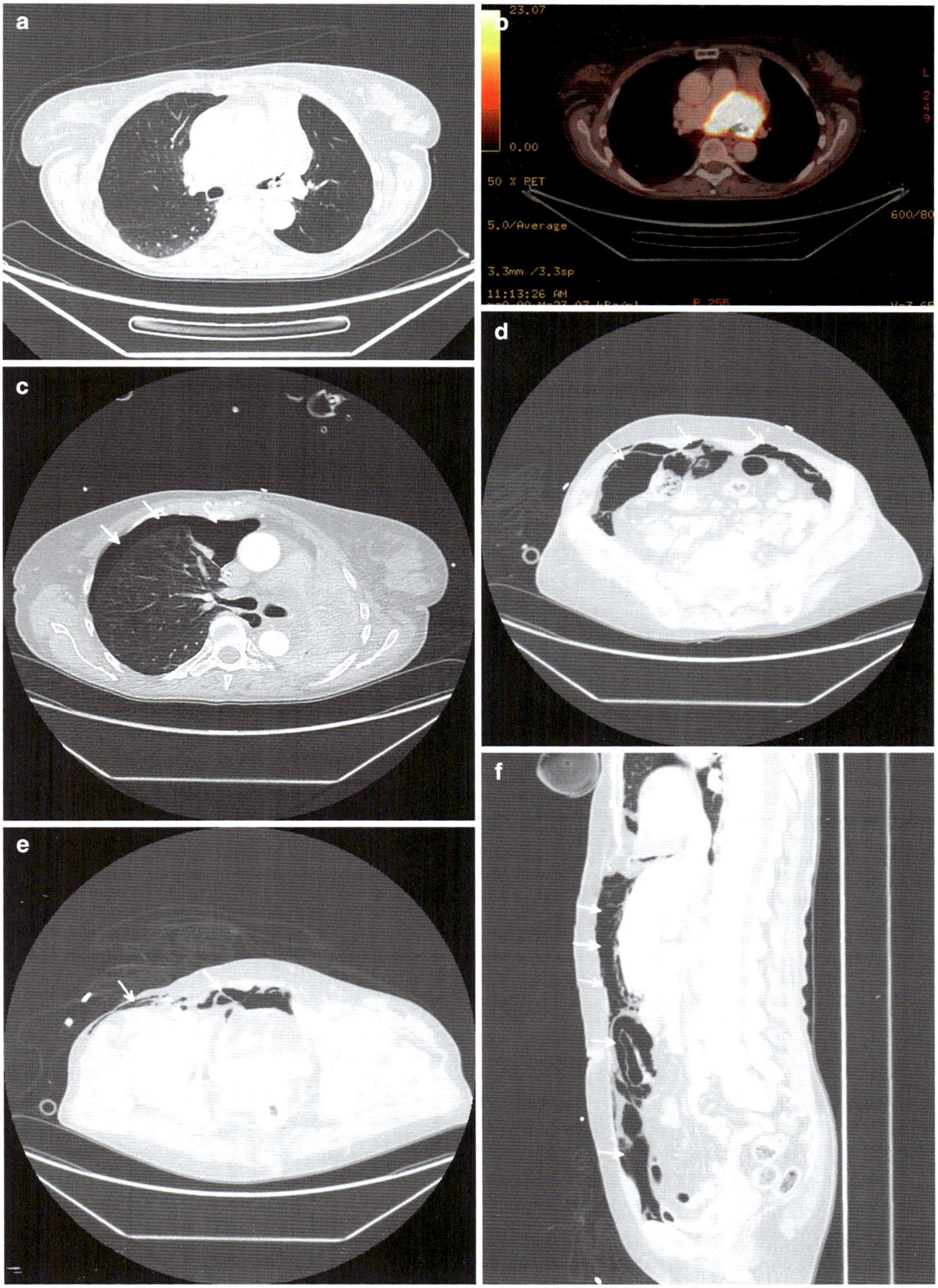
a
b
23.07
0.00
L
50 % PET
5.0/Average
3.3mm /3.3sp
11:13:26 AM
c
d
e
f

5.3 Main Part

Minor soft tissue contusion is usually occult on plain chest radiography. Especially, in obese patients, a haematoma or emphysema can be obscured. Increased density and asymmetry of the soft tissue are hints to a contusion (Mirvis et al. 2014, p. 179). Even small haematoma, appearing unimpressive, can be a marker for serious underlying injury. In up to 32 % of the cases, subcutaneous emphysema can be the first sign of an occult pneumothorax (Ball et al. 2005) which itself might become life threatening, especially during aeromedical transport at altitude or when positive pressure mechanical ventilation is used (Kirkpatrick et al. 2004). As Rothlin et al. detected subcutaneous emphysema by US in 17 % of 70 patients with thoracic pathologic entities, US may also be a reasonable screening tool for this condition (1993).

Tracheobronchial injuries are only found in 1–2 % of blunt chest trauma room patients (Welter and Hoffmann 2013, p. 113) because many patients will already have died from associated injuries before reaching the hospital. The overall estimated mortality is 30 % (Burke 1962; Chesterman and Satsangi 1966; Ecker et al. 1971; Kirsh et al. 1976). Deep cervical emphysema (100 %), paratracheal air (94 %) and pneumothorax (36 %) are radiological manifestations of possible tracheobronchial (Fig. 9) or oesophageal (Fig. 10) injuries. Tracheobronchial ruptures typically proceed transversally, parallel to the cartilage rings (74 %) (Welter and Hoffmann 2013, p. 114) and are usually located within a distance of 2.5 cm from the carina (Welter and Hoffmann 2013, p. 114; Kaewlai et al. 2008, pp. 1559–1561). Consequently, the region around the carina should be a particular reading focus. A persistent pneumothorax in a patient with tube placement and suction indicates a possible injury of the tracheobronchial tree, which should be investigated. The 'fallen lung'sign (Fig. 11), where a lung posterolaterally falls away from the hilum if the patient is supine and inferiorly if the patient is upright, indicates a complete ipsilateral transection of a main bronchus with its accompanying blood vessels. In such cases pneumomediastinum and cervical

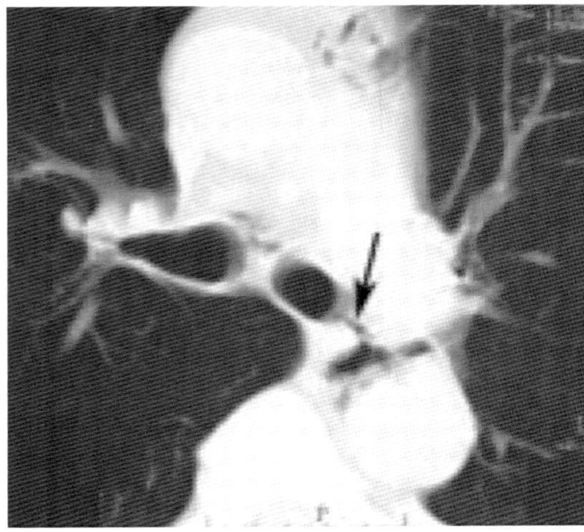

Fig. 9 Bronchial rupture (*arrow*). Axial CT, lung window

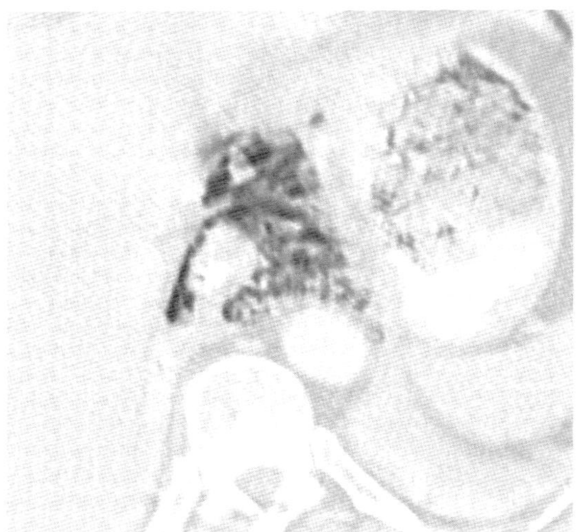

Fig. 10 Oesophagus rupture. Axial CT, lung window

subcutaneous emphysema are typical additional findings (Ball et al. 2005; Kaewlai et al. 2008, pp. 1559–1561). Furthermore, alveolar ruptures can also produce a pneumomediastinum (Fig. 12) via the Macklin effect (Fig. 13), first described by Macklin and Macklin in 1944, where air dissects into the mediastinum along the bronchovascular sheaths. Streaks of air can be seen along the bronchovascular bundles. Most cases of tracheal laceration can be identified with CT (70–100 %) (Kaewlai et al. 2008, pp. 1559–1561; Welter and

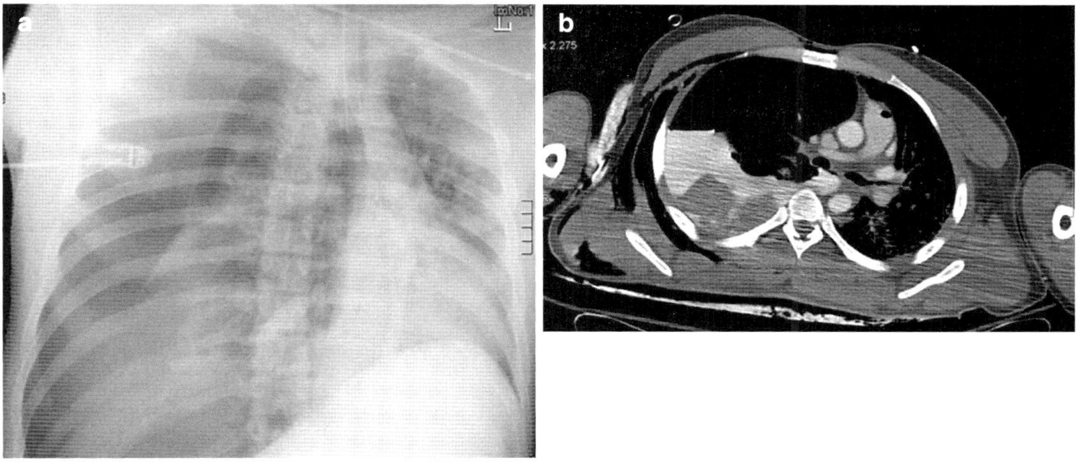

Fig. 11 Fallen lung sign. Polytraumatised patient of unknown age. AP chest radiogram directly after admission (**a**). Note the dorsal position of the lung and the massive tension component to the left side. Axial CE CT with soft tissue window settings (**b**) proofing tension haemopneumothorax, massive bleeding due to complete avulsion of the right hilus and subcutaneous emphysema. Efforts had to be terminated

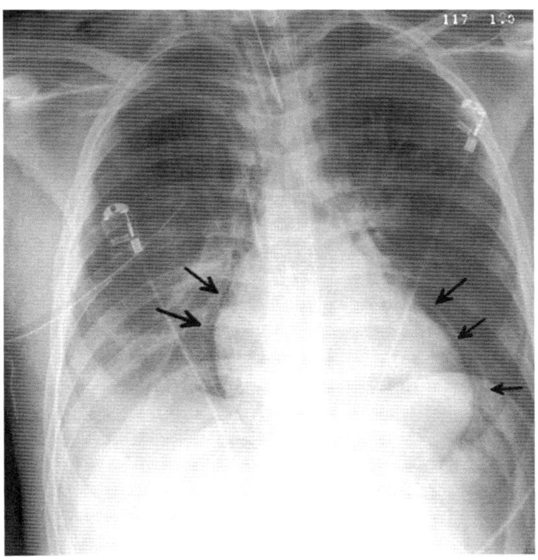

Fig. 12 Pneumomediastinum in AP chest radiogram (*arrows*)

Hoffmann 2013, p. 114). However, the diagnosis of a tracheobronchial tree injury should be confirmed by bronchoscopy. With respect to outcome, airway obstruction, bronchiectasis, pneumonia, abscess and empyema are potential complications (Kaewlai et al. 2008, pp. 1559–1561; Welter and Hoffmann 2013, p. 114).

A high-energy deceleration during a car accident may result in a hematoma of the lower neck and central chest in approximately 16 % of the cases. The presence of such a haematoma, called 'seatbelt sign', may be an indication for neck CT with intravenous contrast to evaluate possible cervical blood vessel injuries (carotid artery injuries 3 %) (Mirvis et al. 2014, p. 179; Rozycki et al. 2002). Vertebral artery injuries occur in about 0.5 % of blunt trauma patients (Nedeltchev and Baumgartner 2005). Especially the combination of a 'seatbelt sign' with a Glasgow Coma Scale <14, an ISS >16 and a fracture of the clavicle and/or first rib should raise particular concern for vascular injuries (Mirvis et al. 2014, pp. 179–183; Rozycki et al. 2002).

5.4 Summary

Even small and unimpressive soft tissue injuries and subcutaneous emphysema can be a marker for serious underlying injuries (e.g. occult pneumothorax in 32 % of patients with subcutaneous emphysema).

Deep cervical emphysema, paratracheal air, pneumomediastinum and pneumothorax (especially persisting pneumothorax after chest tube

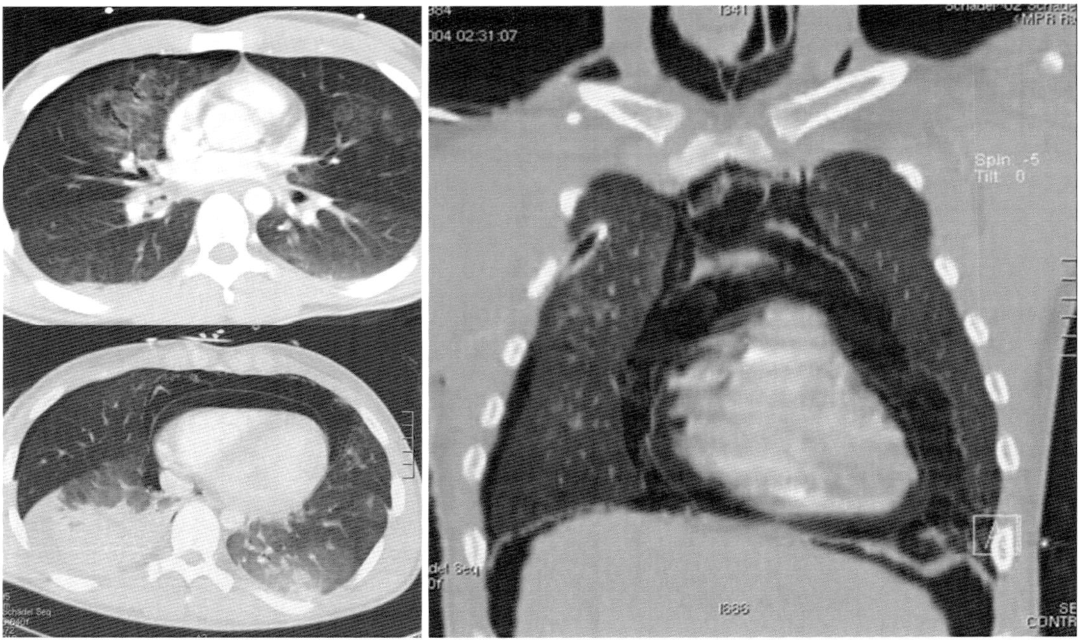

Fig. 13 Macklin effect. Axial and frontal CT reformations, lung window. A rib fracture (not shown) induced distal pulmonary laceration with air dissecting along the bronchovascular sheaths into the mediastinum. Same patient as Fig. 12

placement) are markers for tracheobronchial injuries. These are highly life-threatening conditions (mortality rate 30 %) that mostly appear within a distance of 2.5 cm from the carina.

Tracheal lacerations can be identified with CT in 70–100 % of the cases. However, diagnosis should be confirmed by bronchoscopy.

A 'seatbelt sign' indicates possible cervical blood vessel injuries, which should be ruled out by contrast-enhanced neck CT.

6 Rib Fractures

6.1 Epidemiology of Rib Fractures

Rib fractures are the most common skeletal injury in blunt chest trauma patients. They appear in about 50 % of patients after such an event and in about 10 % of patients after trauma in general (Ziegler and Agarwal 1994; Mirvis et al. 2014, pp. 179–182; Shorr et al. 1987; Henry et al. 2014). Fractures of the first two ribs are associated with thoracic aorta and other thoracic vascular (about 13 %) injuries (Clark et al. 1988; Magu et al. 2009). According to Shalhub et al., arterial haemorrhage after blunt chest trauma is associated with rib fractures in up to 44 % of the cases (Shalhub et al. 2011). Up to 50 % of rib fractures are multiple and, out of these, 8 % are bilateral (Shorr et al. 1987).

The rate of complications, such as pneumothorax, haemothorax, pulmonary contusion, flail chest, pneumonia and atelectasis, rises with the number of fractured ribs (16.4 % for 1–2 fractures, 33.6 % for 3–5 fractures, 52.7 % for 6 or more fractures), according to a study performed by Sirmali et al. (2003).

Flail chest is present in up to 7 % of blunt trauma patients. This condition may induce major haemorrhage or seriously impaired ventilation, and mortality rates – although varying in literature – can be as high as 33 % (Clark et al. 1988; Mirvis et al. 2014, pp. 179–183; Sirmali et al.

2003; Veysi et al. 2003; Kaewlai et al. 2008, p. 1567). Scapula fractures, when detected, should raise awareness of rib injuries, because their presence increases the likelihood of rib fractures (relative risk 3.1; $p<0.01$) and flail chest (relative risk 8.8; $p<0.001$) (Weening et al. 2005). Moreover, rib fractures are predictors for occult pneumothorax (OR = 2.65; 95 % CI = 1.34–5.24; $p=0.005$) (Ball et al. 2005). The overall mortality rate for patients presenting to hospital with rib fractures is approximately 6 % (Sirmali et al. 2003).

6.2 Biomechanics of Rib Fractures

While rib fractures among young adults mainly result from high-energetic trauma, they are often caused by falls from standing height and everyday activities in older adults. For this second group, fall preventing strategies are appropriate and suitable to lower the number of future incidents. Due to the chest wall architecture and the decreased support from muscles and other soft tissue, ribs fracture most often at the lateral aspects (Mirvis et al. 2014, pp. 179–183). The pain experienced from fractures of the bony chest wall, as well as combined direct lung injuries (e.g. pulmonary contusion) or haemorrhage (e.g. from intercostal arteries) may compromise ventilation. These injuries induce shunting and dead space ventilation, which additionally impair oxygenation (Mancini et al. 2014).

6.3 Main Part

Blunt chest trauma is regularly associated with fractures of the bony thorax, which reflect a large amount of energy having been imparted to the chest (Shorr et al. 1987; Henry et al. 2014). Nevertheless, we have to keep in mind that generally and particularly in children, serious trauma can be present in the absence of rib fractures. Skinner et al. investigated the morbidity of children and adults after blunt chest trauma. Compared to adults, children suffered less frequently from rib fractures (20.2 % vs. 42 %) and flail chest (2.4 % vs. 26.3 %), but more often from pulmonary contusion (79.8 % vs. 65.6 %) or associated head injuries (61.9 % vs. 42.3 %) (Skinner et al. 2015).

Isolated rib fractures are rarely life threatening, but bilateral or multiple rib fractures are indicators of severe chest injury with significant morbidity and mortality (Ziegler and Agarwal 1994; Kaewlai et al. 2008, p. 1567). Rib fractures may affect ventilation through laceration of underlying lung parenchyma, paradoxical chest wall motion and pain (Shorr et al. 1987; Henry et al. 2014). A fracture of the first three ribs is an indicator of high-energy trauma since these ribs are short, broad and well-protected by the scapula, clavicles and musculature. The brachial plexus and subclavian blood vessels are located close by and may possibly be injured. On the other hand, fractures of the lower three ribs are associated with trauma of the liver, spleen (Fig. 14), kidneys and lungs (Kaewlai et al. 2008, p. 1567). According to a study performed by Lee et al. including 105,683 trauma patients having been admitted to hospitals in the United States during the years 1984–1986, the presence of three or more rib fractures increased the relative risk of haemothorax/pneumothorax (18.4), spleen injury (6.2) and liver injury (3.6) (Lee et al. 1990). Therefore, rib fractures might be indicators of coexisting thoracic or abdominal trauma (Ziegler and Agarwal 1994; Kaewlai et al. 2008, p. 1567). US and, if the circumstances require, abdominal imaging should be performed to rule out associated injuries if one of the lower three ribs is fractured. If the trauma has not significantly affected the lower three ribs, abdomen or pelvis, a suspicious result in physical exam, laboratory studies or urinalysis will be required to justify the use of advanced imaging of this region, as stated in current guidelines (Henry et al. 2014).

Sirmali et al. developed a rule of thumb for blunt chest trauma patients: according to their findings, three or more rib fractures are an indication for the hospitalisation of patients. Elderly with six or more fractured ribs should be treated in intensive care units (Sirmali et al. 2003). Ball et al. found that 59 % of a group of trauma patients in whom an occult pneumothorax

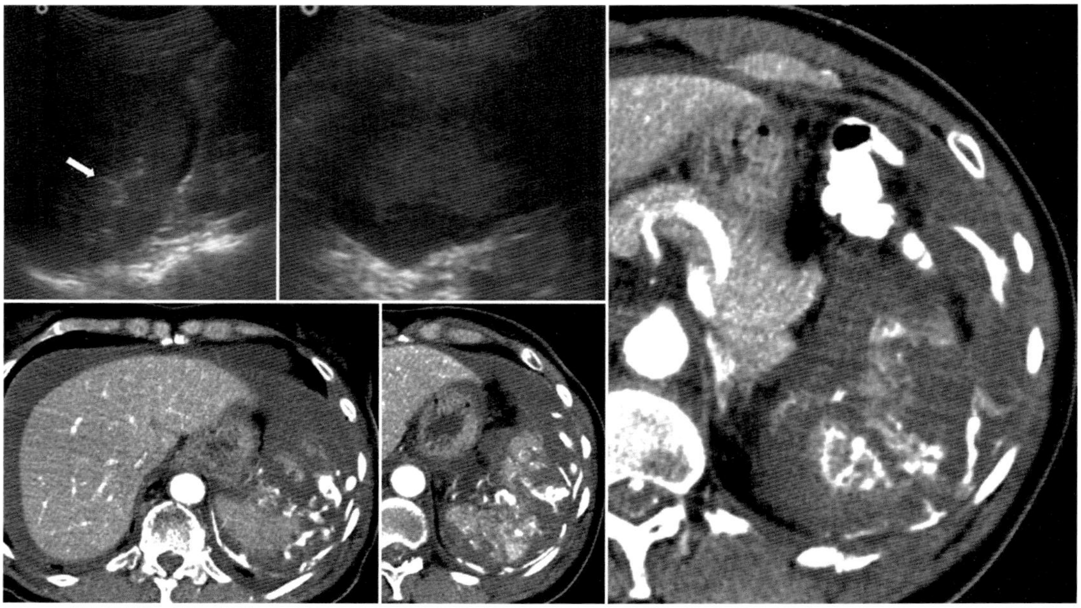

Fig. 14 Splenic haemorrhage (*arrow*) induced by laceration secondary to rib fracture in US and axial CT

(Fig. 15) was evident had coexisting rib fractures, while only 27 % of patients without pneumothorax had rib fractures (Ball et al. 2005). Bulger et al. reported that, according to their findings, the clinician should pay close attention to the number of rib fractures to stratify the expected mortality and morbidity, as the odds ratio rose by 1.19 per fractured rib for death and by 1.16 per fractured rib for pneumonia (Bulger et al. 2000). Pain control is a vital part in patient management to prevent respiratory depression, as well as the development of atelectasis and pulmonary infection. If indicated, epidural analgesia may be superior to intravenous and oral analgesia. Pain from multiple rib fractures can also inhibit weaning a patient from mechanical ventilation (Bulger et al. 2000; Sirmali et al. 2003).

The standard initial, and often the only required, imaging test for disclosing rib fractures in patients after minor trauma is chest radiography in two planes (Henry et al. 2014). It is crucial to weigh up the pros and cons of the available radiological equipment in terms of additional information and specificity against time, radiation burden and costs. Although rib fractures can lead to significant morbidity, it is more important to detect associated complications such as haemothorax (Fig. 16), pneumothorax, pulmonary contusion, flail chest, atelectasis, cardiovascular injury and injuries to solid and hollow abdominal organs. According to the American College of Radiology, chest CT without or with contrast is appropriate for patients with rib or sternal fractures plus at least one of these associated complications identified by clinical examination or other imaging (Henry et al. 2014). When isolated, single fractures, multiple fractures or non-acute fractures have a relatively low morbidity and mortality and are not an indication for chest CT unless malignancy is suspected in the aetiology, and a gain of additional information is expected. Failure to identify isolated rib fractures in uncomplicated cases does not automatically change outcome or patient management. Thus, there is little data to support the use of advanced imaging, even if CT is superior to radiography for detection of these fractures because of its sensitivity of 80–100 % (Henry et al. 2014; Traub et al. 2007; Magu et al. 2009; Bier et al. 2015). However, physicians should always keep in mind that only up to 50 % of rib fractures can be detected with chest radiography (Bulger et al.

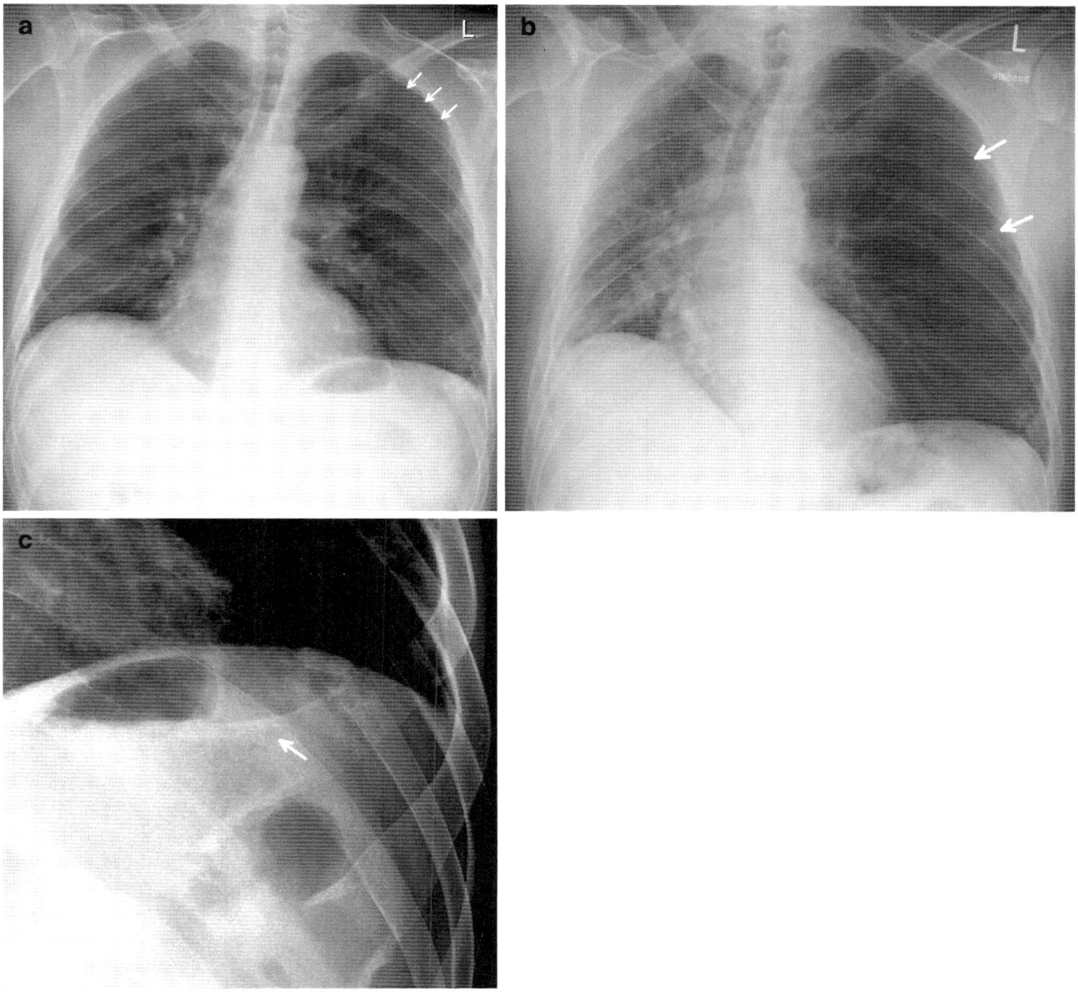

Fig. 15 Pneumothorax extension over the course of time. Initial chest radiogram of a patient with hardly visible pneumothorax (**a**, *arrows*). The patient developed a serious mediastinal shift indicating a tension component with now clearly visible border of the pneumothorax (**b**, *arrows*). A cutout from a lower rib-targeted radiogram revealed a rib fracture (**c**, *arrow*) as the most reasonable cause of the pneumothorax

2000). CT provides significantly more information than chest radiography alone if the patient shows chest wall tenderness, abnormal respiratory effort or reduced air entry. Traub et al. suggest that intubated patients should receive a routine CT chest scan at their first evaluation, as the survey of clinical information is restricted. For a final decision about the use of chest CT, the clinician should consider all clinical features and prior radiological information (Traub et al. 2007).

Fractured ribs may possibly produce a delayed haemothorax (DHX) due to intercostal artery haemorrhage (Fig. 16). DHX is described to appear in 2.1–7.4 % of blunt chest trauma patients. Curfman et al. reported a case of a patient who lost 6500 ml of blood out of one single intercostal artery, 10 days after a traumatic rib fracture while still being in the hospital (Curfman et al. 2015). Pleura-covered parts of the lung may extrude through the chest wall at a locus of traumatic defect, like a rib fracture, causing a traumatic lung herniation. Treatment should be taken into consideration before intubation because positive pressure ventilation can increase this

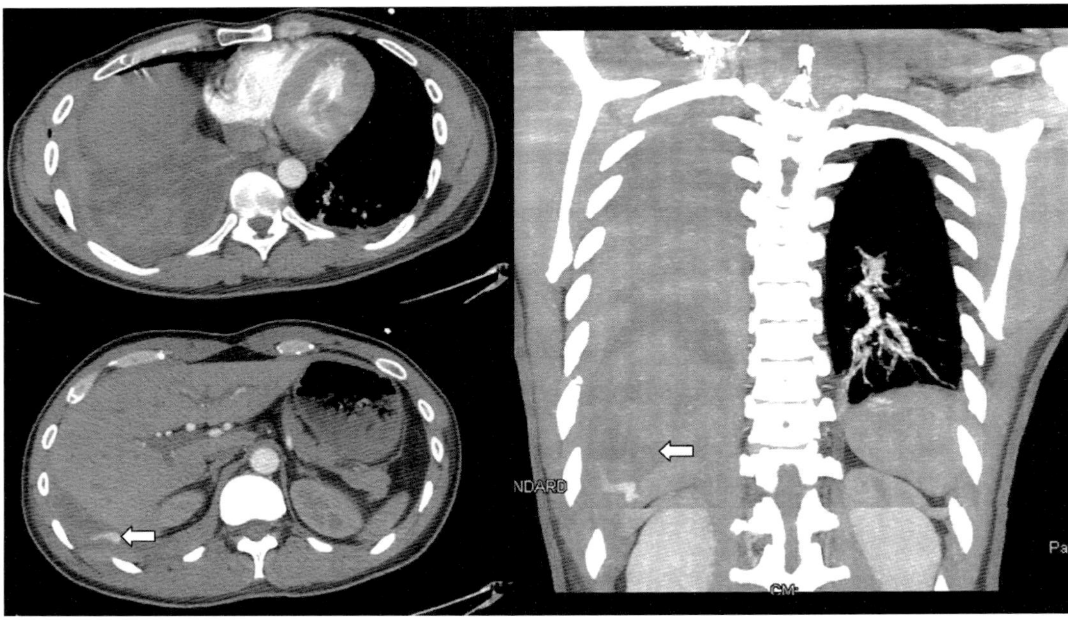

Fig. 16 Active arterial bleeding secondary to a rib fracture, which itself is not shown. The axial images of the chest CT in arterial phase reveal active contrast agent extravasation (*arrows*) leading to a haemothorax of the right side (*left* axial slices; *right* coronal MIP)

condition (Kaewlai et al. 2008, p. 1567). In case of pneumothorax and haemothorax caused by rib fractures, tube thoracostomy can be sufficient as treatment as the pressure from the expanding lungs may possibly stop the bleeding from small loci. Bleeding from major intrathoracic vessels or intercostal arteries usually requires balloon occlusion and thoracotomy (Sirmali et al. 2003).

The infantile chest wall is more elastic than the adult chest wall.

In children, ribs consequently need a higher level of energy transferred to the thorax to fracture. Therefore, children with rib fractures suffer more often from associated haemothorax, pneumothorax, brain injuries, spleen injuries and liver injuries than adults with rib fractures (Kessel et al. 2014). Bulger et al. reported a doubled mortality and thoracic morbidity after blunt chest trauma for elderly patients (65 years and older) in comparison to younger patients, regardless of similar injury patterns and injury severity (Bulger et al. 2000).

Detecting rib fractures in CT can be a quite challenging task. Each rib has a complex shape and extends across numerous sections, while twisting along its longitudinal axis. The sequential rib-by-rib evaluation traversing the whole thorax is tedious and time consuming. Furthermore, fractures can be hard to identify, especially if they are parallel to the section or not dislocated (Ringl et al. 2015). Coronal imaging is more sensitive to detect fractures parallel to axial sections (Cho et al. 2012). Fractures of the ribs are periodically overlooked in radiologic imaging and their detection can be of medical-legal relevance. The major part of the rib fractures missed in CT is located at the anterior arc and over 50 % of missed rib fractures have a buckled shape. They appear equally on both sides of the thoracic cage. Frequently, missed fractures are on the same rib or the neighbouring rib of fractures that have been detected (Cho et al. 2012; Ringl et al. 2015).

Due to often being associated with more severe injuries, the evaluation of rib fractures should take as less time as possible in acute trauma management. Post-processing software for CT data provides an automated recognition and numbering of all ribs, which are displayed – unfolded and rotatable – in one single plane

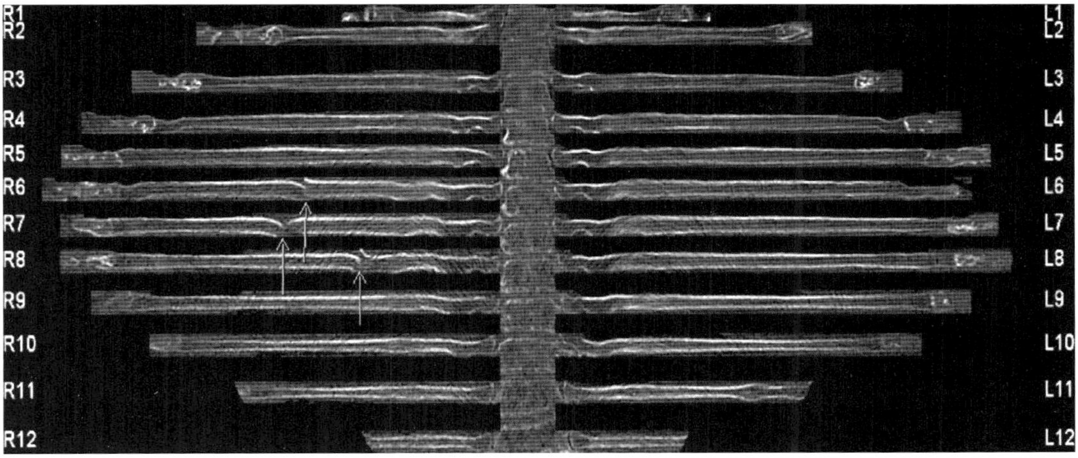

Fig. 17 Unfolded rib display (R1-12 = right ribs, L1-12 = left ribs) of an 88-year-old male patient with traumatic fractures of the sixth, seventh and eighth right rib (*arrows*)

(Fig. 17). 'The unfolded rib display significantly reduces reading time for detection of rib fractures in acute thoracic trauma and does not significantly compromise the diagnostic accuracy' (direct citation Bier et al. 2015). Moreover, the diagnostic accuracy of inexperienced readers (approximately 80 % for multiplanar reformatted images vs. approximately 92 % for unfolded rib images) may even be increased (Bier et al. 2015). Corresponding results were published for the detection of multiple myeloma and metastases from lung cancer (Homann et al. 2015a, b). Bier et al. documented a possible reduction of reading time by approximately 67–80 % (Bier et al. 2015) and a significant enhancement of inter-reader agreement. Manual correction is necessary in cases of incomplete or inaccurate recognition of ribs (Ringl et al. 2015). Furthermore, the utilisation of this technology involves the risk of false-positive findings because of two reasons: first, motion artefacts are harder to identify due to the missing correlation with surrounding tissue and, second, artificial curves caused by the software can be mistaken for buckled fractures (Bier et al. 2015; Homann et al. 2015a). However, these may be easily recognised after completing a short training (Ringl et al. 2015). If included in the standard calculation process of CT imaging, the unfolded rib display may be noticeably useful in the evaluation of the acute trauma patient when saving time is crucial.

Intercostal arteries are regularly exposed between the ribs within the first 6 cm lateral to the spinous process. From this point on, 97 % of intercostal arteries proceed in close local relation to the lower margin of the superior ribs. These ribs serve as shields for intercostal arteries due to their proximity but constitute a threat in case of a fracture (Helm et al. 2013). Rib fractures may tear intercostal, subclavian, axillary and internal mammary arteries and may cause life-threatening intrathoracic bleeding (Fig. 18) with a possible compression of heart and lungs. As a consequence of the increment of the blood density during the clotting process, active haemorrhage usually presents in CT as layers of different attenuation (Mirvis et al. 2014, p. 178). An extravasation of contrast material (attenuation value close to that of an adjacent artery) in CT is evidence of active bleeding (Fig. 19) (Kaewlai et al. 2008, pp. 1561–1565). Treatment can be endovascular (balloon occlusion/covered stent) or open repair. Shalhub et al. found endovascular therapy in case of blunt traumatic injuries to the thoracic outlet arteries to be superior to open repair in terms of operation time (149 min vs. 230 min, $p = 0.03$), blood loss (50 ml vs. 1.225 ml, $p = 0.03$) and morbidity (not statistically significant) (Shalhub et al. 2011).

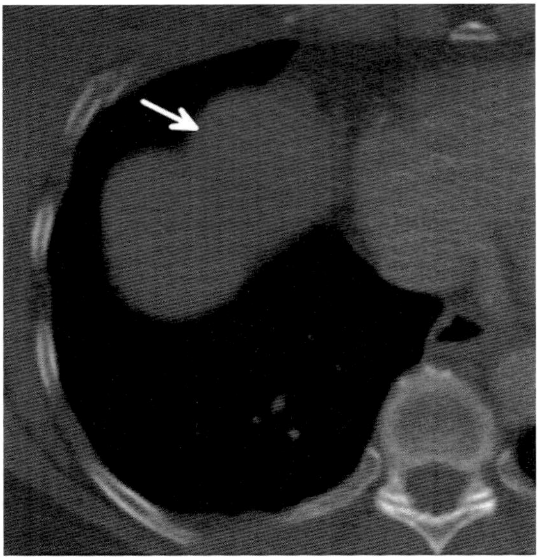

Fig. 18 Traumatic intrathoracic haemorrhage (*arrow tip*) of right internal mammary artery and ipsilateral rib fracture (*arrow base*) in axial CT, bone window settings

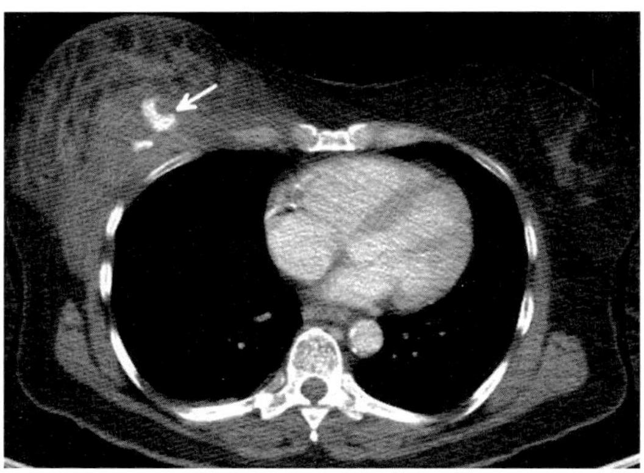

Fig. 19 Intra-mammarian bleeding. Massive soft tissue injury and contrast agent extravasation (*arrow*) as a sign of active haemorrhage of an intercostal artery, axial CT in arterial phase, soft window settings

6.4 Summary

Rib fractures are frequent injuries in patients after blunt chest trauma (50 %) and often associated with injuries to deeper structures. However, such deeper injuries may also be present in the absence of rib fractures.

Fractures of the upper ribs may be associated with injuries of the brachial plexus or subclavian blood vessels, and fractures of the lower ribs are more likely associated with injuries of abdominal organs.

Eighty percent to hundred percent of rib fractures can be identified with CT, and an unfolded display created with post-processing software helps to reduce the reading time by 67–80 % without compromising accuracy.

7 Sternal and Clavicular Fractures

7.1 Epidemiology of Sternal and Clavicular Fractures

In contrast to rib fractures, sternal fractures are rather seldom, appearing in 3–8 % of patients after severe blunt chest trauma (Veysi et al. 2009; Mirvis et al. 2014, p. 183). They should always be interpreted as a sign of a large amount of energy having been transmitted to the chest wall and deeper structures, particularly in combination with a fracture of the scapulae. Seventy percent of sternal fractures affect the body, 16.5 % the manubrium and 12.7 % of fractures are oblique (Schulz-Drost et al. 2015b; Schnyder and Wintermark 2000, pp. 17–20). Among the injuries associated with sternal fractures, which occur in 55–77 % of those patients, are rib fractures (up to 14 %), cardiac contusion (1.5–6 %), cervicothoracic spine injuries (up to 23 %), lung contusion (up to 12 %), flail chest, pericardial effusion and injuries of the internal mammary vessels and their branches, such as the musculophrenic or pericardiophrenic vessels (Schnyder and Wintermark 2000, pp. 17–20; Mirvis et al. 2014, p. 183; Mancini et al. 2014; Knobloch et al. 2006). Due to these grave associated injuries, sternal fractures are related to quite a high mortality of up to 22 % (Schnyder and Wintermark 2000, pp. 17–20). Clavicle fractures account for 2.6–5 % of all fractures (Scheurecker 2015, p. 831). They commonly result from falls or traffic accidents and about half of them occur in children under the age of 10 years (Mirvis et al. 2014, pp. 468–469).

7.2 Biomechanics of Sternal and Clavicular Fractures

Sternal fractures are usually the result of high-energy deceleration or direct blow (up to 84 %) to the anterior chest wall (Kaewlai et al. 2008, p. 1569, Schulz-Drost et al. 2015b). The most common mechanism is the impact of a steering wheel (information of deformity of steering wheel or steering column is valuable), seat belt or airbag to the chest in a motor vehicle collision (Mirvis et al. 2014, p. 183). Other mechanisms may be indirect fractures secondary to a fall on the back or spontaneous fractures as a result of muscle spasms (Schulz-Drost et al. 2015b). Sternal fractures may impair ventilation by contributing to paradoxic chest wall motion in combination with rib fractures (flail chest) (Shorr et al. 1987). Either a blow to the medial clavicle or a blow to the shoulder can lead to sternoclavicular dissection. Whereas a posterior blow to the shoulder often leads to a posterior sternoclavicular dissection, an anterior blow to the shoulder is the appropriate mechanism for an anterior dissection (Kaewlai et al. 2008, p. 1569).

7.3 Main Part

In sternal fractures, the body (70 %) and the manubrium (16.5 %) are most commonly involved (Schulz-Drost et al. 2015a, b; Schnyder and Wintermark 2000, pp. 17–20; Kaewlai et al. 2008, p. 1569). Simple sternal fractures can be seen as isolated injuries that rarely have any consequence, while displaced sternal fractures or sternal fractures with manubriosternal joint disruption regularly are associated with other thoracic, cardiac and spinal injuries. Sternal fractures are best displayed in sagittal or coronal CT because fracture lines are commonly parallel to axial sections. Supine chest radiography often only demonstrates significantly displaced fractures and shows no sign of an existing fracture in up to 84 % of patients (Schnyder and Wintermark 2000, pp. 17–20).

As nearly all of the sternal fractures are accompanied by a hematoma, anterior mediastinal or retrosternal haemorrhage may be the clue to the diagnosis in cases when the fracture is not clearly discernible. The CT density of such a haematoma is close to the value of unenhanced blood and aorta, information in the literature ranges from +20 to +70 HU (primarily depending on the stage of the clotting process). Commonly, there is a preserved fat plane evident between the retrosternal haematoma and the aorta. If the fat border delineation is missing and the retrosternal blood has direct contact to the aortic wall, a traumatic aortic injury is most likely the source of the haematoma. As previously mentioned, sternoclavicular dislocations can occur after blows to the clavicle or to the shoulder. While anterior dislocations are usually evident on palpation and inspection, posterior dislocations may be occult in conventional radiography and clinical examination. CT with contrast can confirm the diagnosis of a suspected posterior sternoclavicular dislocation and evaluate the vascular status. This is obvious in case of aortic injury but also valuable in posterior sternoclavicular dislocations because they are frequently associated with injuries of adjacent blood vessels, trachea and oesophagus. If a sternal fracture is evident, a cardiac evaluation including ECG, cardiac enzymes and troponin should be done to rule out cardiac injury. Most sternal fractures are treated conservatively. In case of nonunion, severe pain or instability, open reduction and internal fixation may be required (Kaewlai et al. 2008, pp. 1561–1562; Feeman 2010; Knobloch et al. 2006, 2008; Mancini et al. 2014; Mirvis et al. 2014, pp. 178–183; Schnyder and Wintermark 2000, pp. 17–20). The recognition of sternal fractures and associated aortic, vascular, pericardial (Fig. 20), cardiac and other thoracic injuries is often crucial in the management of patients with blunt thoracic trauma (Shorr et al. 1987).

Clavicle fractures are categorised with the Allman classification (Allman 1967) in fractures of the proximal third (5 %), middle third (80 %) and

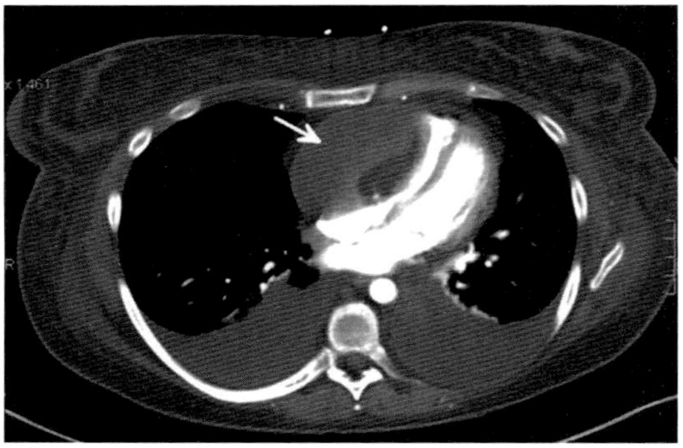

Fig. 20 Traumatic pericardial tamponade (*arrow*). Twenty five-year-old female, axial CT in arterial phase, soft window settings

distal third (15 %) (Mirvis et al. 2014, pp. 468–469). They are usually evaluated with AP and 15° to 25° cephalic tilt apical oblique clavicular radiograms. Complicated and dislocated fractures may need surgical treatment. Preoperative sagittal, coronal and 3D CT reformations are very helpful in this case (Scheurecker 2015, pp. 831–832).

Intravascular aortic stents have revolutionised the treatment of traumatic aortic injury and partially replaced open reduction. This procedure comes along with decreased mortality, complications, operation time and length of stay. The initial CT angiogram is used for the stent-graft placement planning (Mirvis et al. 2014, pp. 204–208). Interventional radiology is a substantial part of radiologic practice. For more information on this topic, we refer to the chapters 'Aortic Injuries' and 'Vascular Chest Emergencies' in this book and the section "The Role of Interventional Radiology" (pp. 235–267) from the book *Emergency Radiology of the Abdomen: Imaging Features and Differential Diagnosis for a Timely Management Approach* (Wirth and Treitl 2012). Furthermore, the book *Problem Solving in Emergency Radiology* (Mirvis et al. 2014) provides a good overview.

7.4 Summary

Sternal fractures are a sign of high-energy deceleration or impact and regularly associated with cardiac and aortic injuries.

Eighty-four percent of sternal fractures are occult on chest radiograms and even with CT non-dislocated fractures can be hard to identify. Retrosternal haemorrhage can be the clue to a sternal fracture.

Clavicle fractures account for 2.6–5 % of all fractures with a portion of 50 % occurring in patients under the age of 10 years. Complicated and dislocated fractures may need surgical treatment, in which case preoperative sagittal, coronal and 3D CT reformations are very helpful.

8 Fractures and Dissection of the Scapula

8.1 Epidemiology of Fractures and Dissection of the Scapula

Fractures and dissection of the scapula are a rather rare condition, occurring in approximately 4–7 % of polytraumatised patients (Kaewlai et al. 2008, pp. 1568–1569; Veysi et al. 2003; Weening et al. 2005). The mean age of the patients ranges from 35 to 45 (Mirvis et al. 2014, pp. 470–471) years and about three out of four patients are male (Weening et al. 2005). The rate of related injuries is very high (75–100 %) (Mancini et al. 2014). Patients with scapula fracture show an average of 3.5 associated injuries, such as rib fractures (27–54 %), cerebral injuries (up to 42 %), clavicle fractures (23–27 %), pulmonary injuries (16–23 %), brachial plexus injuries (8–11 %), arterial injuries (3–11 %), injuries of the thoracic spine (3 %) and adjacent injuries of the shoulder girdle (Schofer et al. 2009; Imatani 1975; McGahan et al. 1980; Salimi et al. 2008; Veysi et al. 2003; Weening et al. 2005; Thompson et al. 1985). According to Schofer et al., scapula fractures may be associated with ipsilateral rib fractures in up to 44 % of the cases (Schofer et al. 2009). In a study including 1164 polytraumatised patients, Veysi et al. found out that the ones presenting with scapula fractures had more severe underlying chest injuries and a significantly higher overall ISS compared to patients without scapula fractures (27.12 ± 15.13 vs. 22.8 ± 14.4, $p = 0.01$).

However, this did not correlate with an increased mortality (Veysi et al. 2003). Weening et al. found the presence of either a pneumothorax (relative risk 3.7; $p<0.001$) or a pulmonary contusion (relative risk 3.5; $p<0.001$) to be significantly more likely in patients with scapula fractures than in control patients (Weening et al. 2005). Data about mortality rates ranges from 2 to 14.3 % (Veysi et al. 2003; Salimi et al. 2008; McGahan et al. 1980; Thompson et al. 1985; Armstrong and Van der Spuy 1984).

8.2 Biomechanics of Fractures and Dissection of the Scapula

The scapula can sustain a high amount of energy in case of an axial compression through the humerus without fracturing, because the energy is distributed via the 'recoil mechanism', described by Rowe (scapula recoils on thoracic cage) (Rowe 1963; Wiedemann 2004). A fractured scapula is definitely a sign for a high-energy transfer, commonly due to motor vehicle collisions (automobile 48–52 %, motorcycle 11–25 %, pedestrian 18–46.7 %) or falls from great heights (12–17.1 %), and one must suspect injuries of deeper structures. Direct force to the scapula (75 % of cases) or indirect transmission of axial force through the humerus are typical mechanisms (Shorr et al. 1987; Kaewlai et al. 2008, pp. 1568–1569; Schofer et al. 2009; Mirvis et al. 2014, pp. 470–471; Imatani 1975; McGahan et al. 1980; Salimi et al. 2008).

Scapulothoracic (ST) dissociation due to major musculoskeletal trauma is a closed complete traumatic forequarter amputation, diagnosed by a pulseless arm and specific radiographic findings. The avulsion of the subclavian, axillary or brachial artery, as well as the avulsion of the brachial plexus can cause major haemorrhage, making the ST dissociation a life-threatening condition (Ebraheim et al. 1987). Furthermore, scapula fractures may be caused by a sudden contraction of the muscles during a seizure or in an electrical accident (Cser and Vajda 1976; Mathews et al. 1983; Wiedemann 2004).

8.3 Main Part

There are various classification systems for scapula fractures. Each one has its raison d'être and provides advantages for specific purposes, but at the same time it has its limitations. The inclusion of a prediction of outcome and treatment option is difficult as they also depend on other factors like fracture displacement, patient-associated conditions or injury of nerves, blood vessels and soft tissue (Harvey et al. 2012; Audige et al. 2014; Bartonicek et al. 2014; Euler et al. 1992; Friederichs et al. 2014; Neuhaus et al. 2014; Schofer et al. 2009; Wiedemann 2004).

The New International Classification of Scapula Fractures (Fig. 21, Table 1), developed by the Orthopaedic Trauma Association (OTA) Classification Committee and the AO Classification Advisory, is a system adjusted to an emergency trauma setting, where clinical communication, documentation, low time consumption and inter-reader agreement are important. The scapula is divided into three segments: processes, fossa and body. Process fractures are subdivided into fractures of the coracoid or acromion. Fossa fractures may be fractures of the rim (1), simple split fractures (2) or complex joint fractures (3). Body fractures are subdivided into simple fractures with one fracture line and either one/no border exit points (1) or two border exit points (2) and fractures with multiple fragments presenting three or more border exits (3) (Harvey et al. 2012; Alton and Gardner 2015).

The utilisation of the Euler and Rüedi classification enables radiologists to give a more detailed characterisation of the morphology, severity and prognosis of scapula fractures. This may be important for decisions between either conservative or operative treatment (Fig. 22, Table 2). Fractures are divided into five groups, three (A, B, C) being extra-articular and two (D, E) being intra-articular. The severity of fracture increases from type A to E and within a specific type with increasing numeric value. Isolated or multifragmentary fractures of the scapula body are classified as type A, fractures of the processes as type B and type C refers to fractures of the scapular neck. Type B fractures are subdivided into

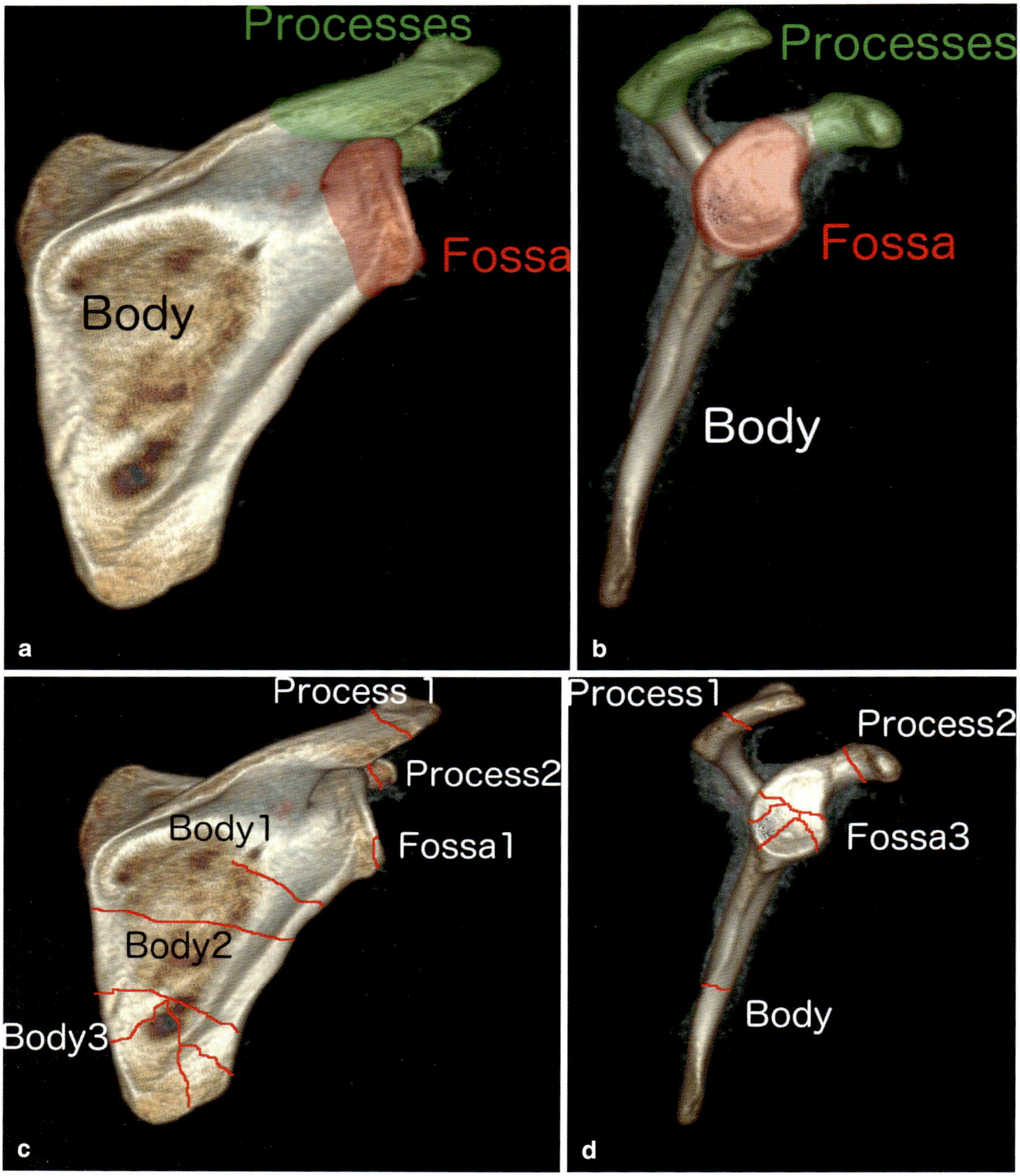

Fig. 21 New International Classification of Scapula Fractures. Dorsal view of fracture areas (**a**): *uncoloured* body, *green* processes, *red* fossa. Glenoidal view of fracture areas (**b**): *uncoloured* body, *green* processes, *red* fossa. Exemplary fracture lines in dorsal view (**c**) and glenoidal view (**d**)

fractures of the spine (B1), coracoid (B2) and acromion (B3). Neck fractures are rarely located at the anatomical neck (C1) but more frequently at the surgical neck (C2). If a fracture of the surgical neck is associated with another injury of the superior shoulder suspensory complex, it is classified as type C3. These fractures may be accompanied by a fracture of the clavicle and acromion (C3a) or by torn coracoclavicular and coracoacromial ligaments (C3b). The ‘coracogleniodal

Table 1 New international classification of scapula fractures

Fossa	
	1. Rim
	2. Simple split fractures
	3. Complex joint fractures
Body	
	1. Simple with a single fracture line and one or no border exit
	2. Simple with one fracture line and two border exit points
	3. Multifragmentary with three or more border exit points
Processes	
	1. Acromion
	2. Coracoid

block' is separated from all stabilising structures in both cases. This condition may clinically present itself as an instable 'floating shoulder'. The suprascapular nerve is particularly in danger when the patient presents with a C2 or C3 fracture, due to the anatomical relation to the incisura scapulae (scapular notch) at the upper margin of the surgical neck. Intra-articular fractures are classified as type D, further subdivided into fractures of the glenoid rim (D1), glenoid fossa (D2) and neck or body fractures with articular involvement (D3). Intra-articular fractures with an associated fracture of the humeral head represent a separate group (type E) (Euler et al. 1992; Wiedemann 2004).

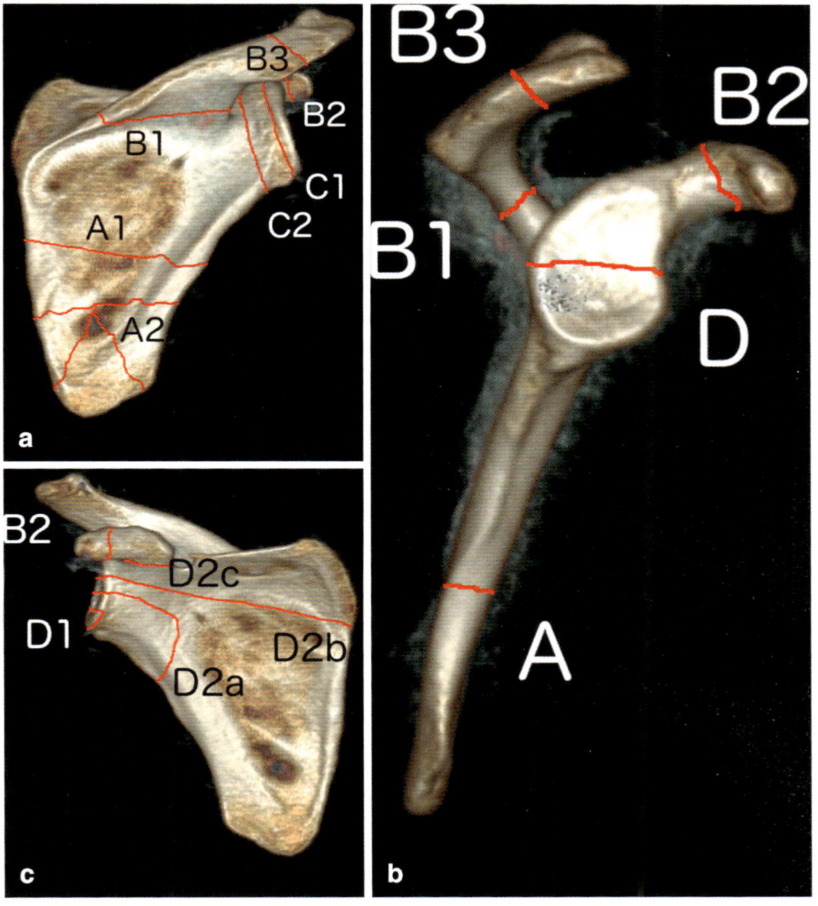

Fig. 22 Euler and Rüedi classification of scapula fractures. Dorsal (**a**), glenoidal (**b**) and ventral (**c**) view

Table 2 Euler and Rüedi classification of scapula fractures

A. Fractures of the scapular body
A1 Isolated
A2 Multifragmentary
B. Fractures of the scapular processes
B1 Spina scapulae
B2 Coracoid
B3 Acromion
C. Fractures of the scapular neck
C1 Anatomical neck
C2 Surgical neck
C3 Surgical neck with
(a) Fractured clavicle and acromion
(b) Torn CC and CA ligaments
D. Articular scapula fractures
D1 Glenoid rim
D2 Glenoid fossa with
(a) Inferior glenoid fragment
(b) Horizontal split of scapula
(c) Coracoglenoid block formation
(d) Comminuted fractures
D3 Combination of neck and body fracture
E. Fracture combination with humeral head fractures

Body (49–89 %) and neck fractures (10–60 %) are more common than glenoid, coracoid or acromion process fractures. A coexisting hematoma may be very small in patients with scapula fractures since the closed fascial compartments can prevent extension (Wiedemann 2004). Thus, the clinical inspection has to be executed carefully not to overlook a scapula fracture. Furthermore, the absence of pain is no exclusion criterion for the existence of a scapula fracture, as a substantial part of patients presents without any pain (28 %) or with only mild pain if the shoulder is heavily stressed (18 %) (Schofer et al. 2009).

The detection of scapula fractures on plain radiographic films can be difficult, and more severe coexisting injuries often disguise clinical symptoms. Thus, these fractures are regularly (more than 30 %) overlooked in the initial trauma workup. CT can reveal intra-articular extension of fractures more precisely. Bartonicek et al. reported that 3D CT reconstructions (Fig. 23) enable the most accurate diagnosis of fractures of the scapula neck (Bartonicek et al. 2014). The

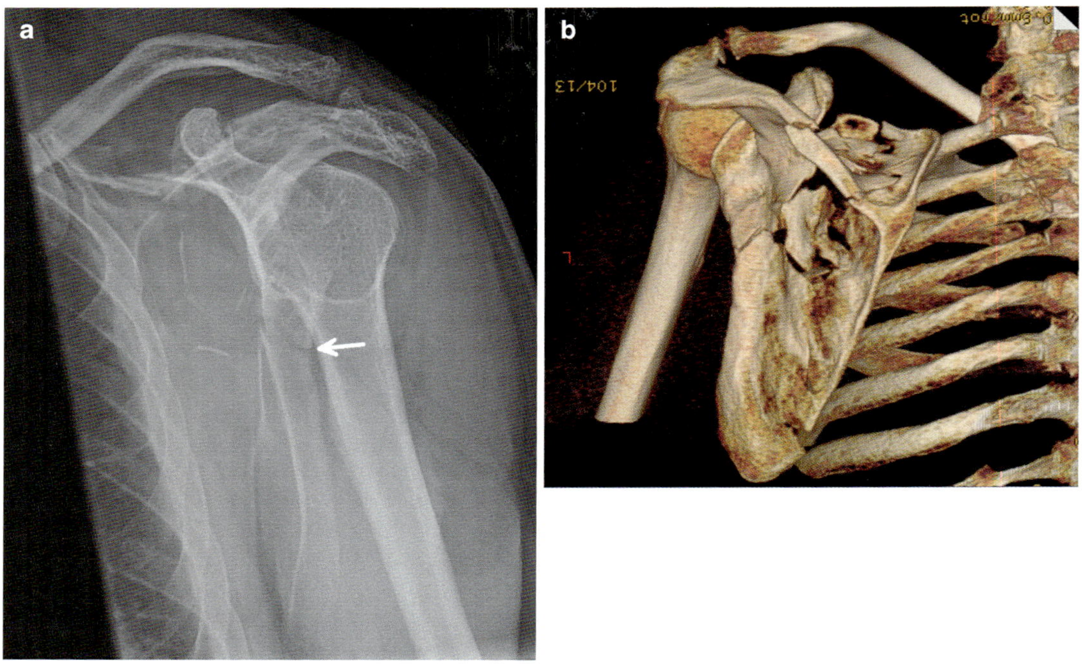

Fig. 23 Scapular fracture. Combined A2 fracture (*arrow*) and B1 fracture (Euler and Rüedi classification) or type 3 body fracture (new international classification, *arrow*) in radiography (**a**) and 3D CT rendering (**b**)

transspinous neck fractures described by Bartonicek are body fractures in keeping with the new international classification of scapula fractures. Displaced glenoid intra-articular fractures and displaced juxtaarticular fractures often require surgical treatment. Nevertheless, up to 88 % of scapula fractures may be treated conservatively with good results in patient outcome. To prevent a loss of shoulder immobility, range-of-motion exercises should be started as soon as possible (Salimi et al. 2008; Mancini et al. 2014; Kaewlai et al. 2008, pp. 1568–1569; Schofer et al. 2009; Wiedemann 2004). According to McGahan et al., up to 50 % of patients with scapula fractures with an indication for operative treatment may have such grave associated injuries that no open reduction can be carried out (McGahan et al. 1980).

Scapula fractures are associated with arterial injuries in 3–11 % of the cases (McGahan et al. 1980; Thompson et al. 1985). As previously mentioned in the section "Rib Fractures", arterial injuries due to blunt trauma can be treated with endovascular approach and by open repair. The endovascular approach is highly successful (for the subclavian artery 94–100 %) and procedure-related complications occur relatively rare (for the subclavian artery 0–22 %) (Shalhub et al. 2011). Mixed procedures may sometimes also be attractive like in the case of fast bleeding control by using a temporary proximal balloon occlusion and subsequent operative refixation of a ruptured artery.

8.4 Summary

Scapula fractures regularly appear after high-energy transfer and are often initially overlooked due to other grave associated injuries.

Scapulothoracic dissociation is a major traumatic injury with the avulsion of the brachial plexus and brachial, axillary or subclavian blood vessels and is life threatening for this reason.

Two examples for common classification systems for scapula fractures are the new international classification and the Euler and Rüedi classification: The New International Classification of Scapula Fractures divides the scapula into fossa, body and processes with further subdivision regarding precise location and severity. In the Euler and Rüedi classification, the scapula is divided into body, processes, neck and articular region. Compared to the new international classification, it is more complex but provides more detailed information and also includes combined fractures.

9 Injuries of the Vertebral Column and Spinal Cord

9.1 Epidemiology of the Vertebral Column and Spinal Cord

Fractures of the thoracolumbar spine occur in up to 18 % of blunt trauma patients (Mirvis et al. 2014, p. 154). Fractures of the cervicothoracic spine may also be associated with sternal fractures as a result of an over-flexion of the trunk (e.g. against a seatbelt) (Fig. 24) (Schnyder and Wintermark 2000, pp. 17–20; Mirvis et al. 2014, p. 183). Turkalj et al. detected vertebral fractures in 27.9 % out of 61 patients with blunt chest trauma (Turkalj et al. 2014). Approximately 16–30 % of all spine fractures are thoracic spine fractures, and about 50 % of patients presented with associated focal neurologic deficits (Lomoschitz et al. 2003).

Worldwide, between 250,000 and 500,000 people suffer a spinal cord injury annually (World Health Organization 2015b). Stephan et al. found spinal cord injury with neurologic deficit to be present in every 13th patient with polytrauma, of which over 50 % suffered from complete cord lesion (Stephan et al. 2015). Such an injury comes along with a two- to fivefold increased risk of dying prematurely, compared with people without spinal cord injuries. Spinal cord injury may be traumatic (90 %) and supported by a pre-existing disease (e.g. cancer) or degeneration. Possible symptoms are the loss of motor or sensory function and more severe failure in the regulation systems of bowel, bladder, blood pressure, heart rate or breathing. In adolescence (15–19 years), females are more at risk, whereas males account for most cases of spinal cord injury in young adulthood (20–29 years). In total,

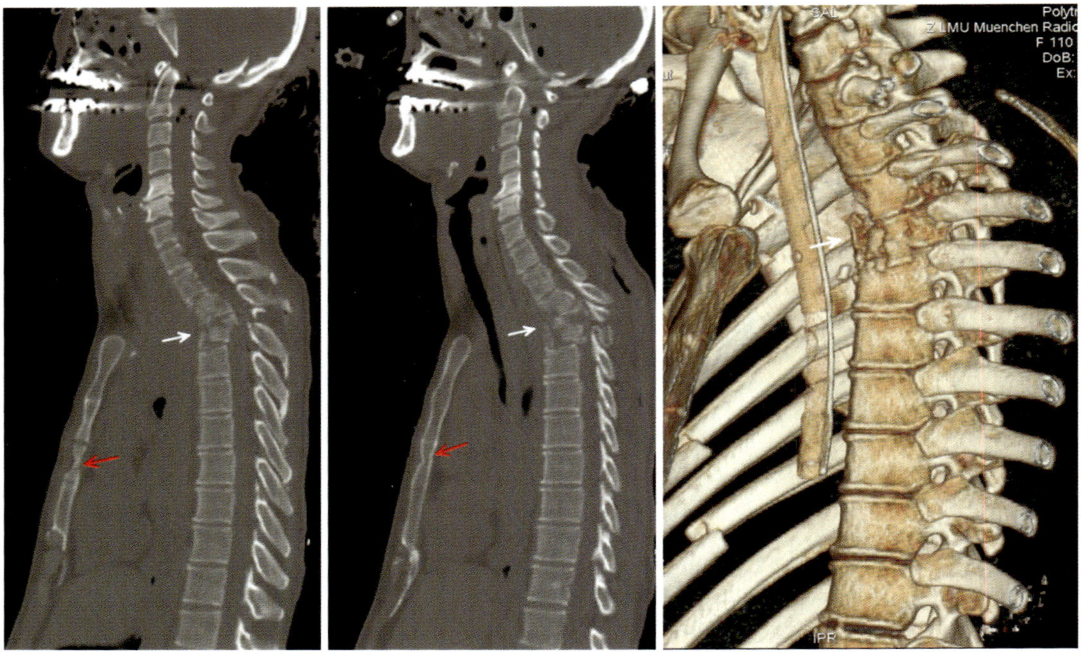

Fig. 24 Vertebral burst fracture of Th3 and Th4 (*white arrows*). Sagittal CT reformation and 3D CT rendering of a polytraumatised patient and an associated sternal fracture (*red arrows*). CT autopsy

the male to female ratio is at least 2:1. Among the possible complications are multi-organ failure, deep vein thrombosis, urinary tract infections, sepsis, muscle spasms, osteoporosis, pressure ulcers, chronic pain, respiratory complications and extended length of hospital stay (Stephan et al. 2015; World Health Organization 2015b). Appropriate rehabilitation therapy is aimed to prevent or alleviate these complications. Approximately 20–30 % of spinal cord injury patients show clinically significant signs of depression, which in turn may reduce the therapy effect. Adequate psychiatric therapy may assist in prevention of the evolution of a vicious circle (World Health Organization 2015b).

9.2 Biomechanics of the Vertebral Column and Spinal Cord Injuries

Vertebral column and spinal cord injuries may be caused by road traffic accidents, falls, crash, acts of violence or related to work or sports (World Health Organization 2015b). Falls (OR, 2.81), crash (OR, 2.80), motor vehicle collision with rollover and/or ejection (OR, 1.11) and unenclosed vehicle crash (OR, 1.08) are the four injury mechanisms that can be seen as high-risk mechanisms for significant spinal injury as they are accountable for 67.4 % of these injuries (Inaba et al. 2015). After vertebral augmentation (e.g. vertebroplasty), a new vertebral fracture is most likely to occur in nearby vertebrae. A connection to osteoporosis is presumable, as vertebral fractures are very common among older men and postmenopausal women (Melton and Kallmes 2006).

Spinal epidural hematoma, associated with coagulopathy, vascular malformations, neoplasms and pregnancy, may occur after spinal trauma and lead to neurologic deficit (Cha et al. 2011).

9.3 Main Part

Clinical findings and radiologic imaging indirectly predict the stability of thoracic and lumbar spine injuries. Widely accepted for this purpose is

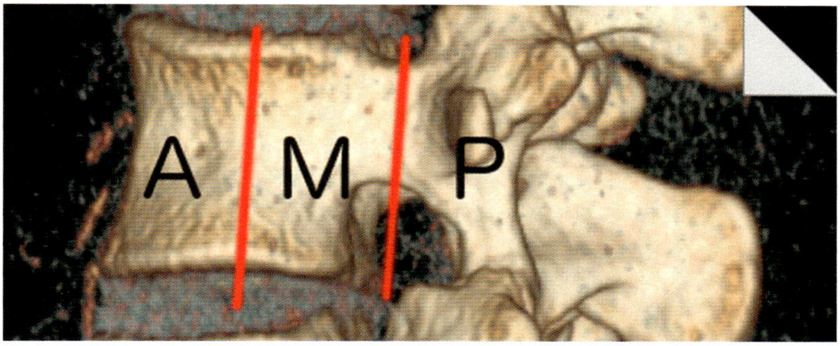

Fig. 25 Denis classification of vertebral fractures. *A* anterior column, *M* middle column, *P* posterior column

the utilisation of the three-column theory, which orthopaedic surgeon Francis Denis publicised in 1982, based on Holdsworth's two-column theory (Denis 1983). The anterior vertebral body, anterior annulus fibrosus and the anterior longitudinal ligament form the anterior column; the middle column includes the posterior wall of the vertebral body, the posterior annulus fibrosus and the posterior longitudinal ligament. The posterior column includes the posterior bony arch and the posterior ligamentous complex (including the interspinous ligaments, the supraspinous ligaments, the capsule and the ligamentum flavum) (Fig. 25). Spinal injuries can be considered as unstable if two or three of these columns are damaged (Fig. 26) with a focus on the middle column (Denis 1983). Denis categorised spinal injuries into four major modes, namely, compression fractures, burst fractures, seat belt-type fractures and fracture dislocation (see Table 3) (Denis 1983). The classification of spinal fractures into stable or unstable can be conducted with the utilisation of multiplanar reformations in computed tomography. Nevertheless, complex fractures or uncertain findings should be evaluated in coronal images (Begemann et al. 2004).

The missed or delayed diagnosis of a spinal injury can result in a disastrous situation and even under strictly precautious management iatrogenic worsening may happen (Mirvis et al. 2014, p. 154; Inaba et al. 2015). Pain (sensitivity 63.3 %, specificity 82.0 %), tenderness to palpation (sensitivity 67.4 %, specificity 77.6 %), deformity (sensitivity 5.3 %, specificity 99.6 %) and neurologic deficit (sensitivity 6.8 %, specificity 99.1 %) are predictors for clinically significant spinal fractures. Nevertheless, these should not be the only criteria to rule out a possible injury, as approximately 21.6 % of patients with clinically significant spinal injury show no suspicious finding in the physical examination (Inaba et al. 2015). In order to develop a clinical decision rule for advanced imaging of the thoracolumbar spine after blunt trauma like the NEXUS and Canadian C-Spine Rules for the cervical spine, Inaba et al. added a high-energy mechanism (see section "Biomechanics of the Vertebral Column and Spinal Cord Injuries") and a patient age ≥60 years to a positive finding in the clinical exam. The combination of these three criteria is 98.9 % sensitive and 29 % specific for clinically significant thoracolumbar spine fractures in blunt trauma patients, and the authors consider the presence of any one of these criteria on its own an indication for advanced imaging (Inaba et al. 2015).

According to the American College of Radiology, a precise evaluation of spinal cord injuries should be performed with the utilisation of MRI if possible, since it is the most accurate tool to display compression of the cord by disc herniation, bone fragments or hematoma (ACR A. C. o. R. 1999).

Little data is available on definite indications for operative treatment of thoracolumbar burst fractures. In their review on existing literature, Pneumaticos et al. consider patients with proven or questioned instability as well as incomplete neurologic deficit and even complete paraplegia to be those who will profit from surgical treatment. Based on the fracture type and the patient's

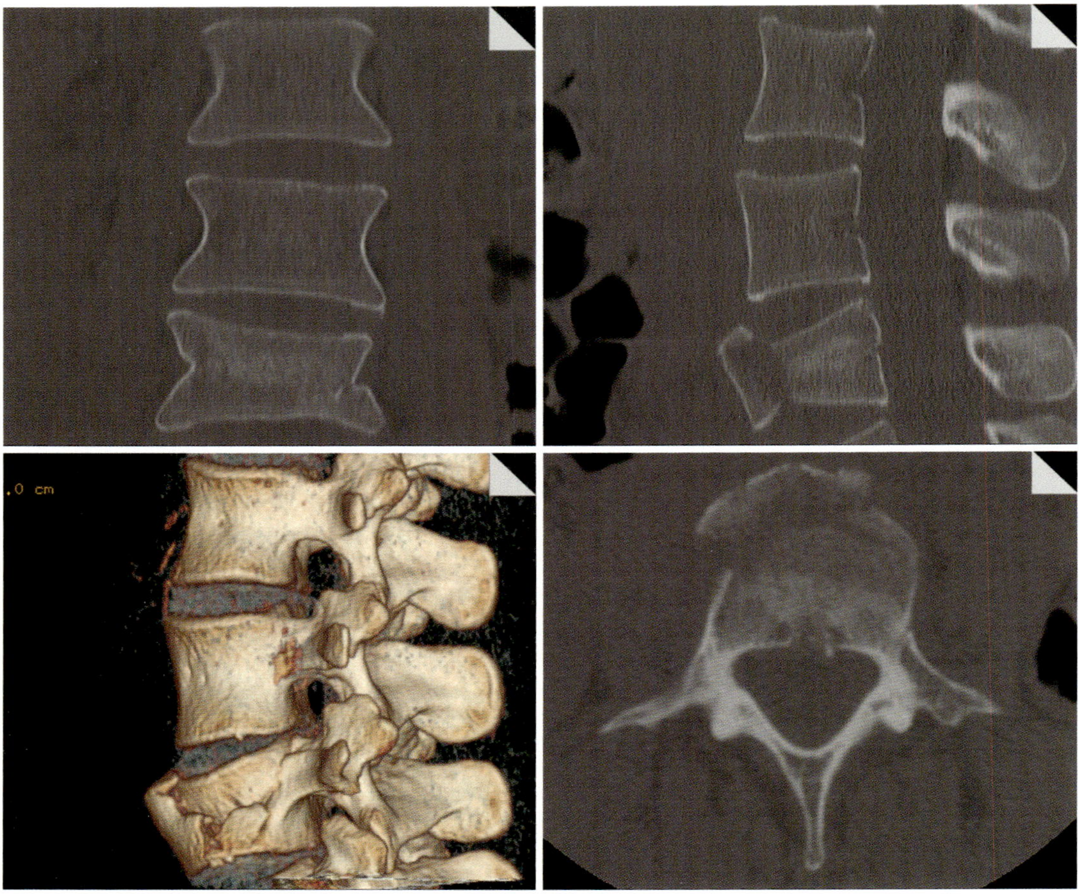

Fig. 26 Vertebral L4 fracture. A 32-year-old woman, CT reformations. The fracture is presumably unstable because of the involvement of the anterior and middle column (three-column theory, Denis)

Table 3 Major types of spinal injuries according to Denis

	Column		
Type of fracture	Anterior	Middle	Posterior
Compression	Compression	None	None or distraction (severe)
Burst	Compression	Compression	None
Seat belt type	None or compression	Distraction	Distraction
Fracture dislocation	Comp./rotation/shear	Dist./rot./shear	Dist./rot./shear

neurological status, anterior, posterior, combined or minimal invasive approaches can be performed (Pneumaticos et al. 2013).

Most patients experience chronic pain after an injury of the spinal cord. In case of a traumatic spinal cord injury, the management of bladder and bowel function is important (World Health Organization 2015b).

9.4 Summary

An important point for treatment and outcome of fractures of the thoracolumbar spine is stability, which is predictable with the utilisation of the three-column theory according to Denis. An injury is considered unstable if two or three columns are involved.

Spinal fractures can be distinguished between compression, burst, seat belt-type and dislocated fractures.

High-energy mechanism, a patient age ≥60 years and a positive finding in the clinical exam (pain, tenderness to palpation, deformity or neurologic deficit) are criteria for a clinical relevant spine fracture, which should be ruled out with the help of CT or MRI.

References

ACR A. C. o. R. (1999) ACR appropriateness criteria-suspected spine trauma [Online]. Available: http://www.acr.org/Search?q=suspectedspinaltrauma. Accessed 5 Feb 2016, 00:58

Allman FL Jr (1967) Fractures and ligamentous injuries of the clavicle and its articulation. J Bone Joint Surg Am 49:774–784

Alton TB, Gardner MJ (2015) Scapular fractures: diagnosis and treatment plan [Online]. Medscape Multispecialty Curr Orthop Pract 26(2). Available: http://www.medscape.com/viewarticle/840138_3. Accessed 4 Jan 2016, 17:36

Armstrong CP, Van Der Spuy J (1984) The fractured scapula: importance and management based on a series of 62 patients. Injury 15:324–329

Audige L, Kellam JF, Lambert S, Madsen JE, Babst R, Andermahr J, Li W, Jaeger M (2014) The AO Foundation and Orthopaedic Trauma Association (AO/OTA) scapula fracture classification system: focus on body involvement. J Shoulder Elbow Surg 23:189–196

Ball CG, Kirkpatrick AW, Laupland KB, Fox DI, Nicolaou S, Anderson IB, Hameed SM, Kortbeek JB, Mulloy RR, Litvinchuk S, Boulanger BR (2005) Incidence, risk factors, and outcomes for occult pneumothoraces in victims of major trauma. J Trauma 59:917–924; discussion 924–925

Barrett-Connor E, Nielson CM, Orwoll E, Bauer DC, Cauley JA (2010) Epidemiology of rib fractures in older men: osteoporotic fractures in men (MrOS) prospective cohort study. BMJ 340:c1069

Barrios C Jr, Pham J, Malinoski D, Dolich M, Lekawa M, Cinat M (2010) Ability of a chest X-ray and an abdominal computed tomography scan to identify traumatic thoracic injury. Am J Surg 200:741–744; discussion 744–745

Bartonicek J, Tucek M, Fric V, Obruba P (2014) Fractures of the scapular neck: diagnosis, classifications and treatment. Int Orthop 38:2163–2173

Battle CE, Hutchings H, James K, Evans PA (2013) The risk factors for the development of complications during the recovery phase following blunt chest wall trauma: a retrospective study. Injury 44:1171–1176

Begemann PG, Kemper J, Gatzka C, Stork A, Nolte-Ernsting C, Adam G (2004) Value of multiplanar reformations (MPR) in multidetector CT (MDCT) of acute vertebral fractures: do we still have to read the transverse images? J Comput Assist Tomogr 28: 572–580

Bier G, Schabel C, Othman A, Bongers MN, Schmehl J, Ditt H, Nikolaou K, Bamberg F, Notohamiprodjo M (2015) Enhanced reading time efficiency by use of automatically unfolded CT rib reformations in acute trauma. Eur J Radiol 84(11):2173–2180

Brink M, Deunk J, Dekker HM, Kool DR, Edwards MJ, VAN Vugt AB, Blickman JG (2008) Added value of routine chest MDCT after blunt trauma: evaluation of additional findings and impact on patient management. AJR Am J Roentgenol 190:1591–1598

Bulger EM, Arneson MA, Mock CN, Jurkovich GJ (2000) Rib fractures in the elderly. J Trauma 48:1040–1046; discussion 1046–1047

Burke JF (1962) Early diagnosis of traumatic rupture of the bronchus. JAMA 181:682–686

Calhoon JH, Trinkle JK (1997) Pathophysiology of chest trauma. Chest Surg Clin N Am 7:199–211

Cha JR, Park KB, Ko SH (2011) Post-traumatic lumbar epidural hematoma with neurology: report of 1 case. Asian Spine J 5:130–132

Chesterman JT, Satsangi PN (1966) Rupture of the trachea and bronchi by closed injury. Thorax 21:21–27

Cho SH, Sung YM, Kim MS (2012) Missed rib fractures on evaluation of initial chest CT for trauma patients: pattern analysis and diagnostic value of coronal multiplanar reconstruction images with multidetector row CT. Br J Radiol 85:e845–e850

Chung JH, Cox CW, Mohammed TL, Kirsch J, Brown K, Dyer DS, Ginsburg ME, Heitkamp DE, Kanne JP, Kazerooni EA, Ketai LH, Ravenel JG, Saleh AG, Shah RD, Steiner RM, Suh RD (2014) American College of Radiology appropriateness criteria for blunt chest trauma. J Am Coll Radiol 11(4):345–351

Clark GC, Schecter WP, Trunkey DD (1988) Variables affecting outcome in blunt chest trauma: flail chest vs. pulmonary contusion. J Trauma 28:298–304

Cser I, Vajda A (1976) Bilateral fracture of the scapulae caused by a convulsive seizure (author's transl). Arch Orthop Unfallchir 86:227–233

Curfman KR, Robitsek RJ, Salzler GG, Gray KD, Lapunzina CS, Kothuru RK, Schubl SD (2015) Massive hemothorax caused by a single intercostal artery bleed ten days after solitary minimally displaced rib fracture. Case Rep Surg 2015:120140

Demirhan R, Onan B, Oz K, Halezeroglu S (2009) Comprehensive analysis of 4205 patients with chest trauma: a 10-year experience. Interact Cardiovasc Thorac Surg 9:450–453

Denis F (1983) The three column spine and its significance in the classification of acute thoracolumbar spinal injuries. Spine (Phila Pa 1976) 8:817–831

Ebraheim NA, Pearlstein SR, Savolaine ER, Gordon SL, Jackson WT, Corray T (1987) Scapulothoracic dissociation (closed avulsion of the scapula, subclavian

artery, and brachial plexus): a newly recognized variant, a new classification, and a review of the literature and treatment options. J Orthop Trauma 1:18–23
Ecker RR, Libertini RV, Rea WJ, Sugg WL, Webb WR (1971) Injuries of the trachea and bronchi. Ann Thorac Surg 11:289–298
Emircan S, Ozguc H, Akkose Aydin S, Ozdemir F, Koksal O, Bulut M (2011) Factors affecting mortality in patients with thorax trauma. Ulus Travma Acil Cerrahi Derg 17:329–333
Euler E, Habermeyer P, Kohler W, Schweiberer L (1992) Scapula fractures – classification and differential therapy. Orthopade 21:158–162
Feeman TG (2010) The mathematics of medical imaging: a beginner's guide. Springer undergraduate texts in mathematics and technology. Springer united states, ISBN10: 0387927123, ISBN13: 9780387927121
Fleming S, Bird R, Ratnasingham K, Sarker SJ, Walsh M, Patel B (2012) Accuracy of FAST scan in blunt abdominal trauma in a major London trauma centre. Int J Surg 10:470–474
Friederichs J, Morgenstern M, Buhren V (2014) Scapula fractures in complex shoulder injuries and floating shoulders: a classification based on displacement and instability. J Trauma Manag Outcomes 8:16
Hager J (2009) BGB § 823 I, Arzthaftungsrecht [Online]. Juris.de. Available: http://www.juris.de.emedien.ub.uni-muenchen.de/jportal/portal/t/12c8/page/jurisw.psml?pid=Dokumentanzeige&showdoccase=1&js_peid=Trefferliste&fromdoctodoc=yes&doc.id=samson-sdg013BGB_P823_I061304&doc.part=C&doc.price=0.0-013.BGB_P823_I.RI_44. Accessed 15 Feb 2016, 15:12
Harvey E, Audige L, Herscovici D Jr, Agel J, Madsen JE, Babst R, Nork S, Kellam J (2012) Development and validation of the new international classification for scapula fractures. J Orthop Trauma 26:364–369
Helm EJ, Rahman NM, Talakoub O, Fox DL, Gleeson FV (2013) Course and variation of the intercostal artery by CT scan. Chest 143:634–639
Henry TS, Kirsch J, Kanne JP, Chung JH, Donnelly EF, Ginsburg ME, Heitkamp DE, Kazerooni EA, Ketai LH, Mccomb BL, Parker JA, Ravenel JG, Restrepo CS, Saleh AG, Shah RD, Steiner RM, Suh RD, Mohammed TL (2014) ACR Appropriateness Criteria(R) rib fractures. J Thorac Imaging 29:364–366
Homann G, Mustafa DF, Ditt H, Spengler W, Kopp HG, Nikolaou K, Horger M (2015a) Improved detection of bone metastases from lung cancer in the thoracic cage using 5- and 1-mm axial images versus a new CT software generating rib unfolding images: comparison with standard (1)(8)F-FDG-PET/CT. Acad Radiol 22:505–512
Homann G, Weisel K, Mustafa DF, Ditt H, Nikolaou K, Horger M (2015b) Improvement of diagnostic confidence for detection of multiple myeloma involvement of the ribs by a new CT software generating rib unfolded images: comparison with 5- and 1-mm axial images. Skeletal Radiol 44:971–979
Huber-Wagner S, Lefering R, Qvick LM, Korner M, Kay MV, Pfeifer KJ, Reiser M, Mutschler W, Kanz KG (2009) Effect of whole-body CT during trauma resuscitation on survival: a retrospective, multicentre study. Lancet 373:1455–1461
Imatani RJ (1975) Fractures of the scapula: a review of 53 fractures. J Trauma 15:473–478
Inaba K, Nosanov L, Menaker J, Bosarge P, Williams L, Turay D, Cachecho R, DE Moya M, Bukur M, Carl J, Kobayashi L, Kaminski S, Beekley A, Gomez M, Skiada D (2015) Prospective derivation of a clinical decision rule for thoracolumbar spine evaluation after blunt trauma: an American Association for the Surgery of Trauma Multi-Institutional Trials Group Study. J Trauma Acute Care Surg 78:459–465; discussion 465–467
Kaewlai R, Avery LL, Asrani AV, Novelline RA (2008) Multidetector CT of blunt thoracic trauma. Radiographics 28:1555–1570
Katrancioglu O, Akkas Y, Arslan S, Sahin E (2015) Spontaneous rib fractures. Asian Cardiovasc Thorac Ann 23:701–703
Kessel B, Dagan J, Swaid F, Ashkenazi I, Olsha O, Peleg K, Givon A, Alfici R (2014) Rib fractures: comparison of associated injuries between pediatric and adult population. Am J Surg 208:831–834
Kirkpatrick AW, Sirois M, Laupland KB, Liu D, Rowan K, Ball CG, Hameed SM, Brown R, Simons R, Dulchavsky SA, Hamiilton DR, Nicolaou S (2004) Hand-held thoracic sonography for detecting post-traumatic pneumothoraces: the Extended Focused Assessment with Sonography for Trauma (EFAST). J Trauma Inj Infect Crit Care 57:288–295
Kirsh MM, Orringer MB, Behrendt DM, Sloan H (1976) Management of tracheobronchial disruption secondary to nonpenetrating trauma. Ann Thorac Surg 22:93–101
Knobloch K, Wagner S, Haasper C, Probst C, Krettek C, Otte D, Richter M (2006) Sternal fractures occur most often in old cars to seat-belted drivers without any airbag often with concomitant spinal injuries: clinical findings and technical collision variables among 42,055 crash victims. Ann Thorac Surg 82:444–450
Knobloch K, Wagner S, Haasper C, Probst C, Krettek C, Vogt PM, Otte D, Richter M (2008) Sternal fractures are frequent among polytraumatised patients following high deceleration velocities in a severe vehicle crash. Injury 39:36–43
Lalande E, Wylie K (2014) Towards evidence-based emergency medicine: best BETs from the Manchester Royal Infirmary. BET 1: ultrasound in the diagnosis of rib fractures. Emerg Med J 31:169–170
Lee RB, Bass SM, Morris JA Jr, Mackenzie EJ (1990) Three or more rib fractures as an indicator for transfer to a Level I trauma center: a population-based study. J Trauma 30:689–694
Locicero J 3rd, Mattox KL (1989) Epidemiology of chest trauma. Surg Clin North Am 69:15–19
Lomoschitz FM, Eisenhuber E, Linnau KF, Peloschek P, Schoder M, Bankier AA (2003) Imaging of chest

trauma: radiological patterns of injury and diagnostic algorithms. Eur J Radiol 48:61–70

Macklin MT, Macklin CC (1944) Malignant interstitial emphysema of the lungs and mediastinum as an important occult complication in many respiratory diseases and other conditions: an interpretation of the clinical literature in the light of laboratory experiment. Medicine 23:281–358

Magu S, Yadav A, Agarwal S (2009) Computed tomography in blunt chest trauma. Indian J Chest Dis Allied Sci 51:75–81

Mancini MC, Talavera F, Karwande SV, Geibel J, Roe BB, Sawyer MAJ, Jablons DM, Kukreja J (2014) Blunt chest trauma: overview, relevant anatomy, workup [Online]. Available: http://emedicine.medscape.com/article/428723-overview. Accessed 9 Oct 2015, 14:54

Mathews RE, Cocke TB, D'Ambrosia RD (1983) Scapular fractures secondary to seizures in patients with osteodystrophy. Report of two cases and review of the literature. J Bone Joint Surg Am 65:850–853

Matsushima K, Frankel HL (2011) Beyond focused assessment with sonography for trauma: ultrasound creep in the trauma resuscitation area and beyond. Curr Opin Crit Care 17:606–612

Mcgahan JP, Rab GT, Dublin A (1980) Fractures of the scapula. J Trauma 20:880–883

Melton LJ 3rd, Kallmes DF (2006) Epidemiology of vertebral fractures: implications for vertebral augmentation. Acad Radiol 13:538–545

Mettler FA, Huda W, Yoshizumi TT, Mahesh M (2008) Effective doses in radiology and diagnostic nuclear medicine: a catalog [Online]. Available: http://pubs.rsna.org/doi/abs/10.1148/radiol.2481071451. Accessed 9 Jan 2016, 18:45

Mirvis SE, Kubal WS, Shanmuganathan K, Soto JA, Yu J (2014) Problem solving in emergency radiology. Elsevier – Health Sciences Division, Saunders; 1 Har/Psc edition 592 pages, ISBN-10: 145575417X, ISBN-13: 978-1455754175

Mueck FG, Wirth K, Muggenthaler M, Kreimeier U, Geyer L, Kanz KG, Linsenmaier U, Wirth S (2016) Radiological mass casualty incident (MCI) workflow analysis: single-centre data of a mid-scale exercise. Br J Radiol 0:20150918, 89:1061. doi:10.1259/bjr.20150918

Nedeltchev K, Baumgartner RW (2005) Traumatic cervical artery dissection. Front Neurol Neurosci 20:54–63

Neuerburg C, Schmidmaier R, Schilling S, Kammerlander C, Bocker W, Mutschler W, Stumpf U (2015) [Identification, diagnostics and guideline conform therapy of osteoporosis (DVO) in trauma patients: a treatment algorithm]. Unfallchirurg 118(11):913–924

Neuhaus V, Bot AG, Guitton TG, Ring DC, Abdel-Ghany MI, Abrams J, Abzug JM, Adolfsson LE, Balfour GW, Bamberger HB, Barquet A, Baskies M, Batson WA, Baxamusa T, Bayne GJ, Begue T, Behrman M, Beingessner D, Biert J, Bishop J, Alves MB, Boyer M, Brilej D, Brink PR, Brunton LM, Buckley R, Cagnone JC, Calfee RP, Campinhos LA, Cassidy C, Catalano L 3rd, Chivers K, Choudhari P, Cimerman M, Conflitti JM, Costanzo RM, Crist BD, Cross BJ, Dantuluri P, Darowish M, De Bedout R, Decoster T, Dennison DG, Denoble PH, Desilva G, Dienstknecht T, Duncan SF, Duralde XA, Durchholz H, Egol K, Ekholm C, Elias N, Erickson JM, Esparza JD, Fernandes CH, Fischer TJ, Fischmeister M, Forigua Jaime E, Getz CL, Gilbert RS, Giordano V, Glaser DL, Gosens T, Grafe MW, Filho JE, Gray RR, Gulotta LV, Gummerson NW, Hammerberg EM, Harvey E, Haverlag R, Henry PD, Hobby JL, Hofmeister EP, Hughes T, Itamura J, Jebson P, Jenkinson R, Jeray K, Jones CM, Jones J, Jubel A, Kaar SG, Kabir K, Kaplan FT, Kennedy SA, Kessler MW, Kimball HL, Kloen P, Klostermann C, Kohut G, Kraan GA, Kristan A, Loebenberg MI, Malone KJ, Marsh L, Martineau PA, Mcauliffe J, Mcgraw I, Mehta S et al (2014) Scapula fractures: interobserver reliability of classification and treatment. J Orthop Trauma 28:124–129

Paffrath T, Lefering R, Flohe S (2014) How to define severely injured patients? – an Injury Severity Score (ISS) based approach alone is not sufficient. Injury 45(Suppl 3):S64–S69

Palvanen M, Kannus P, Niemi S, Parkkari J (2004) Hospital-treated minimal-trauma rib fractures in elderly Finns: long-term trends and projections for the future. Osteoporos Int 15:649–653

Pluskiewicz W, Wilk R, Wielgorecki A, Golba KS, Drozdzowska B (2011) Fracture status in men assessed by quantitative ultrasound measurements at the calcaneus. J Ultrasound Med 30:877–882

Pneumaticos SG, Triantafyllopoulos GK, Giannoudis PV (2013) Advances made in the treatment of thoracolumbar fractures: current trends and future directions. Injury 44:703–712

Raskin MM (2001) Why radiologists get sued [Online]. Medscape Multisecialty Appl Radiol 30(8). Available: http://www.medscape.com/viewarticle/406661. Accessed 2 Jan 2016, 15:54

Reissig A, Copetti R, Kroegel C (2011) Current role of emergency ultrasound of the chest. Crit Care Med 39:839–845

Ringl H, Lazar M, Topker M, Woitek R, Prosch H, Asenbaum U, Balassy C, Toth D, Weber M, Hajdu S, Soza G, Wimmer A, Mang T (2015) The ribs unfolded – a CT visualization algorithm for fast detection of rib fractures: effect on sensitivity and specificity in trauma patients. Eur Radiol 25:1865–1874

Rothlin MA, Naf R, Amgwerd M, Candinas D, Frick T, Trentz O (1993) Ultrasound in blunt abdominal and thoracic trauma. J Trauma 34:488–495

Rowe CR (1963) Fractures of the scapula. Surg Clin North Am 43:1565–1571

Rozycki GS, Tremblay L, Feliciano DV, Tchorz K, Hattaway A, Fountain J, Pettitt BJ (2002) A prospective study for the detection of vascular injury in adult and pediatric patients with cervicothoracic seat belt signs. J Trauma 52:618–623; discussion 623–624

Sajjan SG, Barrett-Connor E, Mchorney CA, Miller PD, Sen SS, Siris e (2012) Rib fracture as a predictor of future fractures in young and older postmenopausal

women: National Osteoporosis Risk Assessment (NORA). Osteoporos Int 23:821–828
Salimi J, Khaji A, Karbakhsh M, Saadat S, Eftekhar B (2008) Scapular fracture: lower severity and mortality. Sao Paulo Med J 126:186–189
Scheurecker G (2015) Traumatic bone and cartilage injuries of the shoulder. Radiologe 55:188–194
Schnyder P, Wintermark M (2000) Trauma of the chest wall. In: Radiology of blunt trauma of the chest, 1st edn. Springer, Berlin/Heidelberg
Schofer MD, Sehrt AC, Timmesfeld N, Stormer S, Kortmann HR (2009) Fractures of the scapula: long-term results after conservative treatment. Arch Orthop Trauma Surg 129:1511–1519
Schulz-Drost S, Oppel P, Grupp S, Krinner S, Langenbach A, Lefering R, Mauerer A (2015a) [Bony injuries of the thoracic cage in multiple trauma : Incidence, concomitant injuries, course and outcome]. Unfallchirurg doi 10.1007/s00113-015-0026-7
Schulz-Drost S, Oppel P, Grupp S, Taylor D, Krinner S, Langenbach A, Hennig F, Mauerer A (2015b) The oblique fracture of the manubrium sterni caused by a seatbelt-a rare injury? Treatment options based on the experiences gained in a level I trauma centre. Int Orthop doi: 10.1007/s00264-015-2801-z
Shalhub S, Starnes BW, Hatsukami TS, Karmy-Jones R, Tran NT (2011) Repair of blunt thoracic outlet arterial injuries: an evolution from open to endovascular approach. J Trauma 71:E114–E121
Shanmuganathan K, Matsumoto J (2006) Imaging of penetrating chest trauma. Radiol Clin North Am 44:38, viii
Shorr RM, Crittenden M, Indeck M, Hartunian SL, Rodriguez A (1987) Blunt thoracic trauma. Analysis of 515 patients. Ann Surg 206:200–205
Sirmali M, Turut H, Topcu S, Gulhan E, Yazici U, Kaya S, Tastepe I (2003) A comprehensive analysis of traumatic rib fractures: morbidity, mortality and management. Eur J Cardiothorac Surg 24:133–138
Skinner DL, DEN Hollander D, Laing GL, Rodseth RN, Muckart DJ (2015) Severe blunt thoracic trauma: differences between adults and children in a level I trauma centre. S Afr Med J 105:47–51
Stephan K, Huber S, Haberle S, Kanz KG, Buhren V, Van Griensven M, Meyer B, Biberthaler P, Lefering R, Huber-Wagner S (2015) Spinal cord injury – incidence, prognosis, and outcome: an analysis of the TraumaRegister DGU. Spine J 15:1994–2001
Thompson DA, Flynn TC, Miller PW, Fischer RP (1985) The significance of scapular fractures. J Trauma 25:974–977
Tillou A, Gupta M, Baraff LJ, Schriger DL, Hoffman JR, Hiatt JR, Cryer HM (2009) Is the use of pan-computed tomography for blunt trauma justified? A prospective evaluation. J Trauma 67:779–787
Tonkopi E, Ross AA (2016) Assessment of effective dose from cone beam CT imaging in SPECT/CT examination in comparison with other modalities. Radiat Prot Dosimetry (Epub ahead of print)
Traub M, Stevenson M, Mcevoy S, Briggs G, Lo SK, Leibman S, Joseph T (2007) The use of chest computed tomography versus chest X-ray in patients with major blunt trauma. Injury 38:43–47
Turkalj I, Petrovic K, Stojanovic S, Petrovic D, Brakus A, Ristic J (2014) Blunt chest trauma – an audit of injuries diagnosed by the MDCT examination. Vojnosanit Pregl 71:161–166
Vevaina J, Bone RC, Kassoff E (2012) Legal aspects of medicine: including cardiology, pulmonary medicine, and critical care medicine. Springer, New York
Veysi VT, Mittal R, Agarwal S, Dosani A, Giannoudis PV (2003) Multiple trauma and scapula fractures: so what? J Trauma 55:1145–1147
Veysi VT, Nikolaou VS, Paliobeis C, Efstathopoulos N, Giannoudis PV (2009) Prevalence of chest trauma, associated injuries and mortality: a level I trauma centre experience. Int Orthop 33:1425–1433
Watts NB, Lewiecki EM, Miller PD, Baim S (2008) National Osteoporosis Foundation 2008 Clinician's Guide to Prevention and Treatment of Osteoporosis and the World Health Organization Fracture Risk Assessment Tool (FRAX): what they mean to the bone densitometrist and bone technologist. J Clin Densitom 11:473–477
Weening B, Walton C, Cole PA, Alanezi K, Hanson BP, Bhandari M (2005) Lower mortality in patients with scapular fractures. J Trauma 59:1477–1481
Welter S, Hoffmann H (2013) Injuries to the tracheobronchial tree. Zentralbl Chir 138:111–116
Wiedemann E (2004) Fractures of the scapula. Unfallchirurg 107:1124–1133
Wilkerson RG, Stone MB (2010) Sensitivity of bedside ultrasound and supine anteroposterior chest radiographs for the identification of pneumothorax after blunt trauma. Acad Emerg Med 17:11–17
Wirth S (2014) Polytraumabefundung: Wenn jede Sekunde zählt. Reiser M, 8. Internationales Symposium Mehrschicht-CT und Aktualisierungskurs Fachkunde Strahlenschutz nach RöV und StrlSchV (inkl. CT-Grundkurs: Protokolle und Anwendungen für Ärzte und MTRAs), Garmisch-Partenkirchen, 22–25 January 2014; [wissenschaftliches Programm]. Eurokongress
Wirth S (2016) Wann brauchen wir notfallmäßig ein MRT? 9. Internationales Symposium Mehrschicht CT, Garmisch-Partenkirchen [Online]. Available: http://www.mehrschicht-ct.org/fileadmin/user_upload/conferences/ct/ct2016/pdf/Programm/ct2016_hauptprogramm.pdf. Accessed 14 Feb 2016, 19:47
Wirth S, Treitl M (2012) The role of interventional radiology. In: Scaglione M, Linsenmaier U, Schueller G (eds) Emergency radiology of the abdomen: imaging features and differential diagnosis for a timely management approach. Springer, Milan/New York
Wirth S, Korner M, Treitl M, Linsenmaier U, Leidel BA, Jaschkowitz T, Reiser MF, Kanz KG (2009) Computed tomography during cardiopulmonary resuscitation using automated chest compression devices – an initial study. Eur Radiol 19:1857–1866
World Health Organization (1994) Assessment of fracture risk and its application to screening for postmeno-

pausal osteoporosis. Report of a WHO Study Group. World Health Organ Tech Rep Ser 843:1–129

World Health Organization (2004) WHO scientific group on the asessment of osteoporosis at primary health care level [Online]. Available: http://www.who.int/chp/topics/Osteoporosis.pdf. Accessed 2 Nov 2015, 18:57

World Health Organization (2015a) Road traffic injuries [Online]. Available: http://www.who.int/mediacentre/factsheets/fs358/en/. Accessed 8 Oct 2015, 15:20

World Health Organization (2015b) Spinal cord injury [Online]. Available: http://www.who.int/mediacentre/factsheets/fs384/en/. Accessed 8 Oct 2015, 15:12

Wuermser LA, Achenbach SJ, Amin S, Khosla S, Melton LJ, 3rd (2011) What accounts for rib fractures in older adults? J Osteoporos 2011:457591

Ziegler DW, Agarwal NN (1994) The morbidity and mortality of rib fractures. J Trauma 37:975–979

Acute Tracheobronchial Injuries

Mariano Scaglione, Roberto Ronza, Claudia Rossi, Maria Teresa Martino, Francesca Iacobellis, Roberto Grassi, and Sujit Vaidya

Contents

Abstract

Tracheobronchial injuries are an unusual clinical entity accounting for 0.2–8 % of all cases of blunt chest trauma. Actually, most patients die before arriving at the emergency department, from either associated injuries to vital structures, hemorrhage, tension pneumothorax, or respiratory insufficiency from an airway injury. Signs and symptoms may be very subtle or nonspecific and therefore clinical diagnosis is easily overlooked. In this chapter, the authors will review the radiological and CT signs of acute tracheobronchial injuries. Furthermore, mechanism of injury, terminology, and clinical issues will be discussed. Finally, management notes and treatment will be illustrated.

1 Introduction

Acute tracheobronchial injury is a rare injury usually related to blunt trauma that involves a partial or complete laceration or puncture of the tracheal or bronchial wall. Death occurs in approximately 30 % of patients with tracheobronchial tears, with 50 % of fatalities occurring within the first hour (Scaglione et al. 2006).

Delayed or missed diagnosis can result in death or severe complications including airway stenosis, atelectasis, pneumonia, bronchiectasis, mediastinitis, sepsis, and decreased pulmonary capacity (Baugartner et al. 1990).

M. Scaglione, MD (✉)
Department of Imaging, Pineta Grande Medical Center, Via Domiziana Km. 30, Castel Volturno 81030, Italy
e-mail: mscaglione@tiscali.it

R. Ronza • C. Rossi • M.T. Martino • F. Iacobellis
R. Grassi
Department of Radiology, Second University of Naples, Piazza Miraglia 2, Naples 80138, Italy

Department of Imaging, Via Domiziana Km. 30, Castel Volturno 81030, Italy

S. Vaidya
Department of Radiology, The Royal London Hospital, Barts and the London NHS Trust, London, UK
e-mail: Sujit.Vaidya@bartshealth.nhs.uk

Med Radiol Diagn Imaging (2016)
DOI 10.1007/174_2016_40, © Springer International Publishing Switzerland

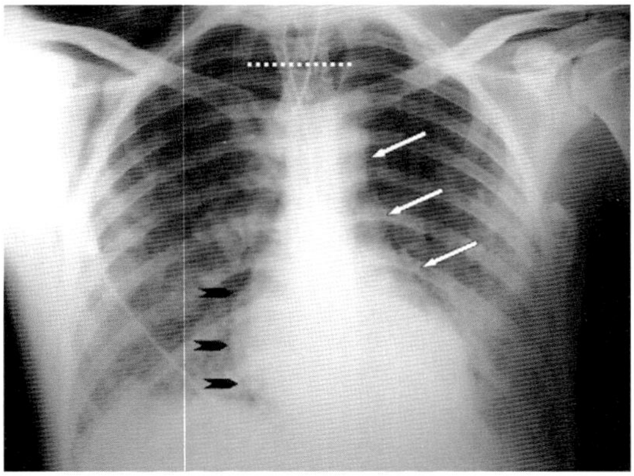

Fig. 1 Penetrating tracheal injury secondary to intubation. Supine chest radiograph shows overdistention of the endotracheal cuff (*dashed line*). Furthermore, left pneumomediastinum (*arrows*), right heart contour outline (*arrowheads*), and bilateral pulmonary contusions are also evident (Reproduced with permission from Elsevier)

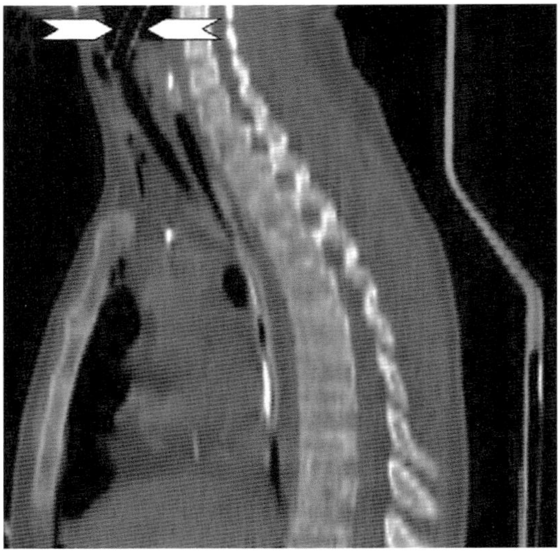

Fig. 2 Cervical tracheal injury secondary to blunt trauma. Parasagittal reformatted 16-row MDCT image depicts displacement of the endotracheal cervical tube (*arrowheads*) through a wall defect consistent with a cervical tracheal injury. This finding was confirmed by bronchoscopy (Reproduced with permission from Elsevier)

Tracheal trauma can result from external or internal injuries. External or penetrating injuries can have devastating effects (Fig. 1), including perforation or transection of the tracheobronchial tree and the esophagus. Penetrating injuries to the thoracic trachea are often associated with heart and great vessel trauma. More than 50 % of gunshot wounds and 10 % of stab wounds involving the tracheobronchial tree distal to the cervical trachea are rapidly fatal (Scaglione et al. 2006).

Internal or non-penetrating injuries may occur secondary to inhalation of noxious fumes or gases, tracheal compression on the rigid vertebral column, or due to aspiration of liquids or foreign bodies. When the tracheobronchial tree is occluded by foreign bodies or there is a sudden chest compression with closed glottis, as in crush or steering wheel injuries, an explosive rupture may occur (Stark 1995).

During recent years, an increase in traffic accident has caused an increase in blunt tracheobronchial injuries, and the most common non-penetrating injury mechanism is the motor vehicle accident. The exact mechanism of intrathoracic, tracheobronchial disruption from non-penetrating trauma is unknown, but these injuries include longitudinal lacerations of the distal trachea or near the carina (usually within 2.5 cm), with complete or partial disruption of the main bronchus (more common, right bronchus) and other lobar bronchi.

2 Mechanism of Injury

The causes of airway injuries are divided into blunt trauma, penetrating trauma, or iatrogenic rupture and into neck (larynx and cervical trachea) or thoracic lesions (chest trachea and bronchi).

Blunt trauma at the neck can cause a hyperextension mechanism that results in tracheal tears and paramedian vertical fractures of the larynx and trachea or lead to complete laryngeal–tracheal separation (Dougenis 2002; Milner 2008); another mechanism is direct blow to the neck injuring the thyroid or cricoid cartilages but also the tracheal rings due to compression against the vertebral column. In a vehicle accident, both mechanisms happen: neck hyperextension from sudden deceleration and direct impact of the neck to the steering wheel or the dashboard: this is the "padded dashboard syndrome" (Nelson 2007) (Fig. 2). Other mechanisms are consequent to improper use of seat belts as a direct blow to the neck in front-on collision or by the sudden increase of intratracheal pressure while the glottis is reflexively closed (Rathlev et al. 2007).

The usual mechanisms of tracheobronchial disruption are (1) excessive pressure in the bronchial tree when the glottis is closed, causing airway blowout at the point of the greatest diameter, i.e, the carina (Laplace's law); in this case, the rupture occurs when the intraluminal pressure exceeds the elasticity of the membranous trachea and bronchi; (2) decrease in the anterior–posterior chest diameter with increase in the lateral diameter; when the lungs are pulled out laterally, the main bronchi and carina become disrupted; and (3) severe and sudden deceleration giving rise to sheer forces that disrupt the airway at the points of relative fixation such as the cricoid cartilage and the carina, similar to the mechanism of traumatic injuries of the thoracic aorta (Huth et al. 1997). In most of cases, probably a combination of these three mechanisms causes the airway lesion (Kiser et al. 2001).

Tracheobronchial injuries are rare in the pediatric population, because the pediatric patient's chest wall is more elastic than the adult's chest wall (Balci et al. 2004). This elasticity decreases when the age increases due to the progressive ossification of the rib cage and the development of increased intercostal muscle tone (Grant et al. 1998). Spontaneous tracheal rupture in a pediatric patient can be secondary to paroxysmal coughing or pernicious vomiting. Non-penetrating tracheobronchial injuries less commonly are secondary to fractures of the regional skeleton of the upper thorax, particularly of the first three ribs.

According to data published by Burack et al., even though only 1 of 188 patients who did not die rapidly on the scene or after the admission to the emergency department had sustained a tracheal injury, it is important for the radiologist to identify this kind of lesion, since missed diagnosis may have fatal consequences (Burack et al. 2007).

Acute injuries of the tracheobronchial tree may be iatrogenic in origin: tracheal intubation, tracheotomy, bronchoscopy or other per-oral intervention (tracheal or esophageal stent placement), and surgery (Paraschiv 2014). The most common cause of iatrogenic tracheobronchial rupture is tracheal intubation, especially when it is performed in stressful, emergency conditions. The site of injury is, preferentially, the posterior membranous wall (Massard et al. 1996; Marty-Ane et al. 1995).

Post-intubation tracheobronchial rupture is an emergency condition, secondary to tube tips placed excessively, cuff over inflation that produces excessive stretching of the membranous wall or by endotracheal tube-repositioning maneuvers without deflating the cuff (Figs. 1 and 3).

Bulging of tracheal wall until tracheal rupture can be a complication of hyperinflated cuff that can lead to ischemic necrosis and subsequent tracheomalacia or strictures, particularly if its diameter exceeds 1.5 times the tracheal diameter (Chen et al. 2001b).

Factors favoring post-intubation tracheal rupture are the lack of experience of the anesthetist; use of double-lumen endotracheal tubes, or a too-thick endotracheal tube; presence of chronic pulmonary disease; and congenital tracheal anomalies.

The conditions most commonly associated with injuries of the trachea in intubation procedure are female gender, age over 50 years old, double-lumen tube, and excessive pressure in the endotracheal cuff (Paraschiv 2014).

A rare complication of blunt chest trauma is the tracheoesophageal fistula that may occur to focal necrosis of the esophageal wall and lead to perforation into the trachea (Stark 1995).

3 Terminology and Clinical Issues

The natural history of blunt tracheobronchial injuries may vary from one patient to another. Many patients immediately die at the trauma scene for acute respiratory insufficiency or within 2 h for associated injuries. A small proportion of patients may present in a delayed fashion, usually within 4 weeks of injury, with hemoptysis, pneumonitis, or both, complicating an obstructed airway (Scaglione et al. 2006). Only rarely do patients present with a healed airway injury years later, typically with dyspnea or the diagnosis of asthma.

Tracheal or main stem bronchi injuries are often not recognized initially, due to its rare incidence, lack or subtle clinical manifestations,

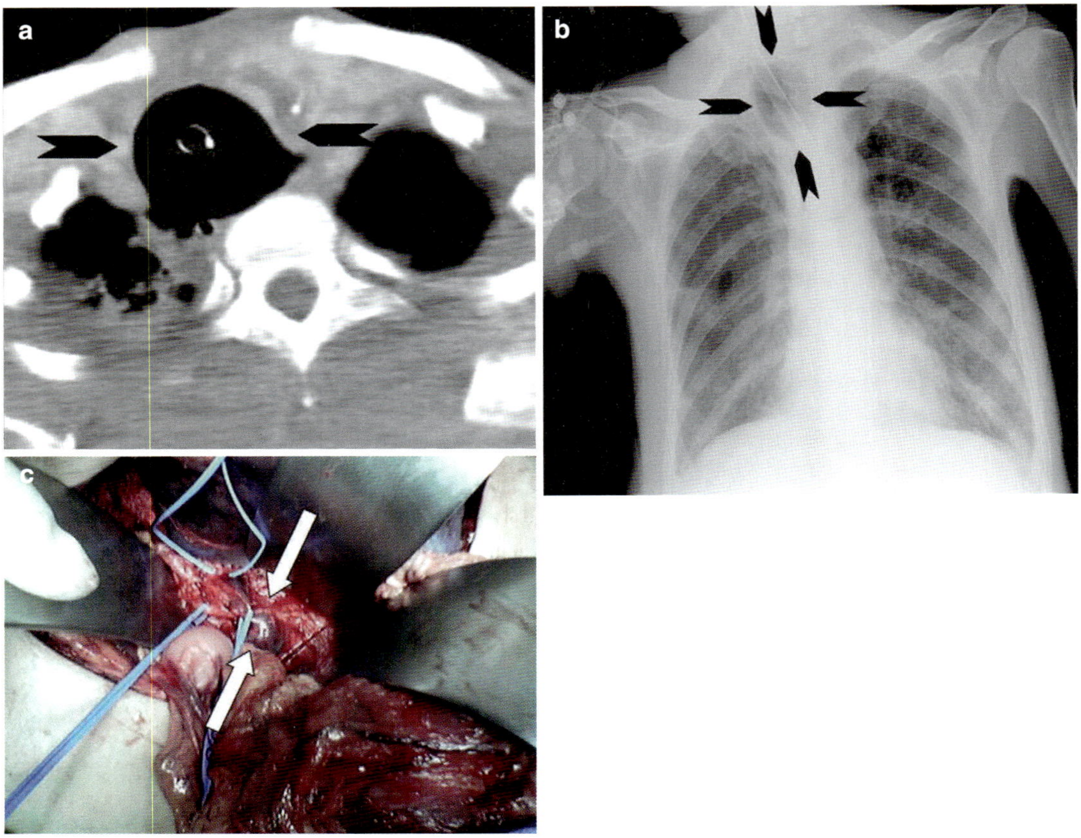

Fig. 3 Penetrating tracheal injury after intubation. (**a**) At the level of the thoracic inlet, chest CT scan shows overdistention of the endotracheal cuff (*arrowheads*). (**b**) Corresponding chest radiograph clearly depicts the same CT finding (*arrowheads*). (**c**) Surgical specimen shows endotracheal cuff herniation through the injured tracheal wall (*arrows*) (Reproduced with permission from Elsevier)

and the much more overt clinical signs of other more common associated injuries (Wiot 1983).

After an acute airway injury, the common symptoms are dyspnea and respiratory distress, hoarseness, or dysphonia. The most common signs of airway injuries are subcutaneous emphysema, pneumomediastinum, pneumothorax, and hemoptysis. These symptoms and signs are nonspecific for this kind of injury. Cervical–thoracic subcutaneous emphysema is the most common finding (65–87 %) (Paraschiv 2014). Pneumothorax, due to the splitting of the mediastinal pleura, occurs in 17–70 %, and the most specific characteristic is the inability to re-expand the lung after chest tube positioning.

A rare clinical manifestation is Hamman's sign, a crackling sound, synchronous with heartbeats, may be heard over the precordium produced by the heart beating against air-filled tissues (Wong and Knight 2006).

4 Imaging

4.1 Radiological Signs

Radiological studies improve the diagnosis of tracheobronchial injuries, especially when the clinical findings are subtle and in the first hours after the injury.

Standard or supine chest and cervical X-rays may reveal early suggestive signs as deep cervical or mediastinal emphysema (92–100 %), pneumomediastinum (85 %), or pneumothorax (40 %).

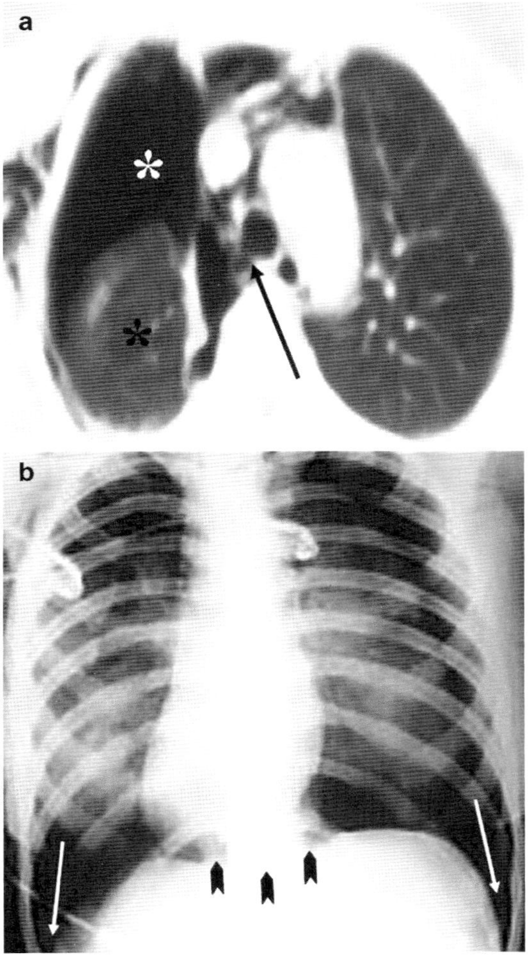

Fig. 4 Blunt bronchial injury (**a**) CT scan shows right-sided subcutaneous emphysema, pneumothorax (*white asterisks*), and pneumomediastinum. The right lung, which is partially collapsed, is detached from the main bronchus (*arrow*) and drops posteriorly (*black asterisk*) in the right hemithorax—the "fallen lung" sign. (**b**) Supine chest X-ray shows the "deep costophrenic sulcus" sign (*arrows*) and the "continuous diaphragm sign" (*arrowheads*) (Reproduced with permission from Elsevier)

These are the most common findings in radiographs. When the pneumomediastinum or pneumothorax is conspicuous, in supine position, the signs of "continuous diaphragm" or "deep costophrenic sulcus" can be appreciated (Fig. 4) due to the redistribution of the air preferentially accumulated over the diaphragmatic structure and anterior to the lungs, respectively (Scaglione et al. 2002).

Other signs suggestive for tracheobronchial injuries include tracheal deformity and overdistended endotracheal balloon cuff (Figs. 1 and 3). On lateral radiographs of the cervical spine, a high position of the hyoid bone associated to deep cervical emphysema can be an important indication of tracheal transection (Polansky et al. 1984).

Defect in tracheal contour, deviation of the endotracheal tube tip, and tube's cuff overdistention or protrusion beyond the edge of the tracheal wall (Chen et al. 2001b) are more specific signs of tracheobronchial rupture.

In some cases, the overdistention of balloon precedes the pneumomediastinum of several hours and may be the first and "small" signs of tracheobronchial injury. A cuff diameter greater than 2.8 cm is an indirect sign of tracheal tear (normal diameter of trachea is 2.7–2.8 cm), excluding other causes: balloon is located in the esophagus, patient is chronically intubated, or preintubation of tracheal enlargement (Rollins and Tocino 1987).

A tracheobronchial lesion may be also seen as a "bayonet sign" when a sharp angulation of the normal tracheal column or of the bronchial lumen occurs (Scaglione et al. 2002).

The "fallen lung" sign may be appreciated when the air leak through the injured tracheobronchial wall leads to lung collapse below the hilus, indicating complete rupture or transection of the main bronchi. This sign was first described by Oh et al. in 1969 and Kumpke in 1970.

A bronchocele/pneumatocele may also be detected after blunt trauma as a consequence of compression–decompression trauma of the chest causing rupture of the small airways and is seen as round radiolucent areas on a chest X-ray (Scaglione et al. 2002; Barbick et al. 2005) (Table 1).

4.2 CT Signs

Chest X-ray may miss some signs of tracheobronchial injuries as about 40 % of pneumothorax or a small amount of extrapulmonary soft tissue air, whereas the CT scan represents the

Table 1 X-ray findings

Specific
Defects in tracheobronchial contours
Deviation of the endotracheal tube tip
Tube's cuff protruding beyond the edge of the tracheal wall
"Bayonet" sign
"Fallen lung" sign
Bronchocele/pneumatocele
Suggestive
Tracheal deformity
Overdistended endotracheal balloon cuff (>2.8 cm)
Subcutaneous cervical or mediastinal emphysema
High position of the hyoid bone associated to deep cervical emphysema
Pneumothorax with "deep costophrenic sulcus" and "continuous diaphragm" signs
Pneumomediastinum
Ingravescent pulmonary atelectasis

gold standard with a sensibility of more than 85 % for diagnosis of injuries and rupture of the tracheobronchial wall. CT allows the direct visualization of the site of tracheobronchial injury, showing focal defects (Fig. 5) or the absence of the wall with "bayonet" or "fallen lung" signs contour deformity or abnormal communication with other mediastinal structures (Lupetin 1997; Baumgartner et al. 1997), overdistention or herniation of the endotracheal cuff (Figs. 6 and 7) with the appearance of "mickey-mouse head" when it occurs through the anterolateral walls of the trachea, displacement of the endotracheal tube, and bronchocele (Figs. 8, 9, 10, and 11) (Chen et al. 2001b, Scaglione et al. 2002).

These findings are not specific for tracheobronchial injuries but are helpful to identify the site of the tracheobronchial tear that needs to be confirmed at bronchoscopy or surgery.

Associated findings, highly suggestive for tracheobronchial injury, are pneumothorax or pneumomediastinum, soft tissue emphysema, and "air leak," particularly if detected at the level of the carina is consistent with main bronchus injury (Scaglione et al. 2006; Savas and Alper 2008) (Table 2).

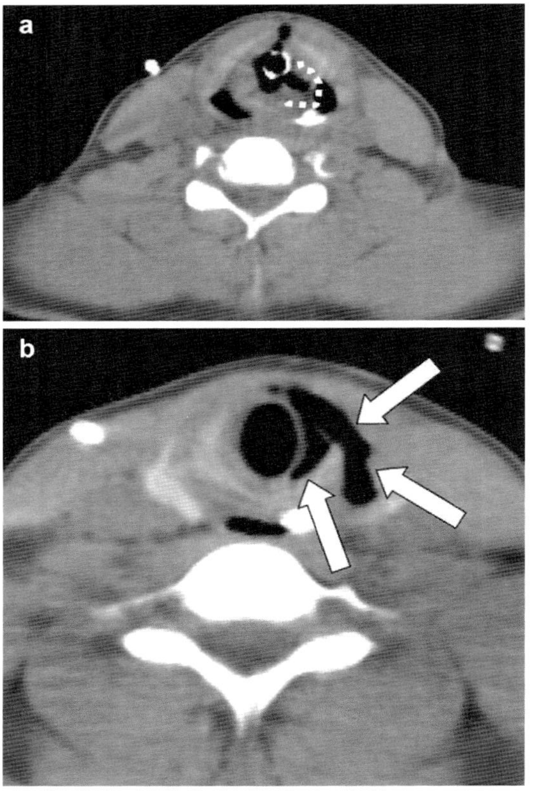

Fig. 5 Cervical tracheal injury secondary to blunt trauma. (**a**) 16-Section MDCT axial source image of the neck (wide window) shows lateral cervical tracheal wall discontinuity (*dashed line*). (**b**) More caudally, "air leak" is clearly evident (*arrows*) (Reproduced with permission from Elsevier)

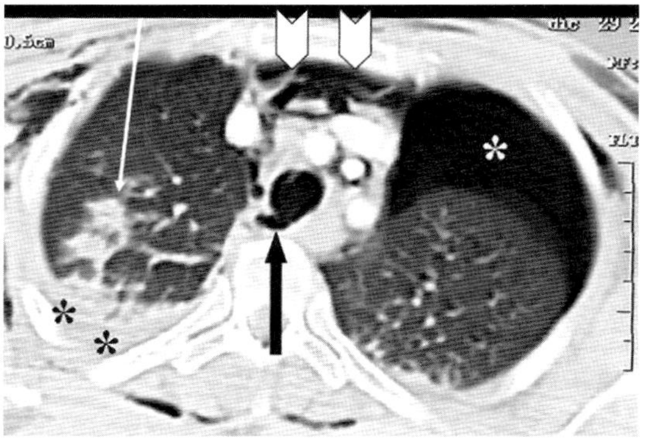

Fig. 6 Blunt tracheal injury after motor vehicle crash. CT demonstrates posterior herniation of the endotracheal cuff (*black arrow*). Furthermore, CT shows diffuse subcutaneous emphysema, right pulmonary contusion (*white arrow*), small pleural effusion (*black asterisks*), pneumomediastinum (*arrowheads*), and left pneumothorax (*white asterisk*) (Reproduced with permission from Elsevier)

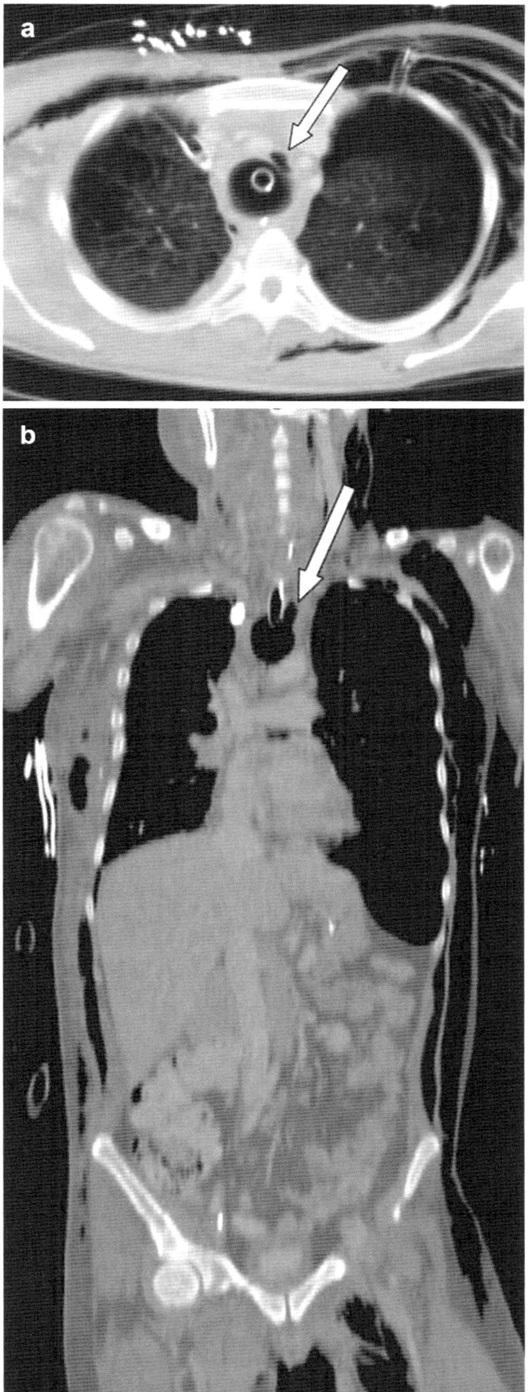

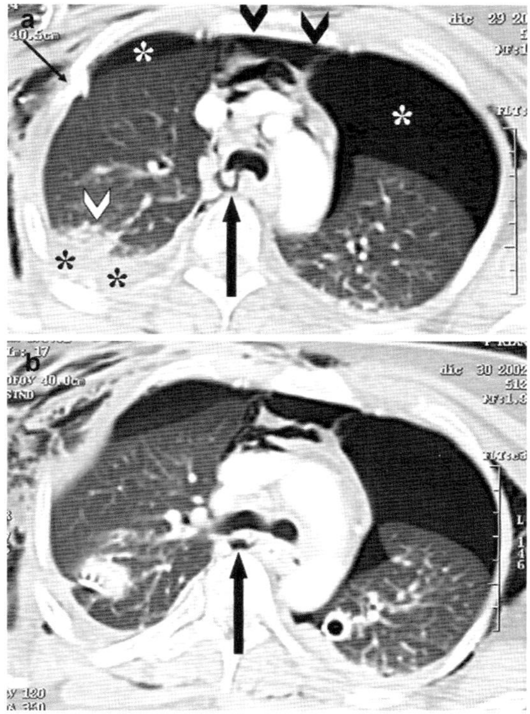

Fig. 8 Blunt bronchial injury after motor vehicle accident. (**a**) At the level of the thoracic carina, in the posterior mediastinum, axial CT scan shows "air leak" (*thick arrow*) in direct connection to the right main bronchus consistent of bronchial injury. This finding was confirmed by bronchoscopy. Associated findings as subcutaneous emphysema, right rib fracture (*small arrow*), pleural effusion (*black asterisks*), small pulmonary contusion (*white arrowhead*), bilateral pneumothorax (*white asterisks*), and pneumomediastinum (*black arrowheads*) are also visible. (**b**) A contiguous, more caudal CT scan also depicts direct "air leak" (*arrow*) and the associated findings (except for the rib fracture) (Reproduced with permission from Elsevier)

Fig. 7 Tracheal injury after blunt trauma (motor vehicle crash). (**a**) 16-Section MDCT axial source image of the neck (lung window) shows overdistention of the endotracheal tube cuff herniated through a tracheal wall defect (*arrow*). Note also massive subcutaneous emphysema and left pneumothorax. (**b**) Coronal reformatted 16-row MDCT scan shows herniation of the endotracheal cuff (*arrow*) and provides a comprehensive evaluation of the spread of the subcutaneous emphysema and the left pneumothorax (Reproduced with permission from Elsevier)

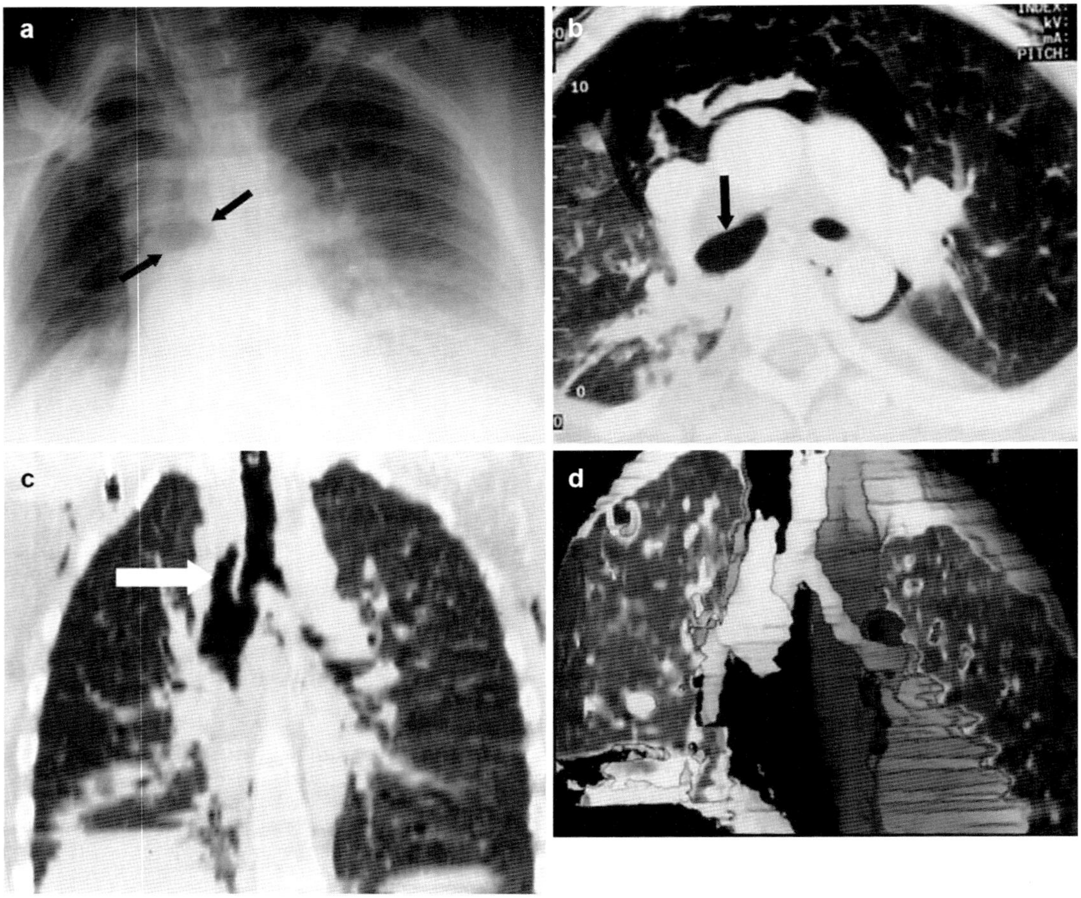

Fig. 9 Blunt bronchial injury after motor vehicle crush. (**a**) Supine chest radiograph shows enlargement of the right main bronchus (*arrows*). (**b**) Axial CT scan confirms the enlargement of the right main bronchus (*arrow*). (**c**) Frontal MIP CT reformation image shows longitudinal extension of injury and also depicts a bronchial pseudodiverticulum (*arrow*). (**d**) SSD reformation image gives optimal representation of the injury surface (Reproduced with permission from Elsevier)

5 Delayed Presentation Injuries

From 5 to 80% of the tracheobronchial injuries can be missed during the first 72 h after the trauma. With time, the bronchus will be filled with fibro-granulation tissue and organizing hematoma resulting either an airway stenosis or a complete obstruction. Tracheal or bronchial stenosis increases the susceptibility to recurrent lung infections leading to bronchiectasis and parenchymal destruction. In the complete airway obstruction, the lung is filled with mucus but protected by infections. Once a delayed tracheobronchial injury is diagnosed, they should be referred to surgery, with different modalities (Chen et al. 2001a; Demir et al 2006).

6 Management and Treatment

After a possible tracheobronchial injury, immediate intubation should be avoided, as attempt to blindly overpass an upper airway injury may

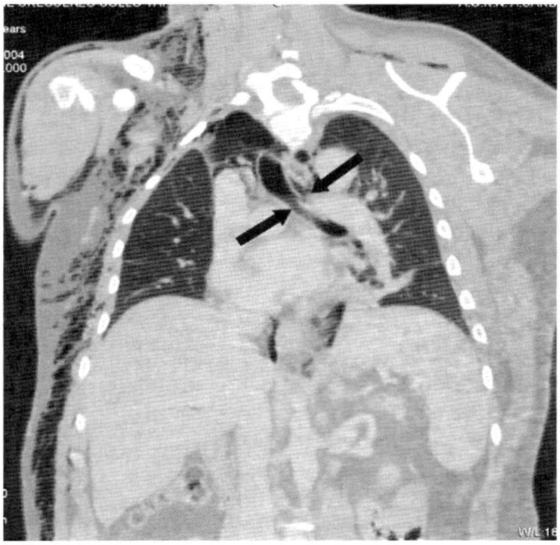

Fig. 10 Bronchial injury after blunt trauma after motor vehicle accident. Coronal reformatted 16-row MDCT scan shows left main bronchus discontinuity (*arrows*) (Reproduced with permission from Elsevier)

worsen the laceration and/or create false passage of the tube (Baumgartner et al. 1997). Therefore, spontaneous breathing of the patient should be preferred until safe airway has been achieved. As bronchoscopy represents the procedure of choice to find the site of the rupture and to make sure that the tube's cuff is inflated beyond the site of the injury, endobronchial intubation over a flexible bronchoscope is the preferred method for diagnosis and management of a tracheobronchial injury (Riley et al. 2004; Karmy-Jones and Wood 2007, Cassada et al. 2000). The rationale for surgery is closing of the airway defect to improve ventilation, preventing mediastinal spillage and infection, and avoiding spontaneous healing complications. Small tears and lacerations should be closed with direct sutures, while complete or partial transections require debridement of the infected and devitalized tissues, trimming of the edges of the injured airway, and end-to-end anastomosis.

Many studies have described the possibility for nonoperative management in patients with post-intubation tracheal lacerations (Conti et al. 2006; Schneider et al. 2007; Jougon et al. 2000;

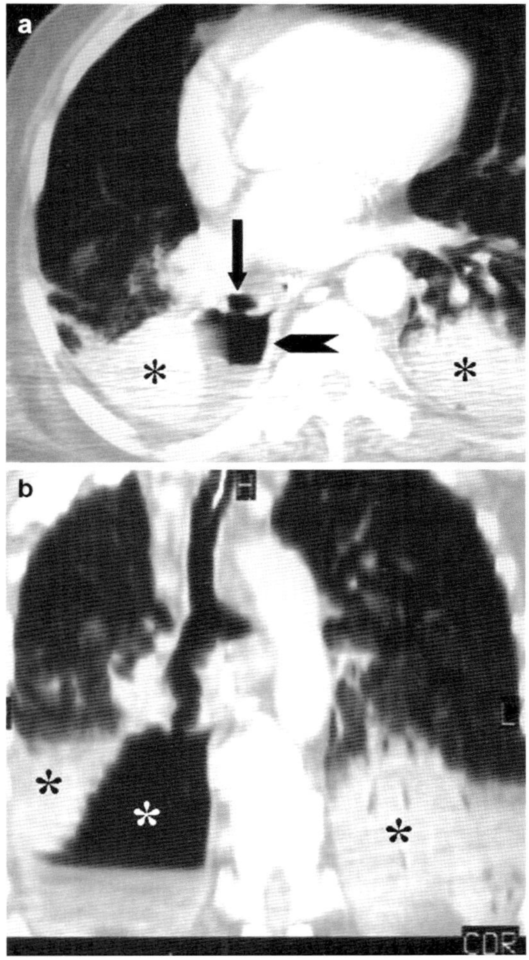

Fig. 11 Penetrating trauma after bronchoscopy. (**a**) CT scan shows right middle bronchus defect (*arrow*) in direct communication with an air-leveled area indicating hydropneumothorax (*arrowhead*). In addition, bilateral pulmonary atelectasis (*asterisks*) is also visible. (**b**) Frontal MPR reformation shows the right middle bronchial discontinuity and the longitudinal extension of the hydropneumothorax (*white asterisk*). Pulmonary atelectasis (*blackasterisk*) (Reproduced with permission from Elsevier)

Lamp 2004). The indications for such management are small lacerations (<2 cm), a tube's cuff inflated distally to the site of the injury, adequate ventilation, reduction or solving of pneumothorax once a chest tube is placed, not increasing subcutaneous emphysema, and absence of infection.

Table 2 CT findings

Specific
Deformity or discontinuity of the tracheobronchial wall
"Bayonet" sign
"Fallen lung" sign
Abnormal communication of tracheal lumen with other mediastinal structures
Herniation of the endotracheal cuff
Displacement of the endotracheal tube
Bronchocele/pneumatocele
Associated
Air leakage around the presumed site of injury
Soft tissue emphysema
Pneumothorax/Pneumomediastinum
Airway stenosis or complete obstruction (late findings)

Even if the prognosis of conservative management is favorable, the patients should be under strict follow-up, and surgery is necessary if airway loss, inadequate ventilation, or signs of infection and sepsis arise.

References

Balci AE, Kazez A, Eren S, Ayan E, Ozalp K, Eren MN (2004) Blunt chest trauma in children: review of 137 cases. Eur J Cardiothorac Surg 26:387–392

Barbick B, Cothren CC, Zimmerman MA, Moore EE (2005) Posttraumatic pneumatocele. J Am Coll Surg 200(2):306–307

Baugartner F, Shepperd B, De Virgilio C et al (1990) Tracheal and main bronchial disruptions after blunt chest trauma: presentation and management. Ann Thorac Surg 50:569–574

Baumgartner FJ, Ayres B, Theuer C (1997) Danger of false intubation after traumatic tracheal transection. Ann Thorac Surg 63:227–228

Burack JH, Kandil E, Sawas A, O'Neill PA, Sclafani SJ, Lowery RC, Zenilman ME (2007) Triage and outcome of patients with mediastinal penetrating trauma. Ann Thorac Surg 83(2):377–382

Cassada DC, Munyikwa MP, Moniz MP, Dieter RA Jr, Schuchmann GF, Enderson BL (2000) Acute injuries of the trachea and main bronchi: importance of early diagnosis. Ann Thorac Surg 69:1563–1567

Chen D, Han L, Hu Y, Yin H, Zhao H, Li H (2001a) Diagnosis and treatment of bronchial rupture from blunt thoracic trauma. Chin Med J (Engl) 114:540–541

Chen JD, Shanmuganathan K, Mirvis SE, Killen KL, Dutton RP (2001b) Using CT to diagnose tracheal rupture. AJR Am J Roentgenol 176:1273–1280

Conti M, Pougeoise M, Wurtz A, Porte H, Fourrier F, Ramon P, Marquette CH (2006) Management of postintubation tracheobronchial ruptures. Chest 131: 412–418

Demir A, Olcmen A, Kara HV, Dincer SI (2006) Delayed diagnosis of a complete bronchial rupture after blunt thoracic trauma. Thorac Cardiovasc Surg 54:560–562

Dougenis D (2002) Trauma of the tracheobronchial tree. Arch Hellen Med 19:258–269

Grant WJ, Mayers RL, Jaffe RL, Johnson DG (1998) Tracheobronchial injuries after blunt chest trauma in children –hidden pathology. J Pediatr Surg 33(11): 1707–1711

Huth J, Milliken JC, Chen JC (1997) Management of tracheobronchial injuries following blunt and penetranting trauma. Am Surg 63(10):896–899

Jougon J, Ballester M, Choukroun E, Dubrez J, Reboul G, Velly JF (2000) Conservative treatment of postintubation tracheobronchial rupture. Ann Thorac Surg 69: 216–220

Karmy-Jones R, Wood DE (2007) Traumatic injury to the trachea and bronchus. Thorac Surg Clin 17:35–46

Kiser AC, O'Brien SM, Detterbeck FC (2001) Blunt tracheobronchial injuries: treatment and outcomes. Ann Thorac Surg 71:2059–2065

Lamp L (2004) Tracheobronchial injuries. Conservative management. Interact Cardiovasc Thorac Surg 3:401–405

Lupetin AR (1997) Computed tomographic evaluation of laryngotracheal trauma. Curr Probl Diagn Radiol 26:185–206

Marty-Ane CH, Picard E, Jonquet O, Mary H (1995) Membranous tracheal rupture after endotracheal intubation. Ann Thorac Surg 60:1367–1371

Massard G, Rouge C, Dabbagh A et al (1996) Tracheobronchial lacerations after intubation and tracheostomy. Ann Thorac Surg 61:1483–1487

Milner A (2008) The airway in face, head, and neck injury. SAJAA 14:52–57

Nelson LA (2007) Airway trauma. Int Anesthesiol Clin 45:99–118

OH KS, Fleischner FG, Wyman SM (1969) Characteristic pulmonary finding in traumatic complete transection of a main-stem bronchus. Radiology 92:371–372

Paraschiv M (2014) Iatrogenic tracheobronchial rupture. J Med Life 7(3):343–348

Polansky A, Resnick D, Sofferman RA, Davidson TM (1984) Hyoid bone elevation: a sign of tracheal transection. Radiology 150:117–120

Rathlev NK, Mezdon R, Bracken ME (2007) Evaluation and management of neck trauma. Emerg Med Clin North Am 25:679–694

Riley RD, Miller PR, Meredith JW (2004) Injury to the esophagus, trachea and bronchus. In: Moore EE, Feliciano DV, Mattox K (eds) Trauma, 5th edn. McGraw-Hill, New York, pp 539–552

Rollins RJ, Tocino I (1987) Early radiographic signs of tracheal rupture. AJR Am J Roentgenol 148(4): 695–698

Savas R, Alper H (2008) Fallen lung sign: radiographic findings. Diagn Interv Radiol 14:120–121
Scaglione M, Pinto A, Romano L (2002) Traumi chiusi del torace. Gnocchi, Napoli
Scaglione M, Romano S, Rotondo A (2006) Acute tracheobronchial injuries: impact of imaging on diagnosis and management implications. Eur J Radiol 59:336–343
Schneider T, Storz K, Dienemann H, Hoffmann H (2007) Management of iatrogenic tracheobronchial injuries: a retrospective analysis of 29 cases. Ann Thorac Surg 83:1960–1964
Stark P (1995) Imaging of tracheobronchial injuries. J Thorac Imaging 10:206–219
Wiot JF (1983) Tracheobronchial trauma. Semin Roentgenol 18:15–22
Wong EH, Knight S (2006) Tracheobronchial injuries from blunt trauma. ANZ J Surg 76:414–415

Esophageal Injuries

Antonio Pinto, Carlo Liguori, Teresa Cinque,
Nicola Gagliardi, and Luigia Romano

Contents

Abstract

Esophageal injuries are uncommon but should be considered in accident victims with penetrating wounds; lower cervical or upper thoracic trauma, following instrumentation; foreign body ingestion; or heavy emesis.

Esophageal injuries may coexist with important associated airway or vascular injuries that should be actively excluded.

Traditionally, water-soluble contrast medium esophagography has been considered a crucial procedure for diagnosing esophageal rupture. Recently, multidetector-row computed tomography (MDCT) is often used as the first imaging modality to identify esophageal trauma and to map contained esophageal injuries that will be treated conservatively.

1 Introduction

Esophageal injuries include penetrating injuries, blunt traumatic perforation, iatrogenic perforation, foreign body impaction or perforation, as well as spontaneous perforation.

Patients usually present with vomiting, chest pain, and subcutaneous emphysema, but these signs occur late in the disease, and when present, they are not easily recognized due to the low prevalence of the condition (Backer et al. 1990). Prompt evaluation is vital as mortality rates exceed 90 % in cases of unrecognized perforation

A. Pinto (✉) • C. Liguori • T. Cinque
N. Gagliardi • L. Romano
Department of Radiology, Cardarelli Hospital, Naples, Italy
e-mail: antopin1968@libero.it

Med Radiol Diagn Imaging (2016)
DOI 10.1007/174_2016_50, © Springer International Publishing Switzerland

(Goudy et al. 2002). Iatrogenic causes of perforation are most common accounting for 33–75.5 % of cases (Duncan and Wong 2003).

Early and accurate diagnosis of esophageal trauma is critical, because the consequences of missed esophageal injury are devastating with potential progression to fulminant mediastinitis and septic shock. Delay in treatment beyond 24 h after onset may adversely affect prognosis (De Lutio di Castelguidone et al. 2006).

Evaluation of injuries of the esophagus may include chest and/or lateral neck radiograph, water-soluble contrast esophograms, flexible pharyngoscopy/laryngoscopy (Goudy et al. 2002), and MDCT. Particularly, emergent flexible endoscopy has been used for the assessment of traumatic injury of the esophagus in patients with penetrating injury to the thorax or neck (Srinivasan et al. 2000).

Computed tomography (CT) is considered the most accurate method for detecting paraesophageal manifestations of traumatic injury of the esophagus including mediastinal collections, abscesses, and effusions (Rubesin and Levine 2003).

2 Mechanism of Injury

Esophageal tears resulting from blunt chest trauma are extremely rare since the esophagus is well protected in the mediastinum, occurring in less than 1 % of blunt trauma cases (Lee et al. 1996). Blunt esophageal injuries may result from a blow to the neck or a burst-type force (Strauss et al. 2007). Injuries to the thoracic esophagus are associated with a far higher mortality than injuries of the cervical esophagus (Makhani et al. 2014).

Esophageal lesions resulting from blunt trauma include mucosal dissection, intramural hematoma, full-thickness laceration with perforation, and complete rupture or transaction (Ghahremani 1994). If perforation occurs, mortality can exceed 50 % due to mediastinal and pleural infection leading to sepsis and multiorgan failure (Griffiths et al. 2009). This is especially due to the characteristics of the esophageal wall. The thin wall, lack of supporting adventitia, and relatively poor blood supply make the esophagus exceedingly susceptible to perforation (Young et al. 2008). Furthermore, the loose areolar connective tissue and lack of serosa make it unable to prevent the spread of infection and inflammation (Onat et al. 2010). This unique anatomical configuration also allows bacteria and digestive enzymes easy access to the mediastinum, leading to mediastinitis, empyema, sepsis, and multiorgan failure. Cultures from the mediastinum in the case of transmural perforations are polymicrobial containing streptococcus, staphylococcus, bacteroides, and pseudomonal species (Burnett et al. 1990).

Esophageal injury should be suspected in cases of penetrating transmediastinal injury in which the wound trajectory or a projectile fragment is found to be close to the esophagus. Firearms are responsible for the majority (~80 %) of esophageal injuries, with knife wounds accounting for most of the remaining injuries. The cervical esophagus is most commonly involved (56 % of cases), followed by the thoracic (30 %) and abdominal (17 %) esophagus. Combined injuries to multiple segments of the esophagus are rare in transmediastinal injury (3 % of cases) (Gunn et al. 2014).

Intramural hematoma of the esophagus can develop spontaneously or can result from hypocoagulable states or as a complication of direct injury during endoscopic procedures or as consequence of direct trauma or ingested matter (De Lutio di Castelguidone et al. 2005). Dissecting intramural hematomas are considered part of the range of emetogenic esophageal injury between the superficial Mallory–Weiss tears and the complete esophageal perforation in the Boerhaave syndrome (Grassi et al. 1995).

A blow to the neck typically results in cervical esophageal injuries, whereas a burst-type force may cause distal esophageal injuries. The latter mechanism is similar to that which causes a postemetic esophageal rupture. Distal esophageal tears usually occur along the left side of the esophageal wall, where less protection is afforded by the pleural lining and the heart (Kaewlai et al. 2008). Intraluminal pressure increase is a frequent cause of esophageal perforation. This increase may occur for iatrogenic causes, such as during stricture dilation as in achalasia or, spontaneously, as in Boerhaave syndrome. In these cases, the distal left posterior wall is the most common site of rupture, which results in a pneumomediastinum and left pleural effusion (Gagliardi et al. 2015).

3 Imaging

3.1 Radiological Signs

Radiographic detection of esophageal injuries relies on the presence of indirect radiological signs including subcutaneous or muscular, thoracic or cervical emphysema, a widened mediastinum, pneumomediastinum, pneumopericardium, left-sided pneumothorax, pleural effusion, an abnormal course of a nasogastric tube when it is inserted, and a left lower lobe atelectasis (Ghahremani 1994). Water-soluble contrast medium esophagography is very useful for detecting the presence of leakage of orally administered contrast material (Fig. 1).

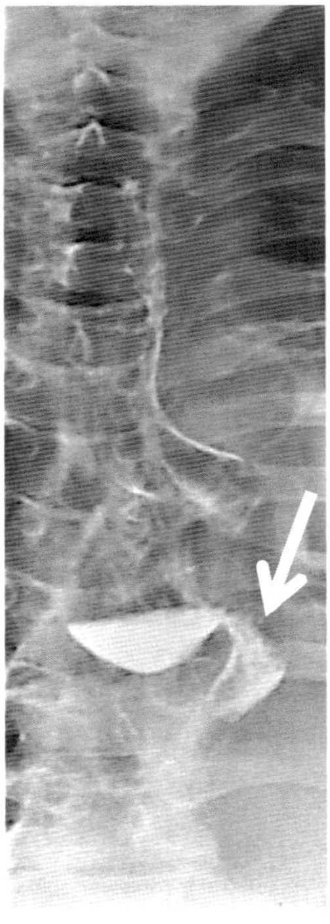

Fig. 1 Thoracic esophageal injury. Water-soluble contrast medium esophagography: leakage of orally administered contrast material (*arrow*)

In patients with penetrating transmediastinal injury, the most common chest radiographic findings of esophageal perforation are left pleural effusion and cervical or mediastinal soft tissue emphysema. Because the radiographic signs of esophageal injury lack sensitivity and specificity, evaluation with CT, esophagography, or esophagoscopy is necessary (Gunn et al. 2014).

In patients with perforation caused by endoscopy or intubation, chest and lateral neck radiographs may show the presence of linear air collections in the mediastinum, fascial planes of the neck and supraclavicular regions, as well as soft tissue swelling in the retropharyngeal region due to hematoma, edema, or abscess (Ghahremani 1994).

The esophagus is a common site for impaction of foreign bodies that are accidentally or purposefully swallowed. Patients who have esophageal foreign bodies can be classified into four groups: pediatric patients, psychiatric patients and prisoners, patients who have underlying esophageal disease, and edentulous adults (Pinto et al. 2012).

Foreign bodies can sometimes be demonstrated with plain radiographs of the neck or conventional barium esophagogram, but these procedures may fail to show the foreign bodies if they are thin, small, or only faintly radiopaques. Fish bones and chicken bones are the most commonly ingested sharp foreign bodies causing problems in their detection with plain radiographs being obscured by overlying tissues (Pinto et al. 2004).

According to some authors (Flynn et al. 1989), the gold standard for diagnosing an esophageal rupture is iodine, water-soluble contrast medium esophagography, which has a specificity close to 100% but only a moderate sensitivity of approximately 75%. In addition to diagnosis, this method helps to determine the location of the perforation but has some disadvantages, such as being operator-dependent and unusable in critically ill patients.

3.2 CT Signs

In patients with clinically suspected esophageal injuries, CT displays the same indirect signs as conventional radiology and more specific signs,

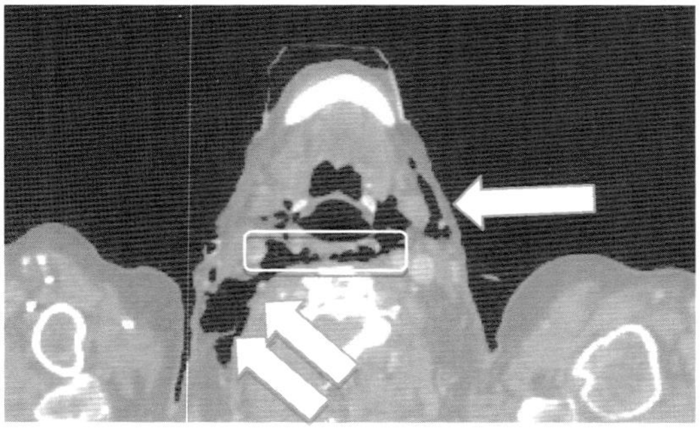

Fig. 2 MDCT demonstrates extensive cervical esophageal wall injury (*rectangle*) with soft tissues emphysema localized at the level the left submandibular space (*arrow*) and of the right cervical lateral wall (*arrows*)

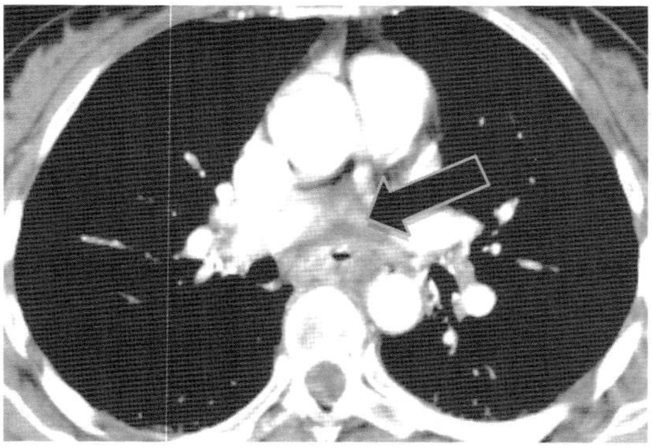

Fig. 3 MDCT examination showing esophageal wall thickening associated with periesophageal edema and fluid (*black arrow*)

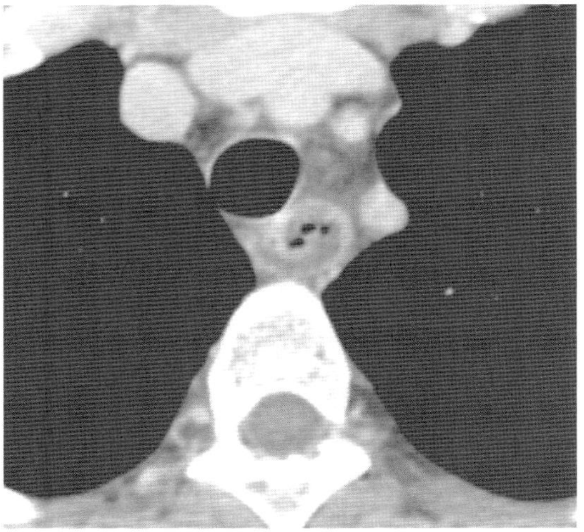

Fig. 4 MDCT demonstrates the presence of periesophageal fluid and small bubble gas

such as a localized esophageal wall thickening, mucosal hyperemia, mucosal dissection, an esophageal hematoma, as well as periesophageal air, edema, and fluid (De Lutio di Castelguidone et al. 2005) (Figs. 2, 3, 4, and 5). In patients with suspected perforation caused by foreign body ingestion (Fig. 6), CT can demonstrate such foreign bodies and exhibit superior images compared to plain radiographs, can visualize secondarily induced inflammatory changes in the adjacent structures, and can suggest the site of esophageal perforation.

In cases of traumatic esophageal perforation, MDCT is very useful for detecting the presence of pneumomediastinum, mediastinitis, hydropneumothorax, or leakage of orally administered contrast material (Fig. 5) into the mediastinum or pleural space. Moreover, in cases of injury caused by firearms, at MDCT, air bubbles, bullet fragments, or bone fragments located adjacent to the esophagus in the mediastinum suggest esophageal perforation. Thickening or discontinuity of the esophageal wall and extravasation of oral contrast material into the mediastinum are direct MDCT signs of esophageal perforation that have a higher specificity (Dosios et al. 2000).

Due to particular anatomic direction of the esophagus, multiplanar reformatted images allow a better identification of the extent of perforation and their complications and also the possible involvement of adjacent structures.

4 Management and Treatment

Review of the literature revealed that esophageal perforations are frequently diagnosed late and that the associated mortality is high (Brinster et al. 2004). Early diagnosis reduces mortality. However, suspicion is first necessary for early diagnosis. When esophageal rupture is suspected, diagnosis is often determined with contrast esophagography, chest radiograph, MDCT, or upper gastrointestinal system endoscopy.

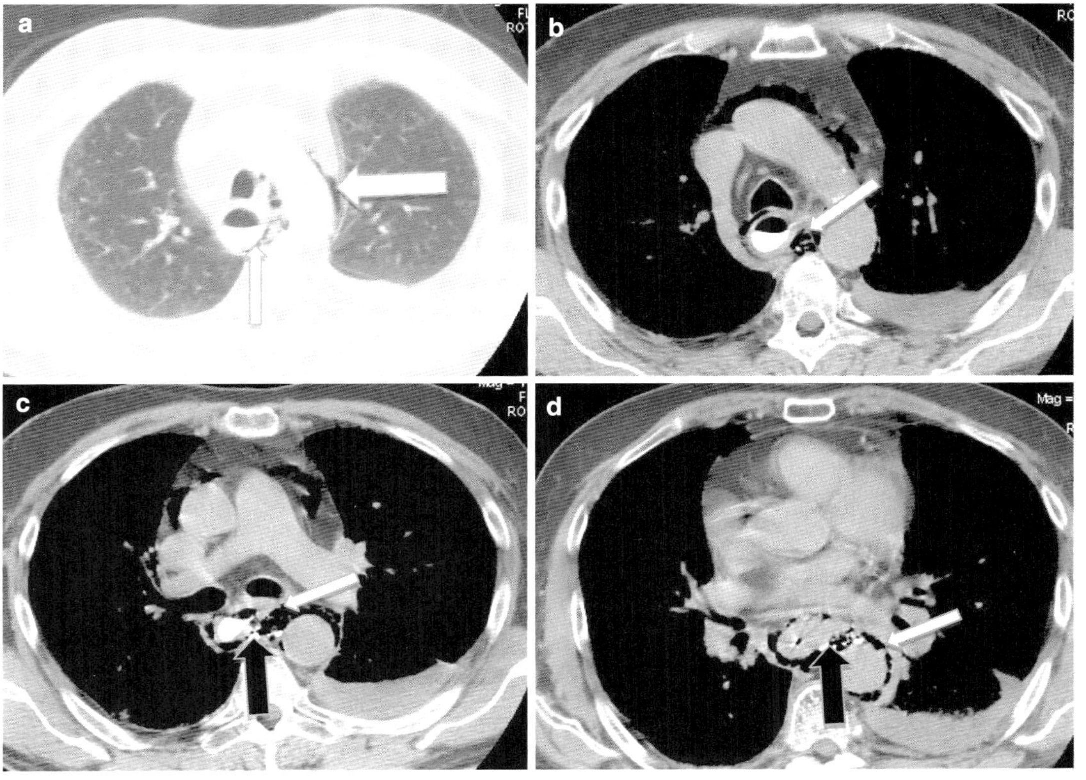

Fig. 5 Perforation of the thoracic esophagus. MDCT shows the presence of pneumomediastinum (**a**, *large arrow*), left pleural effusion, periesophageal air (**a–d**, *small arrow*), and leakage of orally administered contrast material (**c**, **d**, *black arrow*)

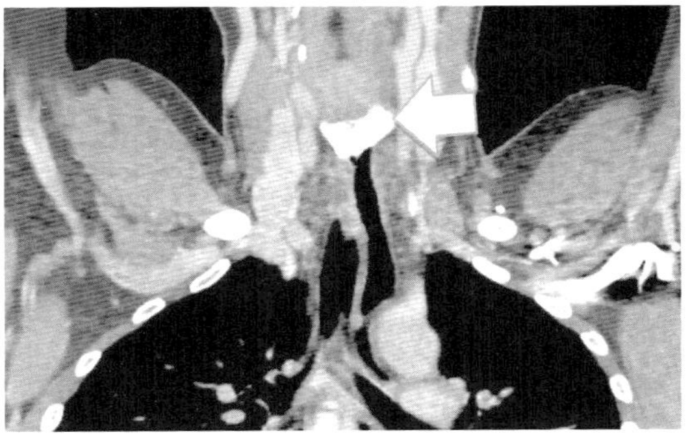

Fig. 6 MDCT shows a foreign body (chicken bone, *arrow*) impacted at the level of cervical esophagus without signs of esophageal perforation

Imaging algorithms and the decision for surgical exploration depend on the stability of the patient, on the region of the cervicothoracic injury, and on the presence of minor or significant signs of vascular, airway, or digestive trauma (LeBlang and Nunez 1999).

The treatment for esophageal perforation has been traditionally immediate surgery.

However, much attention has focused on conservative therapeutic options, especially with the development of effective antibiotics, improved parenteral alimentation, nonoperative methods of irrigation and drainage, and a stronger emphasis on early diagnosis. Overall early diagnosis and appropriate treatment with either conservative or aggressive surgical therapy may account for the improved outcomes in a potentially fatal condition.

Under this context, MDCT may play a significant role in therapeutic decisions by mapping the air and fluid leaks resulting from esophageal perforation and by demonstrating non-contained air or fluid leaks and foreign bodies (Reeder et al. 1995, Asensio et al. 1997).

References

Asensio JA, Berne J, Demetriades D, Murray J, Gomez H, Falabella A, Fox A, Velmahos G (1997) Penetrating esophageal injuries: time interval of safety for preoperative evaluation – how long is safe? J Trauma 43:319–324

Backer CL, LoCicero J III, Hartz RS, Donaldson JS, Shields T (1990) Computed tomography in patients with esophageal perforation. Chest 98:1078–1080

Brinster CJ, Singhal S, Lee L, Marshall MB, Kaiser LR, Kucharczuk JC (2004) Evolving options in the management of esophageal perforation. Ann Thorac Surg 77:1475–1483

Burnett CM, Rosemurgy AS, Pfeiffer EA (1990) Life-threatening acute posterior mediastinitis due to esophageal perforation. Ann Thorac Surg 49:979–983

De Lutio di Castelguidone E, Pinto A, Merola S, Stavolo C, Romano L (2005) Role of spiral and multislice computed tomography in the evaluation of traumatic and spontaneous oesophageal perforation. Our experience. Radiol Med 109:252–259

De Lutio di Castelguidone E, Merola S, Pinto A, Raissaki M, Gagliardi N, Romano L (2006) Esophageal injuries: spectrum of multidetector row CT findings. Eur J Radiol 59:344–348

Dosios TJ, Salemis N, Angouras D, Nonas E (2000) Blunt and penetrating trauma of the thoracic aorta and aortic arch branches: an autopsy study. J Trauma 49: 696–703

Duncan M, Wong RK (2003) Esophageal emergencies: things that will wake you from a sound sleep. Gastroenterol Clin North Am 32:1035–1052

Flynn AE, Verrier ED, Way LW, Thomas AN, Pellegrini CA (1989) Esophageal perforation. Arch Surg 124: 1211–1214

Gagliardi N, Stavolo C, De Gennaro A (2015) Esophageal perforation: assessment with Multidetector row Computed Tomography. In: Romano L, Pinto A (eds), Imaging of alimentary tract perforations, pp 23–27, Springer International Publishing, Switzerland

Ghahremani GG (1994) Esophageal trauma. Semin Roentgenol 29:387–400

Goudy SL, Miller FB, Bumpous JM (2002) Neck crepitance: evaluation and management of suspected upper aerodigestive tract injury. Laryngoscope 112:791–795

Grassi R, Romano L, Diettrich A, Rossi G, Pinto A (1995) Incomplete Boerhaave syndrome of the cervical esophagus. Aktuelle Radiol 6:360–362

Griffiths EA, Yap N, Poulter J, Hendrickse MT, Khurshid M (2009) Thirty-four cases of esophageal perforation: the experience of a district general hospital in the UK. Dis Esophagus 22:616–625

Gunn ML, Clark RT, Sadro CT, Linnau KF, Sandstrom CK (2014) Current concepts in imaging evaluation of penetrating transmediastinal injury. Radiographics 34:1824–1841

Kaewlai R, Avery LL, Asrani AV, Novelline RA (2008) Multidetector CT of blunt thoracic trauma. Radiographics 28:1555–1570

LeBlang SD, Nunez D (1999) Helical CT of cervical spine and soft tissue injuries of the neck. Radiol Clin North Am 37:515–532

Lee S, Mergo PJ, Ros PR (1996) The leaking esophagus: CT patterns of esophageal rupture, perforation and fistulization. Crit Rev Diagn Imaging 37:461–490

Makhani M, Midani D, Goldberg A, Friedenberg FK (2014) Pathogenesis and outcomes of traumatic injuries of the esophagus. Dis Esophagus 27:630–636

Onat S, Ulku R, Cigdem KM, Avci A, Ozcelik C (2010) Factors affecting the outcomes of surgically treated non-iatrogenic traumatic cervical esophageal perforation: 28 years of experience at a single center. J Cardiothorac Surg 5:46

Pinto A, Muzj C, Stavolo C, Pepe M, Cinque T, Romano L (2004) Pictorial essay: foreign body of the gastrointestinal tract in emergency radiology. Radiol Med 107:145–154

Pinto A, Muzj C, Gagliardi N, Pinto F, Setola FR, Scaglione M, Romano L (2012) Role of imaging in the assessment of impacted foreign bodies in the hypopharynx and cervical esophagus. Semin Ultrasound CT MRI 33:463–470

Reeder LB, DeFilippi VJ, Ferguson MK (1995) Current results of therapy for esophageal perforation. Am J Surg 169:615–617

Rubesin SE, Levine MS (2003) Radiological diagnosis of gastrointestinal perforation. Radiol Clin North Am 41:1095–1115

Srinivasan R, Haywood T, Horwitz B, Buckman RF, Fisher RS, Krevsky B (2000) Role of flexible endoscopy in the evaluation of possible esophageal trauma after penetrating injuries. Am J Gastroenterol 95:1725–1729

Strauss DC, Tandon R, Mason RC (2007) Distal thoracic oesophageal perforation secondary to blunt trauma: case report. World J Emerg Surg 2:8

Young CA, Menias CO, Bhalla S, Prasad S (2008) CT features of esophageal emergencies. Radiographics 28:1541–1553

Blunt Traumatic Aortic Injury

Ferco H. Berger and Diederick W. De Boo

Contents

F.H. Berger, MD (✉)
Department of Radiology and Nuclear Medicine, VU University Medical Centre, De Boelelaan 1118, Amsterdam, PK 0 X 126, 1081, HZ, Netherlands
e-mail: fhberger@gmail.com

D.W. De Boo, MD, PhD, EBIR
Department of Radiology, Amsterdam Medical Center – University of Amsterdam, Meibergdreef 9, Amsterdam 1105, AZ, Netherlands
e-mail: dwdeboo@gmail.com

Abstract

Blunt or penetrating trauma to the chest can cause injury to the aorta and its major branching arteries. These injuries are still the second most lethal condition in blunt trauma patients, after head injuries, and need urgent detection and treatment. In this chapter, we will specifically discuss aortic and proximal branch vessel injuries resulting from blunt trauma mechanisms. These are almost invariably resulting from high-impact trauma, usually with rapid deceleration forces. Patients sustaining blunt traumatic aortic injury (BTAI) usually have many concomitant injuries, that will distract from scrutinizing the aorta. This chapter will help radiologist understand BTAI and be a valuable partner in the resuscitation team, both in diagnosis and treatment of BTAI.

1 Introduction

Blunt or penetrating trauma to the chest can cause injury to the aorta and its major branching arteries. These potentially life-threatening conditions need urgent detection and treatment. In this chapter, we will specifically discuss aortic and major vessel injuries resulting from blunt trauma mechanisms. Thousands of peer-reviewed scientific publications are available, indicating the interest and debate on a very dynamic topic. Many terms are used in literature to indicate traumatic injury to the aorta, including but not limited to: blunt aortic

Med Radiol Diagn Imaging (2016)
DOI 10.1007/174_2016_41, © Springer International Publishing Switzerland

injury (BAI), traumatic thoracic aortic injury (TTAI), acute traumatic aortic injury (ATAI), acute thoracic aortic trauma (ATAT), traumatic aortic rupture (TAR) and blunt traumatic aortic rupture (BTAR). We elect to use *blunt traumatic aortic injury* (BTAI), since it indicates blunt trauma as the mechanism and encompasses all injuries within the spectrum. We will give an overview of important issues and our experience with BTAI.

Blunt traumatic injury to the aorta and/or major branching vessels almost invariably results from high-impact trauma, usually with rapid deceleration forces, further detailed in the next section on mechanisms of injury. A well-documented study by Parmley et al. in 1958 demonstrated that around 85 % of victims sustaining BTAI die on the scene or shortly thereafter (Parmley et al. 1958). Improvements in vehicle safety profiles, prehospital care and rapid diagnosis may have improved survival rates. However, this cannot definitively be concluded from the literature over the past six decades. In a study on 881 blunt traumatic fatalities performed in Los Angeles, USA, in 2005, in 304 victims undergoing full autopsy, BTAI was present in 104 (34 %) (Teixeira et al. 2011). Unfortunately, this study does not state the total number of polytrauma patients to give the incidence of BTAI in a population including victims deceased on scene.

A fairly recent large study performed on data collected in the National Trauma Databank in the USA from 2000 to 2005 does have relevant figures on trauma victims transported to hospitals (thus excluding death on scene) (Arthurs et al. 2009). In this study, 3.114 out of 1.1 million trauma patients had BTAI, resulting in an incidence of BTAI in patients alive on scene of 0.3 %. In keeping with literature, the mean age was 41 (±20) and 72 % were males, and the mean injury severity score was 40 (±17). Of this cohort, 113 (4 %) died during transportation to and 599 (19 %) died during triage in the hospital. Of the 2.402 patients surviving transportation and triage, 31 % had major concomitant head injury and 29 % had major abdominal injury (Arthurs et al. 2009).

A meta-analysis with a total of 7258 patients from 90 articles found the following rates of concomitant injuries: orthopaedic fractures in 70 %, thoracic injury in ~50 %, abdominal injury in 40 % and head injury in 37 % (Antonopoulos et al. 2014). In the study by Arthurs et al., two-thirds of patients could not undergo attempts to repair the injury, mostly due to other injuries, and BTAI was found to be an independent prognosticator for poor outcome (Arthurs et al. 2009). The figures in this large study are in keeping with literature in the fact that BTAI despite its relative rarity is still second only to head injury as a cause of death in polytrauma patients. Even compared to matched cohorts with comparable concomitant injuries, BTAI increases risk of mortality fourfold, overall mortality being 55 % (Arthurs et al. 2009).

In patients reaching the hospital with BTAI that can actually receive treatment for their aortic injury, survival rates thereafter are high, in somewhat dated reports form 2008 being estimated in the range of 70–90 % (Steenburg et al. 2008; Demetriades et al. 2008). Further improvement may have occurred since, although, given the concomitant injuries, it is unlikely that survival will ever be close to 100 %. Recent decades have seen important changes in treatment of BTAI, which we will address in a later section. Part of these changes have to do with much more sensitive imaging modalities and more aggressive imaging strategies after trauma, depicting aortic injuries that in more remote decades would not have been picked up.

Despite the fact that patients may survive, associated morbidity will influence most patients' lives after the traumatic incident. Fully independent feeding will be achieved by 72 %, locomotion by 33 % and expression by 80 %, lower numbers than in cohorts matched for other injuries (Arthurs et al. 2009). This is another indication of the severity of trauma and its impact on life after such an injury.

2 Mechanism of Injury

Since Parmley et al. first published a large cohort of patients in 1958, studies have consistently shown BTAI to be the result of high-impact trauma. Motor vehicle accidents (MVAs), motorcycle and airplane crashes, pedestrians struck by vehicles and falls from height make up the vast majority of cases (Parmley et al. 1958; Teixeira et al. 2011; Antonopoulos et al. 2014; Challoumas

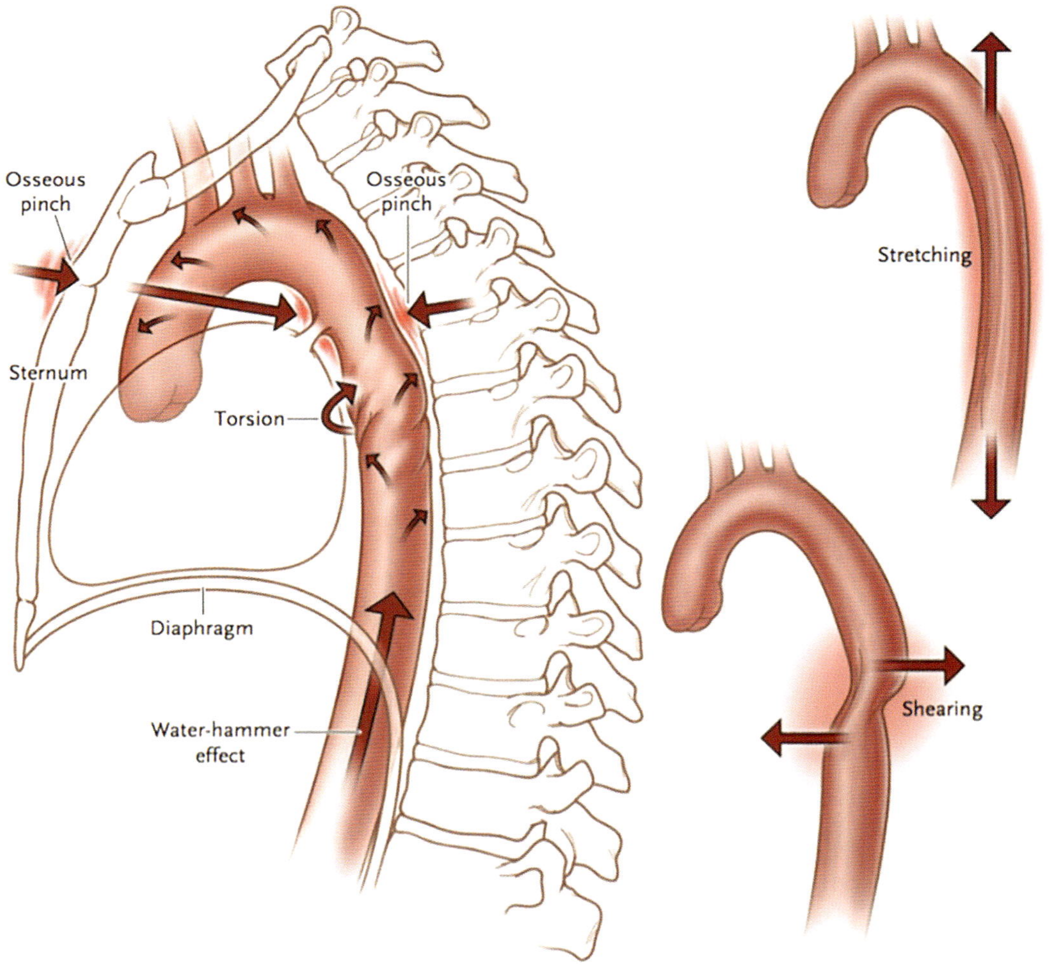

Fig. 1 Theories of blunt traumatic aortic injuries (From 'Blunt Aortic Injury' Neschis DG et al. (2008) NEJM 359:1708–1716. Copyright © (2008) Massachusetts Medical Society. Reprinted with permission of the Massachusetts Medical Society)

and Dimitrakakis 2015; Lin et al. 2016; Fabian et al. 1997; Burkhart et al. 2001).

Injury to the aortic wall is likely a result of any or a combination of the following potential mechanisms, as described by Parmley et al. and others (Parmley et al. 1958; Burkhart et al. 2001; Mosquera et al. 2013; Crass et al. 1990; Cohen et al. 1992; Lundevall 1964; Baqué et al. 2006) (Fig. 1). Direct compression or the so-called osseous pinch may result from the aorta being pinched between the vertebrae and the anterior thoracic skeleton (sternum, clavicles and ribs) (Crass et al. 1990, 1992). Direct penetration from fractured ribs, sternum or vertebrae may also occur. Other mechanisms have their effect in a more indirect manner. Stretching of the aorta from displacement of vertebrae may cause aortic wall injury more remote to the osseous injury site, the so-called 'stretch' injury. Extreme pressure in the aortic lumen by compression on the abdomen or lower chest may also cause injury, a mechanism known as the 'water-hammer' effect. The water-hammer effect, proposed by Lundevall, results when the flow of a noncompressible fluid is occluded dramatically, which leads to high-pressure waves being reflected back along the vessel wall (Lundevall 1964). At the aortic root, the ligamentum arteriosum attachment and the diaphragmatic crus, the aorta is connected to other tissues, increasing regional strain by different deceleration characteristics of the joined tissues. The final mechanism potentially contributing to injury is torsion, which indicates rotational forces of the aorta along its longitudinal axis. A theory about elevated aortic pressure due to compression of the left ventricle that was proposed in the first decades of the twentieth century has since been dismissed by other scientists (Baqué et al. 2006).

Depending on the forces in play, the aorta injury site can be the root, ascending aorta, arch, isthmus, descending aorta or even abdominal aorta (less common). Multiple studies in deceased and surviving patients show the aortic isthmus is the most common location of injury. However, since studies are not inclusive of all blunt trauma-related fatalities, there may be a shift in numbers with more injuries potentially occurring at the aortic root. A considerable number of patients has aortic injury at multiple sites, in the autopsy series by Teixeira et al. amounting up to 18 % (Teixeira et al. 2011) (Fig. 2). In that study, 2 % of injuries were located at the aortic root, 3 % at the ascending aorta and 11 % at the arch. Mention is warranted for the other upper thoracic major vessels, especially the aortic

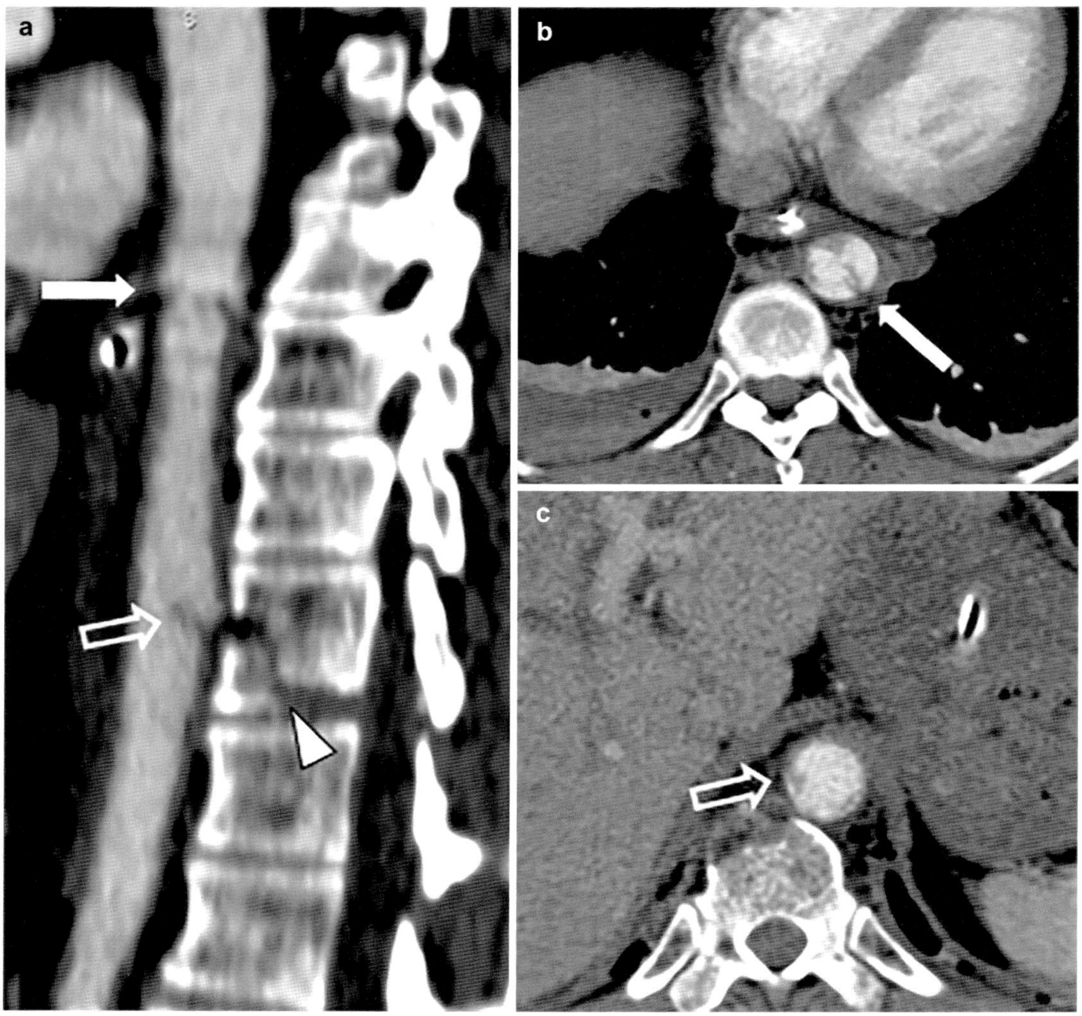

Fig. 2 Example of multilevel blunt traumatic aortic injury on sagittal CTA (**a**) with corresponding axial CTA slides (**b**, **c**). The proximal intimal injury (*solid white arrow*) was most likely caused by a stretch mechanism; the distal intimal flap (*open white arrow*) may have been caused by stretch and/or direct impact from the nearby vertebral fracture (*arrow head*)

arch branches, which can be injured in isolation. In a small sample study by Chen et al., 38 % of injuries involved the proximal aortic arch branching vessels (Chen et al. 2001). Even though the percentage likely is lower, injury to these vessels is important to diagnose and treat if necessary.

3 Terminology and Clinical Issues

The diagnostic and treatment process in polytrauma patients usually takes place in multidisciplinary teams with members of varying level of experience. In combination with stress because of time concerns and multitude of injuries, clear communication is paramount. Therefore, the most important point to make about terminology is that all members of the resuscitation team, including radiology staff, should align the vocabulary used throughout the institution. This also includes which of the many classification schemes is used to grade the injury.

As described in the introduction, many different terms are used in literature to indicate traumatic injury to the aorta after blunt trauma. Further confusion may arise with other terminologies in this setting. Specific terms to be aware of with regard to diagnosis and treatment are mediastinal haematoma, peri-aortic haematoma, minimal aortic injury, pseudo-aneurysm and secondary signs of injury (SSI). We will describe these terms here to minimize confusion.

Mediastinal haematoma is used to describe haematoma within the mediastinum with a fat plane preserved around the aortic adventitia. These haematomas are not considered to be associated to aortic injury, but originate from other sources of bleeding, like mediastinal veins or fractures of vertebrae or sternum (Forman et al. 2013; Raptis et al. 2015) (Fig. 3).

Peri-aortic haematoma is used to describe haematoma directly bordering the aortic adventitia (i.e. loss of peri-aortic fat plane) and either confined to the direct peri-aortic region or

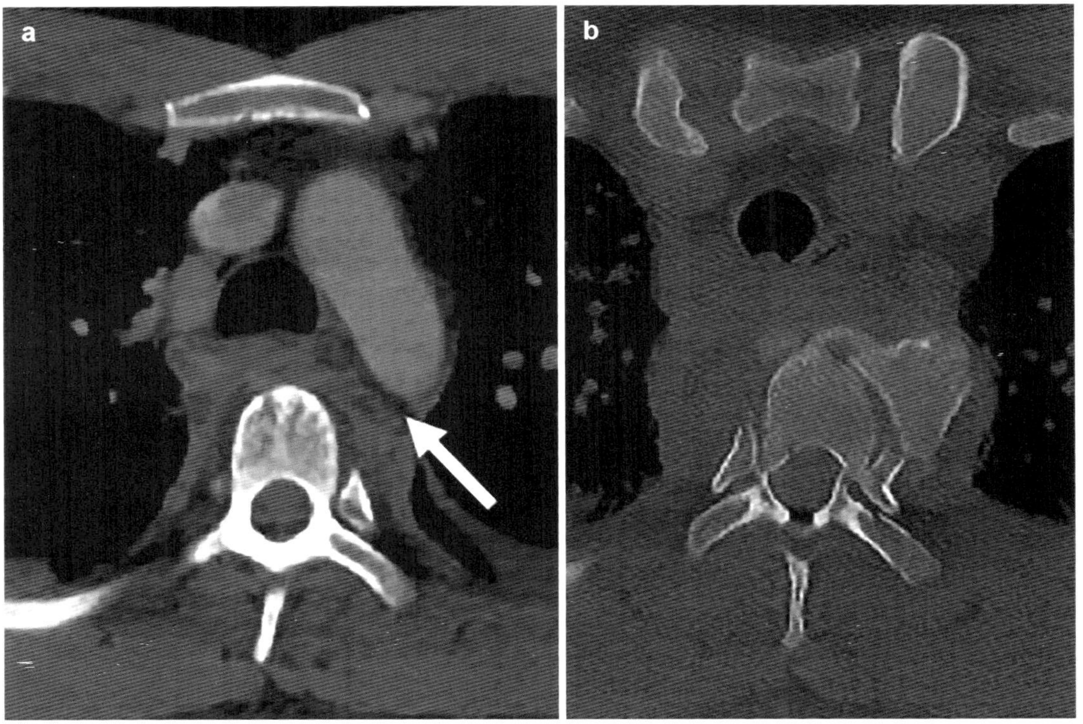

Fig. 3 Example of mediastinal haematoma (**a**) due to thoracic vertebral body fracture dislocation (**b**). Note the fat plane between the aorta and mediastinal haematoma (*arrow*). The fat plane allows to differentiate more distant mediastinal haematoma from peri-aortic haematoma

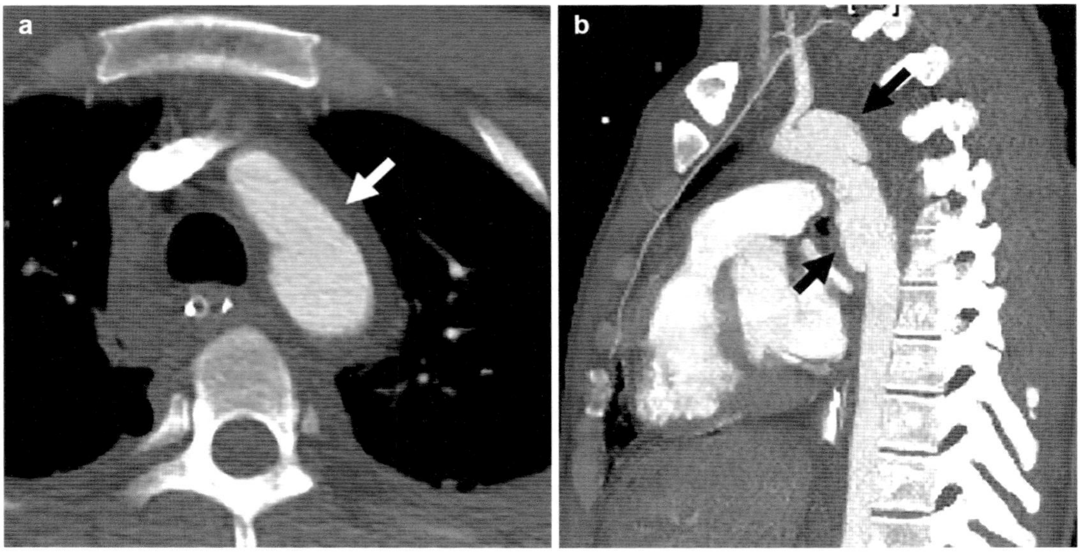

Fig. 4 Axial (**a**) and sagittal-oblique (**b**) CTA demonstrating peri-aortic haematoma (*solid white arrow*) directly abutting the aortic adventitia (loss of peri-aortic fat plane), caused by a long, bilobar pseudo-aneurysm (*solid black arrows*)

extending beyond into the mediastinum (Fig. 4). Although previously reported to occur as a false-positive indirect sign of aortic injury (Steenburg and Ravenel 2008), advances in modern CT techniques pick up previously undetected small injuries. If peri-aortic haematoma is present, the aorta should be scrutinized for presence of injury. If peri-aortic haematoma is absent, this nearly excludes higher-grade aortic injury. However, lesser grade injury is still possible if peri-aortic haematoma is absent, around 21–22 % of such cases occurring without surrounding haematoma (Forman et al. 2013; Aladham et al. 2010).

Minimal aortic injury (MAI, also known as *minor aortic injury*) is a term used to describe a lesser grade of aortic injury that may resolve with conservative measures, including monitoring, blood pressure control and repeat CT. However, multiple groups that publish on the topic define the term differently. The definition ranges from injuries in which outer aortic wall contour is preserved to those including pseudo-aneurysms of up to 50 % of the normal aorta diameter (Forman et al. 2013; Caffarelli et al. 2010; Rabin et al. 2014a).

Pseudo-aneurysm relates to an aortic injury in which there is (near) complete loss of aortic wall integrity resulting in a regular or an irregular deformity of the outer wall of the aorta (Fig. 5). Especially if there is surrounding haematoma with mass effect on the mediastinum, there is a high chance of rupture (Rabin et al. 2014a, b).

Secondary signs of injury (SSI) were recently defined in a study that sought parameters for successful nonoperative management of BTAI as pseudo-coarctation, extensive mediastinal haematoma (with mass effect) and large left haemothorax (Rabin et al. 2014a, b) (Fig. 6). They concluded that grade 3 aortic injuries (pseudo-aneurysms involving more than 50 % the circumference of the aorta in their study) with SSI needed urgent repair, whereas those without SSI could undergo delayed repair (Rabin et al. 2014a). The use of SSI therefore seems to aid management decisions.

3.1 Classification of BTAI

To grade blunt traumatic aortic injury, several classification systems have been published, the first of which was by Parmley et al. in 1958 on the basis of a large autopsy study (Parmley et al. 1958). Gavant et al. published the first classification system based on CT images in 1999, very comprehensive but somewhat difficult to use (Gavant and Helical 1999). In 17 years since, six more groups published classification systems with different degree of variation, namely, Simeone et al. (2006), Azizzadeh et al. (2009),

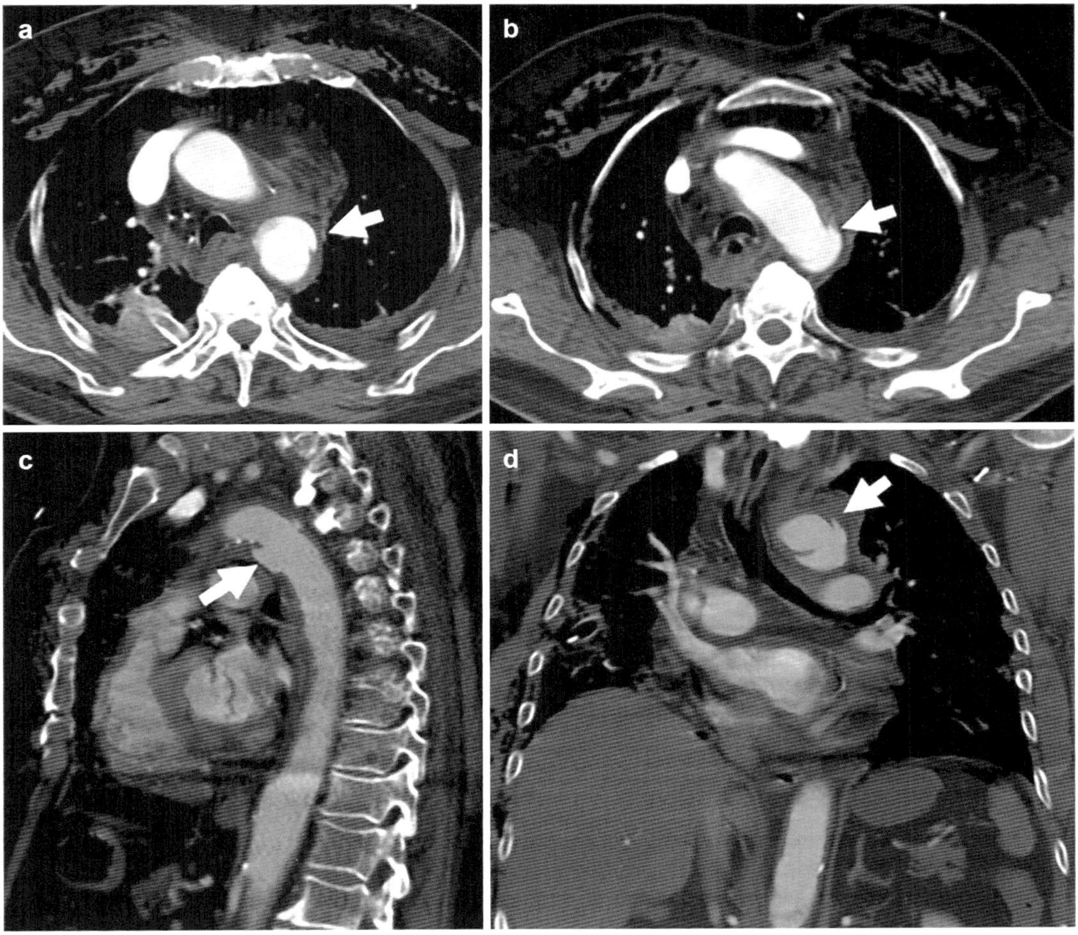

Fig. 5 Axial (**a**, **b**), sagittal (**c**) and coronal (**d**) CTA of a 57-year-old man involved in an MVA. Images depict a proximal thoracic aortic pseudo-aneurysm (*arrows*). Moderate peri-aortic haematoma and extensive subcutaneous emphysema are also present (not marked)

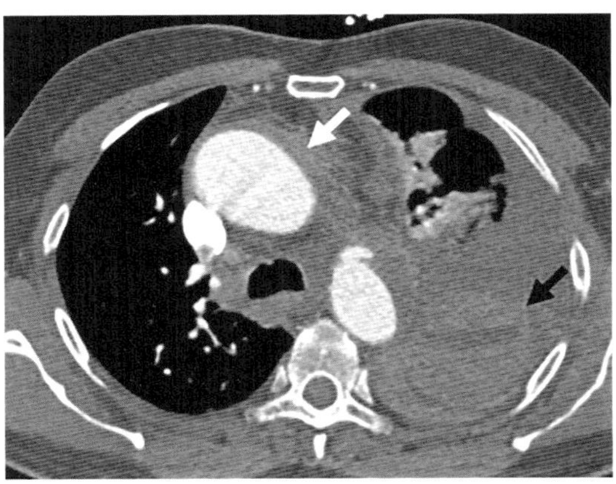

Fig. 6 Example of BTAI with peri-aortic haematoma bordering the ascending (*solid white arrow*) and descending thoracic aorta with large left-sided haemothorax, caused by BTAI at the aortic isthmus. Note the different densities indicating cloth formation (*solid black arrow*)

Caffarelli et al. (2010), Lamarche et al. (2012), Starnes et al. (2012) and Rabin et al. (2014a). The multitude of different classification systems likely reflects local experiences with treatment choices, as well as the rapid improvement of CT technology and endovascular stent grafts used for treatment. In 2011, the Society for Vascular Surgery published clinical practice guidelines for endovascular repair of BTAI (Lee et al. 2011), using the classification system by Azizzadeh et al. (2009). However, this was before other classification systems were published. The Vancouver Simplified classification system in the study by Lamarche et al. found better interobserver agreement than the Simeone and Gavant classifications, the reason for which we like to use it (Lamarche et al. 2012). As mentioned before, the

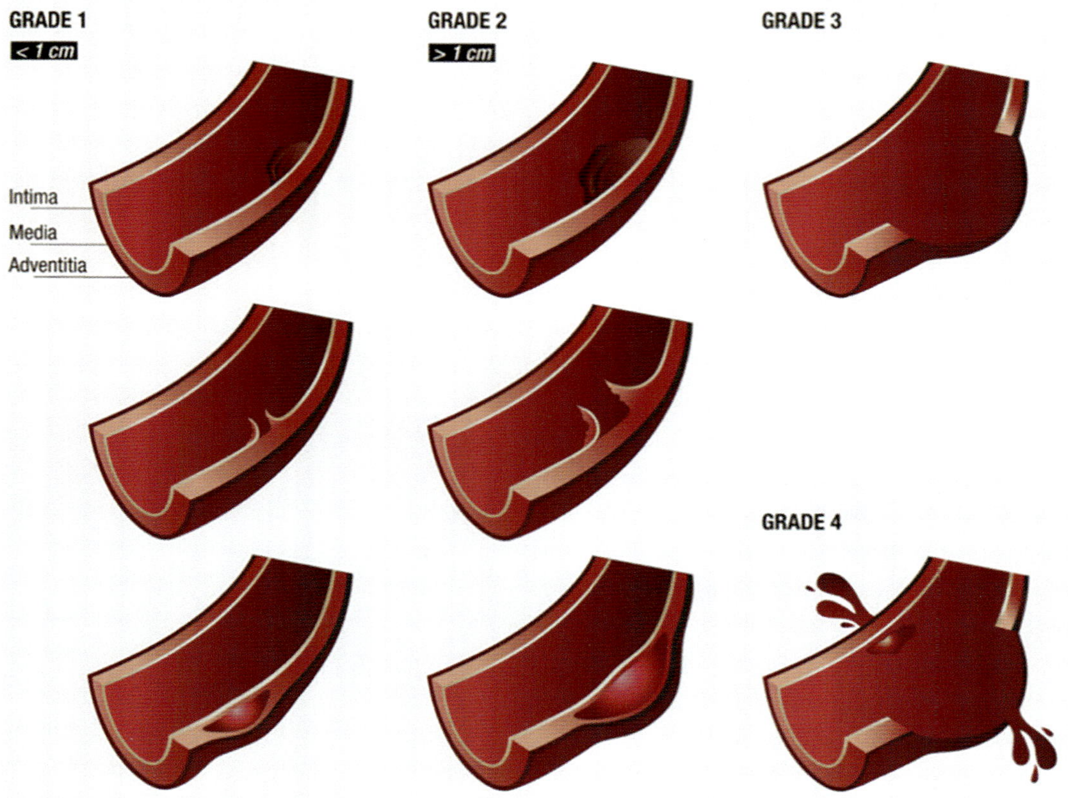

Fig. 7 Vancouver classification of blunt traumatic aortic injury. Grade 1 injuries (luminal thrombus, intimal flap or intramural haematoma) are less than 1 cm; if larger than 1 cm, injuries are grade 2; aortic pseudo-aneurysms are grade 3; and grade 4 are injuries with active contrast extravasation indicating ongoing haemorrhage (From Lamarche et al. (2012), Reply to the Editor, copyright 2012. Reprinted with permission from Elsevier)

most important issue for all team members involved in caring for BTAI patients remains to make sure to use the same terminology and classification.

The Vancouver classification, like most other classifications, has four grades (Fig. 7). Grade 1 and grade 2 essentially have preserved outer aortic contours and consist of luminal thrombus, intimal flap and/or intramural haematoma, these lesions in grade 1 being smaller than 1 cm and in grade 2 larger than 1 cm. Grade 3 and grade 4 lesions demonstrate abnormality of the outer wall of the aorta, with grade 3 lesions being pseudo-aneurysms of any size and grade 4 lesions showing frank contrast extravasation. Given the fact that some publications show good results of conservative management as treatment for smaller pseudo-aneurysms, caregivers may elect to use other classification systems.

3.2 Clinical Issues

Clinical symptoms and signs are non-specific for BTAI, nor sensitive. Patients may have chest pain, back pain or difficulty breathing, and signs include external chest wall injuries, systemic hypotension, concomitant upper limb hypertension with lower limb hypotension or a substantial difference in blood pressures between the right and left brachial arteries (present in up to 50 % of patients with BTAI). Some patients may present initially with no clinical signs but rapidly develop hemodynamic instability (Steenburg et al. 2008;

Raptis et al. 2015). Factors negatively influencing prognosis are a systolic blood pressure <90 mmHg and hypothermia with $T<35$ °C and injury severity score (ISS) >25 (Arthurs et al. 2009).

As stated before, blunt traumatic aortic injury invariably is the result of high-energy trauma to the chest and most often is not confined to this anatomic area. In most cases, significant concomitant injuries are present. Depending on the severity of the aortic injury, the hemodynamic stability of the patient and the severity of the other injuries, treatment priorities have to be decided. If possible, repair of BTAI should be delayed for favourable outcome, especially in concomitant head injuries (Fox et al. 2015; Rabin et al. 2014b). This will also increase the time to carefully evaluate the extent of other injuries. If aortic injury and traumatic brain injury coexist, research has shown that the most unstable injury should be prioritized to immediate care. It also suggests that intracranial haemorrhage is not a contraindication to endovascular aortic stenting or an absolute contraindication to systemic anticoagulation during this procedure (Fox et al. 2015; Kitagawa et al. 2013).

To predict which patients need urgent repair instead of delayed repair, Harris et al. proposed a new aortic injury score to predict early rupture (Harris et al. 2015). From their study, they conclude that a patient is at high risk of early rupture if any two of the following three factors are present: lactate >4 mM, posterior peri-aortic haematoma >10 mm or lesion/normal aortic ratio >1.4 (meaning an aortic diameter more than 40 % increased compared to the nearest normal aortic diameter). Whether these criteria are better predictors of the need of urgent repair of grade 3 injuries than the secondary signs of injury (SSI) defined by Rabin et al. (2014a, b) (see before) remains to be seen. Likely, the criteria of both study groups overlap, but these findings will help select patients that need urgent instead of delayed treatment.

4 Imaging

Post-intravenous contrast CT angiography (CTA) is the standard diagnostic test for detection of thoracic aortic and branch vessel injury (Fox et al. 2015). The sensitivity is 96 %, specificity is 100 % and negative predictive value 99.9 %. These percentages are by far superior when compared to plain chest radiography, transoesophageal echography (TEE) or conventional arch aortography (Steenburg and Ravenel 2008). Furthermore, CTA is very accurate in detection of most other chest injuries, which exist with or without the presence of BTAI. However, other imaging modalities can be useful, so we will discuss strengths, weaknesses and findings of those as well.

4.1 Radiography

Although CT is increasingly being used as the primary imaging modality in trauma resuscitation, chest radiography (CXR) in many centres is still used as the first adjunct to the primary survey. Signs seen on plain films are either sensitive or specific, but never both; therefore, utility of CXR in the setting of suspected BTAI is low (Nagy et al. 2000; Cook et al. 2001; Gutierrez et al. 2016). Especially in the case of MAI, modern CTA can demonstrate BTAI without changes to the outer wall of the aorta and even without bordering haematoma, further underscoring the potential to miss these injuries on CXR. However, signs can still be present on a conventional chest X-ray and, if so, prompt for further evaluation with CTA (Fig. 8).

Signs in decreasing order of sensitivity according to Cook et al. are as follows: mediastinal width >8 cm (sens 90 %, spec 30 %), mediastinum-to-chest width ratio >0.25 (sens 90 %, spec 6 %), opacified AP window (sens 90 %, spec 51 %), irregular aortic knob (sens 80 %, spec 68 %), blurred aortic contour (sens 70 %, spec 53 %), nasogastric tube deviation (sens 50 %, spec 91 %) and trachea shifted to patient's right (sens 40 %, spec 86 %) (Cook et al. 2001).

Signs in decreasing order of specificity are as follows: thoracic spine fracture (spec 93 %, sens 11 %), first rib fracture (spec 91 %, sens 10 %), NG tube deviation (spec 91 %, sens 50 %), depressed left main bronchus (spec 90 %, sens 10 %), wide left paraspinal line (spec 90 %, sens 29 %), clavicle fracture (spec 87 %, sens 0 %), trachea shift to patient's right (spec 86 %, sens 40 %), left apical cap (spec 80 %, sens 20 %) and pulmonary contusion (spec 72 %, sens 30 %) (Cook et al. 2001).

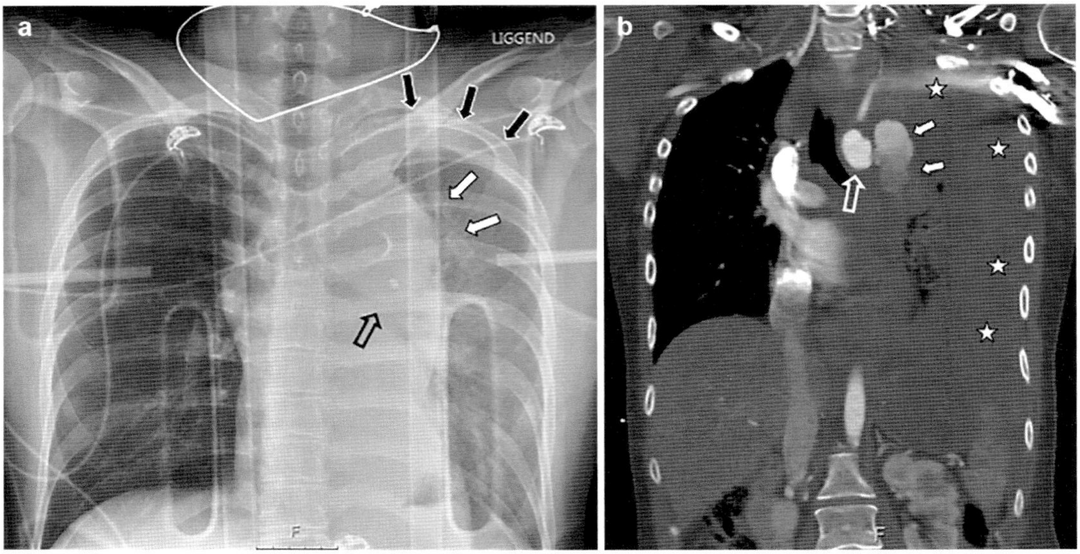

Fig. 8 A 27-year-old woman struck by a car while on moped. Supine AP chest X-ray taken during resuscitation with unsuspected findings consistent with aortic injury (**a**): indistinct aortic contour (*white solid arrows*), depressed left main bronchus (*open black arrow*) and apical cap consistent with haemorrhage extending to the pleural space (*solid black arrows*). Injury was proven with CT (**b**): aortic arch (*open white arrow*) demonstrates frank extravasation (*solid white arrows*) into the pleural cavity (*white asterisks*), consistent with grade 4 injury. Note the homogenous low density of the haemothorax, indicating hyperacute exsanguination with lack of time to form cloth. Patient did not survive to treatment

Rather than spending a lot of time analysing all separate findings and measurements, a general assessment of the mediastinum and decision to 'normal' or 'abnormal' results in better sensitivity and interobserver agreement (Ho et al. 2002). If the only abnormality seen on an initial screening supine anteroposterior CXR is mediastinal width more than 8 cm, it can be worthwhile repeating the CXR standing and posteroanterior, in which case, 38 % of exams will be normal (Schwab et al. 1984). However, we fully agree with Raptis et al. and others that patients with an abnormal CXR, patients with high index of suspicion for BTAI or patients with chest pain out of proportion to their known injuries after appropriate trauma need to proceed to CTA of the chest (Raptis et al. 2015; Fox et al. 2015).

4.2 Angiography/Aortography

The publication of the Eastern Association for the Surgery of Trauma (EAST) practice management guideline for the diagnosis and management of blunt aortic injury in 2000 still defined angiography as the 'gold standard' for the diagnosis of BTAI. However, the workgroup already acknowledged that 'CT scanning is taking more of a role, especially for screening' (Nagy et al. 2000). Since their publication, rapid developments of CT techniques have rendered CTA more sensitive than conventional angiography, mostly due to the detection of extra-luminal abnormalities, either confined to the aortic wall or beyond. This has caused the same society to revise their guidelines, which in their publication in 2015 strongly recommend CT with intravenous contrast for the diagnosis of BTAI (Fox et al. 2015). Angiography is of course still used if endovascular treatment for BTAI is undertaken (Fig. 9).

4.3 Abdominal and Transthoracic Ultrasound

During trauma resuscitation, many centres will include an ultrasound scan according to the focussed abdominal sonography in trauma

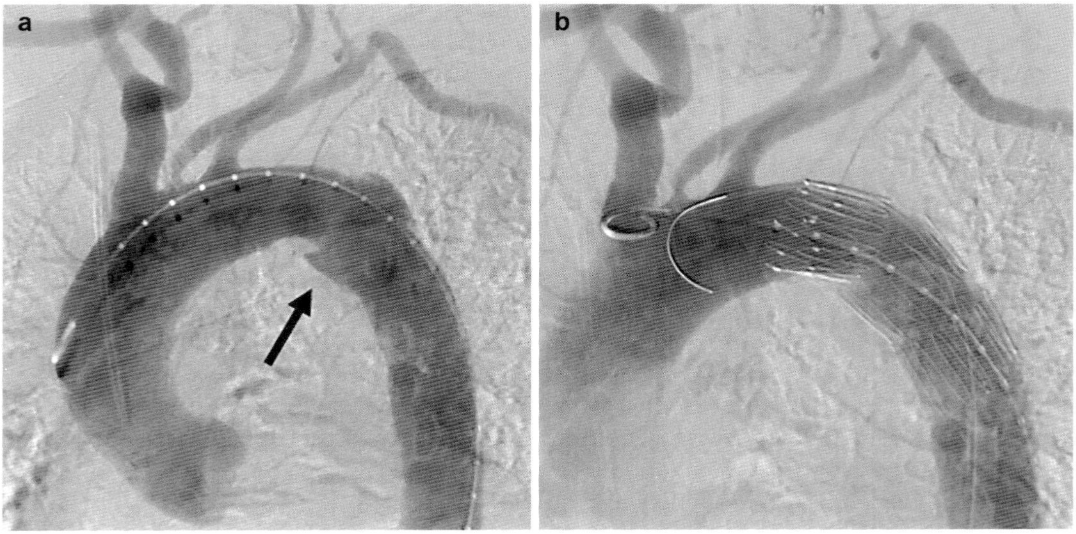

Fig. 9 Thoracic aorta angiogram in left anterior oblique view before (**a**) and after TEVAR (**b**) for aortic pseudoaneurysm at the isthmus (*arrow*)

(FAST) as an adjunct to the primary survey. A FAST examination essentially is a quickly performed ultrasound to demonstrate the presence or absence of free intraperitoneal fluid by evaluating the four abdominal quadrants. In addition, one can look for presence of pericardial effusion, pleural effusion and/or pneumothorax in a reasonably quick and reliable fashion, the so-called extended FAST (e-FAST). Although e-FAST could demonstrate a secondary sign of injury in BTAI, notably large left haemothorax, or demonstrate pericardial effusion, the aorta itself usually is poorly visualized and can only be examined below the diaphragm. The same holds true for transthoracic ultrasound.

4.4 Transesophageal Echocardiography (TOE or TEE)

Already in 2008, Demetriades et al. found that between 1997 and 2007, there had been a near elimination of transoesophageal echocardiography for the diagnosis of BTAI, dropping from nearly 12 % of BTAI patients receiving TOE in 1997 to 1 % in 2007 (Demetriades et al. 2008). The primary use currently is to evaluate cardiac dysfunction and injury or hemodynamic state and response to treatment. TOE can be used to evaluate the descending aorta, being reasonably sensitive for traumatic aortic injury in that location but overall only moderately sensitive (Patel et al. 2003; Rippey and Royse 2009). In hemodynamically unstable patients, transoesophageal echocardiography can be used as bedside test, and the probe can remain in place even in the operating theatre.

4.5 Intravascular Ultrasound (IVUS)

In two papers by Williams et al. in the early 1990s, the use of IVUS is discussed as a tool to be used in equivocal angiographic results for BTAI (Williams et al. 1992; Williams et al. 1993). The limitation of this technique as an initial diagnostic test due to practical restrains was already discussed in their second paper and has not been altered since. Malhotra et al. as well as Patel et al. demonstrated better sensitivity compared to angiography especially for picking up MAI, before the era of CTA as a gold standard (Patel et al. 2003; Malhotra et al. 2001). A more recent paper again proved IVUS to be better than angiography in patients where CTA findings were equivocal. Therefore, the authors advocated the use of IVUS in potential TAI patients in whom angiography is being considered (Azizzadeh et al. 2011). However, the nature of the procedure requires vascular access, with another option to rule out aortic injury being a repeat CTA, with or without ECG triggering. If a patient is managed with endovascular stent-graft placement, IVUS has been shown to be useful for selection of stent-graft size (Wallace et al. 2015; Shi et al. 2015). Compared to the acute CTA, IVUS during the procedure of stent placement demonstrates a larger aortic diameter, possibly reflecting intravascular hypovolemia during resuscitation at initial imaging, necessitating preoperative reassessment of aortic lumen diameter (Wallace et al. 2015).

4.6 Magnetic Resonance Imaging (MRI)

Length of examination time, limited accessibility, non-compliant materials and relatively small bore sizes render MRI unfeasible in the initial assessment of patients with multiple injuries. In patients with equivocal CTA findings for BTAI, an MRI study can be considered if they are hemodynamically stable and also otherwise able to undergo the examination. Fattori et al. published two papers in the mid- to late 1990s on the use of MRI for the diagnosis of acute BTAI and for follow-up in the delay to treatment, demonstrating its feasibility (Fattori et al. 1996; Fattori et al. 1998). The paucity of results when performing literature searches to find the use of MRI in BTAI indicates the limited role for this modality especially in the acute phase, despite the well-documented use in other aortic and major vessel diseases.

4.7 Computed Tomography Angiography (CTA)

As stated before, CTA now is the gold standard for the evaluation of BTAI, given its high accuracy and near-perfect negative predictive value. In these usually severely injured polytrauma patients, the chest will oftentimes be imaged in conjunction with the abdomen and pelvis.

4.8 CT Technique

Different protocols exist to administer iodinated intravenous (IV) contrast material, with either single-bolus, split-bolus or triple-bolus administration being used. To avoid streak artefacts from high concentrations of iodine in the left brachiocephalic vein, IV contrast material should preferably be administered via the right arm whenever possible. Depending on scanner manufacturer and type, an empirically fixed delay or a bolus-triggering mode can be used. The administration of a separate timing bolus before the definitive scan is not commonly chosen in current practice, mostly due to time constrains. Furthermore, with current technical advances in multi-detector computed tomography (MDCT) resulting in high spatial resolution, vascular injuries will be detected even if acquisition phase is past proper arterial phase, which still is the preferred phase of acquisition (Raptis et al. 2015). In our opinion, the radiologist should be present at the acquisition to decide if image quality is satisfactory and to instantaneously order repeat scan or extra phases, especially for the abdomen and pelvis.

When evaluating the aorta, care should be taken to adjust window and level settings as to not mask minimal luminal or mural abnormalities. Specific Hounsfield unit (HU) settings are difficult to give, since the correct window/level setting varies with attenuation values in each scan (depending on kVp, iodine concentration and flow rate of IV contrast administered). In some institutions, a non-contrast scan is obtained prior to the scan with IV contrast to rule out intramural haematoma (IMH), which in our experience is not as important as with aortic dissection protocols. If during the evaluation at the scanner console there is doubt about the presence of IMH, a late-phase CT after 10–15 min can be obtained to evaluate for increased aortic wall attenuation; this however is rarely needed. If uncertainty of aortic injury is caused by artefacts, a repeat scan can be obtained, applying ECG triggering if caused by cardiac pulsation (Fig. 10). Positioning of external lines and arms may further alter image quality.

It is paramount to use thin slices of the original axial dataset for evaluation, and multiplanar

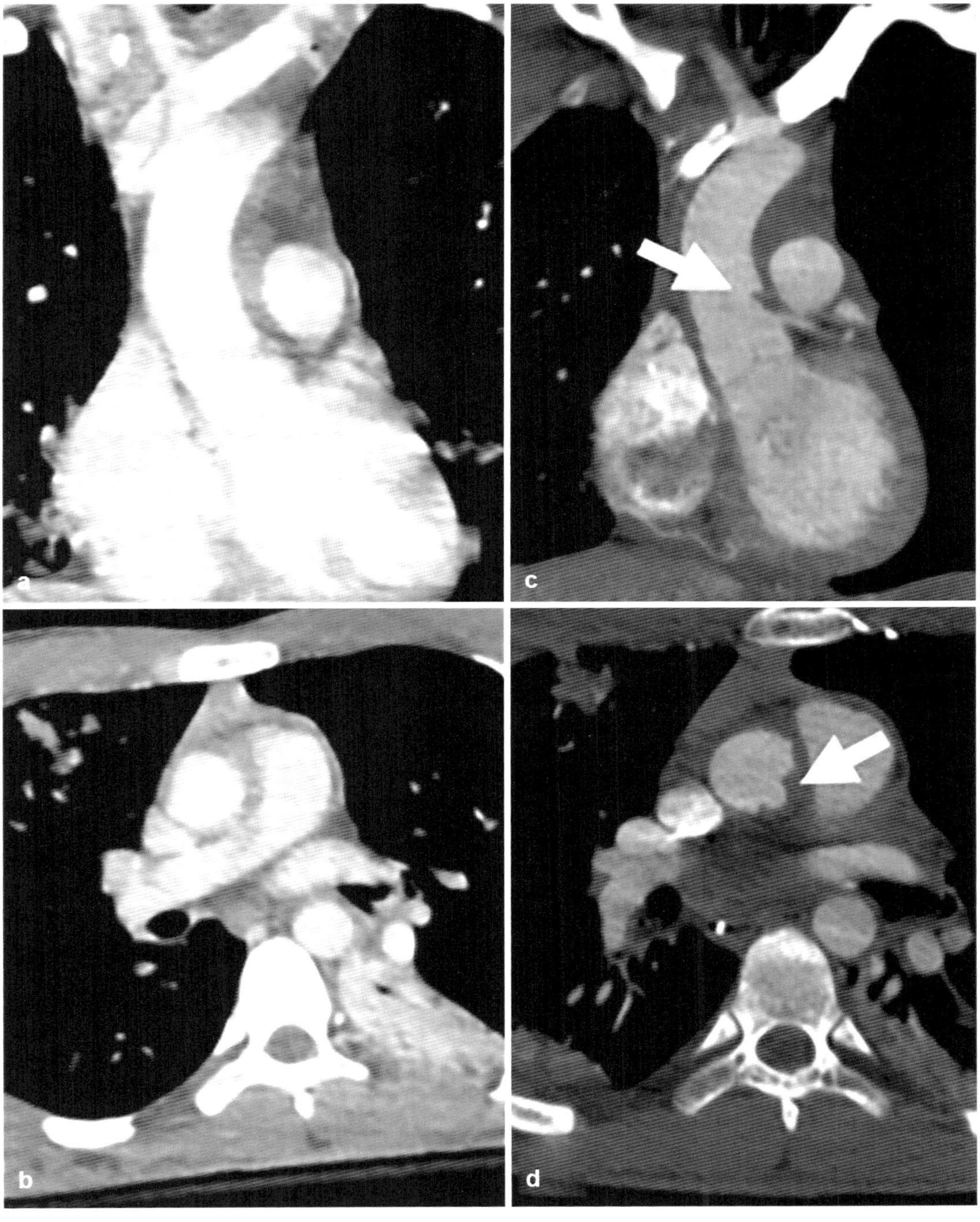

Fig. 10 Initial routine CTA without ECG triggering (**a**, **b**) and follow-up ECG-triggered CTA (**c**, **d**). Small, <1 cm intimal flap with thrombus is identified in the ascending aorta just distal to the origin of the left coronary artery (*arrows*). Although this clinically significant finding was suspected on the initial CTA without ECG triggering, it is appreciated far superiorly on the ECG-triggered CTA

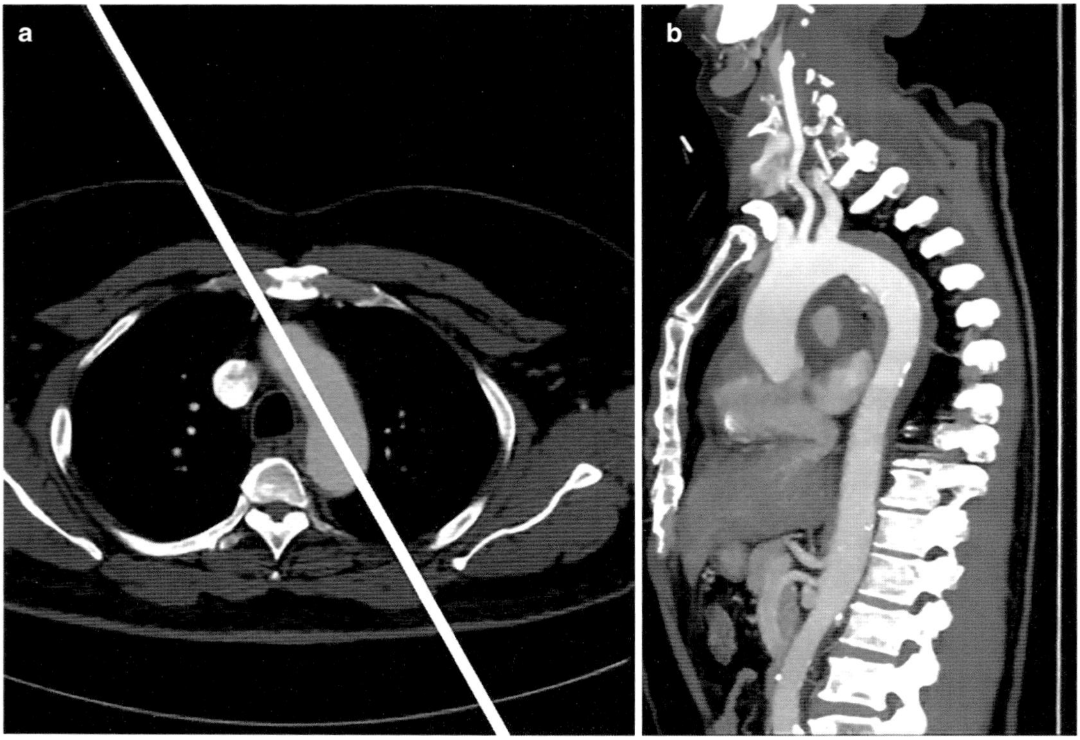

Fig. 11 Axial (**a**) and sagittal-oblique (**b**) or 'candy stick' MPR of the thoracic aortic in the plane along the aortic arch (*white line in* **a**)

reformations (MPRs) should be made, preferably interactively at a workstation or similar server-based software or by MPRs made by technicians according to preset protocols. A sagittal-oblique reconstruction, also referred to as 'candy stick' reconstruction, is especially useful since it shows the entire length of the thoracic (and possibly abdominal) aorta (Fig. 11). Interventional radiologists and surgeons will like the view for the fact that it resembles the oblique view obtained when performing angiography.

4.9 Imaging Findings

Since CT in nearly all cases will be the chosen modality to detect BTAI, we will describe the features of aortic injury here. However, findings on other imaging modalities will be very similar to those seen on CT. After blunt trauma, CT signs of aortic injury can be located at any section of the aorta and can even be present at multiple sites, especially after stretch mechanisms. The most common location to find BTAI on imaging is the aortic isthmus. Signs can be divided in direct and indirect signs of BTAI.

Direct signs are very sensitive and specific for BTAI; however, false positives and false negatives do occur, either caused by technical issues (artefacts) or misinterpretation. Direct signs demonstrate aortic wall changes and make up the grades of aortic injury, irrespective of which classification system is used. Luminal thrombus abutting the intima, an intimal flap and intramural haematoma (IMH) can be seen and depending on size smaller or larger than 1 cm will be grade 1 or grade 2 injuries, respectively (Vancouver classification) (Lamarche et al. 2012). Luminal thrombus abutting the intima oftentimes is demonstrated as a small, round contrast-filling defect on the axial images; however, it can have a more oblong configuration, especially on MPRs (Fig. 12). An intimal flap is a more linear hypodense structure projecting into the lumen of the aorta, connected to the wall (Fig. 13). One very specific and more severe form of intimal flap is circumferential dehiscence of the intima, creating intimo-intimal intussusception, which is demonstrated by a more or less regular circular and linear hypodense line within the aortic lumen (Fig. 14). IMH can be seen as thickening of the aortic wall, separating the intima and adventitia by haematoma in the media. IMHs can be focal or rather long and usually are not circumferential (Fig. 15). If a non-contrast enhanced CT is performed, this portion of the aortic wall will demonstrate increased attenuation (around 40–60 HU), a feature that is less obvious if contrast was given. However, in our experience, the non-contrast scan is not needed to make a confident diagnosis of IMH, given modern-day MDCT resolution.

Grade 3 injuries demonstrate outward contour deviations of the aorta, so-called pseudo-aneurysms, that can be relatively regular or

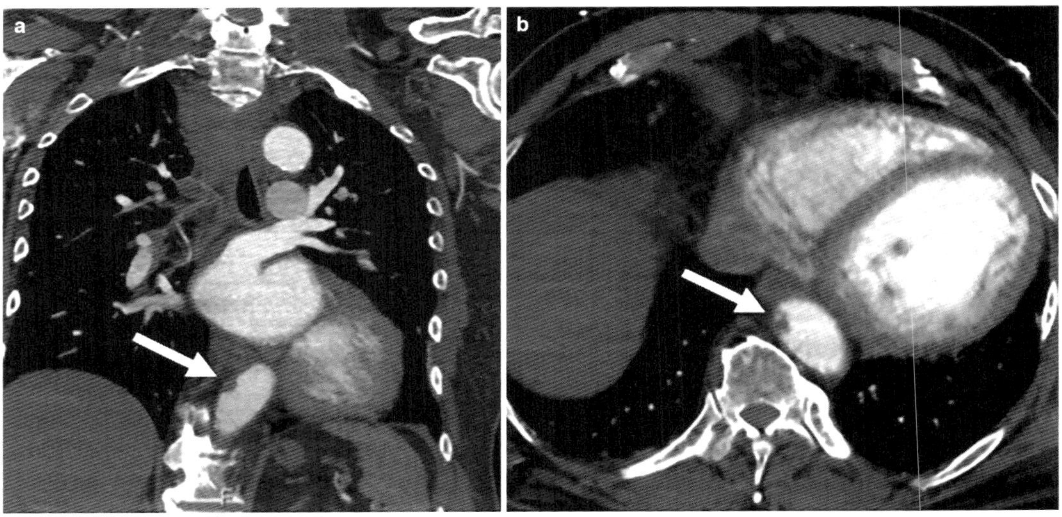

Fig. 12 Coronal (**a**) and axial (**b**) CTA demonstrating a small traumatic aortic intimal injury with thrombus abutting thrombus in the distal descending thoracic aorta (*arrows*)

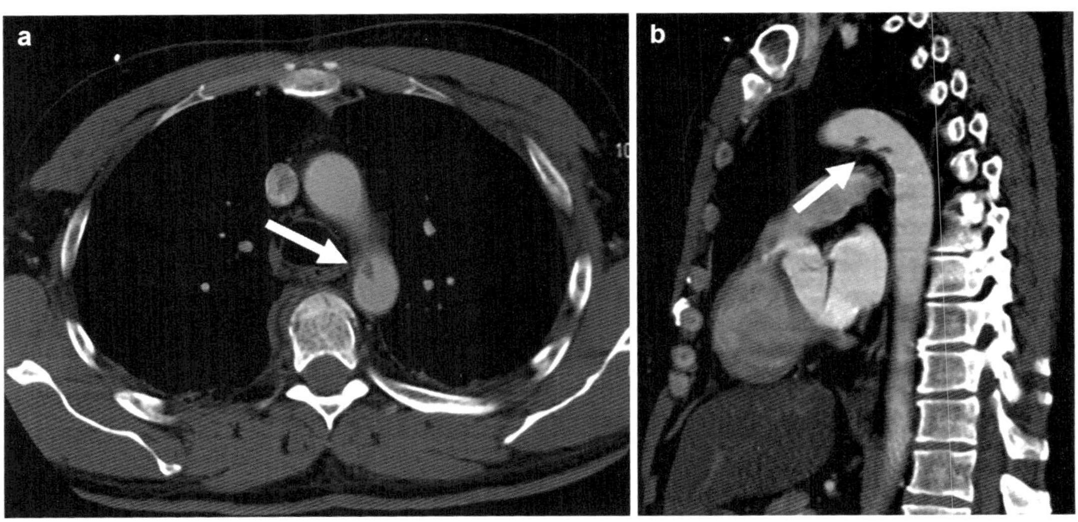

Fig. 13 34-year-old male involved in MVA. Axial (**a**) and sagittal (**b**) CTA reformats show two small intimal flaps at the aortic isthmus (*arrows*) with minimal thrombus at the tips. The injuries healed without invasive therapy (follow-up CTA not shown)

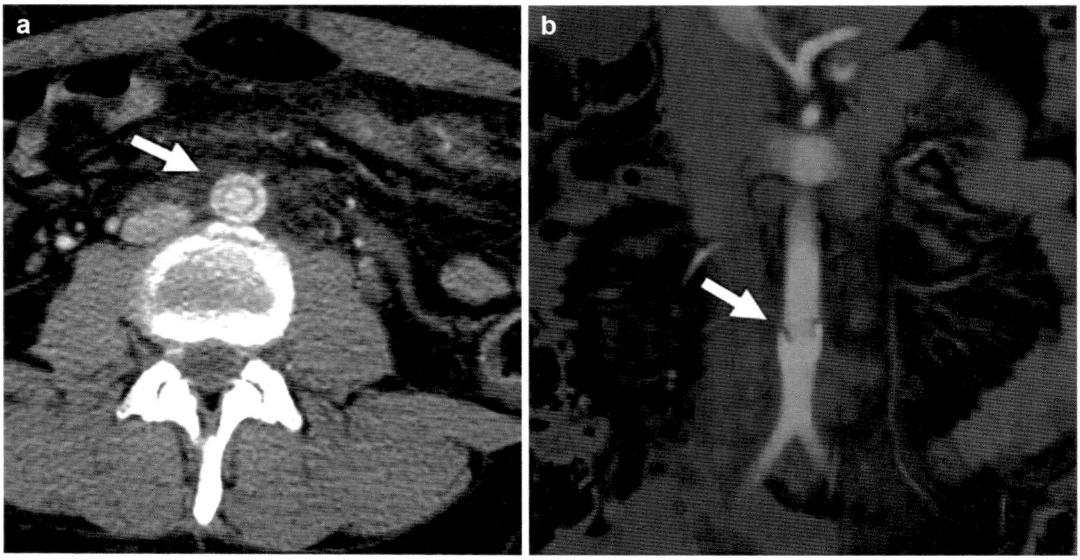

Fig. 14 Pedestrian struck by a car. Axial (**a**) and coronal CTA (**b**) depict an intimo-intimal intussusception at the level of the infra-renal abdominal aorta (*arrow*). Note the peri-aortic haematoma and loss of peri-aortic fat plane (*arrows*)

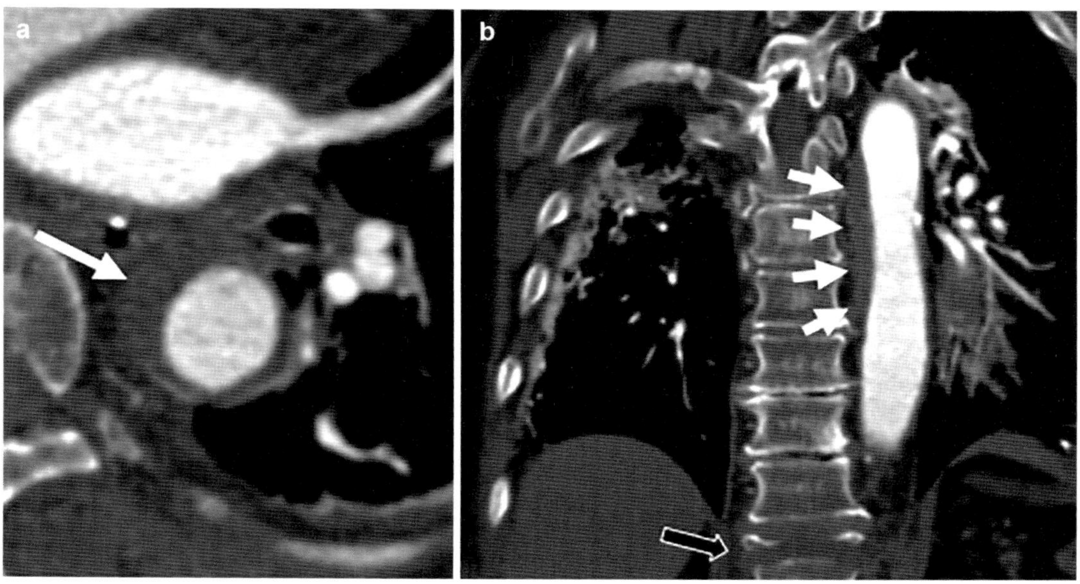

Fig. 15 Long traumatic intramural haematoma (*white arrows*) of the descending thoracic on axial (**a**) and coronal (**b**) CTA. Concomitant thoracic vertebral body fracture and dislocation (*black arrow*)

irregular, the latter likely being more unstable than the former (Figs. 4 and 5). If pseudo-aneurysms are small, they can be difficult to pick up given the orientation in a curved plane in three dimensions, rendering the use of MPRs even more important (Fig. 16). In grade 4 injuries, active extravasation of IV contrast is seen, either from an otherwise fairly normal aorta, or at the site of a (usually irregular) pseudo-aneurysm (Figs. 8 and 17) Needless to say, this is an indication for urgent repair, either by endovascular stent graft or open thoracotomy procedure.

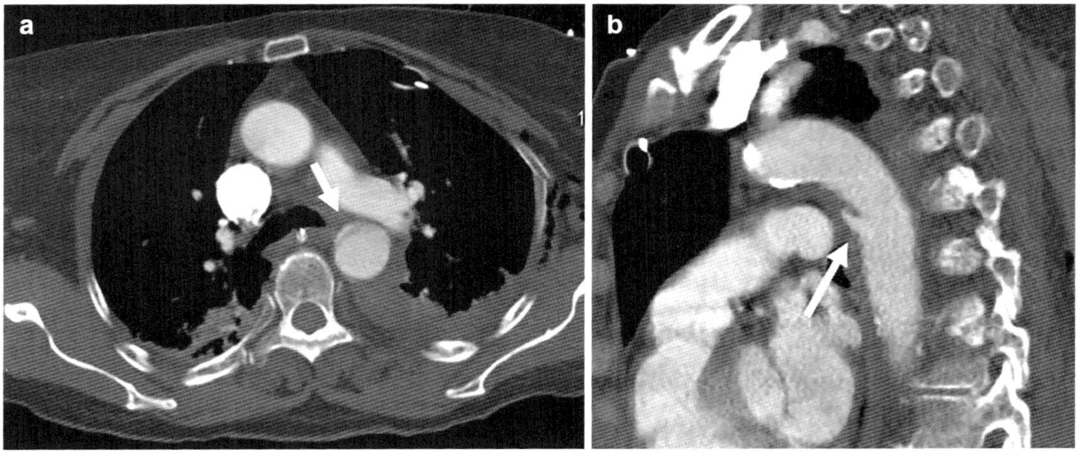

Fig. 16 Small traumatic pseudo-aneurysm (*arrows*) of the thoracic aorta which is harder to detect on axial (**a**) than on the sagittal (**b**) CTA reformat, stressing the need to evaluate all reformats

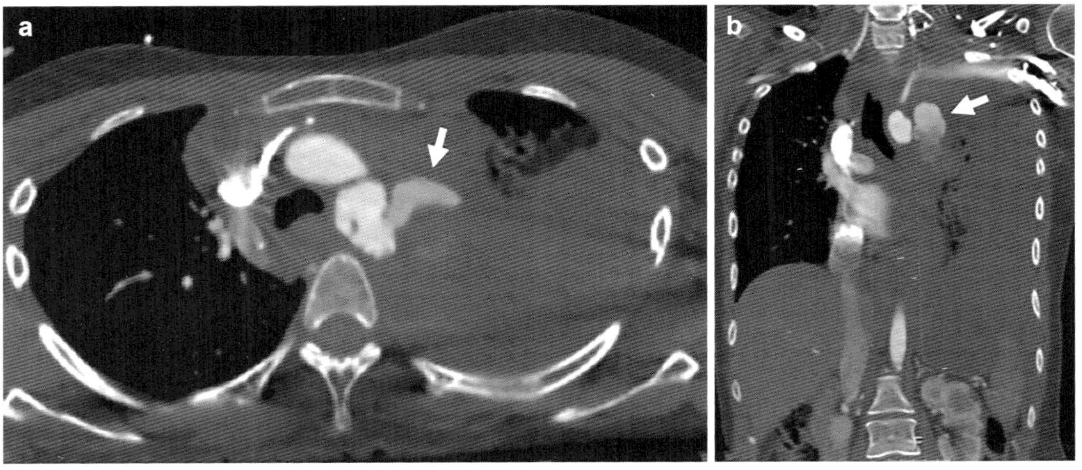

Fig. 17 Axial (**a**) and coronal (**b**) CTA showing traumatic aortic rupture at the level of the arch with active contrast extravasation (*arrow*, same patient as Fig. 8). Large mediastinal haematoma and large left-sided haemothorax. Patient deceased prior to treatment

Indirect signs of aortic injury mostly relate to the bleeding from the aortic injury in the immediate peri-aortic region or beyond. Peri-aortic haematoma, as described before, is haematoma that abuts the aortic adventitia and obliterates the peri-aortic fat plane (Fig. 4) Larger haematomas will extend further into the mediastinum and are slightly hyperdense (40–70 HU). Bleeding from the aortic injury can extend into the pleural space or pericardium, depending on the location of the injury, giving rise to haemothorax or haemopericardium. Usually haemopericardium is homogenously hyperdense, whereas haemothorax can have mixed densities with more hyperdense areas indicating cloth (Fig. 6). However, if pleural effusion has densities similar to fluid (0–20/30 HU), it can be difficult to differentiate hyperacute haematoma from reactive effusion (Fig. 8).

Two *indirect signs* can be seen on abdominal CT and should mandate further investigation of the thoracic aorta. These are obliteration of the retro-crural peri-aortic fat (possibly indicating caudal extension of more cranially located peri-aortic haematoma) (Fig. 18) and otherwise

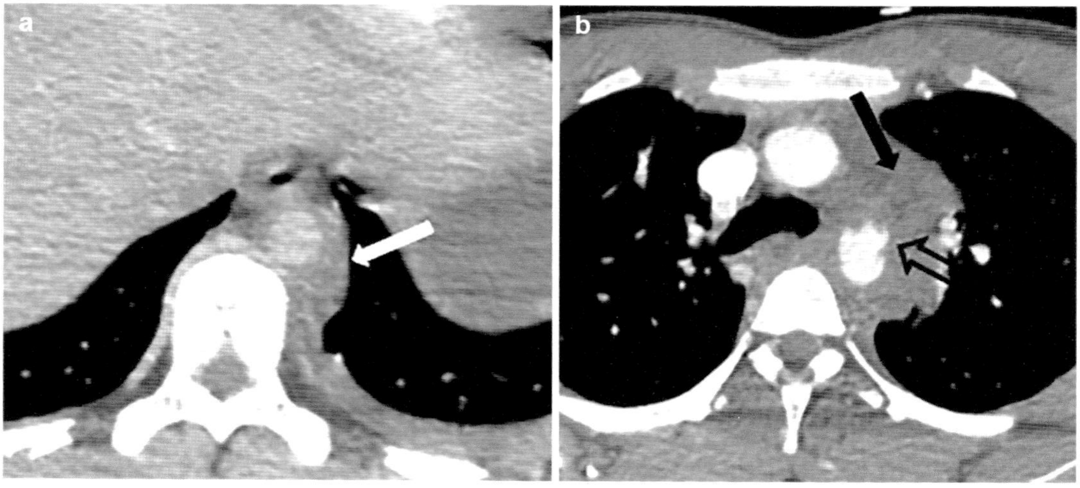

Fig. 18 Example of a retro-crural peri-aortic haematoma (*white arrow*) as can be seen on an abdominal CT as a sign of more proximal BTAI (**a**). In this patient it resulted from peri-aortic haematoma (*solid black arrow*) due to an aortic pseudo-aneurysm (partially shown, *open black arrow*) in (**b**)

unexplained acute renal infracts, especially if bilateral, that can originate from luminal thrombus of more cranially located BTAI.

5 Differential Diagnosis and Pitfalls

In the setting of sustained high-energy trauma, a high index of suspicion for BTAI is warranted. Differential diagnoses that can be mistaken for BTAI mainly reside around the level of the isthmus, namely, a ductus diverticulum, patent ductus arteriosus and aortic spindle. Confusion may also arise more proximally from the nearby superior intercostal vein if opacified by contrast and in younger patients from remaining thymic tissue. Knowing normal anatomy will help discerning these entities from BTAI. A ductus diverticulum is located at the aortic attachment of the ligamentum arteriosum, the former entry to the ductus arteriosus. In contrast with BTAI, a ductus diverticulum has smooth, obtuse angles with the aortic wall, whereas BTAI usually is more irregular and steeply angled and oftentimes has abutting peri-aortic haematoma (Fig. 19) A patent ductus arteriosus is a rarity in itself and therefore a fairly remote option as a differential diagnosis. It can be recognized as a tubular structure with regular contours, where the differential of active contrast extravasation in BTAI usually is irregular and situated within haematoma. Aortic spindles are located just distal to the isthmus and are smooth, regular fusiform mild dilatations of the aorta, again without peri-aortic haematoma (Fig. 19).

Issues related to imaging technique may also cause difficulty in image interpretation, pitfalls mostly being related to artefacts caused by motion and pulsation or due to beam hardening (if the acquisition was performed with arms down). As mentioned before, if IV contrast was administered via the left arm, high concentration of iodine in the left brachiocephalic vein may cause streak artefacts that can hamper assessment of especially the proximal branching vessels. Artefacts can oftentimes be distinguished by evaluation of other structures, such as other vessels or the skin. However, if artefacts are a major concern, a repeat examination with arms up and ECG triggering where possible should be obtained (Fig. 10).

6 Delayed Presentation Injuries

Blunt traumatic injuries to the thoracic aorta and its branch vessels are rare and seldom occur as the sole traumatic entity (Antonopoulos et al. 2014). As mentioned before, patients usually suffer many concomitant injuries and will almost always undergo whole-body MDCT. This modality has an extremely high negative predictive value for blunt traumatic aortic injuries. Although incidence of delayed presentation injuries is unknown, false-negative studies can occur, with missed thoracic aortic injuries following their natural course. Pseudo-aneurysms can be detected incidentally after remote trauma, or they can cause clinical symptoms due to mass effect on surrounding tissues (Fig. 20) or potentially rupture.

7 Proximal Aortic Branch Vessel Injury

In the late 1990s, research demonstrated injuries to the major thoracic branches of the aorta in a considerable number of patients, either with presence of aortic injury, or in isolation. In a well-documented study by Ahrar et al. in 89 patients undergoing angiography for expected BTAI, 17 patients (19 %) had 24 injuries to the aortic arch

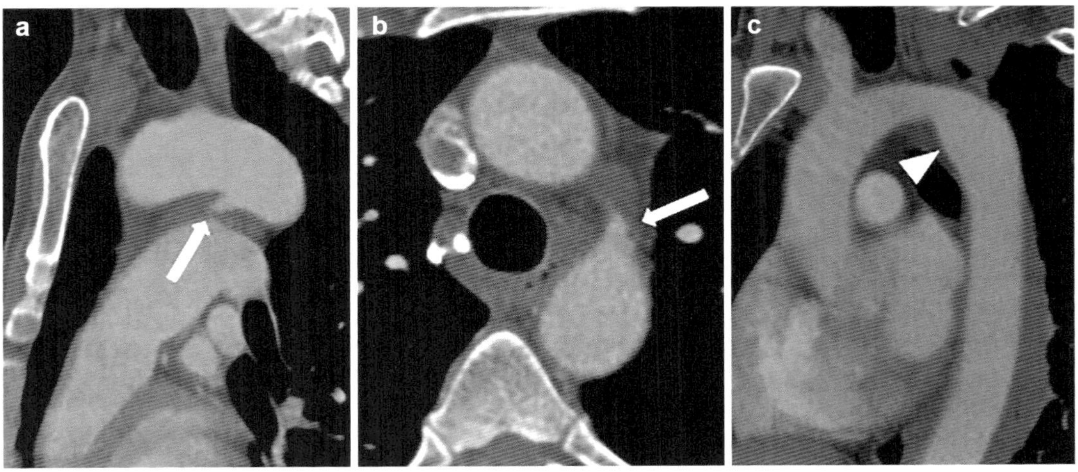

Fig. 19 Anatomic variants that can mimic BTAI; Aortic ductus diverticulum (*arrows*) on sagittal (**a**) and axial CTA (**b**) and aortic spindle (*arrowhead*) on sagittal CTA (**c**)

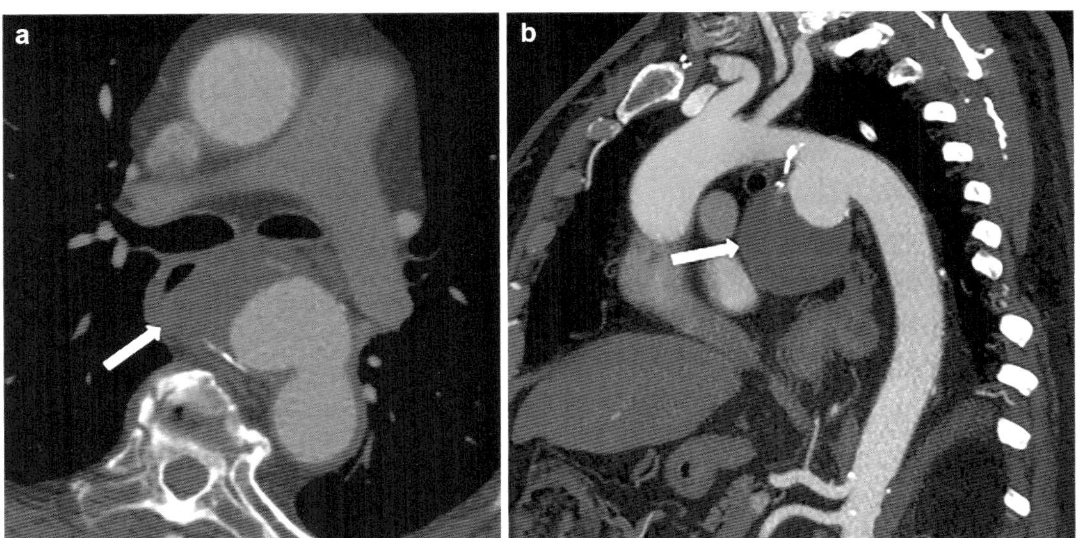

Fig. 20 Partly thrombosed pseudo-aneurysm at the aortic isthmus (*arrow*) compressing the oesophagus (**a**, **b**), with peripheral calcifications as a sign of long-standing entity. This was detected during workup for difficulties swallowing. On questioning, the patient confirmed an MVA in the remote past

branches. In 14 of these 17 patients, the aorta was intact, whereas three patients also had aortic rupture, resulting in 16% of patients having isolated branch vessel injury (Ahrar et al. 1997). The study by Chen et al. revealed aortic branch vessel injuries in one-third of patients who sustained vascular injury from blunt trauma and underwent aortography (Chen et al. 2001). Despite these figures, proximal brachiocephalic arterial injuries due to blunt trauma remain quite rare (Galan et al. 1992; LoCicero and Mattox 1989; Prêtre and Chilcott 1997; Shorr et al. 1987). The innominate artery accounts for 50% of these injuries and is the second most common injured vessel after the thoracic aorta (Prêtre et al. 1997). The left common carotid and left subclavian artery account for the remaining injuries.

Vessel injuries of the innominate and left common carotid artery tend to occur proximal at the vessel origin (Rosenberg et al. 1989; Karmy-Jones et al. 2003; Symbas et al. 2005). Anatomically this is where the vessel is tightly fixed onto the aortic arch, whereas the distal part is more mobile and flexible.

In contrast, blunt subclavian artery injuries are located more distally (Costa and Robbs 1988; Cox et al. 1999). These can be explained by adding the direct force of posterior dislocated clavicles. This mechanism might also explain proximal right common carotid artery injury (Fig. 21).

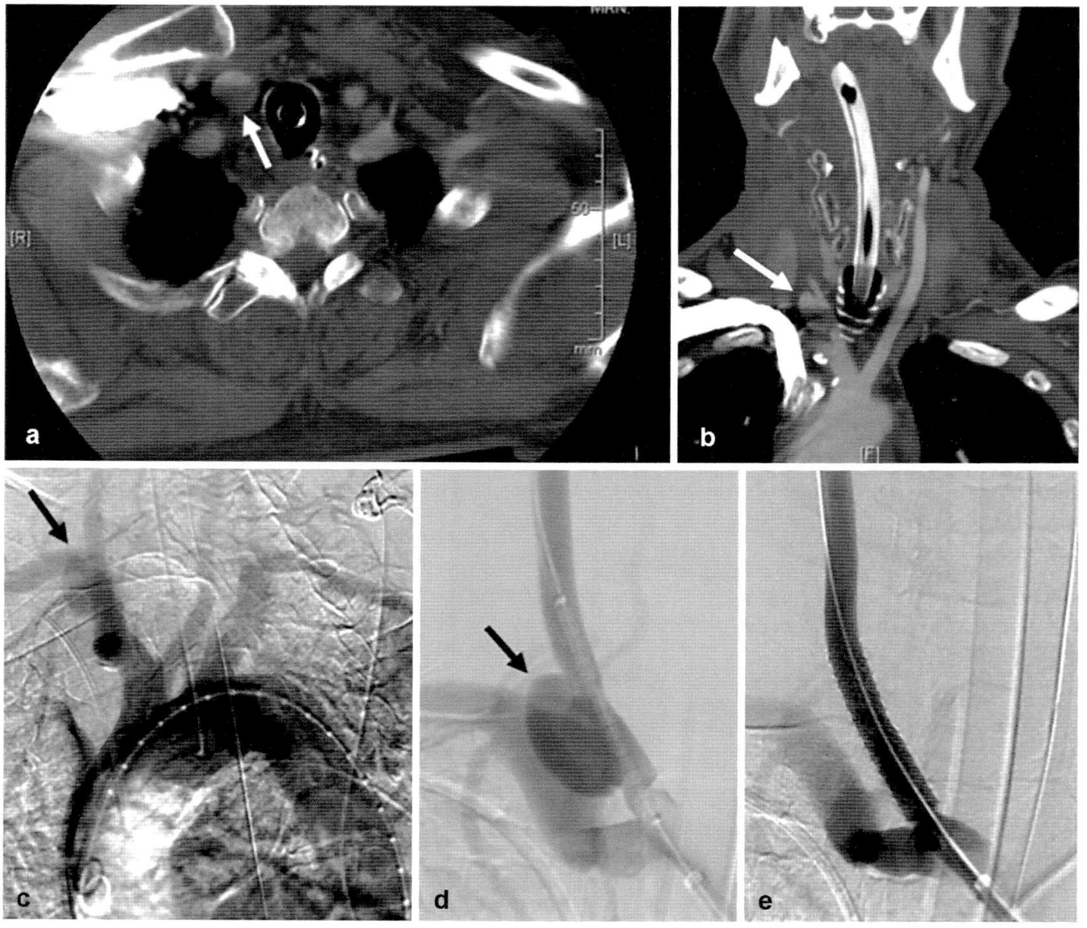

Fig. 21 Axial (**a**) and coronal CTA (**b**) depict a traumatic pseudo-aneurysm of the proximal right common carotid artery (*white arrows*). Mechanism of injury was a posterior dislocation of the medial right clavicle. The pseudo-aneurysm was successfully treated with a covered stent; procedural angiograms show stent placement (**c–e**) to exclude the pseudo-aneurysm (*black arrows*)

Given its proximity to the aortic arch, most injuries are treated surgically, either by primary repair or prosthetic graft interposition. Endovascular management however should always be considered, whether being definite or as a bridge to surgery (Shalhub et al. 2011).

Venous injuries are rarely encountered in isolation after blunt traumatic injuries to the chest.

8 Management and Treatment for BTAI

In the era of arch aortography as the gold standard for diagnosing traumatic injury to the thoracic aorta and its branch vessels, detected injuries were managed surgically or by medical treatment. In the late 1990s, thoracic endovascular aortic repair (TEVAR) was added a third treatment option for BTAI (Semba et al. 1997; Kato et al. 1997; Rousseau et al. 1999). Despite a lack of randomized controlled trials, the available literature demonstrates a superiority of TEVAR in aortic injury-related mortality, stroke and spinal cord injury as compared to open surgical repair (Azizzadeh et al. 2013; Takagi et al. 2008; Pang et al. 2015; Tang et al. 2008). In 2011, the Society for Vascular Surgery published clinical practice guidelines for the treatment of BTAI in which a TEVAR first policy is advocated based on those studies (Lee et al. 2011). They supported the already ongoing shift in management from open surgical repair to TEVAR. However, despite promising short-term outcomes, questions remain regarding long-term durability of TEVAR in the often reasonably young polytrauma patient. Therefore, several trauma centres still perform open repair awaiting long-term outcomes.

With modern CT picking up subtle injuries that went undetected before, many surgeons have now adopted a management approach of BTAI tailored to the specific aortic injury. Minimal aortic injury possibly does not require immediate endovascular or open surgical repair (Malhotra et al. 2001). These patients are managed with aggressive blood pressure control with systolic blood pressure <100 mmHg and heart rates of 60–80 bpm. These aortic injuries are closely followed with serial CTA at 24 h, every 48–72 h for 7 days and after 4 weeks (Fig. 22).

The vascular injuries that require immediate intervention have been clustered in the term severe aortic injury (SAI). Traditionally these included traumatic aortic pseudo-aneurysms and contrast extravasation on CTA. There is however a wide variety on the definitions of MAI and SAI. Consequently, the management of BTAI varies per operator and amongst trauma centres. Recent research shows that an expectant approach is also justified for patients with small traumatic pseudo-aneurysms, previously considered SAI (Caffarelli et al. 2010; Rabin et al. 2014a).

Once the decision for TEVAR is made, thin-slice CTA with multiplanar and three-dimensional reconstruction allows for appropriate visualization of the vascular injuries and planning for TEVAR (Fig. 11). Diagnostic arch aortography in TEVAR planning is obsolete with modern CTA and only performed as part of the TEVAR procedure. Pre-procedure CT images should be assessed for TEVAR eligibility, with absolute contraindication for TEVAR being anatomic ineligibility, mostly due to luminal diameter issues.

The commercially available, on-stock stent grafts require a minimum and maximum diameter and length of the proximal and distal landing zones of the aorta. The diameters vary per manufacturer, but typically range from around 16–46 mm. Under-sizing can lead to failure of proximal and/or distal seal, leading to a type I endoleak. Oversizing also increases the risk of inappropriate sealing due to infolding of the stent graft. A severe complication of oversizing is stent-graft collapse with acute aortic occlusion. Most manufacturers recommend oversizing by 10–20 %.

The diameter of the aorta is influenced by the hemodynamic status of the patient (Chandra et al. 2012; Jonker et al. 2010). Hemodynamically unstable patients have smaller diameters and require more oversizing than hemodynamically stable patients. Care should be taken that the abdominal aorta, iliac and common femoral arteries are of sufficient diameter to deliver the stent graft. The profile of the delivery systems continues to decrease in size, but a minimum of

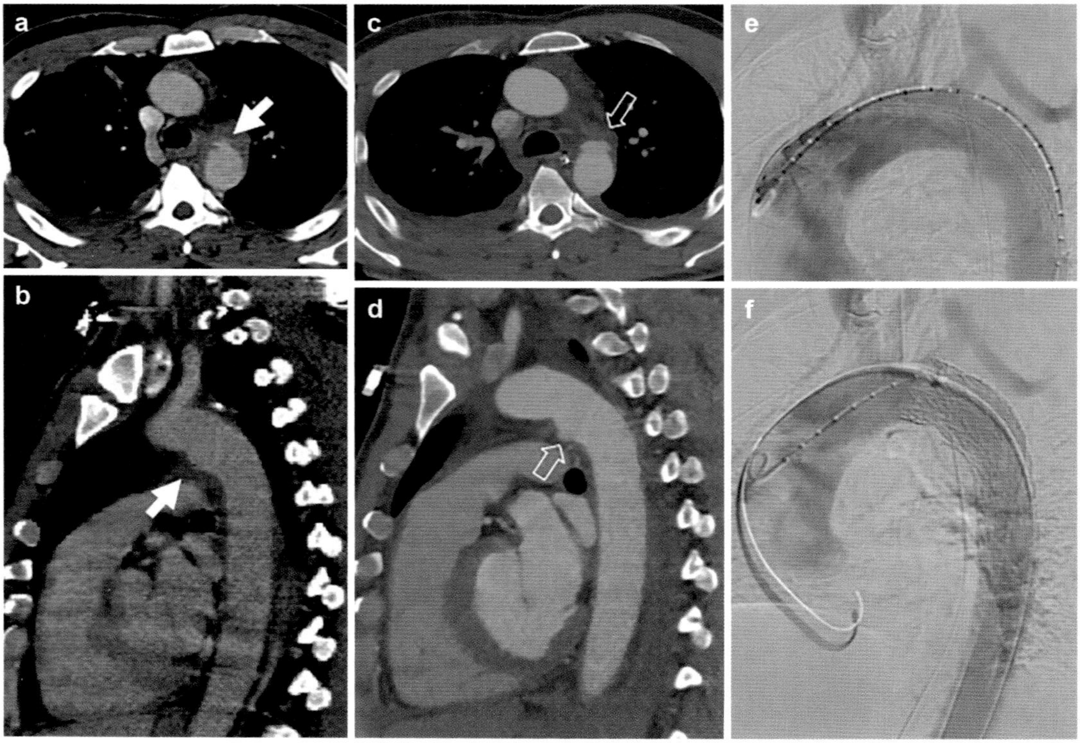

Fig. 22 46-year-old male involved in MVA. Initial CTA (**a**, **b**) demonstrates a small pseudo-aneurysm of the proximal descending aorta (*solid white arrows*) with peri-aortic haematoma. This was treated conservatively with controlled hypotension and close CTA follow-up. CTA at 1-day follow-up (not shown) revealed no interval change. However, CTA at 7 days follow-up (**c**, **d**) showed an increase in size of the pseudo-aneurysm (*open white arrows*). Patient underwent subsequent TEVAR (**e**, **f**)

6–7 mm is recommended. In case of severe aorto-iliac stenosis or occlusions, an abdominal conduit can be used to deliver the stent graft to the thoracic aorta.

Obtaining sufficient proximal seal can require covering of the left subclavian artery (LSA). In the emergency setting, complex endovascular solutions with branched or fenestrated devices are not possible. Re-vascularising the LSA subsequent to covering by TEVAR has long been subject to debate. For TEVAR of aortic aneurysms and dissections, covering of the LSA without revascularization used to be liberally performed. However, more recent published data on TEVAR for aneurysm and type B aortic dissection repair reveal a favourable stroke rate if revascularization is performed prior to TEVAR (Waterford et al. 2016). The Society of Vascular Surgery advocates routine revascularization in elective TEVAR. In patients who need urgent TEVAR with LSA covering, revascularization should be individualized and addressed expectantly on the basis of anatomy, urgency and availability of surgical experience (Lee et al. 2011).

Follow-up imaging after TEVAR aims to diagnose potential adverse events such as device migration, disconnection or endoleak, which might need additional treatment. These have been reported to occur; however, there are no guidelines regarding follow-up imaging after TEVAR for BTAI. Imaging strategies often consist of serial CTA, commonly before discharge for baseline and then at 1, 6 and 12 months followed by annual control. This strategy induces high radiation exposure in a generally young patient population. Long-term data are needed to identify risk factors for potential adverse affects in order to limit this radiation exposure. If patients received an MRI-compatible stent graft, MRI can be used for follow-up, decreasing radiation dose.

References

Ahrar K, Smith DC, Bansal RC, Razzouk A, Catalano RD (1997) Angiography in blunt thoracic aortic injury. J Trauma Inj Infect Crit Care 42(4):665–669

Aladham F, Sundaram B, Williams DM, Quint LE (2010) Traumatic aortic injury: computerized tomographic findings at presentation and after conservative therapy. J Comput Assist Tomogr 34(3):388–394

Antonopoulos CN, Sfyroeras GS, Kallinis A, Kakisis JD, Liapis CD, Petridou ET (2014) Epidemiology of concomitant injuries in traumatic thoracic aortic rupture: a meta-analysis. Vascular 22(6):395–405

Arthurs ZM, Starnes BW, Sohn VY, Singh N, Martin MJ, Andersen CA (2009) Functional and survival outcomes in traumatic blunt thoracic aortic injuries: an analysis of the National Trauma Databank. J Vasc Surg 49(4):988–994

Azizzadeh A, Keyhani K, Miller CC, Coogan SM, Safi HJ, Estrera AL (2009) Blunt traumatic aortic injury: initial experience with endovascular repair. J Vasc Surg 49(6):1403–1408

Azizzadeh A, Valdes J, Miller CC, Nguyen LL, Estrera AL, Charlton-Ouw K et al (2011) The utility of intravascular ultrasound compared to angiography in the diagnosis of blunt traumatic aortic injury. J Vasc Surg 53(3):608–614

Azizzadeh A, Charlton-Ouw KM, Chen Z, Rahbar MH, Estrera AL, Amer H et al (2013) An outcome analysis of endovascular versus open repair of blunt traumatic aortic injuries. J Vasc Surg 57(1):108–114; discussion 115

Baqué P, Serre T, Cheynel N, Arnoux P-J, Thollon L, Behr M et al (2006) An experimental cadaveric study for a better understanding of blunt traumatic aortic rupture. J Trauma Inj Infect Crit Care 61(3):586–591

Burkhart HM, Gomez GA, Jacobson LE, Pless JE, Broadie TA (2001) Fatal blunt aortic injuries: a review of 242 autopsy cases. J Trauma Inj Infect Crit Care 50(1):113–115

Caffarelli AD, Mallidi HR, Maggio PM, Spain DA, Miller DC, Mitchell RS (2010) Early outcomes of deliberate nonoperative management for blunt thoracic aortic injury in trauma. J Thorac Cardiovasc Surg 140(3):598–605

Challoumas D, Dimitrakakis G (2015) Advances in the treatment of blunt thoracic aortic injuries. Injury 46(8):1431–1439

Chandra V, Greenberg JI, Maggio P, Mell MW, Lee JT (2012) Aortic diameter varies in trauma patients: a function of hemodynamic status. J Vasc Surg Elsevier Inc 56(2):586–587

Chen MY, Regan JD, D'Amore MJ, Routh WD, Meredith JW, Dyer RB (2001) Role of angiography in the detection of aortic branch vessel injury after blunt thoracic trauma. J Trauma Inj Infect Crit Care 51(6):1166–1171; discussion 1172

Cohen AM, Crass JR, Thomas HA, Fisher RG, Jacobs DG (1992) CT evidence for the "osseous pinch" mechanism of traumatic aortic injury. AJR Am J Roentgenol 159(2):271–274

Cook AD, Klein JS, Rogers FB, Osler TM, Shackford SR (2001) Chest radiographs of limited utility in the diagnosis of blunt traumatic aortic laceration. J Trauma Inj Infect Crit Care 50(5):843–847

Costa MC, Robbs JV (1988) Nonpenetrating subclavian artery trauma. J Vasc Surg 8(1):71–75

Cox CS, Allen GS, Fischer RP, Conklin LD, Duke JH, Cocanour CS et al (1999) Blunt versus penetrating subclavian artery injury: presentation, injury pattern, and outcome. J Trauma Inj Infect Crit Care 46(3):445–449

Crass JR, Cohen AM, Motta AO, Tomashefski JF, Wiesen EJ (1990) A proposed new mechanism of traumatic aortic rupture: the osseous pinch. Radiology 176(3):645–649

Demetriades D, Velmahos GC, Scalea TM, Jurkovich GJ, Karmy-Jones R, Teixeira PG et al (2008) Diagnosis and treatment of blunt thoracic aortic injuries: changing perspectives. J Trauma 64(6):1415–1418; discussion 1418–1419

Fabian TC, Richardson JD, Croce MA, Smith JS, Rodman G, Kearney PA et al (1997) Prospective study of blunt aortic injury: multicenter trial of the American Association for the Surgery of Trauma. J Trauma Inj Infect Crit Care 42(3):374–380; discussion 380–383

Fattori R, Celletti F, Bertaccini P, Galli R, Pacini D, Pierangeli A et al (1996) Delayed surgery of traumatic aortic rupture. Role of magnetic resonance imaging. Circulation 94(11):2865–2870

Fattori R, Celletti F, Descovich B, Napoli G, Bertaccini P, Galli R et al (1998) Evolution of post-traumatic aortic aneurysm in the subacute phase: magnetic resonance imaging follow-up as a support of the surgical timing. Eur J Cardiothorac Surg 13(5):582–586; discussion 586–587

Forman MJ, Mirvis SE, Hollander DS (2013) Blunt thoracic aortic injuries: CT characterisation and treatment outcomes of minor injury. Eur Radiol 23(11):2988–2995

Fox N, Schwartz D, Salazar JH, Haut ER, Dahm P, Black JH et al (2015) Evaluation and management of blunt traumatic aortic injury: a practice management guideline from the Eastern Association for the Surgery of Trauma. J Trauma Acute Care Surg 78(1):136–146

Galan G, Peñalver JC, París F, Caffarena JM, Blasco E, Borro JM et al (1992) Blunt chest injuries in 1696 patients. Eur J Cardiothorac Surg 6(6):284–287

Gavant ML, Helical CT (1999) grading of traumatic aortic injuries. Impact on clinical guidelines for medical and surgical management. Radiol Clin North Am 37(3):553–574, vi

Gutierrez A, Inaba K, Siboni S, Effron Z, Haltmeier T, Jaffray P et al (2016) The utility of chest X-ray as a screening tool for blunt thoracic aortic injury. Injury 47(1):32–36

Harris DG, Rabin J, Kufera JA, Taylor BS, Sarkar R, O'Connor JV et al (2015) A new aortic injury score

predicts early rupture more accurately than clinical assessment. J Vasc Surg 61(2):332–338
Ho RT, Blackmore CC, Bloch RD, Hoffer EK, Mann FA, Stern EJ et al (2002) Can we rely on mediastinal widening on chest radiography to identify subjects with aortic injury? Emerg Radiol 9(4):183–187
Jonker FH, Verhagen HJ, Mojibian H, Davis KA, Moll FL, Muhs BE (2010) Aortic endograft sizing in trauma patients with hemodynamic instability. J Vasc Surg 52(1):39–44
Karmy-Jones R, DuBose R, King S (2003) Traumatic rupture of the innominate artery. Eur J Cardiothorac Surg 23(5):782–787
Kato N, Dake MD, Miller DC, Semba CP, Mitchell RS, Razavi MK et al (1997) Traumatic thoracic aortic aneurysm: treatment with endovascular stent-grafts. Radiology 205(3):657–662
Kitagawa RS, Van Haren RM, Yokobori S, Cohen D, Beckerman SR, Ahmad F et al (2013) Management of simultaneous traumatic brain injury and aortic injury. J Neurosurg 119(2):324–331
Lamarche Y, Berger FH, Nicolaou S, Bilawich A-M, Louis L, Inacio JR et al (2012) Vancouver simplified grading system with computed tomographic angiography for blunt aortic injury. J Thorac Cardiovasc Surg. 144(2):347–354, 354.e1
Lee WA, Matsumura JS, Mitchell RS, Farber MA, Greenberg RK, Azizzadeh A et al (2011) Endovascular repair of traumatic thoracic aortic injury: clinical practice guidelines of the Society for Vascular Surgery. J Vasc Surg Elsevier Inc 53(1):187–192
Lin C-C, Liu K-S, Chen H-W, Huang Y-K, Chu J-J, Tsai F-C et al (2016) Blunt aortic injury: risk factors and impact of surgical approaches. Surg Today 46(2):188–196. doi: 10.1007/s00595-015-1152-0. Epub 2015 Apr 7
LoCicero J, Mattox KL (1989) Epidemiology of chest trauma. Surg Clin North Am 69(1):15–19
Lundevall J (1964) Traumatic rupture of aorta-with special reference to road accidents. Acta Pathol Microbiol Scand Acta pathologica et microbiologica Scandinavica 62:29–33
Malhotra AK, Fabian TC, Croce MA, Weiman DS, Gavant ML, Pate JW (2001) Minimal aortic injury: a lesion associated with advancing diagnostic techniques. J Trauma Inj Infect Crit Care 51(6):1042–1048
Mosquera VX, Marini M, Muñiz J, Lopez-Perez JM, Gulias D, Cuenca JJ (2013) Aortic injuries in crush trauma patients: different mechanism, different management. Injury 44(1):60–65
Nagy K, Fabian T, Rodman G, Fulda G, Rodriguez A, Mirvis S (2000) Guidelines for the diagnosis and management of blunt aortic injury: an EAST Practice Management Guidelines Work Group. J Trauma Inj Infect Crit Care 48(6):1128–1143
Pang D, Hildebrand D, Bachoo P (2015) Thoracic endovascular repair (TEVAR) versus open surgery for blunt traumatic thoracic aortic injury. Pang D, editor. Cochrane Database Syst Rev. Chichester, UK: John Wiley & Sons, Ltd; 9:CD006642
Parmley LF, Mattingly TW, Manion WC, Jahnke EJ (1958) Nonpenetrating traumatic injury of the aorta. Circulation 17(6):1086–1101
Patel NH, Hahn D, Comess KA (2003) Blunt chest trauma victims: role of intravascular ultrasound and transesophageal echocardiography in cases of abnormal thoracic aortogram. J Trauma Inj Infect Crit Care 55(2):330–337
Prêtre R, Chilcott M (1997) Blunt trauma to the heart and great vessels. N Engl J Med 336(9):626–632
Prêtre R, Chilcott M, Mürith N, Panos A (1997) Blunt injury to the supra-aortic arteries. Br J Surg 84(5):603–609
Rabin J, DuBose J, Sliker CW, O'Connor JV, Scalea TM, Griffith BP (2014a) Parameters for successful nonoperative management of traumatic aortic injury. J Thorac Cardiovasc Surg 147(1):143–149
Rabin J, Harris DG, Crews GA, Ho M, Taylor BS, Sarkar R et al (2014b) Early aortic repair worsens concurrent traumatic brain injury. Ann Thorac Surg 98(1):46–51; discussion 51–52
Raptis CA, Hammer MM, Raman KG, Mellnick VM, Bhalla S (2015) Acute traumatic aortic injury: practical considerations for the diagnostic radiologist. J Thorac Imaging 30(3):202–213
Rippey JC, Royse AG (2009) Ultrasound in trauma. Best Pract Res Clin Anaesthesiol 23(3):343–362
Rosenberg JM, Bredenberg CE, Marvasti MA, Bucknam C, Conti C, Parker FB (1989) Blunt injuries to the aortic arch vessels. Ann Thorac Surg 48(4):508–513
Rousseau H, Soula P, Perreault P, Bui B, d'Othee BJ, Massabuau P et al (1999) Delayed treatment of traumatic rupture of the thoracic aorta with endoluminal covered stent. Circulation 99(4):498–504
Schwab CW, Lawson RB, Lind JF, Garland LW (1984) Aortic injury: comparison of supine and upright portable chest films to evaluate the widened mediastinum. YMEM 13(10):896–899
Semba CP, Kato N, Kee ST, Lee GK, Mitchell RS, Miller DC et al (1997) Acute rupture of the descending thoracic aorta: repair with use of endovascular stent-grafts. J Vasc Interv Radiol 8(3):337–342
Shalhub S, Starnes BW, Hatsukami TS, Karmy-Jones R, Tran NT (2011) Repair of blunt thoracic outlet arterial injuries: an evolution from open to endovascular approach. J Trauma 71(5):E114–E121
Shi Y, Tsai PI, Wall MJ, Gilani R (2015) Intravascular ultrasound enhanced aortic sizing for endovascular treatment of blunt aortic injury. J Trauma Acute Care Surg 79(5):817–821
Shorr RM, Crittenden M, Indeck M, Hartunian SL, Rodriguez A (1987) Blunt thoracic trauma. Analysis of 515 patients. Ann Surg 206(2):200–205
Simeone A, Freitas M, Frankel HL (2006) Management options in blunt aortic injury: a case series and literature review. Am Surg 72(1):25–30
Starnes BW, Lundgren RS, Gunn M, Quade S, Hatsukami TS, Tran NT et al (2012) A new classification scheme for treating blunt aortic injury. J Vasc Surg Elsevier Inc 55(1):47–54

Steenburg SD, Ravenel JG (2008) Acute traumatic thoracic aortic injuries: experience with 64-MDCT. Am J Roentgenol 191(5):1564–1569

Steenburg SD, Ravenel JG, Ikonomidis JS, Schönholz C, Reeves S (2008) Acute traumatic aortic injury: imaging evaluation and management. Radiology 248(3):748–762

Symbas JD, Halkos ME, Symbas PN (2005) Rupture of the innominate artery from blunt trauma: current options for management. J Card Surg 20(5):455–459

Takagi H, Kawai N, Umemoto T (2008) A meta-analysis of comparative studies of endovascular versus open repair for blunt thoracic aortic injury. J Thorac Cardiovasc Surg 135(6):1392–1394

Tang GL, Tehrani HY, Usman A, Katariya K, Otero C, Perez E et al (2008) Reduced mortality, paraplegia, and stroke with stent graft repair of blunt aortic transections: a modern meta-analysis. J Vasc Surg 47(3):671–675

Teixeira PG, Inaba K, Barmparas G, Georgiou C, Toms C, Noguchi TT et al (2011) Blunt thoracic aortic injuries: an autopsy study. J Trauma 70(1):197–202

Wallace GA, Starnes BW, Hatsukami TS, Sobel M, Singh N, Tran NT (2015) Intravascular ultrasound is a critical tool for accurate endograft sizing in the management of blunt thoracic aortic injury. J Vasc Surg 61(3):630–635

Waterford SD, Chou D, Bombien R, Uzun I, Shah A, Khoynezhad A (2016) Left subclavian arterial coverage and stroke during thoracic aortic endografting: a systematic review. Ann Thorac Surg 101(1):381–389

Williams DM, Simon HJ, Marx MV, Starkey TD (1992) Acute traumatic aortic rupture: intravascular US findings. Radiology 182(1):247–249

Williams DM, Dake MD, Bolling SF, Deeb GM (1993) The role of intravascular ultrasound in acute traumatic aortic rupture. Semin Ultrasound CT MR 14(2):85–90

Cardiac Injuries

Ulrich Linsenmaier and Lucas L. Geyer

Contents

U. Linsenmaier, MD, PhD (✉)
Director Institute for Diagnostic and Interventional Radiology, HELIOS Kliniken München West, Associate Professor of Radiology, Ludwig-Maximilians-University Munich (LMU), Past President ESER – European Society of Emergency Radiology, Munich 81737, Germany
e-mail: Ulrich.Linsenmaier@helios-kliniken.de

L.L. Geyer, MD
Institute for Clinical Radiology, LMU Ludwig-Maximilians-University Hospital Munich, Marchioninistr. 15, Munich 81377, Germany
e-mail: Lucas.Geyer@med.lmu.de

Abstract

Cardiac injury due to penetrating or blunt thoracic trauma is relatively rare but associated with significant morbidity and mortality. Many of these injuries have not been characterized fully by diagnostic imaging so far. With the introduction of fast MDCT an established emergent diagnostic modality is now available for heart imaging, that allows the detection and characterization of a large variety of myocardial, pericardial, vascular and mediastinal injuries. Beside the established methods, like cardiac ultrasound and cardiac angiography, it allows now in the emergency setting a thorough morphologic characterization of injuries and its' potential bleeding dynamics. This article reviews the spectrum of blunt and penetrating heart injuries as well as the imaging modalities commonly used in the acute trauma setting.

1 Introduction

Cardiac injury is rare and is related with significant mortality and morbidity. Radiological imaging of cardiac injuries is relatively new, and the majority of the imaging features have not yet been fully evaluated. With the introduction of fast multidetector CT (MDCT), these injuries have increasingly come into the focus of radiology, and CT can now identify a large spectrum of

Med Radiol Diagn Imaging (2016)
DOI 10.1007/174_2016_64, © Springer International Publishing Switzerland

injury patterns. In the acute trauma setting, it is crucial to recognize these findings and to initiate appropriate treatment (Mattox et al. 2012).

Cardiac injuries are caused by work accidents, explosions, falls from height, and also from CPR and assaults. In communities where there is a higher ratio of firearm ownership among the public, the likelihood of penetrating injuries to the heart is higher (Table 1) (Parmley et al. 1958; Tenzer 1985).

In many cases, injuries to the heart lead to immediate death. Typically, the myocardium, pericardium, and the coronary arteries are affected. In blunt trauma, the heart can be compressed between a flexed spine and the sternum; however, shearing forces, twisting, and deceleration trauma have also been described. The mechanically injured heart can be further damaged by hypovolemic shock, arterial hypotension, and resulting myocardial ischemia. In addition, heart function may be impaired by hypoxia from other injuries such as pulmonary contusions, pulmonary lacerations, and pneumothorax as well as multi-organ failure (MOF) (Parmley et al. 1958; Fulda et al. 1991; Orliaguet et al. 2001).

Up to 25 % of deaths from traumatic events are associated with cardiac injuries. The incidence of blunt cardiac injury has risen during the last decades, but early diagnosis and efficient, specific treatment are mandatory and are correlated with increasing survival rates. A major proportion of patients with manifest cardiac injuries die on the scene before they can reach medical treatment. In cardio surgery, new technologies are influencing outcomes, as bypass surgery and the use of intra-aortic balloon devices can assist the cardiac function and thus may help to improve the outcome (Table 2) (Mattox et al. 2012; Co et al. 2011).

Table 1 Cardiac injury – mechanism of injury

In principle, any mechanism with kinetic energy to the thoracic cage may cause blunt cardiac trauma
Typical examples:
Motor-vehicle accident (>20 mph) with compression by the steering wheel
Deceleration trauma
Accidental falls from great heights
Objects of great weight falling directly onto the sternum
Blast and direct forces applied to the chest
Increased abdominal pressure
Cardiopulmonary resuscitation

Table 2 Cardiac injury – clinical presentation

Acute findings	Subacute findings
Complete hemodynamic instability	Tenderness and pain along the anterior chest wall
Congestive heart failure	Dysrhythmias
Cardiopulmonary arrest	New heart murmur
Cardiogenic shock	Pericardial friction rub
Symptoms of pericardial tamponade	

2 Imaging Modalities

2.1 Cardiac Ultrasound (US)

Echocardiography (cardiac US) provides precise evaluation of the existence of pericardial effusions. In addition, small volumes of not more than 25 ml can be detected. Myocardial wall motion and the valvular structures can also be assessed, as well as the left ventricular function. Transesophageal echocardiography (TEE) can also be used to assess the ventricular function in cases of myocardial contusion and was deployed to evaluate the aorta for signs of aortic injury (AI) before reliable CT angiography (CTA) from advanced MDCT scanning became available (Restrepo et al. 2007, 2012). However, TEE is more time-consuming and invasive and is difficult to perform with concomitant injuries, e.g., to the face and cervical spine. Additionally, it is not always available and is operator dependent. Therefore today TEE plays only a minor role in the acute trauma setting.

US findings of acute cardiac injury comprise cardiac wall compression and pulmonary artery compression as well as paradox flow patterns, abnormalities of the ventricular septum, and abnormal swinging motion of the heart itself (Restrepo et al. 2007, 2012).

Alternatively, transthoracic cardiac US can be performed. It is rapid, noninvasive, and efficient. It is reported that even limited training in cardiac US techniques may provide an efficient means of detecting pericardial hemorrhage. Sensitivity is reported to be 90 %, specificity 97 %, and accuracy 96%. Pericardial emergency ultrasound of the heart is an important component of FAST ultrasound (focused assessment with sonography in trauma) (Mattox et al. 2012; Co et al. 2011).

2.2 Conventional Radiography (CR) of the Chest

Supine conventional radiography (CR) of the chest is still a component of the initial trauma workup in the emergency room. However CR is limited to delineate the full spectrum of injuries to the thorax and heart as well. In many cases, however, signs of pneumopericardium, hematothorax, pneumothorax, and mediastinal widening, due to mediastinal hematoma, can be detected. Imaging quality of supine CR of the chest in the emergency setting is often limited and most of the important cardiac injury patterns cannot be detected (Mattox et al. 2012; Co et al. 2011).

2.3 Cardiac Angiography

Angiography of the coronary arteries (syn. cardiac angiography) is not an established component of a typical trauma-imaging workup in the emergency room. However, it is very sensitive and specific in imaging coronary artery injuries, and it can detect even subtle vascular lesions. In addition, it offers the entire spectrum of opportunities for immediate interventional treatments of vascular lesions. It is indicated in all cases of suspected vascular injury and also when ischemia is suspected with ECG changes after trauma, to evaluate patients for traumatic aneurysms, intima dissections, and vascular thrombosis after trauma. Most of these lesions can be detected and can undergo intermediate interventional treatment.

2.4 Multidetector CT (MDCT)

Many patients with suspected multiple trauma undergo a MDCT from head to toe, so-called whole-body CT (WBCT). MDCT is the imaging modality of choice for the evaluation of all kinds of chest trauma and is highly sensitive and specific for the evaluation of lung injuries, pneumothorax, active hemorrhage, pericardial or myocardial injury, pleural and pericardial effusions, hematothorax, and also cardiac herniation and cardiac luxation. MDCT can also depict valvular injuries and papillary muscle rupture as well as avulsion of the aortic and mitral valve (Linsenmaier et al. 2002; Mirvis).

High-quality MDCT is today available in all major trauma centers, it is widely accepted, and MDCT is today the core imaging modality in the major trauma setting. In thoracic and cardiac imaging, MDCT can detect penetrating foreign bodies, it also depicts the track of penetrating objects, and it allows for initiation of a targeted treatment. MDCT has a high sensitivity and accuracy in the detection of pleural and pericardial effusions or pericardial hemorrhage and tamponade. It detects pericardial and myocardial lacerations and also active hemorrhage from the heart. It also depicts luxation and displacement of the heart and has also a high sensitivity for concomitant mediastinal vascular and lung injuries. Due to its high spatial and timely resolution, it delivers isotropic voxel allowing for the calculation of high-resolution multiplanar reconstructions (MPRs). Today small motion and flow artifacts are now much reduced from prior scanner generations. ECG-gated MDCT scanning is an adjunct to the initial whole-body CT (WBCT) in the acute trauma setting. Contrast medium (CM) is administered in all studies, and an extended CM bolus allows for a contrast filling of the right and left heart and the vascular in- and outflow at the same time. Primary axial reconstruction is performed with the thinnest possible slice thickness (ST) of 0.5–0.625 mm; diagnostic axial images are reconstructed at 1–1.5 mm and coronal and sagittal MPRs at 2–3 mm and VRT as well (Fig. 1) (Mirvis; Korner et al. 2009).

2.5 Cardiac Magnetic Resonance Imaging (MR)

Cardiac magnetic resonance imaging (MR) has the ability to assess cardiac anatomy as well as cardiac function; it can visualize signs of myocardial ischemia and myocardial infarction (MI). In myocar-

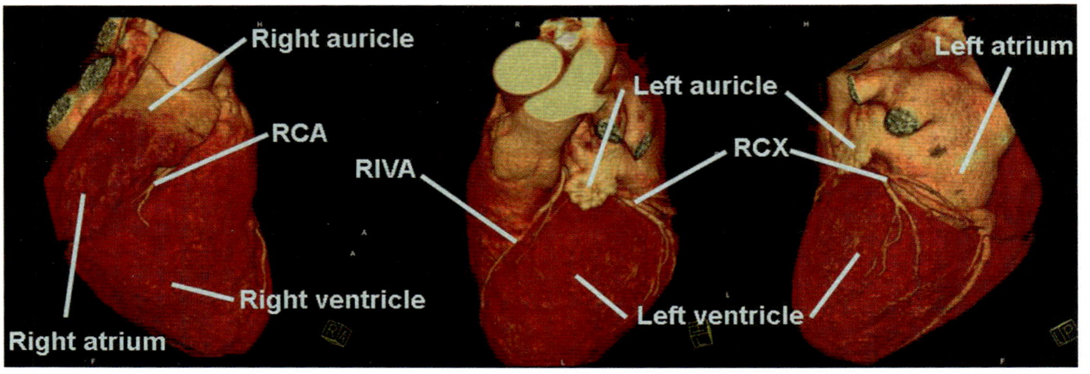

Fig. 1 CT anatomy of the heart ECG-gated cardiac CT in a volume-rendering technique (VRT) for radial display

dial contusions, it can depict abnormal cardiac wall motion and abnormal valve function and can detect edema and ischemia of the myocardium. MRI is not useful in the early and acute trauma workup as availability of 24 h/7 days is limited, the exam is complex to be performed, and the patient monitoring is difficult at the same time. However, if indications are given, it is a valuable noninvasive imaging method in addition to MDCT of the acute setting (Co et al. 2011; Korner et al. 2009).

3 Blunt Cardiac Injuries

Minor injuries are so-called myocardial contusions (syn. cardiac contusion); more severe injuries comprise ruptures of the pupillary muscles, valve injuries, injuries to the coronary arteries, and septal and myocardial injuries as well as cardiac rupture. Most common causes of blunt cardiac injury are high-speed motor-vehicle accidents (MVAs), crush or blast injuries, falls from height, and less common, direct violence or direct impact to the chest or abdomen. Also iatrogenic injuries are reported due to cardiopulmonary resuscitation (CPR). A clinical algorithm is available for management of patients after blunt cardiac trauma (Fig. 2).

3.1 Myocardial Contusion

Myocardial contusion is best defined as motion changes of the cardiac wall when myocardial infarction (MI) could be ruled out. Clinically it can be suspected in cases of significant chest trauma and persistent arterial hypotension despite volume therapy (Embrey; Kaye and O'Sullivan).

Myocardial contusion has to be differentiated from myocardial infarction which can be clinically difficult to distinguish. In myocardial infarction (MI), symptoms are related to a vascular territory, and the tissue at the risk shows a transition zone when in myocardial contusion the tissue at risk is more confined and has a distinct edge. The incidence of myocardial contusion is reported in a wide range with 10–75 %, probably due to inconsistent findings, and a scientific standard for diagnosis is still missing (Mattox et al. 2012; Co et al. 2011; Symbas; Tenzer).

These injuries are also named under the term myocardial contusion (alternatively, myocardial concussion) and are usually best diagnosed by laboratory testing of isoenzyme MB of creatine phosphokinase (CPK-MB), echocardiography, and ECG. The troponin test is an additional laboratory test (CTNI and CTNT >0.1 μg/l), with increased levels of the protein troponin usually observed in patients with cardiac contusions. Typically, patients only undergo monitoring on intermediate care units (Table 3) (Mattox et al. 2012; Co et al. 2011; Symbas; Tenzer).

The introduction of the diagnosis cardiac contusion is controversial as clinical importance, incidence, and morbidity and mortality remained controversial. It is accepted that younger patients with ECG abnormalities after trauma should

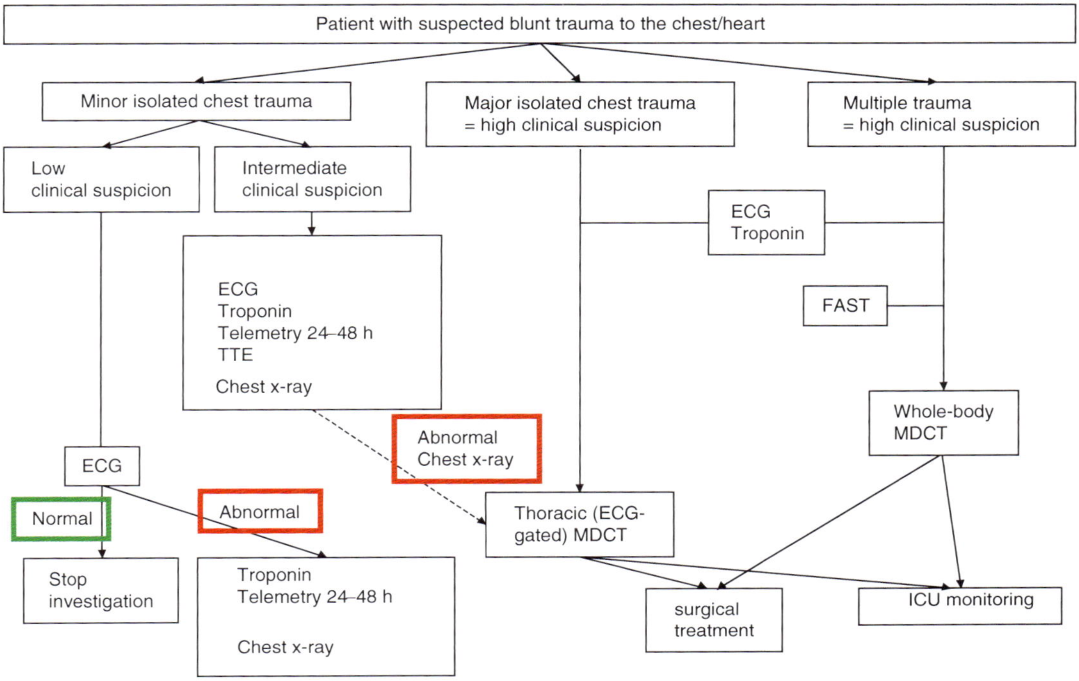

Fig. 2 Clinical algorithm for management of patient with suspected blunt trauma to the heart. The algorithm distinguishes minor isolated chest trauma from major isolated chest trauma and multiple trauma (El-Chami et al. 2008)

Table 3 Cardiac injury – laboratory and ECG diagnosis

Laboratory findings/cardiac enzymes	ECG findings
Cardiac markers are biomarkers measured to assess heart dysfunction: Myoglobin, LDH-1 isozyme, glycogen phosphorylase isoenzyme BB (GPBB), creatine kinase MB, troponin T and I *Creatine kinase* MB (CK MB) has turned out to be nonspecific *Troponin T*: very specific marker for cardiac injury (91 %), but with low sensitivity (31 %) *Troponin I* shows the best correlation of sensitivity and specificity in different trials. In combination with EKG abnormalities, it exhibits 100 % sensitivity for detection of clinically significant blunt cardiac trauma such as cardiogenic shock, dysrhythmias requiring treatment, or structural cardiac abnormalities related to trauma Levels <1.05 μg/L in asymptomatic trauma patients, indicative of cardiac injuries Levels >1.05 μg/L associated with ventricular dysrhythmias and left ventricular dysfunction The remaining cardiac parameters are not relevant for trauma monitoring	The important role of ECG bases on the fact that electrical instability is an important indicator for blunt cardiac trauma ECG is a quickly available tool for the first survey: Hemodynamically stable patients with normal EKG need no further monitoring Significant electrical disorders are suggestive of cardiac injuries especially the presence of any new bundle branch block Other typical findings: persistent sinus tachycardia (most often), atrial fibrillation, ST depression, ST elevation Limitation: present abnormalities are not pathognomonic markers for diagnostic correlations

undergo further evaluation. ECG is a clinical indicator in multiple injured patients as significant cardiac disease is relatively rare in young patients after trauma.

When ECG abnormalities occur, they are significant and need further evaluation. Clinical recommendations comprise that patients after thoracic trauma, as long as they are symptom-free, do not need any surveillance or monitoring; in symptomatic patients, intermediate care or telemetry monitoring is considered to be sufficient (Cachecho et al.; Fabian et al.; McLean et al.).

Pathophysiologically there is a wide range of tissue damage in myocardial contusions, from transmural hemorrhage and tissue necrosis to superficial contusions with different extend of tissue loss. The resulting perfusion defects and myocardial dysfunction most likely result from focal contusion and tissue edema when coronary artery disease is not present. The right heart is more affected due to its position next dorsal to the sternum. Clinical findings comprise ECG changes and elevated cardiac enzymes (creatine phosphokinase and serum cardiac troponin) (Allen and Liedtke; Ghersin et al.).

Clinical symptoms can mimic myocardial infarction, including dyspnea and chest pain; the ECG changes are variable and most cases are uncomplicated. However, a progress to an arrhythmia, cardiac dysfunction, hypotension, and low-output failure as well as myocardial rupture can be observed leading to life-threatening cardiac failure.

Abnormal cardiac wall motion is best diagnosed with echocardiography. In the setting of whole-body computed tomography after trauma (WBCT), there are no specific imaging features reported for myocardial contusion so far. Advanced ECG-gated MDCT enables an anatomic workup including CT angiography (CTA) of the coronary arteries. In addition, it allows for a functional assessment of the heart including assessment of the cardiac wall motion in 4D technique and initial reports on myocardial perfusion. Concomitant injuries of the thorax and mediastinum are present in many cases and can deteriorate the clinical situation (Fig. 3) (Embrey; Kaye and O'Sullivan).

Cardiac MR and positron emission tomography (PET) can delineate the possible extend of the hypoperfused myocardium and can be used for further workup if myocardial contusion is suspected (Co et al. 2011; Kaye and O'Sullivan).

3.2 Injuries to the Pericardium

Pericardial tears can differ in size from millimeters to an extent over the entire pericardium. They are most common at the diaphragmatic surface and the left-sided pericardium. Typically they are

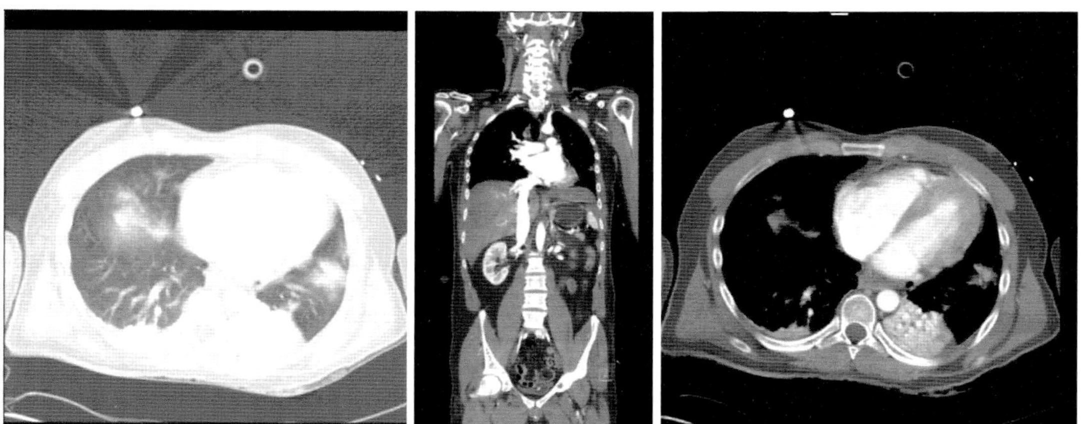

Fig. 3 Myocardial contusion: ungated MDCT of the whole body showing heart dilatation of the right atrium and ventricle, pulmonary contusion and hematothorax, and atelectasis of the left lower lobe. A contrast reflux with retrograde paradox flow in the inferior vena cava (IVC)

result of an increased intra-abdominal pressure or the direct impact to the chest and mediastinum (Fulda et al. 1991; Parmley et al.).

Conventional radiography (CR) may show air in the pericardium (pneumopericardium); pericardial injuries can be complicated by diaphragmatic rupture and cardiac herniation from resulting in severe cardiac failure. However CT findings are by far more sensitive and specific.

Pericardial tears and ruptures are rare injuries, with an incidence of only 0.3–0.5 %. They occur with severe deceleration forces or are due to osseous fragment perforation by fractures to the sternum or the ribs. Pneumopericardium is a complication of pericardial rupture; an air collection is located ventral to the myocardium in the pericardial sac. Pneumopericardium is a sign for pericardial injury. The tear itself can be detected by irregular margins of the pericardium, discontinuity, and interposition of fat or long parenchyma. This can be further complicated by cardiac tamponade and compression. Pneumopericardium is always a sign for pericardial injury; the pericardial tear itself can be detected by irregular margins or discontinuity of the pericardium, but also by interposition of fat or lung parenchyma (Restrepo et al. 2007; Farhataziz and Landay) (Fig. 4).

After pericardial injury MDCT can be used to depict pericardial effusions. In the acute trauma setting, every pericardial effusion has to be evaluated for hemorrhage; MDCT can measure the density of effusions in Hounsfield units (HU) and confirm pericardial hemorrhage and tamponade (Restrepo et al. 2007).

Further complications include the displacement of the heart through the pericardial rupture into the mediastinum or thoracic cavity, showing an empty air-filled pericardium on MDCT. As the vascular structures are stretched or also rotated (also described as volvulus), this can lead to immediate compression of the heart and obstruction of the vascular system. Cardiac luxation describes herniation and compression of the heart, which can result in obstruction of the upper venous inflow over the superior vena cava (SVC). Luxation can occur in up to 28 % of pericardial ruptures, and there is a high associated mortality rate of up to 67 %. An ECG allows observation of a change of the heart axis. Cardiac US is of limited value only. MDCT can be used to diagnose heart displacement as well as the compression and deviation of the myocardium and the heart chambers (Fig. 5) (Moront et al.; Bruschi et al.).

3.3 Injuries to the Heart Valves, Papillary Muscles, Chorda Tendinea, and Septum

Blunt cardiac trauma can result in ruptures of the myocardial septum, the valves, and the papillary muscles. Patients with preexisting heart disease and disorders of these structures are more prone to this type of trauma.

Clinically, these injuries can be associated with acute left ventricular failure and atypical systolic murmurs. Systolic murmur is a sign of valve injury and papillary muscle injuries. In the case of

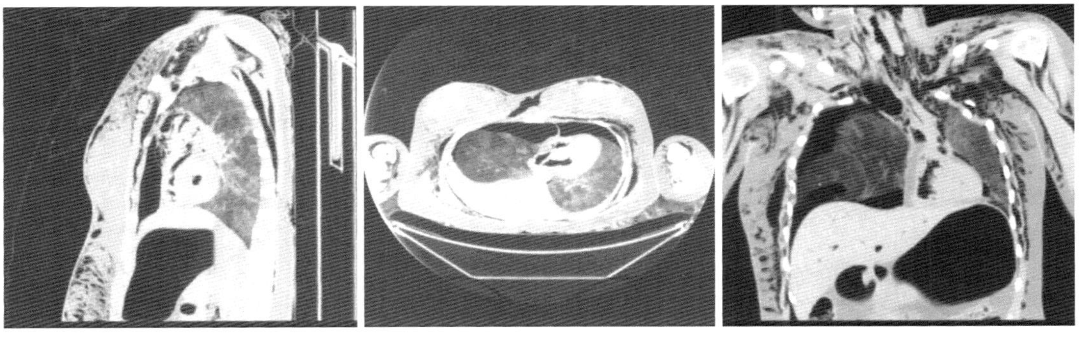

Fig. 4 Pneumopericardium: ungated MDCT showing a pneumopericardium on post-mortem CT (PM CT). There is pathological air collection in the chambers of the heart, pneumomediastinum, soft tissue emphysema, pneumothorax, gastric hyperinflation, and hematothorax

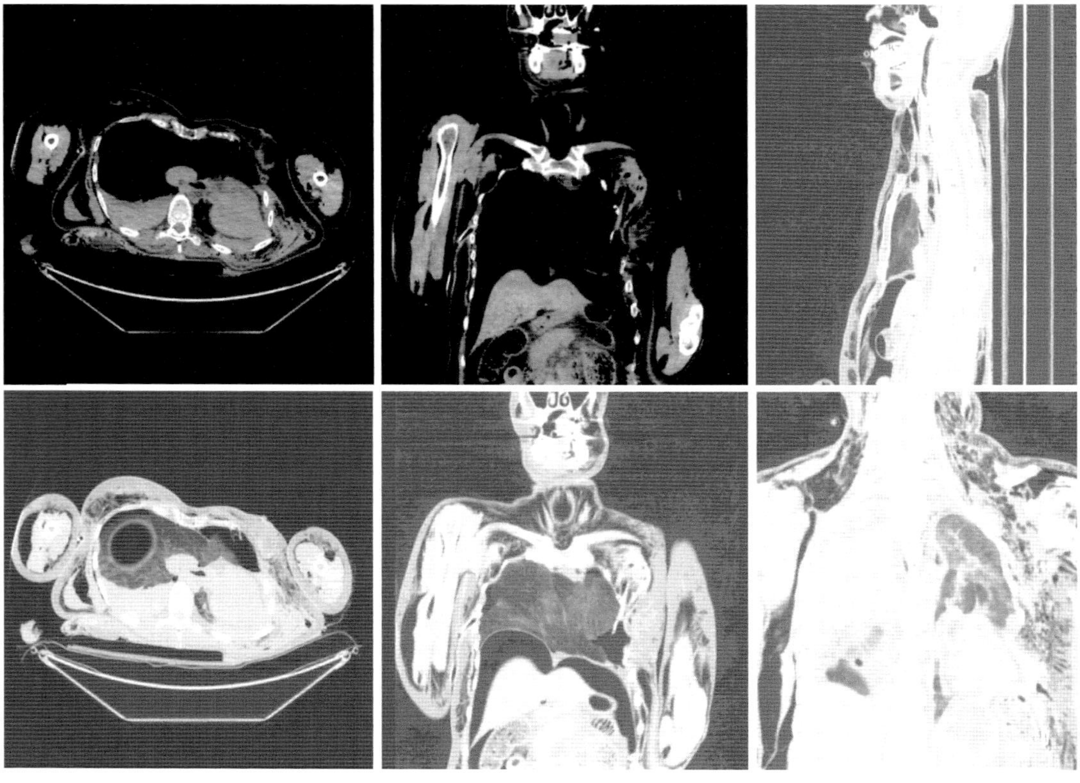

Fig. 5 Cardiac luxation: ungated MDCT case of cardiac herniation where the heart is dislocated from its anatomical position into the left thoracic cavity, lateral to the spine. The so-called black hole in the soft tissue window and "kissing lungs" due to the displacement of the entire heart can be observed in the lung window

severe ventricular failure, operative treatment is mandatory. Injuries to the septum can also result in atypical murmurs. Ruptures of the septum can result in left-right blood shunts, with the clinical symptoms dependent on the extent of the lesion caused. Operative interventions with regard to these injuries are determined by the individual case. Small septal injuries may be treated conservatively; larger defects are subject to surgical repair (Mattox et al. 2012; Moront et al.).

Moront et al. reported a case of injury of the tricuspid valve and the intraventricular septum days after blunt injury, and the patient underwent operative treatment. The ventricular septum ruptures were observed in the muscular septum close to the apex of the heart (Moront et al.).

Parmely et al. reported a series of 546 cases of blunt cardiac trauma and described a 9 % incidence of injuries to the valves. In their series mitral, aortic, and tricuspid valves were involved (Parmley et al. 1958).

An injury of the heart valve and traumatic valvular dysfunction is rare. It can be suspected if pulmonary edema is present after chest trauma. Commonly affected is the aortic valve as common as the mitral and tricuspid valves. The underlying mechanism is an excessive elevation of blood pressure in the heart, but also an elevated intra-abdominal pressure can be transmitted to the heart and affect the cardiac valve and papillary muscles. Commonly observed are injuries of the mitral valve, including rupture of the chorda tendinea and the papillary muscles and aortic valve injuries (Bruschi et al.; Kan and Yang).

Imaging workup comprises usually echocardiography, TEE, and cardiac angiography. But early reports also suggest that MDCT can detect some of these injuries (Lee et al.).

3.4 Injuries to the Coronary Arteries

Intima dissection of the coronary arteries can result in thrombosis and occlusion and subsequent myocardial ischemia. In an elder population with preexisting coronary artery disease (CAD), it may be difficult to distinguish a traumatic occlusion from a non-trauma-associated arteriosclerotic occlusion of the vessel. As a complication arteriovenous (AV) fistulas as well as atrioventricular fistulas of the coronary arteries were described as result of blunt injury; however they are very rare (Mattox et al. 2012).

Diagnostic imaging with MDCT is now possible, and even in non-gated MDCT after trauma, the occlusions of the left coronary artery could be depicted. This is much dependent on the heart frequency and the timely resolution of the non-gated MDCT scanner. And not always the coronary artery main stems can be depicted on non-gated MDCT. The addition of ECG-gated MDCT studies and contrast CTA of the coronary arteries may be an option. However in the emergency setting, gated MDCT of the chest is not a primary choice.

Diagnostic imaging typically comprises card angiography, and interventional recanalization can be intended; revascularization and stent implantation are interventional treatment options.

Coronary artery injuries are relatively rare and account for 2 % of all thoracic injuries. As multiple injuries have been described, the left anterior descending artery (LAD) is most likely affected, also due to its immediate retrosternal location. Clinically signs of myocardial infarction (MI) can be observed in ECG, which can result in hypotension and arrhythmia. Intima dissection and thrombosis are more common, but vascular ruptures with free hemorrhage have also been reported. In ungated MDCT imaging using high spatial and timely resolution, diagnosis can be made; however this is based on single-case reports. If injuries to the coronary arteries are suspected, ECG-gated MDCT with CTA of the coronary arteries is indicated and also the use of triple rule out (TRO) protocols can be used. Immediate interventional treatment is carried out by coronary angiography recanalization and stent treatment (Pretre and Chilcott; Sheikh et al.) (Figs. 6 and 7).

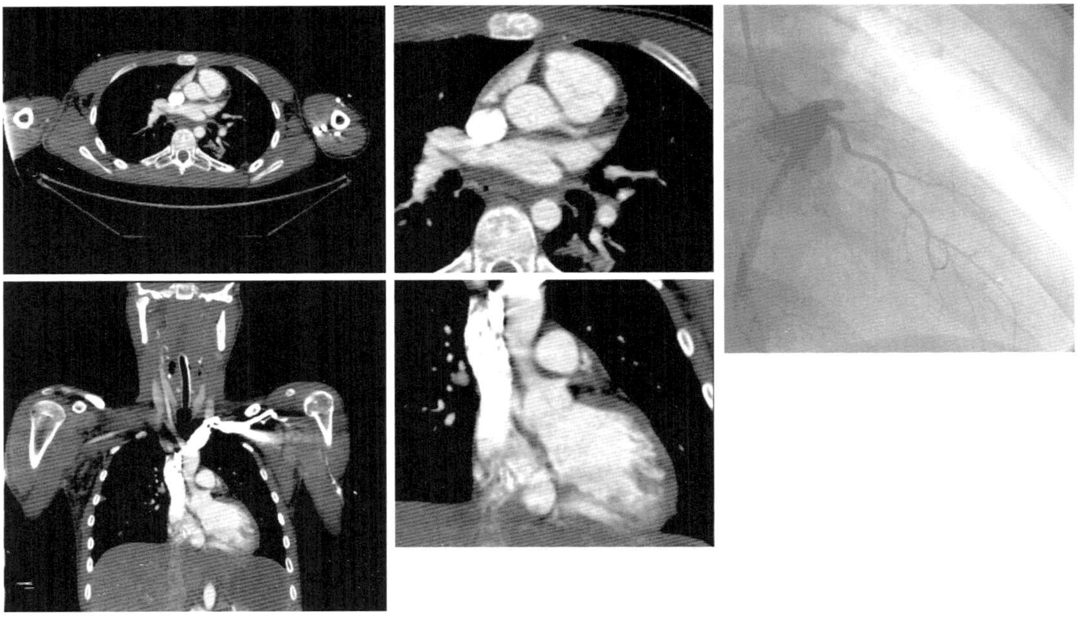

Fig. 6 Injury to the left coronary artery: Dissection of the LAD. Ungated MDCT/WBCT in a patient after polytrauma. Two centimeters from the main stem, an occlusion of LAD can be observed; the interruption of the CM-enhanced LAD with little downstream effusion, coronary angiography confirmed the diagnosis

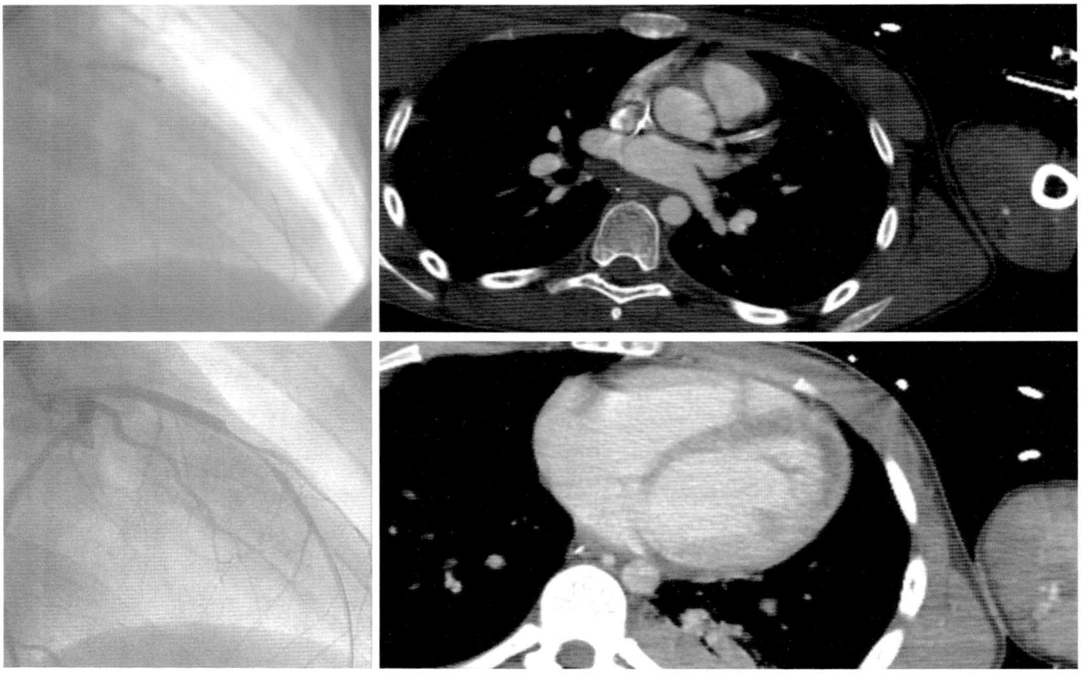

Fig. 7 Recanalization of LAD and stent-graft placement in the LAD, and follow-up CT with hypodense subendocardial rim of the myocardium which is as a correlate of myocardial infarction

Penetrating injuries of the coronary arteries most likely occur in the left anterior descending, coronary artery (LAD) resulting in myocardial dysfunction. However, the majority of coronary artery injuries are more distal. Proximal injuries can be treated by emergent coronary artery bypass surgery and smaller vessels with diameters of less than 1 mm and can result in small infarcts.

3.5 Cardiac Rupture

Cardiac rupture is typically the result of the severe thoracic trauma mostly associated with MVA as well as falls from height and direct blast injuries to the chest. The underlying mechanism of injury has been described as direct force to the chest with increased thoracic pressure and transmission to the heart. Decelerating forces typically affect the borders of mobile and fixed anatomic structures of the heart, also explaining arterial and caval tears. Additionally, severe trauma to the abdomen can be transmitted via vascular structures such as the inferior vena cava (IVC) to the right heart, causing rupture of the heart. Cardiac rupture also occurs as a result of myocardial contusion, traumatic myocardial necrosis, and formation of pseudoaneurysms. Direct force from sternal or costal fractures with penetrating bone fragments can directly perforate the cardiac walls (Mattox et al. 2012).

Many patients have no cardiac function on admission, due to cardiac tamponade, severe hemorrhage, or pericardial tamponade. Diagnosis can be delayed in patients who are stable, and in a series of 24 cases, 16 were delayed by up to 1 h (Patton et al.). In addition, polytrauma and associated injuries make the diagnosis difficult. ECG can show a bundle branch block or deviation of the heart axis in cases of cardiac herniation.

Echocardiography (syn. cardiac ultrasound) can depict pericardial hemorrhage, and it is recommended to decompress the pericardium immediately even under cardiac arrest.

Ultrasound-guided pericardial puncture is an option to confirm the diagnosis.

Clinical treatment is comparable to that for penetrating cardiac injuries. Pericardial decompression is followed by sternotomy, and insertion of an intra-aortic balloon pump is a treatment option (Fulda et al. 1991; Calhoon et al.; Kato et al. 1988; Mattox et al. 1992). It should be considered that in these cases associated injuries are common, and the entire torso and skeleton should be diagnosed by whole-body CT (WBCT). Common associated injuries include aortic injuries, abdominal injuries (up to 43 %), head injuries (up to 51 %) and skeletal injuries (up to 40 %). The outcome is limited; Fulda et al. (Fulda et al. 1991) describe a mortality rate of 48 % in patients with cardiac arrest, and the overall mortality is reported to be up to 76 %. Kato et al. (Kato et al. 1988) report a mortality rate of more than 90 % in a cohort of 63 patients.

Myocardial rupture (cardiac rupture) is rare, and the incidence is reported as 0.1–0.3 % in patients with severe chest trauma. However, it is associated with a high mortality, accounting for 36–56 % of blunt thoracic injuries. Again, the right heart is more prone to injury due to its retrosternal position and the thinner myocardial wall of the right ventricle. In gross hemorrhage it can lead to pericardial tamponade and immediate cardiac arrest, and patient deserves cardiopulmonary resuscitation (CPR) (Co et al. 2011; Kato et al. 1988; Van Horn 2007).

Depending on the presence of a pericardial injury, the hemorrhage is contained in the pericardial sac or can procreate to the mediastinum and the thoracic cavity. The extent of the hemorrhage in an intact pericardium can lead to tamponade. Blunt myocardial rupture occurs with increased central venous pressure (CVP) in the diastole, leading to increased pressure in the ventricle when the atrioventricular valve is closed. Myocardial rupture is lethal in many cases, e.g., in a patient presenting with refractory hypotension and tachycardia (Figs. 8, 9, and 10) (Van Horn 2007).

The mortality of patients undergoing surgery is reported as high as 33 %, but where treatment is successful, a good long-term outcome is reported. MDCT has proven to be able to show complete and incomplete myocardial rupture, while active hemorrhage can be observed by the extravasation of contrast-enhanced blood into the pericardium, mediastinum, or thoracic cavity. Additional use of MR can depict myocardial disorders such as muscular thinning, formation of myocardial scars, and ischemia in cases of infarction more sensitively, but this is not appropriate in the acute setting (Mirvis; Zoni et al.).

4 Penetrating Cardiac Injury

The spectrum of penetrating injuries includes injuries to the atrium and the ventricle, injuries to the vascular structures, injuries to the trachea, bronchi, esophagus, as well as of the bony cage and the thoracic spine. Penetrating transmediastinal injury (TMI) is defined injury that transverses the mediastinum.

In a recent series of 532 penetrating injuries, the right ventricle was involved (35 %), less common are the left ventricle (25 %), right atrium (33 %), left atrium (14 %), and the aorta (14 %) (Demetriades and van der Veen). The right heart is more prone to injury due to its location dorsal to the sternum. In penetrating injuries, the extent and severity of injury depend on the caliber of the penetrating objects. The clinical symptoms can change from asymptomatic and normal ECG to unstable vital signs, hypotension, and cardiac arrest due to cardiac tamponade or active hemorrhage (Elie; Gasparri et al.; Thourani et al.).

Penetrating injury is mostly based on firearms and knives; less common is perforation by bone fragments from sternum or rip fractures. Iatrogenic injury is rare but can be related to accidental cardiac puncture, interventional procedures, or central venous access devices (Mattox et al. 2012; Asensio et al. 1996). As the right ventricle is in direct contact with the interior chest wall, it is more prone for cardiac injury. In a series of 711 patients, the authors reported a distribution of injuries to the right ventricle (40 %) and left ventricle (40 %) being more common than injuries to right atrium (24 %) and left atrium (3 %) (Wall et al. 1997).

The pathophysiology and the clinical outcome are influenced by two main factors, the severity

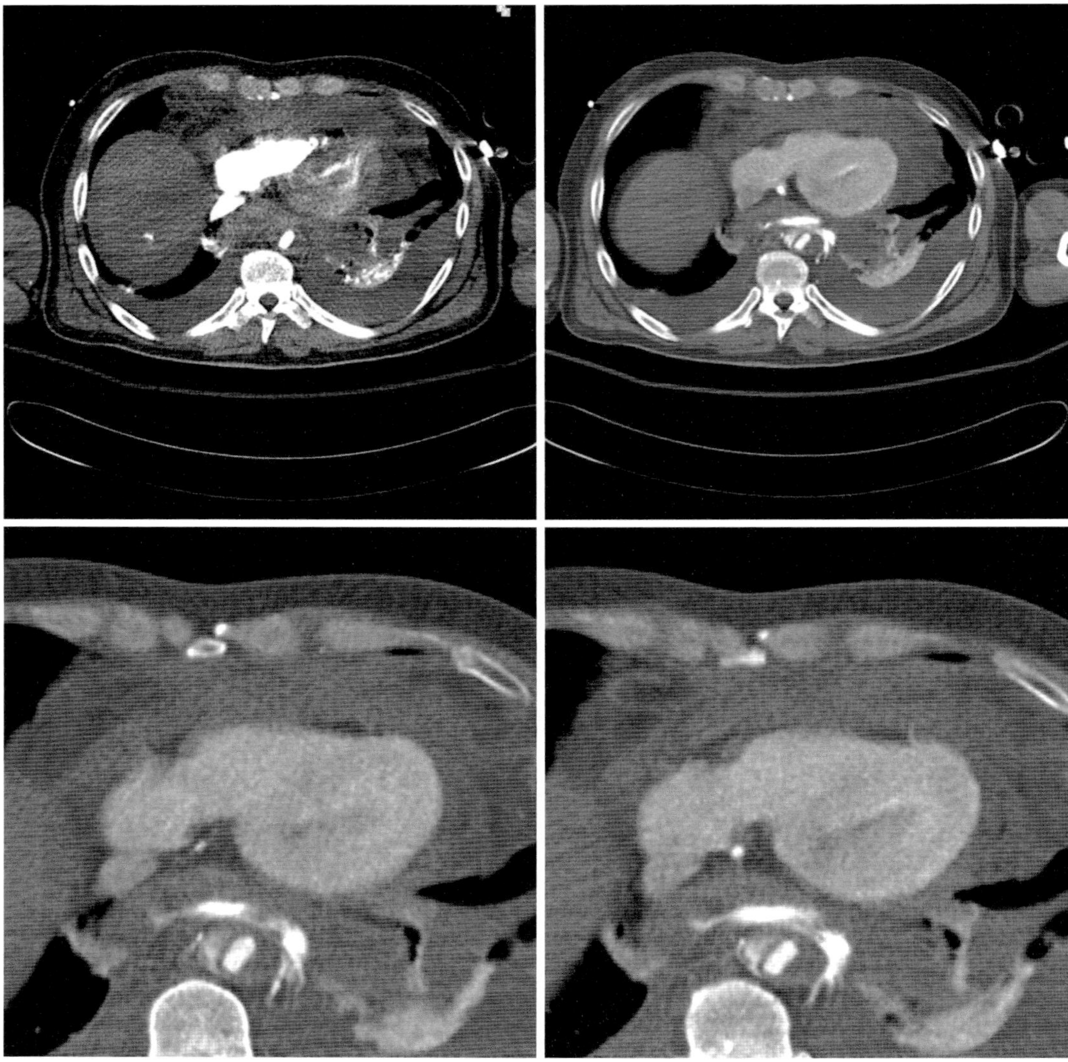

Fig. 8 Cardiac rupture: ungated MDCT with a cardiac chamber rupture. Missing delineation of the myocardium of the right cardiac chambers can be seen, as well as active hemorrhage from the heart to the pericardium with a compression of the heart. The corollary is that hemopericardium-associated injuries comprise hematothorax and acute aortic rupture

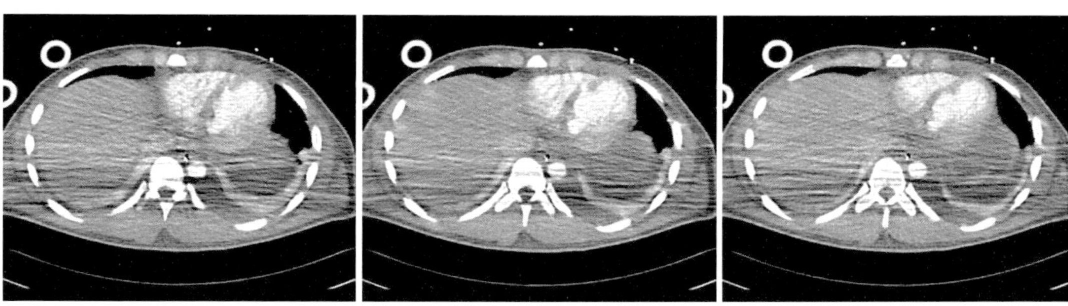

Fig. 9 Cardiac rupture: ungated MDCT whole-body CT of a patient showing a septal injury with septal rupture. The discontinuity of the cardiac septum and the transseptal hemorrhage is depicted

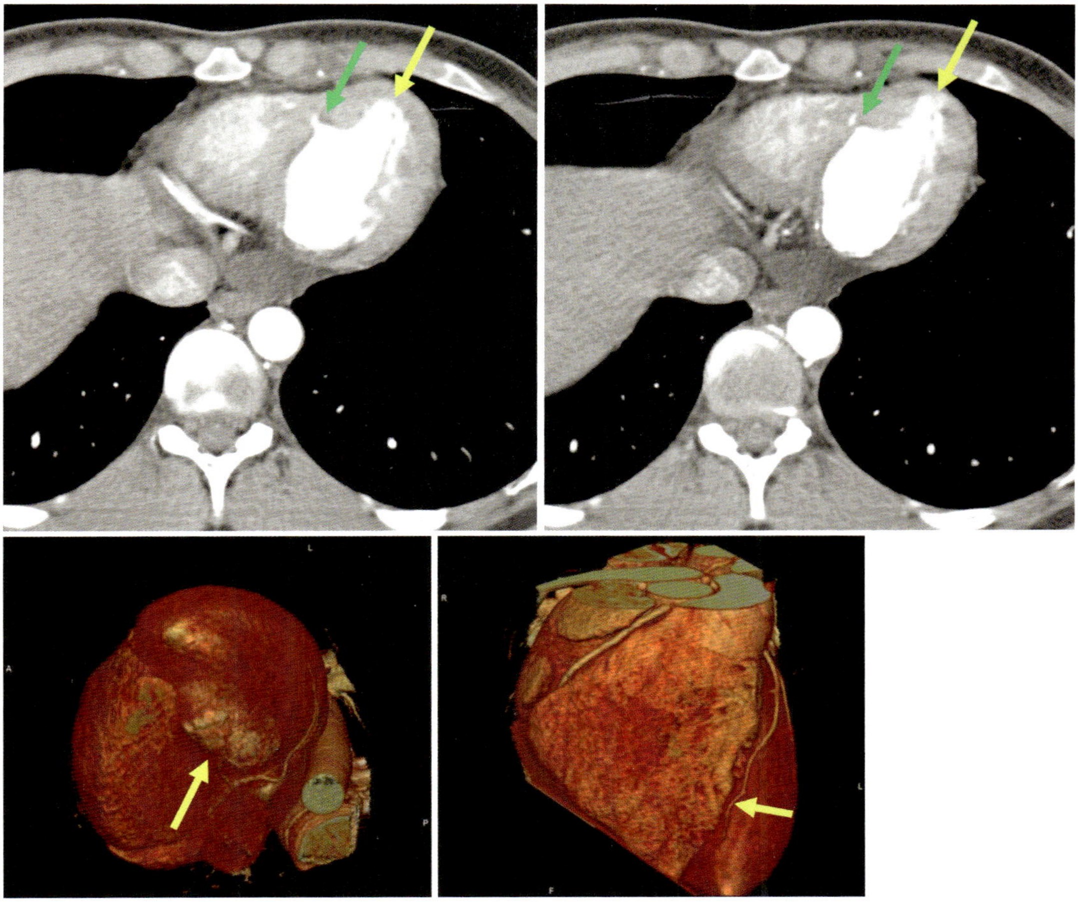

Fig. 10 ECG-gated MDCT of the heart, axial reconstructions, and VRT. The figure shows (**a**) a discontinuity of the intraventricular septum with intraseptal bleeding as a sign of incomplete rupture (*green arrows*) and (**b**) intramyocardial bleeding on the apex of the left ventricle (*yellow arrows*) as a sign of traumatic cardiac aneurysm displaying in the VRT reconstruction

and rate of bleeding and the involvement and extend of pericardial tamponade. Penetrating injuries with small knives are self-limited and can often result uncomplicated with self-healing of the laceration. Up to 90% of patients with small object-penetrating injuries show pericardial tamponade (Symbas).

Clinically, patients present with tachycardia and increased pressure in the ventricular filling as well as paradox pulse, a high drop in systolic blood pressure during inspiration, and increased myocardial contractility. They also exhibit extended neck veins, as well as paradox inspiration and increased CVP; however, the latter can also be associated with pneumothorax, which is a differential diagnosis.

This can result in a compensated status of tamponade; however, under volume replacement the cardiac function and systemic blood pressure can still be kept within the limits. However, even a slight deterioration in pericardial tamponade can result in severe left ventricular-filling defects, immediate systemic hypotension, and cardiac output failure. The myocardial compression also results in ischemia due to compression of the coronary artery flow – leading to an uncompensated cardiac tamponade (Mattox et al. 2012).

Larger wounds or gunshot injuries result in hemorrhage from the cardiac chambers and, in many cases, associated injuries causing further blood loss and leading to clinical deterioration. Myocardial injuries to the left ventricle or right ventricle can be self-sealing, but the atrium is in greater danger, as there is less muscular substance. Direct injuries to the coronary artery can result in rapid pericardial tamponade. Penetrating injuries to the septum or the heart valves are less common.

Patients suffering from penetrating cardiac trauma who can be brought directly to the operating theater have a survival rate of 97 % for stab and 71 % for gunshot injuries. Of patients undergoing emergency thoracotomy, only 14 % survive; for those arriving at the hospital without cardiac function, the survival rate is only 7.8 %. Milham et al. report an overall mortality rate of 47 % in a sample of 2,253 patients (Mattox et al. 2012).

Imaging is often limited to CR of the chest if patients are hemodynamically unstable. CR can depict foreign bodies, pneumopericardium, an enlarged heart figure, and mediastinal widening, as well as concomitant lung injuries (Gunn et al. 2014).

Cardiac US is the most established imaging method; it can be quickly performed and it is repeatable to monitor hemorrhage to establish an early and quick diagnosis of penetrating cardiac injury. Cardiac ultrasound can demonstrate hemorrhage to the pericardium with or without cardiac tamponade by a subxiphoid view. Ultrasound signs of cardiac tamponade include pericardial effusion, cardiac tamponade, and diastolic compression of the atrium due to the increased pericardial pressure, dilatation of the inferior vena cava, and right ventricular diastolic collapse (Gunn et al. 2014; Gunn 2012).

In a study of 225 patients, US showed a sensitivity of 100 %, a specificity 96 %, and accuracy was 97.3 %. The average time from fast ultrasound to surgery was 12.1 ± 5 min, highlighting the importance of early and fast ultrasound in this group of patients (Rozycki et al.).

MDCT is performed whenever possible; it can show directly the entry point and the wound track of projectile-specific organ injury findings. It allows for a thorough diagnosis of the mediastinal organs including the esophagus, trachea, and the arterial and venous system as well as direct heart and lung injuries. MDCT can locate the position of foreign bodies and allow for an assessment of active bleeding in imaging (Gunn et al. 2014; Gunn 2012).

MDCT is indicated in patients who are hemodynamically stable or who recompensate after fluid resuscitation. The detection of active bleeding is usually an immediate indication for surgical treatment. In subacute findings, patients can also be further evaluated by bronchoscopy and esophagography.

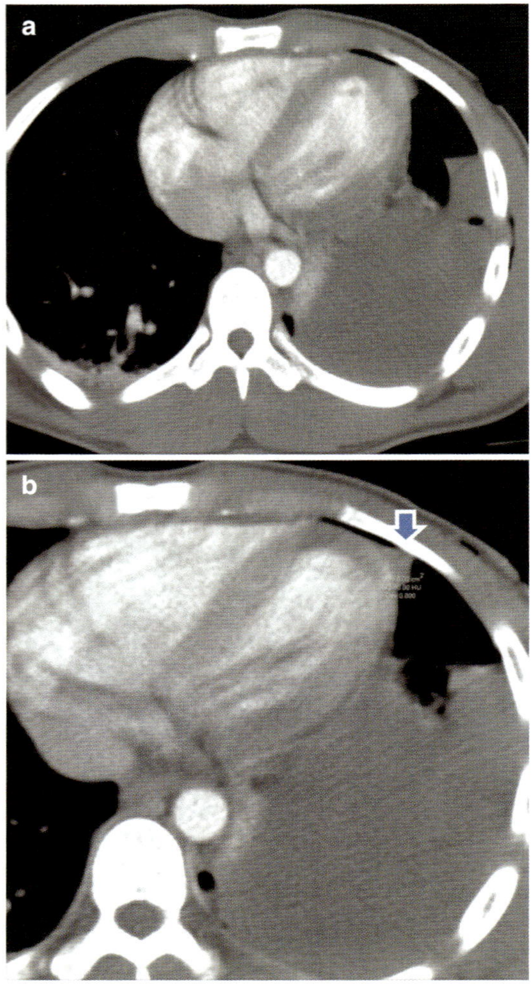

Fig. 11 Ungated MDCT of the heart, axial reconstructions. The figure shows (**a**) a stab wound to the left ventricle with perforation of the myocardium and (**b**) the bleeding site at the apex of the heart and a large left-sided hemopneumothorax (Images are courtesy of Professor Stuart Mirvis MD, University of Maryland, R Adams Cowley Shock Trauma Center, Baltimore, MD, USA ©)

Penetrating vascular injuries are located frequently in the ascending aortic arch and proximal great vessel. The mortality rate after penetrating aortic injury is 90–100 %. Patients typically undergo immediate surgery. MDCT findings include active vascular hemorrhage, formation of pseudoaneurysms, and vascular occlusions (Gunn 2012; Dosios et al. 2000). Gunn et al. recommend correlating all bullet entry points with the exit points and the number of visible bullets in the body (Gunn et al. 2014).

Projectiles can also embolize and transverse vascular structure and airways, the esophagus, and pleural cavity. Smaller projectiles have been reported to enter the aorta and embolize in the systemic circulation. Penetrating cardiac injury is often lethal, with mortality rates ranging from 3 to 81 % (Kang et al. 2009; Schmelzer et al. 1989). Again, the right heart is more prone to injury due to its anterior position.

MDCT has a reported sensitivity of 76.9 % and specificity of 99.7 % for penetrating cardiac injury where hemopericardium and pneumopericardium were observed as signs of injury; sensitivity is up to 100 %. MDCT can depict injuries to the coronary arteries, cardiac veins, valvular complex extravasation of blood, and mediastinal and lung injuries. There is evidence that MDCT is useful in the evaluation of penetrating cardiac injury (Figs. 11 and 12) (Gunn et al. 2014; Mollberg et al. 2012).

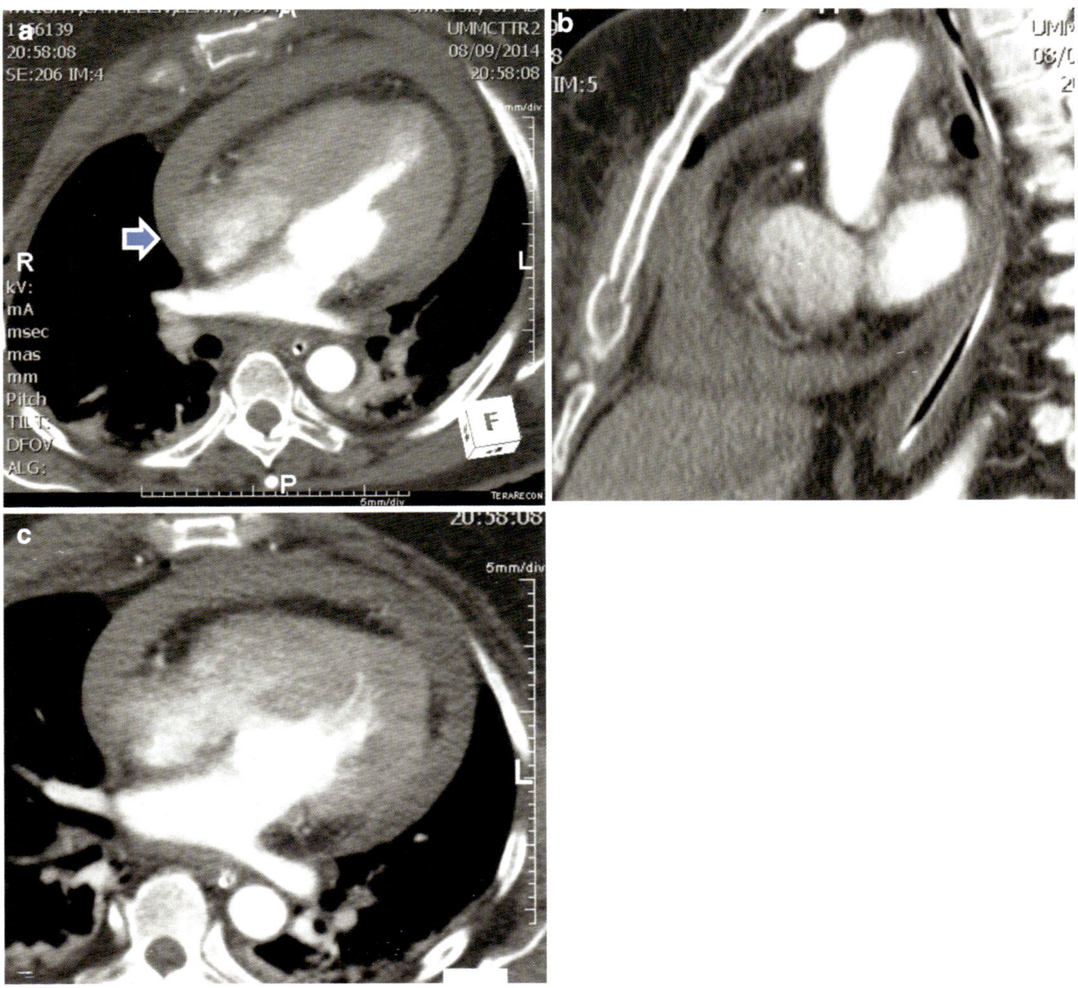

Fig. 12 Ungated MDCT of the heart, axial, and sagittal reconstructions. The figure shows (**a**, **c**) a stab wound through the sternum into the right ventricle with large pericardial hematoma and (**b**) active bleeding from the right ventricle and a heart compression by pericardial hemorrhage (Images are courtesy of Professor Stuart Mirvis MD, University of Maryland, R Adams Cowley Shock Trauma Center, Baltimore, MD, USA ©)

MR imaging has been used in stable patients to distinguish ventricular aneurysms for flow quantification of septal defects (Co et al. 2011; Plurad et al. 2013). Emergency thoracotomy should be performed in cases of prolonged resuscitation and a lack of response to volume therapy (Mattox et al. 2012).

5 Trauma Scoring

To date, no MDCT or imaging-based trauma score exists for the grading of cardiac injury.

To assess the severity of cardiac injury, clinical and anatomic parameters are evaluated, with various scoring systems in clinical practice. The most common is CVRS (cardiovascular-respiratory score), which is a predictor for the probability of survival and correlates with the severity of injury (Asensio et al. 1996; Asensio et al.). A further scoring system is the Organ Injury Scale developed by the AAST (American Association for the Surgery of Trauma), which provides a scaling of injury (severity scores) for individual organs (Table 4) (Mattox et al. 2012).

Associated injuries such as coronary artery dissections, active bleeding, and involvement of more than one heart chamber – or a delay in diagnosis and treatment – worsen the probability of survival (Table 5) (Mattox et al. 2012; Mattox et al.).

Table 4 Cardiac injury – cardiac injury organ scale

Grade I
Blunt cardiac injury with minor ECG abnormality (nonspecific ST- or T- wave changes, premature atrial or ventricular contraction or persistent sinus tachycardia)
Blunt or penetrating pericardial wound without cardiac injury, cardiac tamponade, or cardiac herniation
Grade II
Blunt cardiac injury with heart block or ischemic changes without cardiac failure
Penetrating tangential cardiac wound up to but not extending through the endocardium without tamponade
Grade III
Blunt cardiac injury with sustained or multifocal ventricular contractions
Blunt or penetrating cardiac injury with septal rupture, pulmonary or tricuspid incompetence, papillary muscle dysfunction, or distal coronary artery occlusion without cardiac failure
Blunt pericardial laceration with cardiac herniation
Blunt cardiac injury with cardiac failure
Penetrating tangential myocardial wound up to but not through the endocardium with tamponade
Grade IV
Blunt or penetrating cardiac injury with septal rupture, pulmonary or tricuspid incompetence, papillary muscle dysfunction, or distal coronary artery occlusion producing cardiac failure
Blunt or penetrating cardiac injury with aortic or mitral incompetence
Blunt or penetrating cardiac injury of the right ventricle, right or left atrium
Grade V
Blunt or penetrating cardiac injury with proximal coronary artery occlusion
Blunt or penetrating left ventricular perforation
Stellate injuries <50 % tissue loss of the right ventricle, right or left atrium
Grade VI
Blunt avulsion of the heart
Penetrating wound producing >50 % tissue loss of a chamber

Developed by the American Association for the Surgery of Trauma (AAST) (1994) (Mattox et al. 2012)

Table 5 Cardiac injury – concomitant injuries in multiple trauma

Pleural space: pneumothorax, hematothorax
Lungs: pulmonary contusion, pulmonary laceration, traumatic lung herniation
Mediastinum: pneumomediastinum
Airways: bronchial laceration, tracheal lacerations, Macklin effect
Esophagus tear
Thoracic vessels: injuries to the aorta, great thoracic vessels, and internal mammary artery
Diaphragm rupture
Chest wall: sternal, clavicular or rib fracture, flail chest, sternoclavicular dislocations
Fractures of the thoracic spine

References

Allen RP, Liedtke AJ (1979) The role of coronary artery injury and perfusion in the development of cardiac contusion secondary to nonpenetrating chest trauma. The Journal of trauma 19(3):153–156

Asensio JA, Berne JD, Demetriades D, Chan L, Murray J, Falabella A et al (1998) One hundred five penetrating cardiac injuries: a 2-year prospective evaluation. The Journal of trauma 44(6):1073–1082

Asensio JA, Stewart BM, Murray J, Fox AH, Falabella A, Gomez H et al (1996) Penetrating cardiac injuries. Surg Clin North Am 76(4):685–724

Bruschi G, Agati S, Iorio F, Vitali E (2001) Papillary muscle rupture and pericardial injuries after blunt chest trauma. European journal of cardio-thoracic surgery: official journal of the European Association for Cardio-thoracic Surgery 20(1):200–202

Cachecho R, Grindlinger GA, Lee VW (1992) The clinical significance of myocardial contusion. The Journal of trauma 33(1):68–71; discussion -3

Calhoon JH, Hoffmann TH, Trinkle JK, Harman PK, Grover FL (1986) Management of blunt rupture of the heart. The Journal of trauma 26(6):495–502

Co SJ, Yong-Hing CJ, Galea-Soler S, Ruzsics B, Schoepf UJ, Ajlan A et al (2011) Role of imaging in penetrating and blunt traumatic injury to the heart. Radiographics Rev Publ Radiol Soc N Am Inc 31(4):E101–E115

Demetriades D, van der Veen BW (1983) Penetrating injuries of the heart: experience over two years in South Africa. The Journal of trauma 23(12):1034–1041

Dosios TJ, Salemis N, Angouras D, Nonas E (2000) Blunt and penetrating trauma of the thoracic aorta and aortic arch branches: an autopsy study. J Trauma 49(4):696–703

El-Chami MF et al (2008) Blunt cardiac trauma. J Emerg Med 35:127–133

Elie MC (2006) Blunt cardiac injury. The Mount Sinai journal of medicine, New York 73(2):542–552

Embrey R (2007) Cardiac trauma. Thoracic surgery clinics 17(1):87–93, vii

Fabian TC, Cicala RS, Croce MA, Westbrook LL, Coleman PA, Minard G et al (1991) A prospective evaluation of myocardial contusion: correlation of significant arrhythmias and cardiac output with CPK-MB measurements. J Trauma 31(5):653–659; discussion 9–60

Farhataziz N, Landay MJ (2005) Pericardial rupture after blunt chest trauma. J Thorac imag 20(1):50–52

Fulda G, Brathwaite CE, Rodriguez A, Turney SZ, Dunham CM, Cowley RA (1991) Blunt traumatic rupture of the heart and pericardium: a ten-year experience (1979-1989). J Trauma 31(2):167–172; discussion 72–73

Gasparri MG, Lorelli DR, Kralovich KA, Patton JH, Jr (2000) Physical examination plus chest radiography in penetrating periclavicular trauma: the appropriate trigger for angiography. J Trauma 49(6):1029–1033

Ghersin E, Khoury A, Litmanovich D, Lorber A, Halberthal M, Engel A et al (2005) Comprehensive multidetector computed tomography assessment of severe cardiac contusion in a pediatric patient: correlation with echocardiography. J Comput Assist Tomo 29(6):739–741

Gunn ML (2012) Imaging of aortic and branch vessel trauma. Radiol Clin North Am 50(1):85–103

Gunn ML, Clark RT, Sadro CT, Linnau KF, Sandstrom CK (2014) Current concepts in imaging evaluation of penetrating transmediastinal injury. Radiographics Rev Publ Radiol Soc N Am Inc 34(7):1824–1841

Kan CD, Yang YJ (2005) Traumatic aortic and mitral valve injury following blunt chest injury with a variable clinical course. Heart (British Cardiac Society) 91(5):568–570

Kang N, Hsee L, Rizoli S, Alison P (2009) Penetrating cardiac injury: overcoming the limits set by nature. Injury 40(9):919–927

Kato S, Nagata Y, Ota T, Sahara T, Kato R, Tsuchioka H (1988) Successful repair of right atrial rupture due to nonpenetrating trauma of the chest. Kyobu Geka Jpn J Thorac Surg 41(11):913–915

Kaye P, O'Sullivan I (2002) Myocardial contusion: emergency investigation and diagnosis. Emergency medicine journal EMJ 19(1):8–10

Korner M, Reiser M, Linsenmaier U (2009) Imaging of trauma with multi-detector computed tomography. Radiologe 49(6):510–515
Lee H, Ruzsics B, Schoepf UJ, Stewart EA, Costello P, Glenn JL et al (2009) New-onset heart failure caused by spontaneous papillary muscle rupture: diagnosis with dual-source computed tomographic coronary angiography. J Thorac Cardiovasc Surg 137(1):e19–21
Linsenmaier U, Krotz M, Hauser H, Rock C, Rieger J, Bohndorf K et al (2002) Whole-body computed tomography in polytrauma: techniques and management. Eur Radiol 12(7):1728–1740
Mattox KL, Beall AC Jr, Jordan GL Jr, De Bakey ME. Cardiorrhaphy in the emergency center. (0022–5223 (Print))
Mattox KL, Flint LM, Carrico CJ, Grover F, Meredith J, Morris J et al (1992) Blunt cardiac injury. J Trauma 33(5):649–650
Mattox KL, Moore EE, Feliciano DV (2012) Trauma, 7th edn. McGraw Hill, New York
McLean RF, Devitt JH, Dubbin J, McLellan BA (1991) Incidence of abnormal RNA studies and dysrhythmias in patients with blunt chest trauma. J Trauma 31(7):968–970
Mirvis SE (2004) Diagnostic imaging of acute thoracic injury. Seminars in ultrasound, CT, and MR 25(2):156–179
Mollberg NM, Wise SR, De Hoyos AL, Lin FJ, Merlotti G, Massad MG (2012) Chest computed tomography for penetrating thoracic trauma after normal screening chest roentgenogram. Ann Thorac Surg 93(6):1830–1835
Moront M, Lefrak EA, Akl BF (1991) Traumatic rupture of the interventricular septum and tricuspid valve: case report. J Trauma 31(1):134–136
Orliaguet G, Ferjani M, Riou B (2001) The heart in blunt trauma. DCOM- 20010830(0003–3022 (Print))
Parmley LF, Manion WC, Mattingly TW (1958) Nonpenetrating traumatic injury of the heart. Circulation 18(3):371–396
Patton AS, Guyton SW, Lawson DW, Shannon JM (1981) Treatment os severe atrial injuries. Am J Surg 141(4):465–471
Plurad DS, Bricker S, Van Natta TL, Neville A, Kim D, Bongard F et al (2013) Penetrating cardiac injury and the significance of chest computed tomography findings. Emerg Radiol 20(4):279–284
Pretre R, Chilcott M. Blunt trauma to the heart and great vessels. (0028–4793 (Print))
Restrepo CS, Lemos DF, Lemos JA, Velasquez E, Diethelm L, Ovella TA et al (2007) Imaging findings in cardiac tamponade with emphasis on CT. Radiographics Rev Publ Radiol Soc N Am Inc 27(6):1595–1610
Restrepo CS, Gutierrez FR, Marmol-Velez JA, Ocazionez D, Martinez-Jimenez S (2012) Imaging patients with cardiac trauma. Radiographics Rev Publ Radiol Soc N Am Inc 32(3):633–649
Rozycki GS, Feliciano DV, Schmidt JA, Cushman JG, Sisley AC, Ingram W et al (1996) The role of surgeon-performed ultrasound in patients with possible cardiac wounds. Annals of surgery 223(6):737–744; discussion 44–46
Schmelzer V, Mendez-Picon G, Gervin AS (1989) Case report: transthoracic retrograde venous bullet embolization. J Trauma 29(4):525–527
Sheikh M, Ben-Nakhi A, Shukkur AM, Sinan T, Al-Rashdan I (2009) Accuracy of 64-multidetector-row computed tomography in the diagnosis of coronary artery disease. Medical principles and practice: International journal of the Kuwait University, Health Science Centre 18(4):323–328
Symbas PN (1991) Cardiothoracic trauma. Current problems in surgery 28(11):741–797
Symbas PN. Traumatic heart disease. (0146–2806 (Print))
Tenzer ML (1985) The spectrum of myocardial contusion: a review. J Trauma 25(7):620–627
The American Association for the Surgery of Trauma (1994) Injury scoring scales. http://www.aast.org/library/traumatools/injuryscoringscales.aspx
Thourani VH, Feliciano DV, Cooper WA, Brady KM, Adams AB, Rozycki GS et al (1999) Penetrating cardiac trauma at an urban trauma center: a 22-year perspective. The American surgeon 65(9):811–816; discussion 7–8
Van Horn JM (2007) A case study of right ventricular rupture in an elderly victim of motor vehicle crash: incorporating end-of-life care into trauma nursing. J Trauma Nurs Off J Soc Trauma Nurses 14(3):136–143
Wall MJ Jr, Mattox KL, Chen CD, Baldwin JC (1997) Acute management of complex cardiac injuries. J Trauma 42(5):905–912
Zoni A, Arisi A, Corradi D, Ardissino D (2003) Images in cardiovascular medicine. Magnetic resonance imaging of impending left ventricular rupture after acute myocardial infarction. Circulation 108(4):498–499

Traumatic Diaphragmatic Injuries

A. Olsen, R. Nicola, C. Raptis, and M. Patlas

Contents

A. Olsen, DO • R. Nicola, MS DO
Department of Imaging Science, Division of Emergency Imaging, University of Rochester, 601 Elmwood Ave, Rochester, NY 14642, USA
e-mail: refky_nicola@urmc.rochester.edu

C. Raptis, MD
Mallinckrodt Institute of Radiology, Washington University School of Medicine, 510 S Kings highway Blvd, Campus Box 8131, St Louis, MO 63110, USA

M. Patlas, MD (✉)
Division of Emergency/Trauma Radiology, Department of Radiology, McMaster University, 237 Barton Street East, Hamilton, ON, Canada
e-mail: patlas@HHSC.CA

Abstract

Diaphragmatic injuries are uncommon injuries in the chest, thus they can easily be missed by the radiologist and surgeon. Therefore, a high index of suspicion is important for an early diagnosis and to avoid any complications. Multidetector computed tomography is the modality of choice for the diaphragmatic injuries. On MDCT, there are direct and indirect signs of diaphragmatic injuries. In this chapter we discuss the findings associated with blunt as well as penetrating diaphragmatic injuries with an emphasis on the role of the radiologist in making the diagnosis.

1 Introduction

Traumatic injuries to the diaphragm are caused by blunt or penetrating trauma, either to the chest or abdominal wall. Regardless of the etiology, these injuries require treatment to avoid the serious complications of obstruction or strangulation of herniated viscera. As nonoperative management

Med Radiol Diagn Imaging (2016)
DOI 10.1007/174_2016_42, © Springer International Publishing Switzerland

increases and fewer initially occult cases of diaphragmatic injury are diagnosed intraoperatively, the imaging diagnosis of these injuries has become increasingly more important (Fair et al. 2015). Despite the importance of recognizing these injuries, detecting diaphragmatic injuries is still a diagnostic challenge for many radiologists and trauma surgeons (Reber et al. 1998; Hanna et al. 2008).

Penetrating diaphragmatic injuries are commonly caused by gunshot or stab wounds. There is no definite predilection for the side of diaphragmatic injury among victims of gunshot wounds (Patlas et al. 2015). Serious injuries from stab wounds are more common on the left than on the right, which is probably due to protective effect from the liver on the right hemidiaphragm, a greater proportion of right-handed assailants, and a relative underdiagnosis of subtle right diaphragmatic injuries (Patlas et al. 2015).

Surgery has long played a significant role in the management of patients presenting with penetrating thoracoabdominal injuries; however, selective nonoperative management is increasingly recommended for these patients, with good outcomes in the setting of both blunt and penetrating traumas (Croce et al. 1995; Iochum et al. 2002; Como et al. 2010; Dreizin et al. 2015). There is a growing trend for conservative management of blunt traumatic patients. As nonoperative management of traumatic patients increases, it is possible that some diaphragmatic injuries which were once only identified intraoperatively will only be detected radiologically or after complications of diaphragmatic injury arise. This trend in the shift of the management strategy will require a need for greater vigilance by radiologists for subtle signs of diaphragmatic injury.

The radiologic detection of diaphragmatic injuries is difficult because many physicians are unfamiliar with the scope of diaphragmatic injuries and their imaging findings (Hanna et al. 2008; Desir and Ghaye 2012). Many imaging signs have been described for the detection of these injuries; however, some patients present with only one or a few of the many known signs. As such, being familiar with the radiologic signs of diaphragmatic injury is essential for the practicing radiologist, especially in the emergency setting.

Frequently, significant or life-threatening thoracic and abdominal injuries can distract the radiologist from the more subtle findings of diaphragmatic injuries. The key to a successful radiologic diagnosis of diaphragmatic injury is to have a high degree of suspicion based on clinical setting and to develop a familiarity with the classic imaging findings of traumatic diaphragmatic injury (Guth et al. 1995).

Although some animal models suggest spontaneous healing of small diaphragmatic defects, there are no published reports of a human diaphragmatic injury healing without surgery (Shatney et al. 2003; Desir and Ghaye 2012). Physiologic negative intrathoracic pressures during unassisted ventilation and the constant motion of the diaphragm likely impede healing of diaphragmatic injuries and can result in delayed herniation of intra-abdominal contents (Desir and Ghaye 2012). In cases of missed diaphragmatic injury, reports indicate potential for delayed complications of visceral herniation with potential for obstruction or strangulation, with mortality of approximately 30–60 % in cases of visceral strangulation (Murray et al. 1996; Desir and Ghaye 2012; Panda et al. 2014; Dreizin et al. 2015). Therefore, it is essential that these injuries be detected as early as possible.

2 Anatomic and Developmental Considerations

The diaphragm is a thin musculotendinous sheet with a concave undersurface and apertures allowing passage of transdiaphragmatic structures. The largest of these are the hiatuses of the inferior vena cava, esophagus, and aorta. The caval hiatus is located at the T8–T9 intervertebral disk level to the right of the central tendon. The inferior vena cava is adherent to its margin (Standring 2016). The esophageal hiatus is at the level of the tenth vertebral body. The esophagus is not directly continuous with the muscle of the esophageal hiatus (Standring 2016). The aortic hiatus is an osseo-aponeurotic aperture at the lower level of the twelfth vertebral body, passing outside of the diaphragmatic muscle fibers adjacent to the vertebral column, and is not affected by their contraction (Standring 2016).

Congenital areas of weakness may be present between diaphragmatic muscle fibers that insert on the sternum and the ribs (sternocostal triangles) and between the fibers that insert on the ribs and the lumbar vertebrae (lumbocostal triangles). These areas of weakness are likely responsible for non-traumatic Morgagni and Bochdalek hernias (Thomas Sadler et al. 2003). In addition, the interface between the embryologic septum transversum (originating anteriorly) and the pleuroperitoneal folds corresponds to potential areas of inherent weakness in the posterolateral diaphragm, which may be predisposed to rupture in the setting of high-energy abdominal trauma (Desir and Ghaye 2012).

3 Mechanism of Injury

In the USA, penetrating diaphragmatic injuries are twice as common as blunt diaphragmatic injuries (Fair et al. 2015). Penetrating injuries are due to knife and gunshot wounds and tend to result in smaller diaphragmatic injuries, typically on the order of 1 or 2 cm in length (Iochum et al. 2002; Desir and Ghaye 2012). The small size of the corresponding diaphragmatic defect may also lead to difficulty directly appreciating these injuries on imaging studies (Desir and Ghaye 2012). Because of the small size of defects generally seen in penetrating diaphragmatic injuries, herniation of abdominal contents is uncommon after penetrating diaphragmatic injury (Dreizin et al. 2015). Penetrating injuries may injure any organs or structures in line with the trajectory of the wound and as such may vary widely in distribution (Iochum et al. 2002) but commonly involve liver and hollow viscus (Fair et al. 2015).

Penetrating diaphragmatic injuries from stabbings occur more frequently on the left than the right (Patlas et al. 2015). This is theorized to result from the higher number of right-handed assailants who face their victim at the time of injury (Panda et al. 2014). Another factor that may contribute to the relative frequency of left-sided penetrating diaphragmatic injuries is the protection which the liver provides and whose absence on the left results in areas of weakness in the left hemidiaphragm (Panda et al. 2014).

Blunt diaphragmatic injuries are most commonly the result of motor vehicle accidents, but other causes include falls and severe blows to the body. It has been proposed that multiple mechanisms of injury may be involved in a blunt diaphragmatic injury, which may be differentiated by the direction of greatest impact at the time of injury. A frontal impact on the abdomen is proposed to increase intra-abdominal pressure, resulting in subsequent upward force from intra-abdominal contents moving toward the relatively low-pressure thorax (Iochum et al. 2002; Desir and Ghaye 2012). Lateral impacts have been proposed to injure the diaphragm through shear forces (Iochum et al. 2002; Desir and Ghaye 2012). Other factors such as fractured ribs or the phase of the respiratory cycle may also play a role in the mechanism of blunt diaphragmatic injury (Rees et al. 2005; Desir and Ghaye 2012). In contrast to the small size of penetrating diaphragmatic injuries, blunt diaphragmatic injuries tend to be large (>10 cm) (Iochum et al. 2002). Perhaps not surprisingly, left hemidiaphragmatic injuries are associated with splenic injuries, and right hemidiaphragmatic injuries are associated with hepatic injuries.

Diaphragmatic injury will essentially never occur in isolation. Penetrating diaphragmatic injuries are associated with liver injury (53.6 %), splenic injury (29.1 %), pulmonary injury (28.1 %), stomach injury (26.6 %), hemothorax (26.2 %), and pneumothorax (20.4 %) (Fair et al. 2015). Blunt diaphragmatic injuries are associated with pulmonary injury (48.7 %), splenic injury (44.8 %), liver injury (39.7 %), pneumothorax (30 %), and hemothorax (21.5 %) (Fair et al. 2015). Other injuries commonly associated with blunt diaphragmatic injury include renal, aortic, cardiac, and osseous injuries, such as spinal, pelvic, and rib fractures (Iochum et al. 2002; Desir and Ghaye 2012; Fair et al. 2015). The coincident injuries seen in association with blunt diaphragmatic injury, for instance, result in mortality of approximately 12–42 % (Iochum et al. 2002; Desir and Ghaye 2012).

The proportion of left-sided to right-sided diaphragmatic injuries is higher after blunt trauma with frontal impact; however, relative numbers of right and left diaphragmatic injury are similar after posterior impacts (Desir and Ghaye 2012). Side impacts typically result in injury on the side of impact (Desir and Ghaye 2012). The increased frequency of left-sided blunt diaphragmatic injuries is attributed to the protective effect of the liver on the right hemidiaphragm and the vulnerability of an unprotected area of congenital weakness of the left diaphragm (Desir and Ghaye 2012). Some of the difference in frequency of left and right injuries may also be due to underdiagnosis of subtle right-sided injuries (Killeen et al. 1999; Patlas et al. 2015). The left hemidiaphragm runs next to abdominal fat that makes its contour more visible, while the right hemidiaphragm may be difficult to distinguish from the higher-attenuation hepatic parenchyma (Killeen et al. 1999; Iochum et al. 2002; Desir and Ghaye 2012).

4 Epidemiology

The relative frequency of penetrating and blunt diaphragmatic injuries varies, with significantly higher numbers of penetrating injuries seen in several large studies (Hammer et al. 2014; Fair et al. 2015; Gao et al. 2015). Some smaller studies have included a greater number of blunt diaphragmatic injuries than penetrating diaphragmatic injuries, which may be due to their small sample size or possibly because the frequency of gunshot wounds and stabbings is proportionally lower in their study populations (Panda et al. 2014; Leung et al. 2015).

Penetrating diaphragmatic injuries are more common among young men, with males making up 91.4 % of cases in the USA (Fair et al. 2015). The average age of US patients diagnosed with penetrating diaphragmatic injuries is 31 years (standard deviation of 13 years) (Fair et al. 2015). The relatively high proportion of men presenting with penetrating diaphragmatic injury is probably due to the fact that men are more likely than women to be involved in stabbings and shootings (Hanna et al. 2008). Penetrating diaphragmatic injuries are reported in 10–42 % of penetrating thoracoabdominal traumas (Spann et al. 1995; Bodanapally et al. 2009; Yucel et al. 2015).

Blunt diaphragmatic injuries are also more common among men (Fair et al. 2015). Men comprised 67.9 % of blunt diaphragmatic injuries in a recent study of over 3700 diaphragmatic injuries in the USA, with an average age of 44 years (standard deviation of 19 years). Blunt thoracoabdominal trauma results in diaphragmatic injury in 0.8–8.0 % of cases (Iochum et al. 2002; Desir and Ghaye 2012). When compared to patients with penetrating diaphragmatic injuries, patients with blunt diaphragmatic injuries have longer stays in intensive care, longer ventilator requirements, and higher mortality (19.8 % vs. 8.8 %) (Fair et al. 2015).

5 Radiographic Evaluation

Even with the increasing use of MDCT imaging, first-line trauma imaging is usually a portable chest radiograph. There are numerous limitations of chest radiographs such as lack of patient cooperation, the use of portable equipment, and suboptimal patient positioning (Iochum et al. 2002). Despite these factors, initial radiographic evaluation may successfully render a diagnosis of diaphragmatic injury. The sensitivity of initial radiographs has a wide range of reported values, from 17 to 65 % (Iochum et al. 2002; Patlas et al. 2015). The reported sensitivity of chest radiograph for right-sided diaphragmatic injuries (approximately 17 %) is lower than for left-sided injuries (approximately 27–60 %) (Iochum et al. 2002).

The most valuable signs of diaphragmatic rupture seen on chest radiography are definite visualization of abdominal viscera above the diaphragm (with or without a focal constriction of herniated viscera as they pass through the violated diaphragm, the collar sign) and visualization of the tip of a nasogastric tube above the diaphragm (Gelman et al. 1991; Desir and Ghaye 2012). The sensitivity for an NG tube crossing the left diaphragm on chest radiograph has a sensitivity of approximately 44–64 % (Gelman et al. 1991; Guth et al. 1995).

Another finding that is highly suggestive of diaphragmatic injury is the unexplained elevation of a hemidiaphragm. In the setting of blunt abdominal trauma, a 4 cm elevation of either hemidiaphragm is correlated with injury to that hemidiaphragm; however, some authors suggest a higher cutoff of 6 cm from the contralateral diaphragm (Gelman et al. 1991; Guth et al. 1995; Desir and Ghaye 2012).

Unfortunately, most patients with a traumatic diaphragmatic injury present with nonspecific findings on chest radiography, such as obscured outline of the injured hemidiaphragm, mild elevation of the affected hemidiaphragm, mediastinal shift to the contralateral side, and sequela of trauma such as effusions, pneumothorax, or rib fractures (Gelman et al. 1991; Guth et al. 1995; Desir and Ghaye 2012, Patlas, Leung et al. 2015).

If a patient cannot be imaged by CT (either because their condition is too unstable to allow transport to the scanner or due to a lack of availability of CT scanning), serial chest radiographs may be useful, especially after extubation (Gao et al. 2015). Because of the artificially increased intrathoracic pressures while undergoing positive pressure ventilation, herniation of intra-abdominal contents into the thorax may be delayed or prevented until after extubation. For this reason, comparison between radiographs should be made from before and after cessation of positive pressure ventilation when possible in patients unable to be imaged by CT (Gao et al. 2015).

Although chest radiographs may be diagnostic for diaphragmatic injuries, they are generally inferior to CT images in their evaluation, with sensitivity not greater than 65 % (Gelman et al. 1991; Patlas et al. 2015). One potential pitfall in the diagnosis of diaphragmatic injuries by chest radiography is a normal-appearing (false-negative) radiograph in the setting of acute diaphragmatic injury, which may be present in 15 % of patients presenting with diaphragmatic rupture (Guth et al. 1995).

Differential considerations must be kept in mind when nonspecific findings are present in the setting of acute thoracoabdominal trauma. Congenital hernias can also mimic traumatic herniation. Eventration of abdominal contents into the thoracic cavity can be mistaken for an acute finding if not recognized as nontraumatic. Other differential considerations for subtle abnormalities on chest radiographs may include atelectasis, pleural effusion, hemothorax, pulmonary contusion, pulmonary laceration, or phrenic nerve palsy (Gelman et al. 1991; Guth et al. 1995; Iochum et al. 2002).

6 CT Evaluation

Evaluation with MDCT is increasingly common, as are powerful workstations which allow review of reformatted images in a timelier manner. The maturation of CT technology, including MDCT, has improved CT scan sensitivity for blunt diaphragmatic injury from approximately 60 % with conventional CT scans to 77–100 % with MDCT, with MDCT specificity of approximately 93–98 % (Desser et al. 2010; Magu et al. 2012). The sensitivity of MDCT for penetrating diaphragmatic injuries is approximately 73–100 %, with specificity of approximately 50–92 % (Bodanapally et al. 2009; Dreizin et al. 2015).

7 CT Signs of Blunt Diaphragmatic Injury

Regarding blunt diaphragmatic rupture, Desir and Ghaye have classified signs into three groups: direct, indirect, and signs of uncertain or controversial origin (Desir and Ghaye 2012). Signs of blunt diaphragmatic injuries are described below using this classification.

Direct signs of blunt diaphragmatic rupture include the following:

- *Visualized diaphragmatic defect* – A visualized defect of the diaphragm may demonstrate muscular retraction and thickening of diaphragmatic muscular fibers near the defect. A diaphragmatic injury is most easily visualized directly when air or fat abuts the diaphragm. This sign's reported sensitivity and specificity range from approximately 17 to 90% and 90 to 100%, respectively, in the setting of blunt trauma (Desir and Ghaye 2012; Hammer et al. 2014):
  - *Pitfalls*: Eventration of the diaphragm may make the diaphragm imperceptible in some individuals (Desser et al. 2010). Fluid or soft tissue attenuation material (hemothorax, pleural effusion, ascites, lung consolidation, etc.) in contact with the diaphragm may obscure a true diaphragmatic injury; however, this may be less common when scanned by MDCT with a greater number

of detectors (Chen et al. 2010; Patlas et al. 2015). Additionally, approximately 6% of asymptomatic adults will have evidence of nontraumatic diaphragmatic defects, which mimic a focal injury in the setting of acute trauma (Iochum et al. 2002).

- *Dangling diaphragm sign* (Desser et al. 2010) – The appearance of this sign overlaps with visualization of a diaphragmatic defect, as described above. This less commonly described sign refers to visualization of the free edge of the torn diaphragm curling inwards on itself, which appears as a comma-shaped soft tissue structure. Thickening of this free flap of the diaphragm has also been reported. Sensitivity and specificity of the dangling diaphragm sign are reported as 54 and 98%, respectively (Desser et al. 2010):
  - *Pitfalls*: This sign's pitfalls are similar to those of the visualized diaphragmatic defect.
- *Absent diaphragm* – The diaphragm may be absent in the area of a diaphragmatic injury. When the diaphragm or a portion of the diaphragm is not visualized after acute injury, abdominal contents are commonly herniated. Absence of the visualized diaphragm has a reported sensitivity and specificity of 18–43% and 91%, respectively (Desir and Ghaye 2012):
  - *Pitfalls*: This sign's pitfalls are similar to those of the visualized diaphragmatic defect.

Indirect signs of blunt diaphragmatic rupture may be the only evidence to suggest a blunt diaphragmatic injury:

- *Herniation through a defect* – Herniation of abdominal contents into the abdomen may occur in the setting of trauma or as the result of either congenital or acquired diaphragmatic hernias. Abdominal contents may herniate into either the pleural or, less likely, the pericardial space. Reported sensitivity of herniated abdominal contents after blunt trauma is higher on the left than on the right (42–91% on the left, 8–50% on the right), while specificity is reportedly at 98–100% (Desir and Ghaye 2012):
  - *Pitfalls*: Diaphragmatic hernias (e.g., Bochdalek or Morgagni hernias) are potential mimics of this sign, especially if prior imaging is not available to demonstrate the stable nature of the hernia.
- *Collar sign* – This sign refers to a waist-like band constricting herniated abdominal contents as they pass from the abdomen to the thoracic cavity through the sometimes-not-visualized diaphragmatic defect. This sign may be best appreciated on reformatted sagittal or coronal images. Overall sensitivity and specificity for blunt diaphragmatic injury are reported as 44–63% and 98–100%, respectively, with sensitivity lower on the right (50%) than on the left (78%) (Killeen et al. 1999):
  - *Pitfalls*: Prior trauma or diaphragmatic slips may result in atypical contours of abdominal organs and may be mistaken for a collar sign (Desir and Ghaye 2012). The collar sign may also be present in congenital or acquired hernias. Motion artifact has caused an artifactually narrowed appearance of upper abdominal organs and the diaphragm, though this motion artifact is less likely with faster scan times.
- *Hump and band signs* – These signs are a subset of the collar sign, primarily used in evaluating the right diaphragm. The "hump" being referenced is a focal outpouching of the liver which has herniated above the injured right diaphragm. The "band" refers to an area of hypoattenuation within the liver at the level of the diaphragmatic defect on contrast-enhanced studies (Rees et al. 2005). It is hypothesized that compression from the rim of the damaged diaphragm results in a rim of relative hypoperfusion of the liver at the site of herniation (Rees et al. 2005). Both the hump and band signs are best appreciated on coronal and sagittal reformatted images. While specificity for these signs has not been determined, sensitivity of the hump sign is reported to be 50–83%, and sensitivity of the band sign is reported to be 33–42% (Rees et al. 2005; Chen et al. 2010):
  - *Pitfalls*: Similar to the collar sign, prior hepatic laceration or fracture or diaphragmatic slips may be mistaken for a positive

hump sign (Desir and Ghaye 2012). Also, because of their subtle nature when compared to the collar sign, these signs may be missed if only axial views are reviewed. They are more apparent on sagittal and coronal reformatted images. A congenitally high right hemidiaphragm may also mimic a hump sign.

- *Dependent viscera sign* – When supine, the left hemidiaphragm normally suspends the stomach, spleen, and bowel above the posterior chest wall, while the right hemidiaphragm normally suspends the liver away from the posterior chest wall, each separated by posteroinferior portions of the lungs. When abdominal viscera are herniated into the pleural space, this support is no longer present, and the herniated abdominal contents can fall against the posterior chest wall (Cantwell 2006). In the setting of blunt trauma, sensitivity for this sign is reported as 54–90 %, with a reported specificity of practically 100 % (Bergin et al. 2001; Desser et al. 2010; Desir and Ghaye 2012):
  - *Pitfalls*: Patients with congenital or hiatal hernias may demonstrate this sign without acute injury. This sign has been reported to have a low sensitivity for small ruptures, atypically configured or anteriorly located ruptures or when pleural effusion is present (Bergin et al. 2001; Cantwell 2006; Desir and Ghaye 2012).
- *Abdominal contents peripheral to the diaphragm or lung* – When the normal contour of the diaphragm is well visualized, abdominal contents may be seen outside this contour. If abdominal contents are seen outside the normal contour of the diaphragm, they will have herniated into the thoracic cavity. Sensitivity and specificity are not reported for this sign (Desir and Ghaye 2012):
  - *Pitfalls*: In the unlikely situation that the diaphragm was inverted (such as from a large effusion), this relationship may be abnormal (Desir and Ghaye 2012).
- *Elevated abdominal organs* – Because many processes may result in discrepancies of the apparent heights of the right and left hemidiaphragm, unilateral elevation of abdominal organs into the thoracic cavity is insufficient to diagnose diaphragmatic rupture. When seen in conjunction with other features suggesting diaphragmatic rupture, elevation of abdominal organs into the thoracic cavity may help reassure the correct diagnosis. Although other values have also been suggested, a significant correlation has been shown between a 4 cm elevation of the right relative to the left hemidiaphragm and right-sided rupture. Overall sensitivity and specificity for a 4 cm diaphragmatic asymmetry are reported to be 50–83 % and 89–99 %, respectively (Desir and Ghaye 2012):
  - *Pitfalls*: Mimics of this sign may include phrenic nerve injury, atelectasis, or subpulmonic effusion.
- *Concomitant pneumothorax with pneumoperitoneum or hemothorax with hemoperitoneum* – With the presence of either air or blood in both the thoracic and abdominal cavities, one should strongly consider diaphragmatic injury in the setting of trauma. Effusion or ascites may also pass between the thoracic and abdominal cavities in the setting of a damaged diaphragm (Desir and Ghaye 2012):
  - *Pitfalls*: It may be difficult to prove that the combination of pneumothorax with pneumoperitoneum or hemothorax with hemoperitoneum does not represent synchronous injuries within both cavities (Desir and Ghaye 2012).

Signs of uncertain or controversial origin:

- *Thickening of the diaphragm* – Muscular fibers of the diaphragm may retract and thicken after diaphragmatic injury. The thickening of the diaphragm can vary in appearance, and no standard measurements for diaphragmatic thickness are established. In the setting of blunt diaphragmatic injury, overall sensitivity has been reported as 56–75 %, and specificity is reported to be approximately 95 % (Desir and Ghaye 2012):
  - *Pitfalls*: The diaphragm may be congenitally thickened due to unequal distribution of muscular fibers during embryologic migration. Additionally, blood or fluid

accumulated near the diaphragm such as a retroperitoneal hematoma may mimic thickening of the diaphragm and incorrectly suggest a diaphragmatic injury (Nchimi et al. 2005; Desir and Ghaye 2012).

- *Diaphragmatic and peridiaphragmatic extravasation of contrast* – Arterial contrast extravasation from the diaphragm is highly specific for diaphragmatic injury. Although sensitivity is low (reported between 0 and 12 %), specificity is reported between 93 and 98 % (Nchimi et al. 2005; Desser et al. 2010):
  - *Pitfalls*: This sign is nonspecific because extravasation of contrast can be difficult to localize to the diaphragm (and to exclude bleeding of adjacent organs) (Desir and Ghaye 2012).
- *Fractured rib or ribs* – Rib fractures can suggest injury to the diaphragm by their size, position, and location. The relative location of a rib fragment may indicate it has crossed the surface of the adjacent diaphragm. Sensitivity and specificity of rib fractures in diagnosing diaphragmatic injury are unknown (Desir and Ghaye 2012).

8 CT Signs of Penetrating Diaphragmatic Injury

In the setting of penetrating trauma, contiguous injury to organs above and below the diaphragm is the most useful and accurate sign, with sensitivity and specificity of 82–100 % and 82–83 %, respectively (Bodanapally et al. 2009; Panda et al. 2014; Dreizin et al. 2015).

Direct visualization of a diaphragmatic defect in the setting of penetrating trauma has a broad range of reported sensitivities (7–100 %) (Panda et al. 2014; Dreizin et al. 2015); however, specificity is consistently high, reported in the range of 90–100 % (Bodanapally et al. 2009; Dreizin et al. 2015).

Thickening of the diaphragm near the area of penetrating injury, presumably due to retraction of muscle fibers from the site of injury, has a reported sensitivity of approximately 48–83 %, with specificity reported near 70 % (Bodanapally et al. 2009; Panda et al. 2014).

Although penetrating diaphragmatic injuries typically result in small diaphragmatic defects, a penetrating injury may result in a large diaphragmatic defect based on its trajectory. Any of the signs related to the larger blunt diaphragmatic injuries can be seen in the setting of a large defect. Because of this, signs related to herniation (collar sign, dependent viscera sign, herniation of abdominal contents into the thoracic cavity) tend to have low sensitivities and high specificities in the setting of penetrating trauma, as discussed below.

The collar sign also has low sensitivity in the range of 0–24 %, with specificity reported near 100 % (Bodanapally et al. 2009; Panda et al. 2014; Dreizin et al. 2015).

The dependent viscera sign may theoretically be seen in large defects associated with penetrating trauma, but was not reported in two recent studies (Bodanapally et al. 2009; Dreizin et al. 2015).

Sensitivity of herniation of abdominal fat or viscera into the thoracic cavity in the setting of penetrating trauma is approximately 7–17 %, and specificity approaches 100 % (Bodanapally et al. 2009; Patlas et al. 2015).

Concurrent hemothorax and hemoperitoneum have a sensitivity of 50 % and a specificity of 95 % for penetrating abdominal injuries (Nchimi et al. 2005).

The reported sensitivity for the dangling diaphragm sign is 0–17 %, without reported specificity (Panda et al. 2014; Dreizin et al. 2015). In describing the dangling diaphragm sign, Desser et al. acknowledged that it would be less likely in penetrating trauma (Desser et al. 2010).

Active extravasation of contrast in or along the diaphragm has a sensitivity of 8 % and a specificity of 100 % (Dreizin et al. 2015).

9 Additional Pitfalls in CT Imaging

Although herniation of intra-abdominal contents is not needed to diagnose diaphragmatic injury, it does represent a potential complication of both blunt and penetrating diaphragmatic injuries. As was previously mentioned, herniation of abdominal viscera into the thoracic cavity can be prevented or delayed due to positive pressure ventilation. Positive pressure ventilator assistance is commonly needed as part of the supportive measures implemented after major trauma.

Additionally, herniation or eventration of abdominal organs such as the liver, spleen, or bowel through a thinned diaphragm may mimic a traumatic injury and should be correlated to prior imaging if available (Iochum et al. 2002). In cases of eventration, close examination of the margins of the diaphragm may demonstrate a faint line that corresponds to the thinned diaphragm overlying the eventrated organs.

10 MRI Evaluation

The use of MRI in an acute trauma setting is usually impractical because of patient hemodynamic instability and resuscitative medical equipment incompatibility. MRI can be successfully used in cases of equivocal initial imaging in hemodynamically stable patients, late presentation of a diaphragmatic injury, or suspicion of a chronic diaphragmatic injury (Killeen et al. 1999; Barbiera et al. 2003).

One benefit of using MRI to evaluate the diaphragm is the ability to image directly in coronal and sagittal planes without needing to rely on reconstructions, as is the case with CT (Killeen et al. 1999; Iochum et al. 2002). Directly imaged sagittal and coronal planes allow appreciation of the contrast between the mediastinal or the abdominal fat and the low-signal band of the diaphragm itself. Diaphragmatic injuries can be diagnosed by visualization of diaphragmatic defects directly or by visualizing herniation of fat across the diaphragm. It has been suggested that T1 imaging in sagittal and coronal planes may be enough to clearly contrast the fat of the mediastinum and abdominal cavity to the hypointense band of the diaphragm and may be sufficient to diagnose defects of the diaphragm (Shanmuganathan et al. 1996; Killeen et al. 1999).

As with CT, MR imaging signs of diaphragmatic injury include disruption of the diaphragmatic contour or intrathoracic herniation of abdominal contents, such as viscera or fat (Iochum et al. 2002; Barbiera et al. 2003). At least one small series has demonstrated the ability to diagnose diaphragmatic injuries as small as 1 cm (Barbiera et al. 2003).

Many of the same findings described in the above CT signs of diaphragmatic injury may apply equally well to MR imaging. Diaphragmatic discontinuity and herniation of fat or viscera have been commonly reported together in cases detected with MR imaging (Shanmuganathan et al. 1996; Barbiera et al. 2003). Any of the signs which rely on the physical relationships of the thoracic and abdominal organs (e.g., the collar sign, directly visualized defect of the diaphragm, herniation of abdominal viscera into the thoracic cavity, or diaphragmatic extravasation of contrast) may be equally applicable to MR and CT imaging; however, the sensitivity and specificity of these signs in MR imaging have not yet been clarified. In a small series of patients with equivocal imaging findings, the sensitivity and specificity of MRI in detecting diaphragmatic injuries were both 100 % (Shanmuganathan et al. 1996).

11 Ultrasound

Little has been published on the sonographic diagnosis of diaphragmatic rupture; however, there are case reports that suggest its potential during focused assessment with sonography in trauma (FAST) exams (Blaivas et al. 2004; Kirkpatrick et al. 2006; Gangahar and Doshi 2010). Findings during FAST or modified FAST exams which have been demonstrated in the setting of proven traumatic diaphragmatic injuries include elevation of the diaphragm, poor diaphragmatic excursion, replacement of the expected sliding of the lung by the liver in the lower chest (liver sliding sign), or organs being either obscured or apparently absent on FAST exam due to anatomic distortions in the setting of herniation (Rip's absent organ sign) (Blaivas et al. 2004; Kirkpatrick et al. 2006; Gangahar and Doshi 2010). No significant statistical data on the sonographic diagnosis of diaphragmatic injury is available.

Potential pitfalls with sonographic evaluation of the diaphragm in the acute setting include non-acute causes of diaphragmatic dysfunction and eventration of the diaphragm (Blaivas et al. 2004; Kirkpatrick et al. 2006). The nonvisualization of organs is also a nonspecific finding in ultrasonography and can be attributable to other causes such as COPD, obesity, or dextrocardia (Gangahar and Doshi 2010).

Conclusion

Diaphragmatic injuries are caused by penetrating and blunt trauma, both of which are frequently associated with additional traumatic injuries. Both radiologists and surgeons, especially in the setting of life-threatening injuries, miss diaphragmatic injuries. A missed diaphragmatic injury puts a patient at risk of delayed injury and complications such as strangulation, with potentially disastrous consequences. Selective nonoperative management is becoming more common in management of both blunt and penetrating trauma. In order to ensure that diaphragmatic injuries are not missed, radiologists should be familiar with the signs or diaphragmatic injury and should have a high degree of suspicion in the setting of blunt or penetrating trauma. Comparison to prior imaging may help differentiate chronic or congenital mimics of diaphragmatic injury. The proliferation of MDCT and increasing use of multiplanar reconstructions have also made the evaluation for diaphragmatic injuries more accurate and reliable and should always be employed.

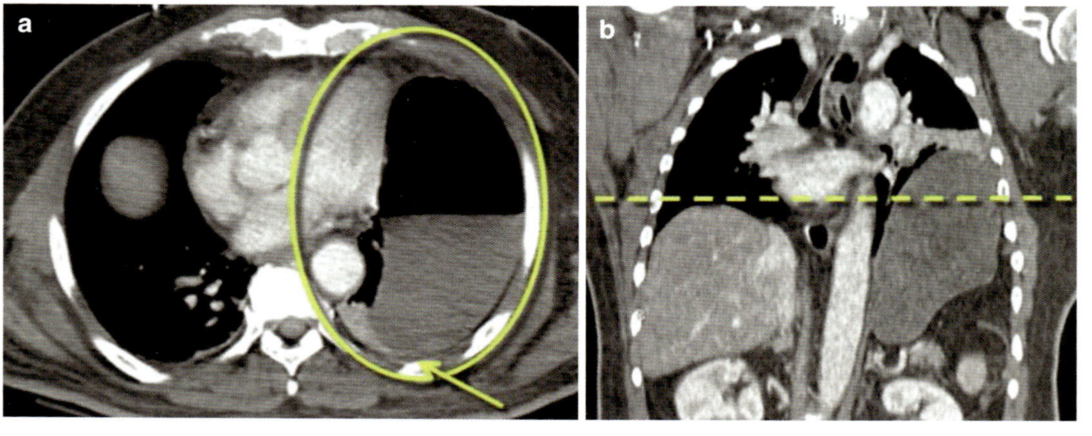

A 62-year-old man who was struck by a car: Computed tomography (CT) images demonstrate the absence of the interposition of lungs between the upper abdominal contents and the chest wall consistent with the *dependent viscera sign* (arrow). There is *intrathoracic herniation* of abdominal viscera as demonstrated by visualization of abdominal organs within the pleural space (circle). Additionally, coronal reconstructions demonstrate *elevation of left-sided abdominal contents* above the left diaphragmatic dome (line)

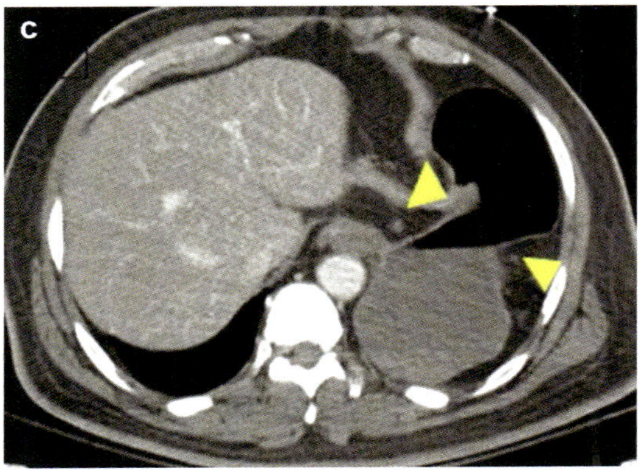

A 62-year-old man who was struck by a car: Computed tomography (CT) image demonstrates the tear in the diaphragm results in a waist-like constriction of the stomach (image C arrowheads). These findings are representative of the *collar sign*. The patient's CT findings of a left diaphragmatic rupture were confirmed at surgery

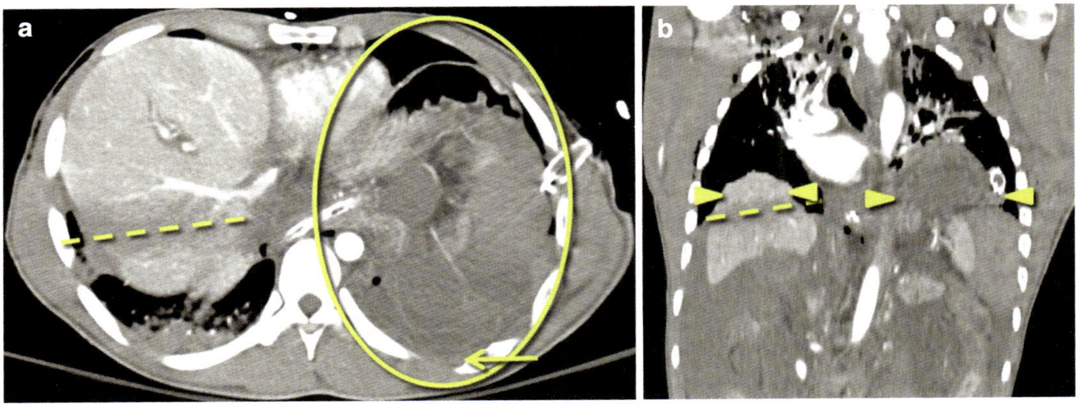

A 25-year-old who suffered a motor vehicle collision: CT images demonstrate a linear band of hypoattenuation through the liver, the *band sign* (images A and B, dashed line). Once again, we see abdominal organs located within the left pleural space (image A, circle) and the *dependent viscera sign* (image A, arrow). Abdominal contents are located *above the level of the diaphragm* (image B, arrowheads). The patient's CT findings of bilateral diaphragmatic rupture were confirmed at surgery. Bilateral diaphragmatic injury can occur in 5–8 % of cases of blunt trauma with diaphragmatic injury. Consequently, a careful inspection of the contralateral hemidiaphragm should be pursued once a diaphragmatic injury is found

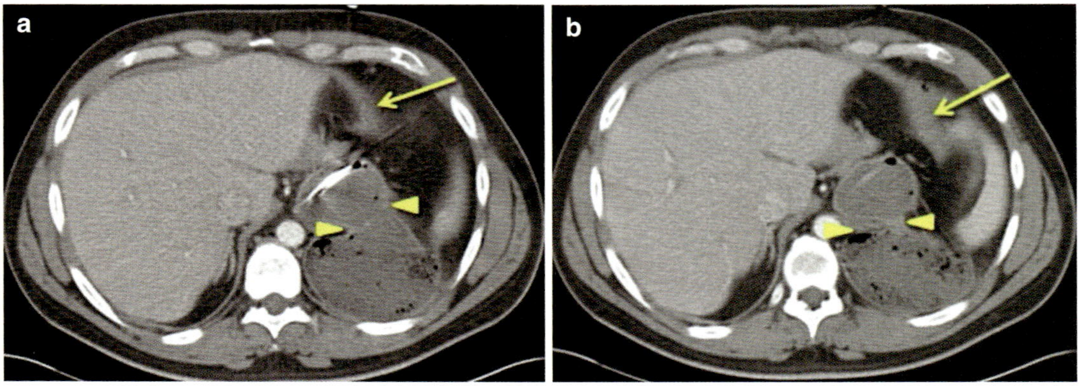

A 33-year-old in motor vehicle collision: Axial CT images demonstrate the *dangling diaphragm sign* as evidenced by the inward curling of the diaphragm from its normal course (images A and B, arrows). Additionally, there is *thickening* of the injured diaphragm (images A and B, arrows). The *collar sign* is also present (images A and B, arrowheads)

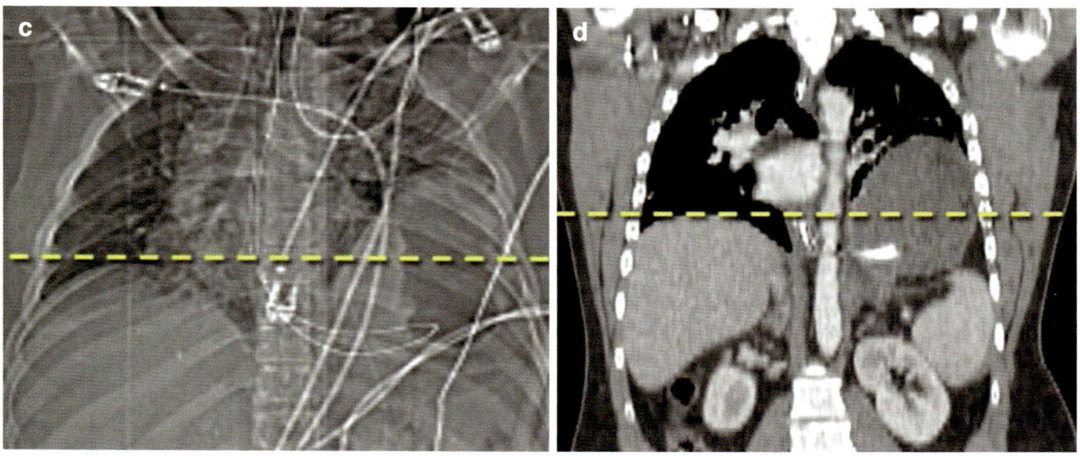

A 33-year-old in motor vehicle collision: The topogram demonstrates apparent elevation of the left hemidiaphragm (image C, dashed line). The coronal CT reformations confirm *elevated abdominal organs* within the left thorax ≥4 cm above the level of the level of the right diaphragmatic dome (image D, dashed line). Diaphragmatic rupture was confirmed at surgery

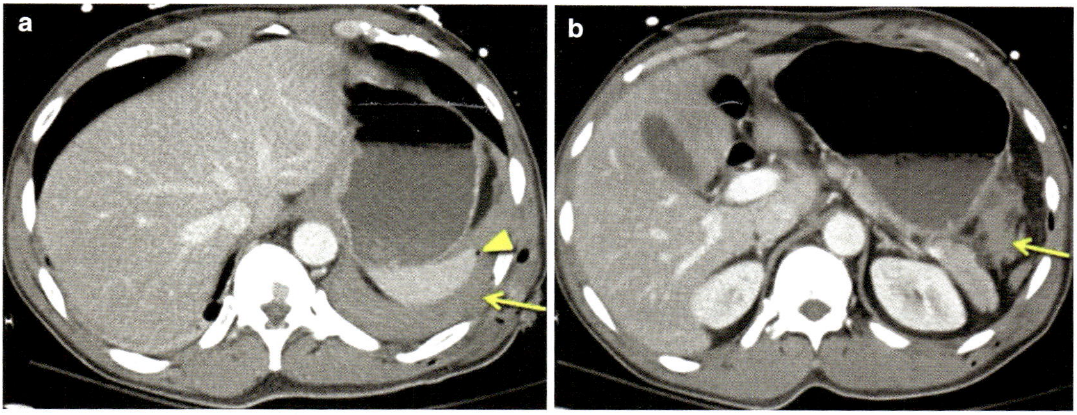

A 47-year-old man stabbed in the left flank: Axial CT images demonstrate *contiguous injuries above and below the diaphragm* which raise the suspicion of diaphragmatic injury. There is a left hemothorax (image A, arrow), hemoretroperitoneum with blood tracking along the gastrosplenic ligament (image B, arrow), and a focus of free gas abutting the spleen (image A, arrowhead)

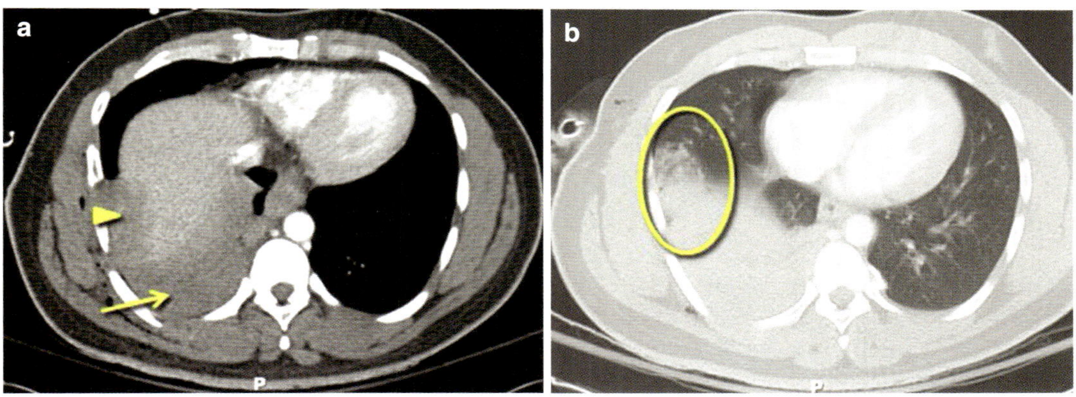

A 34-year-old man with gunshot wound to the right chest: Axial CT images demonstrate a pulmonary contusion (image B, circle), hemothorax (image A, arrow), and hepatic laceration (image A, arrowhead). *Contiguous injury* on both sides of the diaphragm suggests diaphragmatic injury

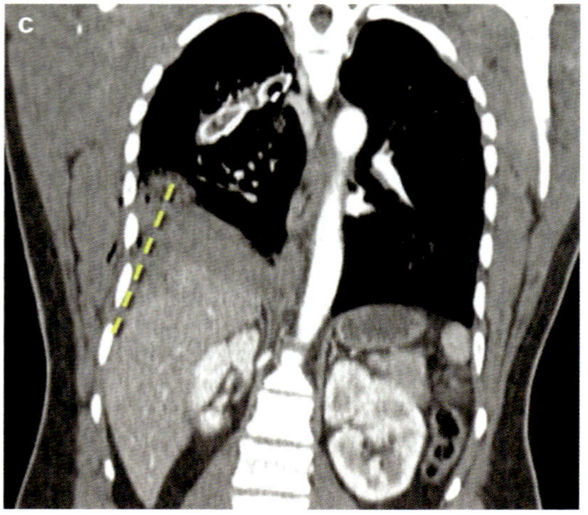

A 34-year-old man with gunshot wound to the right chest: Multiplanar reconstruction demonstrates the *wound tract* (image C, dashed line) traversing the right hemidiaphragm with injuries on both sides of the diaphragm. This case illustrates the value of coronal images to find the wound tract. The patient's diaphragmatic injury was confirmed at surgery

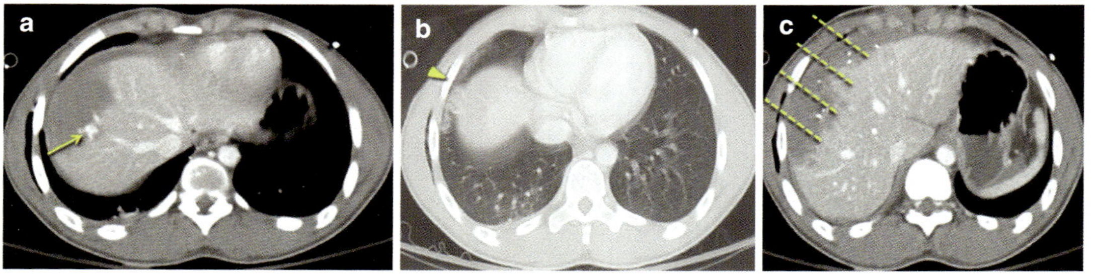

A 21-year-old man with gunshot wound to the right chest: Axial CT image shows a liver laceration with active extravasation of contrast (image A, arrow) and an associated subcapsular hematoma. Axial lung windows demonstrate a pulmonary contusion (image A, arrowhead) and trace pneumothorax. Illustrative *wound tracts* of metallic shot pellets traverse the right hemidiaphragm. No diaphragmatic discontinuities are seen on CT, but these findings are consistent with diaphragm laceration

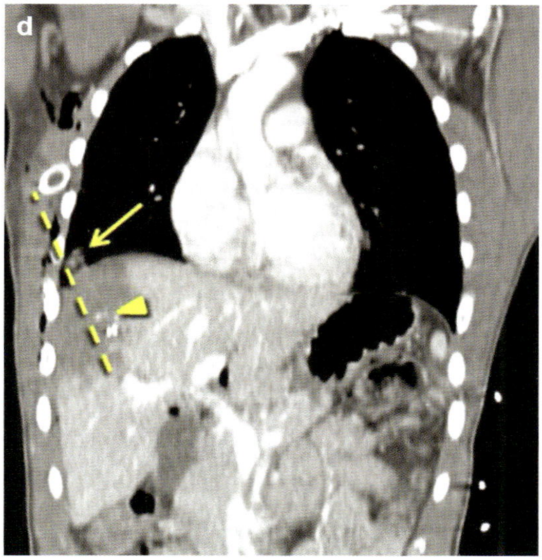

A 21-year-old man with gunshot wound to the right chest: Once again we see the benefit of multiplanar reformations. Coronal images show that the *wound tract* (dashed line) courses through the right hemidiaphragm. *Contiguous injury* above and below the right hemidiaphragm was also demonstrated as lung injury from the bullet tract can be seen above the diaphragm (arrow) and active extravasation within the liver is seen along the path of the shot (arrowhead). Right diaphragmatic injury was confirmed at surgery

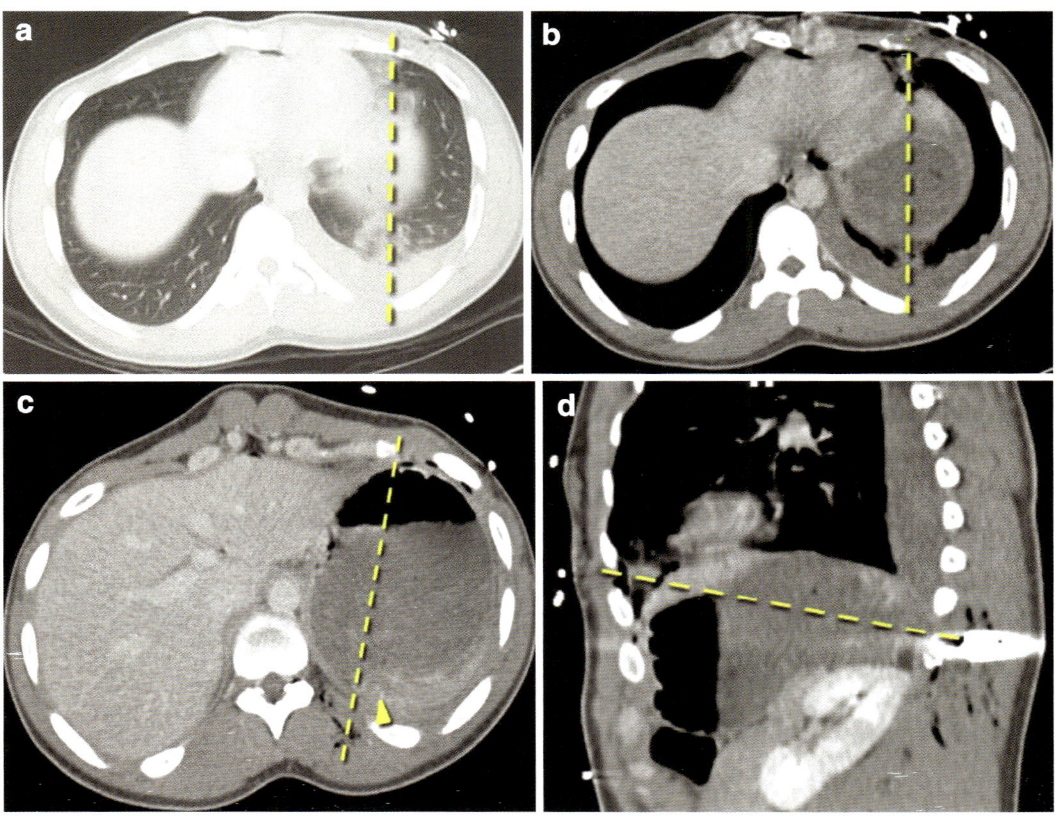

A 28-year-old man with a gunshot wound to the left upper quadrant: Axial images demonstrate pulmonary contusion. The *bullet tract* (images A and B, dashed line) traverses the left hemithorax and left upper quadrant. The *wound tract* (image C, dashed line) also courses inferiorly through the abdomen, and there is evidence of hemoperitoneum (arrowhead). *Contiguous injuries* above and below the diaphragm are concerning for diaphragmatic injury. Sagittal reformations show the *wound tract* (image D, dashed line) coursing from above the diaphragm into the abdomen. Left diaphragmatic injury was confirmed at surgery

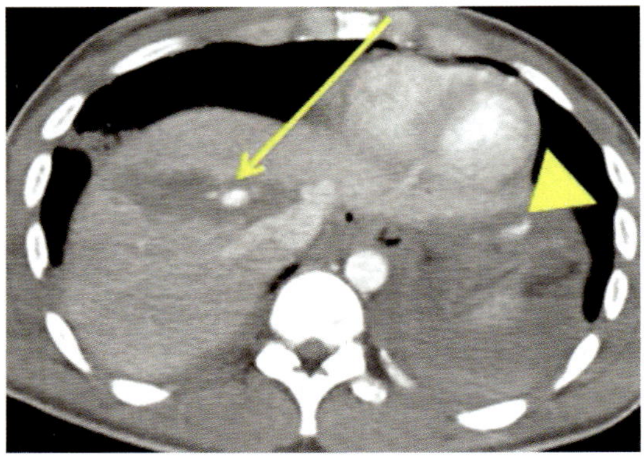

GSW with tract through the upper abdomen; image shows active extravasation from hepatic laceration (arrow) and below the left hemidiaphragm (arrowhead)

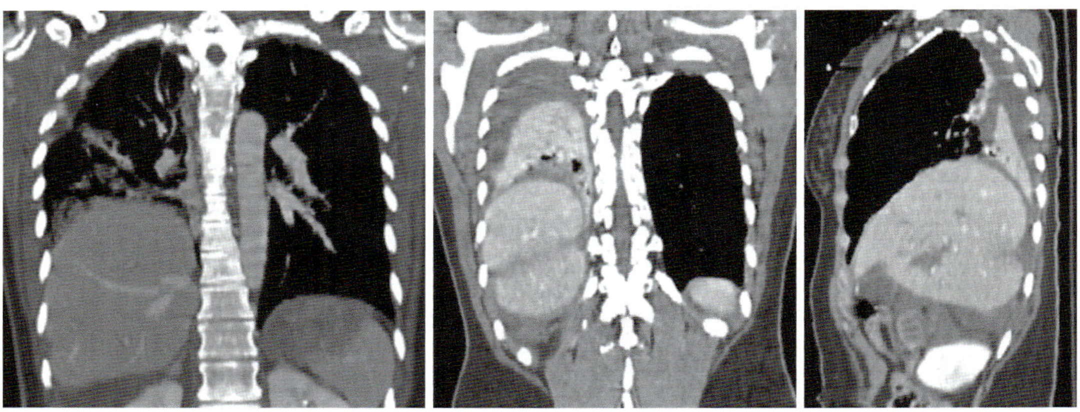

MVC with large right diaphragmatic defect, herniation of the liver into the left thorax, band, and collar signs

References

Barbiera F, Nicastro N, Finazzo M, Lo Casto A, Runza G, Bartolotta TV, Midiri M (2003) The role of MRI in traumatic rupture of the diaphragm. Our experience in three cases and review of the literature. Radiol Med 105(3):188–194

Bergin D, Ennis R, Keogh C, Fenlon HM, Murray JG (2001) The "dependent viscera" sign in CT diagnosis of blunt traumatic diaphragmatic rupture. AJR Am J Roentgenol 177(5):1137–1140

Blaivas M, Brannam L, Hawkins M, Lyon M, Sriram K (2004) Bedside emergency ultrasonographic diagnosis of diaphragmatic rupture in blunt abdominal trauma. Am J Emerg Med 22(7):601–604

Bodanapally UK, Shanmuganathan K, Mirvis SE, Sliker CW, Fleiter TR, Sarada K, Miller LA, Stein DM, Alexander M (2009) MDCT diagnosis of penetrating diaphragm injury. Eur Radiol 19(8):1875–1881

Cantwell CP (2006) The dependent viscera sign. Radiology 238(2):752–753

Chen HW, Wong YC, Wang LJ, Fu CJ, Fang JF, Lin BC (2010) Computed tomography in left-sided and right-sided blunt diaphragmatic rupture: experience with 43 patients. Clin Radiol 65(3):206–212

Como JJ, Bokhari F, Chiu WC, Duane TM, Holevar MR, Tandoh MA, Ivatury RR, Scalea TM (2010) Practice management guidelines for selective nonoperative management of penetrating abdominal trauma. J Trauma 68(3):721–733

Croce MA, Fabian TC, Menke PG, Waddle-Smith L, Minard G, Kudsk KA, Patton JH Jr, Schurr MJ, Pritchard FE (1995) Nonoperative management of blunt hepatic trauma is the treatment of choice for hemodynamically stable patients. Results of a prospective trial. Ann Surg 221(6):744–753; discussion 753–745

Desir A, Ghaye B (2012) CT of blunt diaphragmatic rupture. RadioGraphics 32(2):477–498

Desser TS, Edwards B, Hunt S, Rosenberg J, Purtill MA, Jeffrey RB (2010) The dangling diaphragm sign: sensitivity and comparison with existing CT signs of blunt traumatic diaphragmatic rupture. Emerg Radiol 17(1):37–44

Dreizin D, Bergquist PJ, Taner AT, Bodanapally UK, Tirada N, Munera F (2015) Evolving concepts in MDCT diagnosis of penetrating diaphragmatic injury. Emerg Radiol 22(2):149–156

Fair KA, Gordon NT, Barbosa RR, Rowell SE, Watters JM, Schreiber MA (2015) Traumatic diaphragmatic injury in the American College of Surgeons National Trauma Data Bank: a new examination of a rare diagnosis. Am J Surg 209(5):864–868; discussion 868–869

Gangahar R, Doshi D (2010) FAST scan in the diagnosis of acute diaphragmatic rupture. Am J Emerg Med 28(3):387.e381–383

Gao JM, Du DY, Li H, Liu CP, Liang SY, Xiao Q, Zhao SH, Yang J, Lin X (2015) Traumatic diaphragmatic rupture with combined thoracoabdominal injuries: difference between penetrating and blunt injuries. Chin J Traumatol 18(1):21–26

Gelman R, Mirvis SE, Gens D (1991) Diaphragmatic rupture due to blunt trauma: sensitivity of plain chest radiographs. AJR Am J Roentgenol 156(1):51–57

Guth AA, Pachter HL, Kim U (1995) Pitfalls in the diagnosis of blunt diaphragmatic injury. Am J Surg 170(1):5–9

Hammer MM, Flagg E, Mellnick VM, Cummings KW, Bhalla S, Raptis CA (2014) Computed tomography of blunt and penetrating diaphragmatic injury: sensitivity and inter-observer agreement of CT Signs. Emerg Radiol 21(2):143–149

Hanna WC, Ferri LE, Fata P, Razek T, Mulder DS (2008) The current status of traumatic diaphragmatic injury: lessons learned from 105 patients over 13 years. Ann Thorac Surg 85(3):1044–1048

Iochum S, Ludig T, Walter F, Sebbag H, Grosdidier G, Blum AG (2002) Imaging of diaphragmatic injury: a diagnostic challenge? RadioGraphics 22(Suppl 1): S103–S116

Killeen KL, Mirvis SE, Shanmuganathan K (1999) Helical CT of diaphragmatic rupture caused by blunt trauma. AJR Am J Roentgenol 173(6):1611–1616

Kirkpatrick AW, Ball CG, Nicolaou S, Ledgerwood A, Lucas CE (2006) Ultrasound detection of right-sided diaphragmatic injury; the "liver sliding" sign. Am J Emerg Med 24(2):251–252

Leung VA, Patlas MN, Reid S, Coates A, Nicolaou S (2015) Imaging of Traumatic Diaphragmatic Rupture: Evaluation of Diagnostic Accuracy at a Level 1 Trauma Centre. Can Assoc Radiol J 66(4):310–317

Magu S, Agarwal S, Singla S (2012) Computed tomography in the evaluation of diaphragmatic hernia following blunt trauma. Indian J Surg 74(4):288–293

Murray JG, Caoili E, Gruden JF, Evans SJ, Halvorsen RA Jr, Mackersie RC (1996) Acute rupture of the diaphragm due to blunt trauma: diagnostic sensitivity and specificity of CT. AJR Am J Roentgenol 166(5): 1035–1039

Nchimi A, Szapiro D, Ghaye B, Willems V, Khamis J, Haquet L, Noukoua C, Dondelinger RF (2005) Helical CT of blunt diaphragmatic rupture. AJR Am J Roentgenol 184(1):24–30

Panda A, Kumar A, Gamanagatti S, Patil A, Kumar S, Gupta A (2014) Traumatic diaphragmatic injury: a review of CT signs and the difference between blunt and penetrating injury. Diagn Interv Radiol 20(2):121–128

Patlas MN, Leung VA, Romano L, Gagliardi N, Ponticiello G, Scaglione M (2015) Diaphragmatic injuries: why do we struggle to detect them? Radiol Med 120(1):12–20

Reber PU, Schmied B, Seiler CA, Baer HU, Patel AG, Buchler MW (1998) Missed diaphragmatic injuries and their long-term sequelae. J Trauma Inj Infect Crit Care 44(1):183–188

Rees O, Mirvis SE, Shanmuganathan K (2005) Multidetector-row CT of right hemidiaphragmatic rupture caused by blunt trauma: a review of 12 cases. Clin Radiol 60(12):1280–1289

Shanmuganathan K, Mirvis SE, White CS, Pomerantz SM (1996) MR imaging evaluation of hemidiaphragms in acute blunt trauma: experience with 16 patients. AJR Am J Roentgenol 167(2):397–402

Shatney CH, Sensaki K, Morgan L (2003) The natural history of stab wounds of the diaphragm: implications for a new management scheme for patients with penetrating thoracoabdominal trauma. Am Surg 69(6):508–513

Spann JC, Nwariaku FE, Wait M (1995) Evaluation of video-assisted thoracoscopic surgery in the diagnosis of diaphragmatic injuries. Am J Surg 170(6):628–630; discussion 630–621

Standring S (2016) Diaphragm and phrenic nerves. Gray's anatomy. S. Standring, Elsevier, UK, pp 970–975

Thomas Sadler JL, Langman J, Sadler-Redmond SL, Sulik KK (2003) Langman's medical embryology. Lippincott Williams & Wilkins, Philadelphia, PA

Yucel M, Bas G, Kulali F, Unal E, Ozpek A, Basak F, Sisik A, Acar A, Alimoglu O (2015) Evaluation of diaphragm in penetrating left thoracoabdominal stab injuries: the role of multislice computed tomography. Injury 46(9):1734–1737

Part II

Nontraumatic, Nonvascular Chest Emergencies

Infection

P. Agarwal, L. Romano, H. Prosch, and G. Schueller

Contents

P. Agarwal • H. Prosch
Department of Biomedical Imaging and Image-guided Therapy, Vienna General Hospital, Medical University of Vienna, Währingergürtel 18-22, 1090 Vienna, Austria

L. Romano
Department of Emergency Radiology, Cardarelli Hospital, Naples, Italy

G. Schueller (✉)
Assoc. Prof. Dr. Gerd Schueller MBA, Academic Health, Rietgrabenstrasse 76b, CH-8152 Opfikon, Switzerland

1 Community-Acquired Pneumonia

1.1 Introduction

Community-acquired pneumonia (CAP) is a frequent lower respiratory tract infection.

It is highly influenced by the geographic area and the population.

The microorganisms may reach the lower respiratory tract from inhaled air or from infected oropharyngeal secretions (Vincent et al. 1995). Droplet transmission from human to human is another usual mode of spread of the pulmonary infection, especially in immunocompetent patients and young children.

Clearance by mucociliary system can filter infective organisms 5–10 nm in diameter, so that microorganisms between 1 and 2 nm can reach the alveolar tissue. The alveolar infection depends on the balance between the virulence of the microorganism and body defenses due to cellular phagocytosis. There are several factors

Med Radiol Diagn Imaging (2016)
DOI 10.1007/174_2016_38, © Springer International Publishing Switzerland

predisposing to the development of CAP as cardiovascular diseases, diabetes, uremia, immunodeficiency, obstructive pulmonary chronic disorders with mucociliary clearance insufficiency, and age.

Alcoholic patients and people with poor oral hygiene are particularly sensitive to develop pulmonary infections (Barlettand Finegold 1974).

The clinical presentation of pneumonia is frequently represented with sudden symptoms as high fever, cough, purulent expectoration, and deep chest pain. Neutrophilia is common.

CAP is classified into three main groups: lobar pneumonia, bronchopneumonia, and interstitial pneumonia (Bhalla and Mc Loud 1998).

Lobar pneumonia appears in the lung parenchyma periphery and then diffuses up to the hilum. It is generally limited to one pulmonary segment or lobe.

Bronchopneumonia occurs when infectious microorganisms produce acute bronchial mucosal inflammation and spread through the airway into the alveolar spaces determining pulmonary consolidation.

Interstitial pneumonia is determined by the infection of pulmonary interstitium and is mainly caused by viral organism.

The same organism may produce several different patterns that depend on the balance between the microorganism charge and the body immunity defenses.

The spectrum of bacteria responsible for CAP includes *Streptococcus pneumoniae*, *Haemophilus influenzae*, *Staphylococcus aureus*, *Mycoplasma pneumoniae*, *Chlamydia pneumoniae*, *Legionella pneumophila*, and *Klebsiella pneumoniae* (American Thoracic Society 1995; Marom et al. 1999; De Paso 1991).

Among the types of CAP, *S. pneumoniae* is the most frequent causing bacteria, and it is associated with a high mortality rate in the elderly and childhood.

Haemophilus influenzae also is one of the most frequent bacteria causing CAP, because it frequently colonizes the human upper respiratory tract, especially the nasopharynx, and is considered to form part of the normal respiratory flora. It is also an important cause in the acute exacerbation of chronic obstructive pulmonary infectious disease (Kofteridis et al. 2009).

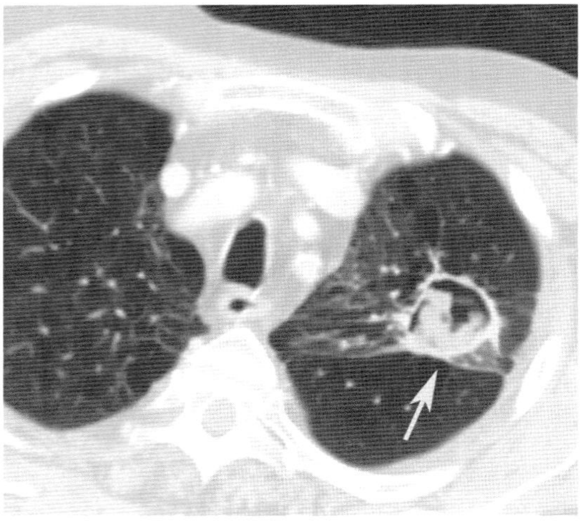

Fig. 1 Fungal abscess (*white arrow*) in diffuse pulmonary emphysema. Post-contrast CT axial scan demonstrates large air-containing dishomogeneous focal area, with peripheral-enhanced irregular wall, characteristic of fungal abscess, with underlying pulmonary emphysema

The viruses that most commonly cause pneumonia are respiratory syncytial virus, herpes simplex, parainfluenza virus, influenza virus, adenovirus, and cytomegalovirus.

The funguses that most commonly cause pneumonia are *Pneumocystis*, *Aspergillus*, and *Candida*.

Pulmonary emphysema and bronchiectasis are frequently seen in patients with CAP because chronic obstructive pulmonary disease is a predisposing factor for developing pulmonary infection (Reittner et al. 2000a) (Fig. 1).

1.2 Lobar Pneumonia

Depending on the severity of the pulmonary alveolar tissue involvement, the pattern of the infection may be patchy or homogeneous. The consolidation is usually confined to one lobe, although multilobar involvement is not uncommon (Fig. 2). Because the bronchial tree is not involved, there is no volume loss of the inflamed pulmonary segment or lobe.

Lobar pneumonia is characterized by the filling of alveolar spaces by edema full of white and inflammatory cells. The inflammation generally begins at the lung mantle and then diffuses to the entire lobe through Kohn pores and peripheral small

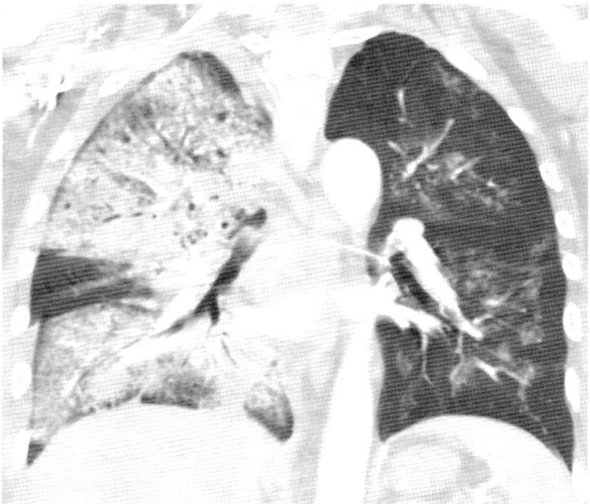

Fig. 2 Bilateral pneumonia. CT coronal scan demonstrates lobar consolidation of *right upper* and *lower lobes* with no volume loss and bulging of interlobar fissure. On the other side, there are lobular areas of consolidation. Air bronchograms within the consolidation areas are preserved

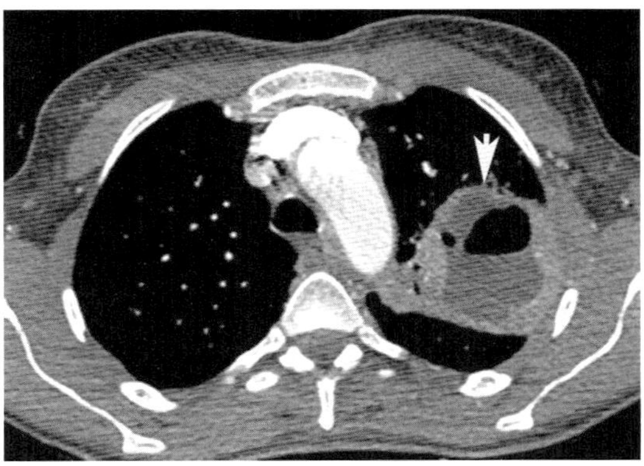

Fig. 3 Lung abscess. Post-contrast CT axial scan demonstrates large focal area of decreased attenuation with air-fluid level, with rim enhancement, characteristic of lung abscess (*arrow*) of the left upper lobe

airways; usually it is limited by an interlobar fissure. The air bronchograms within the consolidation area are preserved (Fig. 2). Nodular pneumonia is frequently caused by fungal infections and is prevalent in young or immunocompromised patients.

The pneumonia could be complicated with cavitation and abscess (Fig. 3), necrosis of the inflamed lung parenchyma, and loculated empyema (Muller et al. 2007).

Abscesses develop in up to 30% of cases, are usually solitary, and typically have an irregular wall. They could rupture into the pleural space

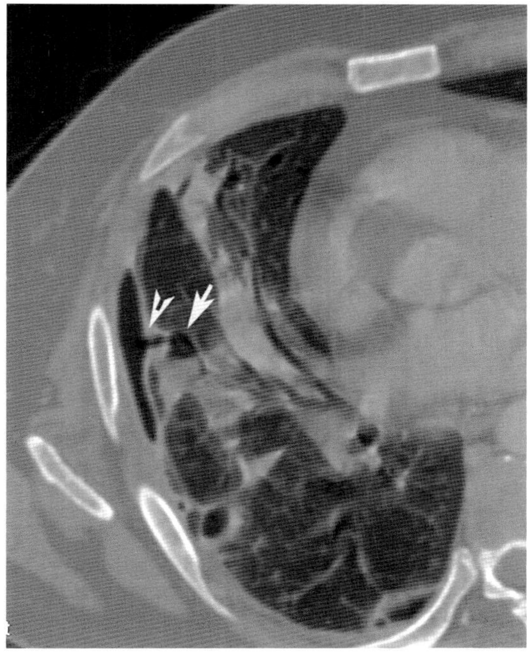

Fig. 4 Post-contrast CT axial scan demonstrates a small air-containing pulmonary cavity with fluid level (*arrow*) ruptured into the pleural space (*arrow tip*) with a small left pneumothorax

with the development of pneumothorax and empyemas (Fig. 4). Abscesses may also erode into bronchial tree and produce air-containing cavities with fluid levels. The consequent bronchial aspiration and diffusion of infection can determine patchy consolidation or nodules in dependent portions of both the lungs (Fig. 5). The consolidations are usually multilobar and bilateral in distribution.

A large solitary abscess or primary lung abscess can develop in a patient without underlying lung inflammation as a consequence of aspiration of oropharyngeal secretions in combination with impairment of systemic defense condition.

Necrotizing pneumonia, generally determined by Gram-negative bacteria, produces exfoliated pulmonary tissue within a cavity or diffuses microabscesses secondary to thrombosis of the vessel that supply the consolidation. Sometimes necrotizing pneumonia consists of a fulminant process associated with focal areas of necrosis that results in abscesses that can coalescence, resulting in large cavities that may exhibit thick fibrotic walls if they are chronic. There are large

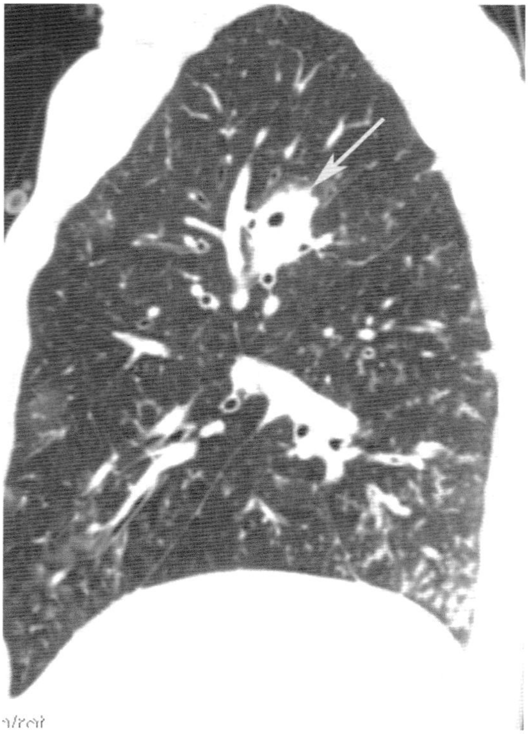

Fig. 5 CT sagittal scan demonstrates multiple nodules in dependent portions of the lung

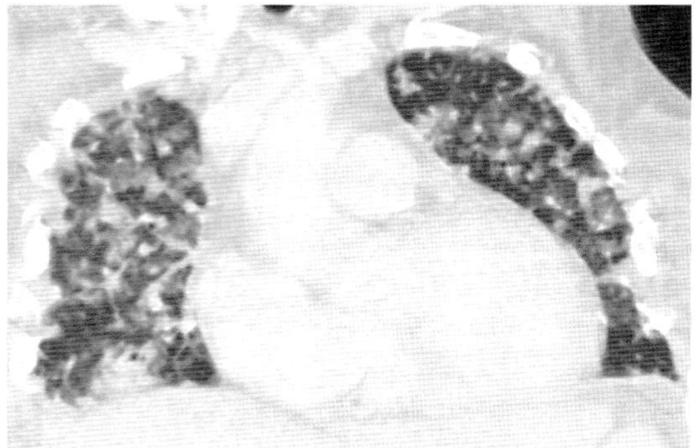

Fig. 6 Bronchopneumonia. CT coronal scan demonstrates multiple, bilateral, centrilobular nodules

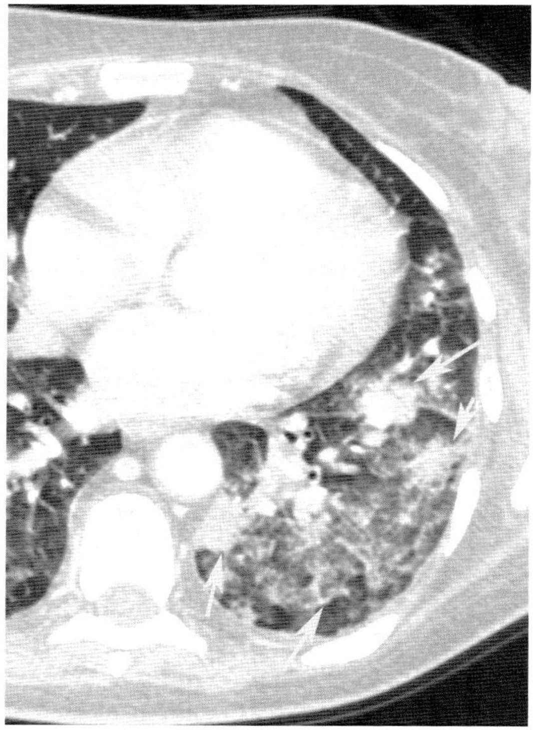

Fig. 7 Bronchopneumonia. CT axial scan demonstrates multiple, lobular (*arrow*), patchy, confluent consolidation areas of the left lower lobe

cavities with concomitant small cavities frequently associated with empyema (Winer-Muram et al. 1993). This feature is frequent in immunocompromised patients.

1.3 Bronchopneumonia

Bronchopneumonia or lobular pneumonia is characterized by a peribronchiolar inflammation with thickening of peripheral bronchial wall, the diffusion of inflammation to the centrilobular alveolar spaces, and development of nodules (Fig. 6). From the centrilobular tissue, the inflammation can spread to lobular (Fig. 7) or subsegmental areas giving a consolidation. The areas of consolidation may be patchy or confluent, multilobar, unilateral, or bilateral (Fig. 8). Because the process involves the airways, it can determine a loss of volume of the affected pulmonary segment (Ito et al. 2009).

1.4 Interstitial Pneumonia

Interstitial pneumonia is frequently caused by virus.

The viral pneumonia begins with the destruction and exfoliation of the respiratory ciliated and

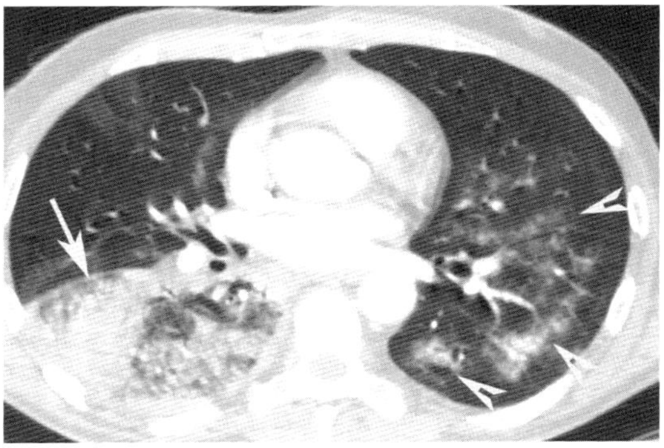

Fig. 8 Bronchopneumonia. CT axial scan demonstrates multiple confluent areas of consolidation (*arrow*) of the right lower lobe and patchy lobular areas of consolidation of the left lower lobe (*arrow tips*)

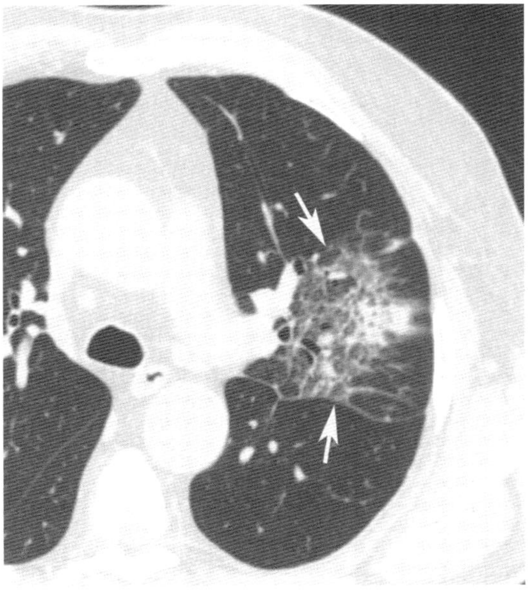

Fig. 9 Interstitial pneumonia. CT axial scan evidences that the lingular interstitial septa, bronchial and bronchiolar walls are thickened for an inflammation process (*arrows*). There is also a central lobular consolidation with patchy appearance

mucous cells. The interstitial septa and the bronchial and bronchiolar walls become thickened for the inflammation process and lymphocyte interstitial infiltrates (Fig. 9). The consequent interstitial pneumonia has often a patchy appearance, frequently with coalescence, involving predominantly the peribronchial portions of the

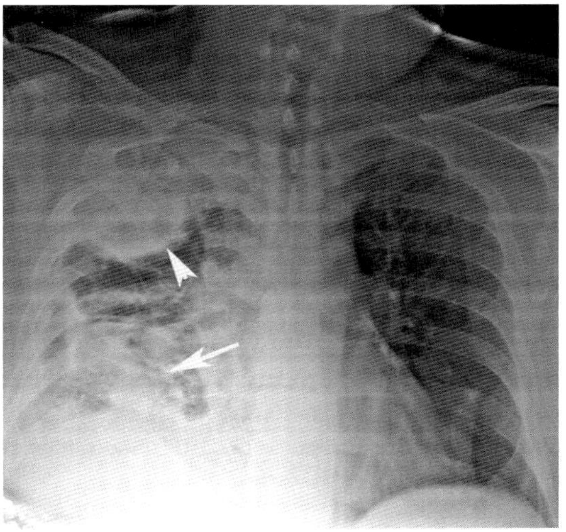

Fig. 10 Chest radiograph shows a right upper lobe opacity (*arrow tip*) and a nonhomogeneous consolidation of the right lower lobe (*arrow*)

pulmonary lobules (Shiley et al. 2010). With the progression of inflammation, the alveolar sacs fill with exudate that could be hemorrhagic. As consequence a hyaline membrane can develop in alveolar spaces.

The pneumonia can heal completely, but sometimes a chronic interstitial fibrosis can occur.

1.5 Radiographic Features

Chest radiography represents an important initial examination in all patients suspected of having pulmonary infection and for monitoring response to therapy.

Its role is to identify the pulmonary opacities (Fig. 10), their internal characteristics and distribution, pleural effusion, and presence of other complications as abscesses and pneumothorax.

Radiographic manifestations depend on the immune status of the patient and the presence of preexisting lung chronic alterations as emphysema, chronic bronchitis, and bronchiectasis and vary somewhat among the various species of causing microorganisms.

The most common radiographic findings include hazy ground-glass opacities, confluent or patchy airspace consolidations, cavitations, and

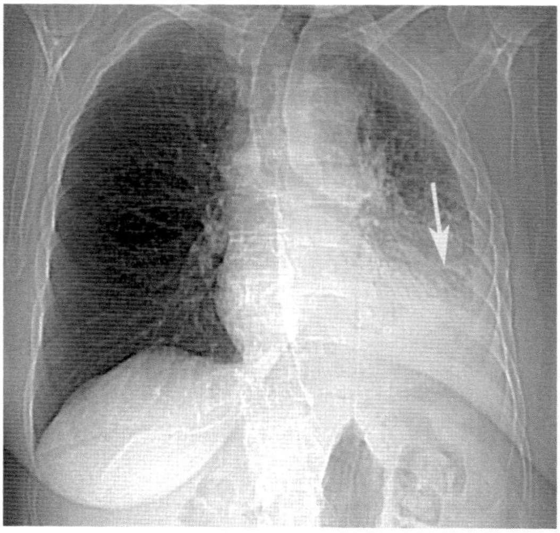

Fig. 11 Posteroanterior chest radiograph shows dense left lower lobe airspace consolidation (*arrow*) with pleural fluid

poorly defined linear or reticular-nodular opacities (Chastre et al. 1998).

These alterations may involve mainly the perihilar regions, lower lung zones, or upper lung zones. They are usually unilateral but may involve both lungs. Other findings are pleural effusion and hilar adenopathy.

In some cases, the radiographic findings are suggestive or consistent with the diagnosis of pneumonia and are sufficiently specific in proper clinical context to preclude the need for additional imaging (Fig. 11) (Franquet 2001).

However, the bedside plain film, the projection effects, and the poor density resolution frequently limit the value of radiography as a diagnostic tool. Radiographic features are sometimes nonspecific, and the relatively low diagnostic accuracy of chest radiography can be improved with CT.

1.6 Computed Tomography Findings

CT has been shown to be more sensitive than x-ray plain film and provide additional information that affects diagnosis or management in up to 70 % critically ill patients (Heussel et al. 1997).

High resolution CT allows accurate assessment of airspace inflammation (Okada et al. 2012).

The distribution of parenchymal alterations is based on the evidence of their localization at CT scan. If the primary opacity is predominantly located in the inner third of the lungs, the pathology is classified as having a central distribution. A peripheral opacity is defined as a lesion localized in the outer third of the lungs. Zonal predominance is classified as either upper or lower. In the upper lung zone predominance, the alteration is located above the level of the tracheal carina, whereas in the lower zone predominance, it is located below the upper zone.

The CT findings include nodules, interlobular septal thickening, intralobular reticular opacities, ground-glass opacities, tree-in-bud pattern, lobar-segmental consolidation, lobular consolidation, abscesses, pneumatocele, pleural effusion, pericardial effusion, mediastinal and hilar lymphadenopathies, airway dilatation, and emphysema.

Nodules measure from 3 to 10 mm and are divided into three types: centrilobular nodules that are small nodules in centrilobular location, peribronchovascular nodules that are relatively larger nodules associated with the peribronchovascular bundle, and "random nodules" that are not associated with centrilobular structures or bronchovascular bundle.

The centrilobular nodules reflect a peribronchial inflammation with a centrilobular distribution (Fig. 12).

They are defined as a dot-like opacities localized inside the center of a secondary pulmonary lobule. They are present around the peripheral pulmonary arterial branches or 3–5 mm from the pleura, interlobular septa, or pulmonary veins.

Nodules that are present in the bronchovascular bundle are called peribronchovascular nodules (Fig. 13).

Hemorrhagic pulmonary nodules have a central area of soft tissue attenuation surrounded by a halo of ground-glass attenuation (Primack et al. 1994).

Pulmonary hemorrhage in association with nodules occurs in patients with herpes simplex virus, candidiasis, and cytomegalovirus pneumonia (Thurlbeck et al. 1991)

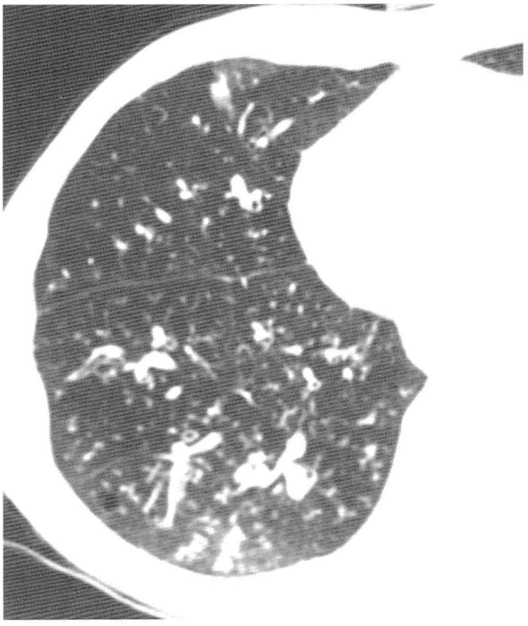

Fig. 12 CT axial scan evidences multiple centrilobular nodules and peribronchial inflammation with centrilobular distribution

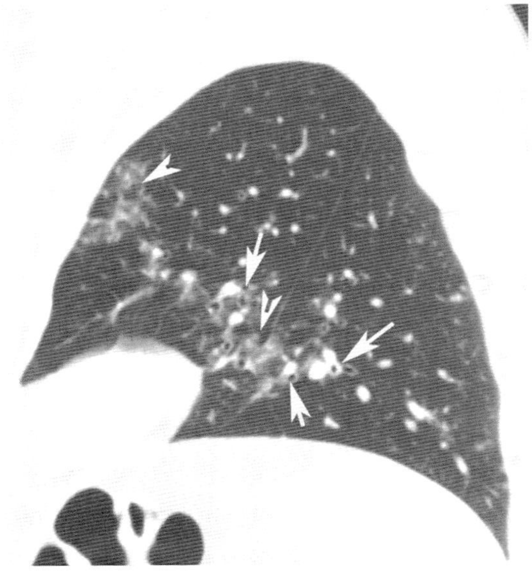

Fig. 13 Peribronchovascular nodules. CT sagittal scan shows small nodules (*arrow tips*) in the bronchovascular bundle and peribronchial inflammation (*arrows*)

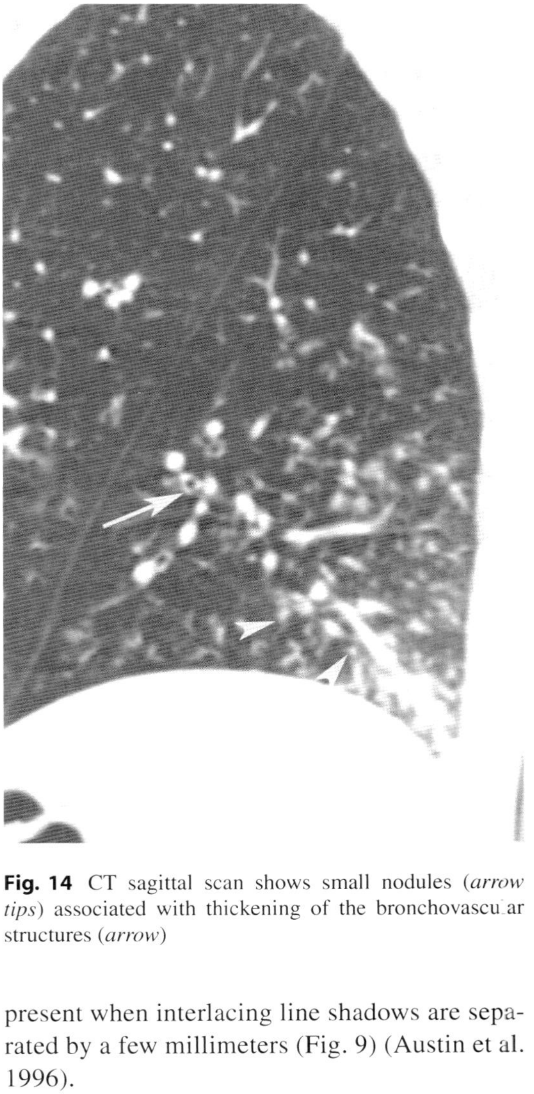

Fig. 14 CT sagittal scan shows small nodules (*arrow tips*) associated with thickening of the bronchovascular structures (*arrow*)

Interlobular septal thickening are defined as abnormal widening of the interlobular septa. Intralobular reticular opacity is considered to be present when interlacing line shadows are separated by a few millimeters (Fig. 9) (Austin et al. 1996).

It is frequently associated with bronchial wall thickening. Thickening of the bronchovascular structures is defined as an apparent thickening of the bronchovascular bundle in comparison with the unaffected lung parenchyma (Fig. 14).

Ground-glass opacity was defined as hazy increased opacity with preservation of bronchial and vascular markings (Fig. 15). It is present particularly in pneumocystis and cytomegalovirus infections (Fig. 16).

Tree-in-bud pattern may be seen in a variety of bacterial, mycobacterial, fungal, and viral infections and consists of centrilobular branching tubular structures, bronchovascular bundle

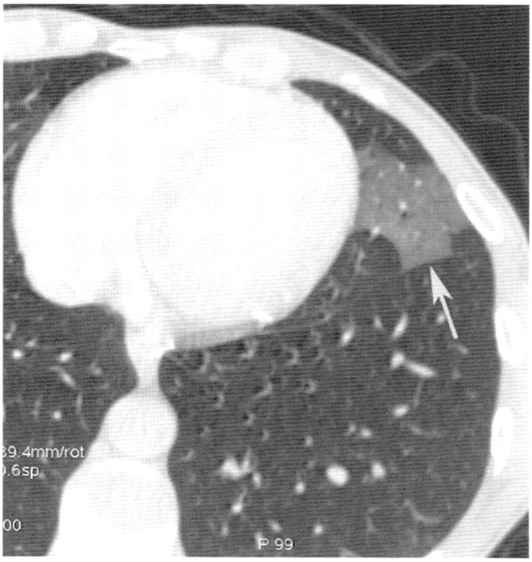

Fig. 15 Ground-glass opacity. CT axial scan evidences a lingular ground-glass opacity (*arrow*) with preservation of bronchial and vascular markings

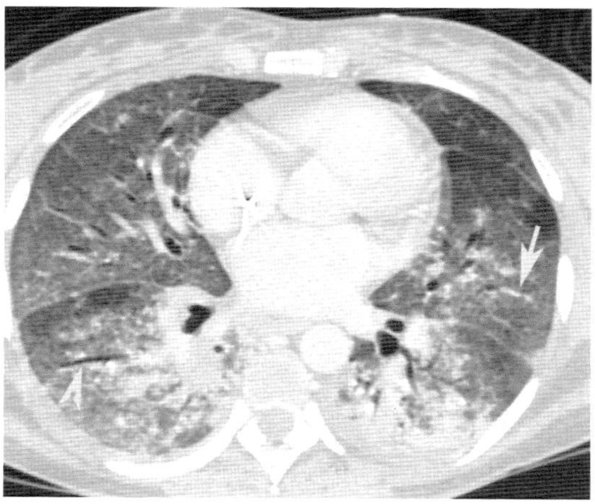

Fig. 16 CT axial scan demonstrates multiple, confluent, bilateral ground-glass opacities with preservation of bronchial (*arrow tip*) and vascular (*arrow*) markings

thickening, and nodules and reflects the presence of bronchiolar inflammation and filling of the bronchiolar lumen by inflammatory exudate (Fig. 17) (Aquino et al. 1996).

Airspace consolidation is considered to be present when homogeneous increases in pulmonary parenchymal attenuation obscured the margins of vessels and airway walls (Fig. 2) (Hansell et al. 2008).

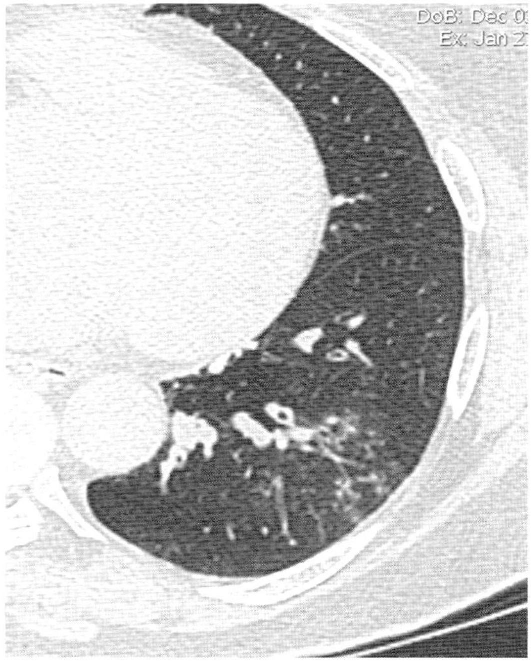

Fig. 17 Tree in bud. CT axial scan demonstrates centrilobular branching tubular structures, bronchovascular bundle thickening, nodules that reflect the presence of bronchiolar inflammation, and filling of the bronchiolar lumen by inflammatory exudate

The CT findings in viral pneumonia are based on the evidence of small patchy opacities that can coalescence (Fig. 18), composed of multiple, poorly defined 2–3 mm nodules; multilobar involvement is frequent. Bronchial wall and peribronchial thickening frequently spread outward from the hila. Hilar adenopathy and pleural effusion are common.

The abscess can drain into a bronchus that leads to the classic air-fluid level, present in up to 72 % of cases (Fig. 3). The complete drainage of the cavity can lead to a pneumatocele.

Pneumatocele is a frequent consequence of an abscess drained in the lumen of a bronchus; it is a gas-filled area with a thin wall that may increase and can get ruptured into the pleural space, causing a pneumothorax. It can also heal completely, fading from the periphery to form a tiny thin-walled air-cyst or a linear scar.

Pleural effusion is better detected with CT than with radiography and is often associated with a high risk of empyema that requires prompt early drainage.

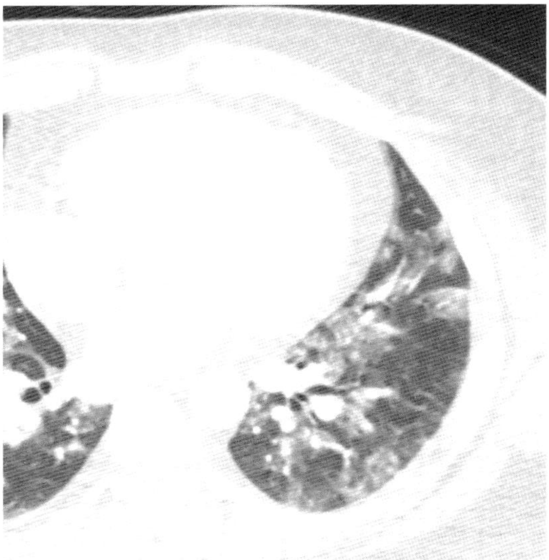

Fig. 18 Viral pneumonia CT axial scan evidences small patchy opacities of the left lower lobe

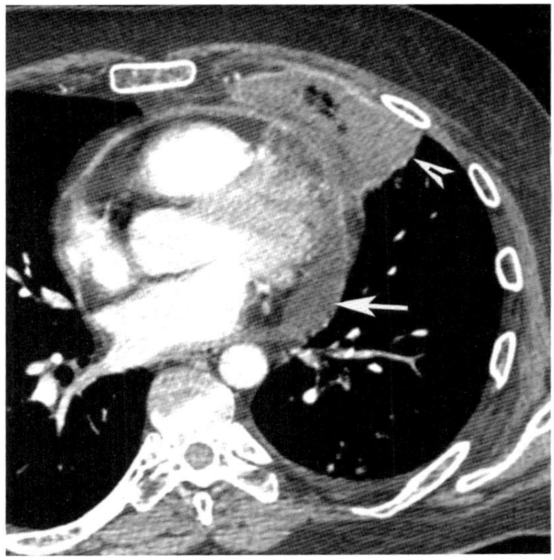

Fig. 19 Pulmonary abscess associated with purulent pericarditis. Post-contrast CT axial scan demonstrates a prepericardial lung abscess (*arrow tip*) of the left lower lobe associated with thickening of the pericardium and pericardial effusion (*arrow*)

Purulent pericarditis is a relatively rare and a rapidly fatal complication of pneumonia. The consequent development of cardiac tamponade may be rapid. At the beginning, heart size may be normal at chest radiograph, whereas CT can demonstrate early the pericardial effusion that requires prompt drainage for avoiding cardiac compression (Fig. 19) (Naidich et al. 1983).

Mediastinal and hilar lymphadenopathies are evaluated when the minimal diameter of a lymph node is larger than 10 mm. Lymph node enlargement is very frequent in pneumonia and generally involves the paratracheal, tracheobronchial, and subcarinal mediastinal chains.

Airway dilatation predisposes to pneumonia and is considered to be present if the bronchial size exceeded that of the near pulmonary artery.

Pulmonary emphysema is frequently associated with pneumonia and is defined as scattered or diffuse areas of low attenuation without internal vascular structures in comparison with normal pulmonary parenchyma (Fig. 1).

1.7 Conclusion

Pneumonia is the first leading cause of death due to infection worldwide (Vilar et al. 2004a).

Many Gram-positive, Gram-negative bacteria, funguses, and viruses can cause the infectious pulmonary disease, and the severity of pneumonia depends on the balance between the microorganism charge, the body immunity defenses, and the quality of the underlying pulmonary tissue.

Among the types of CAP, *S. pneumoniae* is the most frequent causing bacteria, has a tendency to develop antibiotic resistance, and is associated with a high mortality rate in the elderly and childhood (Musher et al. 2002).

Radiographically pneumonia is divided into three patterns: lobar pneumonia, bronchopneumonia, and interstitial pneumonia (Muller et al. 2007).

Chest x-ray film is routinely performed for the initial evaluation of patients with suspect pulmonary infection, and it is considered the recommended tool for the diagnosis of CAP. However, chest x-ray film not always evidences all the findings of pneumonia, and it is limited by the interobserver variability in interpretation.

Especially in not clear or even negative chest radiography pattern, in patients with clinical symptoms, CT is recommended, for its high spatial resolution and the ability to evidence very early and minimal pulmonary alterations indicative of pneumonia.

2 Atypical Infections

2.1 Definition

Community-acquired pneumonias have been traditionally divided into "typical" and "atypical" pneumonias. The main aim of such a classification was to help the clinician narrow the differential diagnosis and choose an appropriate therapy based on the likely offending organism (Murray and Mason 2010).

Typical pneumonia is characterized by infection with bacteria such as *Streptococcus pneumoniae*, *Klebsiella pneumoniae*, and *Haemophilus influenzae*. It presents with symptoms such as acute onset of high grade fever with chills, cough with purulent expectoration, and pleuritic chest pain. Further evaluation of these patients reveals an elevated white blood cell count, elevated CRP, and lobar or segmental consolidation on imaging studies (Murray and Mason 2010).

Atypical pneumonia, as the name explains, does not show these *typical* features. An early use of this term in the literature dates back to 1938 when cases of patients who presented with milder symptoms and protracted course came to notice (Reimann 1938). These patients had more generalized symptoms like malaise, body pains, and low-grade fever with dry cough and flu-like symptoms. The causative organism could not be cultivated on regular media or stained with regular staining methods. Mycoplasma was first isolated in 1944 and was attributed as the etiology of primary atypical pneumonia (Eaton et al. 1944). However, several other organisms cause atypical symptoms.

Although originally used to signify any infection that was unusual in presentation, atypical pneumonia is now a broad term that includes infections caused by common organisms like *Mycoplasma pneumoniae*, *Chlamydia pneumoniae*, and *Legionella pneumophila* and viruses (Marrie et al. 1981). Atypical, however, does not mean that they are rare; they account for almost 15–20 % of the cases of CAP (Arnold et al. 2007). *Mycoplasma pneumoniae* is the most common cause of atypical pneumonia followed by *Chlamydia pneumoniae* and *Legionella pneumophila* (Arnold et al. 2007). Apart from these conventional pathogens, there are emerging infections with newer organisms like *Hantavirus*, human metapneumovirus that can also cause atypical pneumonia. In view of the current radiological discussion and similar radiological appearances shared by mycoplasma and various viruses, we will also be discussing some additional infections in this chapter, which, although not considered routinely under the heading of "atypical pneumonia," are atypical enough to justify their inclusion here.

2.2 General Features

Infections with many, if not all, atypical organisms share some common features. Mycoplasma, chlamydia, and viruses have many similarities in their pathology, clinical, and radiological features. Grossly, these pathogens cause predominant histological changes in the respiratory epithelium and in the peribronchial interstitium (Müller et al. 2007; Müller 2003). The ensuing bronchiolitis and alveolitis are characterized by infiltration of the epithelium with mononuclear cells and presence of neutrophilic exudate in the lumen of the airways. These changes are predominantly seen in the terminal and respiratory bronchioles and manifest radiologically as peribronchial nodules (Müller et al. 2007; Müller 2003).

Bronchiolitis with exudate in the lumen of the airways is seen on radiographs as reticulonodular pattern and on CT as tree-in-bud nodules. As the nodules enlarge, they involve the entire secondary pulmonary lobule and are seen as "lobular" consolidation: these features are typical of bronchopneumonia pattern. Further extension into segmental and patchy lobar consolidation may be seen in advanced stages, and this may be difficult to distinguish from bacterial infection. Partial filling of the airways gives rise to ground-glass opacities (Müller et al. 2007).

Some infections like influenza and hantavirus cardiopulmonary syndrome, on the other hand, cause rapidly progressive pneumonia with diffuse alveolar damage (Kim et al. 2002).

The clinical course of atypical pneumonias is generally subacute, the WBC counts are generally normal, and the imaging features are heterogeneous and nonspecific.

2.3 Radiological Aspects

Diagnosis of pneumonia requires a combination of clinical, microbiological, and radiological features. Chest radiograph is usually sufficient to confirm the diagnosis. It also helps in follow-up of the patients and evaluation of the response to treatment. CT scans are not routinely recommended but are helpful in case of doubtful features on chest radiographs, when no adequate response to the treatment is noted and when complications or underlying pathology is suspected (Vilar et al. 2004b). CT scan can be further helpful in suggesting an etiological diagnosis. In indeterminate cases, CT-guided procedures come in as problem-solving tools for the correct diagnosis.

2.4 Bacteria

2.4.1 Mycoplasma Pneumonia

Mycoplasma pneumoniae is a common cause of community-acquired pneumonia, particularly in young children. It is the smallest free-living organism, measuring approximately 125–150 microns in size which is similar to that of myxovirus (Marrie et al. 2012). Lack of cell wall makes them highly pleomorphic.

Mycoplasma pneumoniae was first isolated from the sputum of a patient with "atypical pneumonia" by Eaton et al. and was initially considered to be a virus due to its ability to pass through bacterial filters. Subsequent studies led to its identification as bacteria (Cunha 2010).

Mycoplasma pneumonia is commonly seen in young children and adolescents and shows a declining incidence in adults (Meyer Sauteur et al. 2016). It spreads through droplet spread or direct contact. The incubation period is around 1–2 weeks (John et al. 2001).

Clinical symptoms resemble a viral infection and are characterized by mild symptoms like dry cough, headache, malaise, and low-grade fever (John et al. 2001). In view of these mild symptoms, it is also called as "walking pneumonia" (Meyer Sauteur et al. 2016). However, sometimes severe infection and extrapulmonary manifestations may also be seen. In one study by Marrie et al., common extrapulmonary manifestations were thrombocytosis, hemolysis, Guillain-Barré syndrome, and pulmonary hemorrhage (Marrie et al. 2012). In asthmatic patients, it can cause an acute exacerbation of asthma and present with acute dyspnea.

Typically, the WBC counts remain in the normal range. A secondary bacterial infection is likely when they are elevated (John et al. 2001).

An attempt to suggest the offending organisms on radiology can be worthwhile for two main reasons: firstly, infection with these cell wall-deficient bacteria calls for treatment with antibiotics other than the usual cell wall synthesis inhibitors like penicillin, which are otherwise suitable for typical infections with pneumococcus. Laboratory tests take time, pending, which a radiological diagnosis can prove helpful in clinical decision making. Secondly, in appropriate settings, radiological features, although not highly specific, can be suggestive of the diagnosis in many cases.

The chief pathology is acute cellular bronchiolitis with bronchial wall inflammation, peribronchial infiltrates of lymphocytes and macrophage, and intraluminal exudative fluid (Pipavath et al. 2005; Muller and Miller 1995). This is seen radiologically as thickening of bronchial wall and centrilobular nodules.

Radiographic features of mycoplasma are generally nonspecific and resemble viral pneumonias closely. Reticulonodular infiltrates in one or more lobes are seen on radiographs (John et al. 2001) (Fig. 20). Various studies have highlighted lower lobe predominance (John et al. 2001; Guckel et al. 1989). Bilateral peribronchial

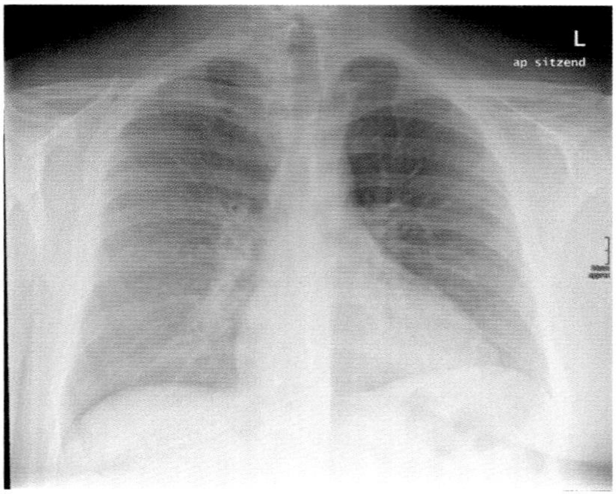

Fig. 20 A 21-year-old man with mycoplasma pneumonia: chest radiograph showing enlarged left hilar shadow. Reticulonodular opacities in the right lower lung field

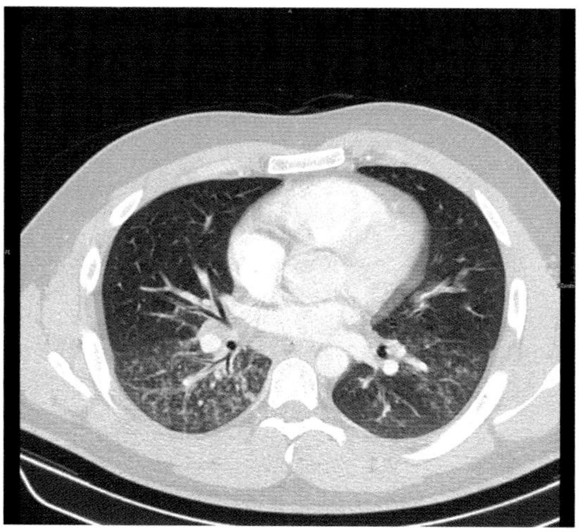

Fig. 21 Same patient as in Fig. 20: CT scan showing centrilobular nodules, tree-in-bud, and bronchial wall thickening in both lower lobes

infiltrates may also be seen. Patchy consolidation may be seen; however, dense lobar consolidation as in typical bacterial pneumonias is less likely (Eaton et al. 1944).

Mycoplasma pneumoniae pneumonia presents itself on computed tomography (CT) like bronchopneumonia. Centrilobular nodules are the most common findings on CT (Reittner et al. 2000b) (Fig. 21). They coalesce and form consolidations. Consolidations and ground-glass opacities with patchy involvement of the secondary pulmonary lobules and interspersed sparing of some lobules are typical (Reittner et al. 2000b). A combination of bronchial wall thickening and centrilobular nodules with bronchopneumonia can be highly suggestive of mycoplasma. CT helps to demonstrate the nodules and bronchial wall thickening better than radiographs, thereby helpful in pointing toward the diagnosis. Pleural effusions are less commonly encountered, seen in around 20 % of the cases, and when present are transient (John et al. 2001; Hsieh et al. 2007).

2.4.2 *Chlamydia pneumoniae*

Chlamydias are obligate intracellular bacteria that possess a cell wall. They exist in two forms: a smaller extracellular elementary body and a larger intracellular form called the reticulate body (Webb et al. 2011). Three species of chlamydia area known:

Chlamydia trachomatis typically causes ocular infection (trachoma) and sexually transmitted disease but may cause pneumonia in infants who are born to infected mothers.

Chlamydia psittaci is a pathogen in birds (causing psittacosis) and may cause respiratory infections in humans. The mode of infection is through aerosols containing bacteria generated from infected birds (Knittler and Sachse 2015).

Chlamydia pneumoniae was the third species to be discovered, first isolated in 1968 during trachoma vaccine trail and accounts for an estimated 10 % of the CAP cases (Kuo et al. 1995). It is a common cause of atypical pneumonia.

Transmission of infection occurs through respiratory secretions. Incubation period is several weeks.

Symptoms tend to be protracted and are subacute in onset. Prolonged cough and low-grade fever are typical features. Initial prodromal phase of upper respiratory tract symptoms like pharyngitis and hoarseness of voice are not uncommon.

The infection is typically mild, and extrapulmonary symptoms are less common in comparison to mycoplasma infection. It has also been implicated in coronary artery disease.

CT features consist of bronchopneumonia with consolidation, GGO, peribronchial thickening, and nodules, similar to mycoplasma infection. However, pleural effusions are more common in patients with *Chlamydia pneumoniae*, bronchial wall thickening and centrilobular nodules more common in mycoplasma infection (Okada et al. 2005). Some studies described increased prevalence of emphysema and bronchial dilatation in *Chlamydia pneumoniae* pneumonia; COPD is an important risk factor for chlamydia (Hahn 1999; Karnak et al. 2001).

2.4.3 *Legionella pneumophila*

Legionella pneumonia is an atypical pneumonia, first discovered in 1976 due to an outbreak in a convention in Philadelphia (Fraser et al. 1977). The source of infection was later narrowed down to the cooling system of the air conditioner with circulating water which acts like a conducting medium for the bacteria.

It is a Gram-negative obligate intracellular bacterium that is a parasite of freshwater protozoans. It tends to colonize in various water facilities and causes outbreaks of infection when aerosols containing the bacteria are inhaled (Fields et al. 2002). In humans, it infects the macrophages, where it resides and multiplies.

Legionella pneumophila is described to cause two diseases: Legionnaires' disease which is a severe multisystemic infection and pneumonia with a long incubation period from 2 to 10 days and Pontiac fever which is a mild clinical illness with flu-like symptoms and a short incubation period of 36 h. *Legionella pneumophila* serogroup 1 accounts for most of the cases (Fields et al. 2002).

Legionnaires' disease varies from mild to severe disease requiring ICU care. It tends to cause electrolyte abnormalities, typically hyponatremia and hypophosphatemia, the presence of which must raise the suspicion of this infection. Presenting symptoms are usually constitutional like fever, myalgias, headache, confusion, and diarrhea which are seen early in the course of the disease, and then nonproductive cough appears later (Tsai et al. 1979).

Radiological features are usually nonspecific and resemble bacterial lobar pneumonia.

Radiographs show patchy peripheral consolidations initially. Airspace consolidation due to alveolitis is typical. Bilateral, multilobar, and multisegment consolidation and ground-glass opacities are the most common radiological features on CT (Yagyu et al. 2003). Centrilobular nodules and diffuse peribronchial thickening characteristic of mycoplasma and chlamydia are less commonly encountered in legionella (Kim et al. 2007). Cavitation may be seen occasionally in immunosuppressed individuals and patients on high steroids (Fairbank et al. 1991). Pleural effusions are seen in up to half of the patients and are usually mild or moderate. Delayed clearing up of the infiltrates and residual fibrosis may occasionally be seen.

2.5 Viruses

Lower respiratory tract infections can be caused by various viruses, and it is estimated that approximately 10% of infections in CAP are due to viral etiology (ref). Along with the various radiological features, knowledge of the clinical history can be invaluable in narrowing the differential diagnosis. For example, in immunocompetent host, influenza virus is commonly implicated as an offender. In immunosuppressed individuals, however, the usual inciting organisms are herpes, cytomegalovirus, and adenovirus (Kim et al. 2002).

Viruses can be divided into (a) RNA viruses, myxoviruses (influenza, RSV, measles), coronavirus, and hantavirus, and (b) DNA viruses, adenovirus and herpes group including CMV and varicella zoster.

2.5.1 Influenza Virus

Influenza virus belongs to the family *Orthomyxoviridae* and is a single-stranded RNA virus. It has three predominant serotypes: influenza A, B, and C. Influenza A is responsible for majority of the epidemics and pandemics. Influenza virus A and B may cause pneumonia, while C causes only sporadic mild infections (Webb et al. 2011).

Infection with influenza virus is usually self-limiting. It favors secondary bacterial infection through various mechanisms like altering the respiratory epithelium. Diabetes mellitus, pregnancy, extremes of age, immunosuppression,

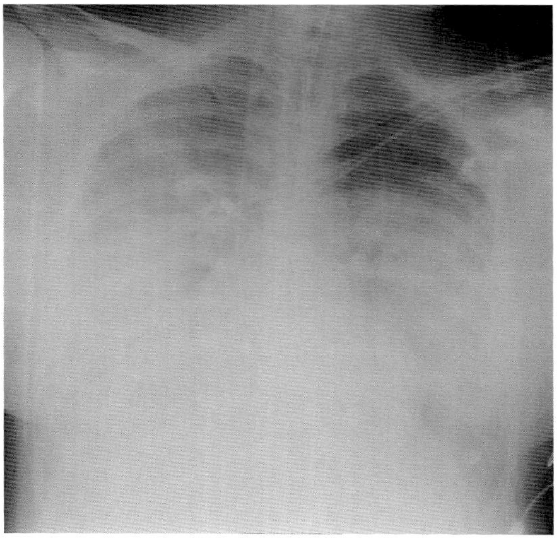

Fig. 22 A 29-year-old man with H1N1 pneumonia: chest radiograph showing extensive areas of consolidation in both lungs with only a relative sparing of the left upper lung field

and underlying pulmonary or cardiac conditions are some of the factors that predispose to a fulminant infection and pneumonia, and death within 24 h may be seen in extreme cases (Oikonomou et al. 2003). Such an infection is characterized histologically by diffuse alveolar damage.

Radiological features are varied and consist of segmental areas of consolidation which may be unilateral or bilateral (Fig. 22). Pleural effusions are rare. On CT, ground-glass opacities, centrilobular tree-in-bud nodules, and patchy consolidations may be seen (Oikonomou et al. 2003).

2.5.2 Respiratory Syncytial Virus

It is an RNA virus belonging to *Paramyxoviridae* family. Almost all infants are infected with RSV by 2 years of age (Drysdale et al. 2016). RSV typically causes upper respiratory tract infections, otitis media, bronchiolitis, asthma-/viral-induced wheezing, and pneumonia. Bronchiolitis may be seen in up to 80 % of the cases (Drysdale et al. 2016). In immunocompromised individuals, it can cause severe pneumonia with high mortality (Mayer et al. 2014).

In addition to bronchial wall thickening and peribronchial nodules, typical features of RSV infection on radiography are air-trapping and hyperinflation due to bronchiolitis (Müller et al. 2007). CT reflects the features of bronchopneumonia and bronchiolitis. Multifocal consolidations/GGO with tree-in-bud nodules may be seen interspersed with areas of air-trapping (Mayer et al. 2014).

2.5.3 Measles

It is a febrile illness with rash caused by an RNA virus belonging to *Paramyxoviridae* family. It spreads from one person to another through droplet spread. The clinical manifestations are more severe in adults and immunocompromised hosts.

Bronchial wall thickening, centrilobular nodules, GGO, and interlobular septal thickening are seen on CT, and the features are nonspecific (Franquet 2011).

2.5.4 SARS-Coronavirus

Coronaviruses, commonly implicated in cold, are RNA viruses of *Coronaviridae*. In 2002, a new strain caused an outbreak in China which spread rapidly throughout the world (Peiris et al. 2003). This was called SARS-coronavirus (severe acute respiratory syndrome). Transmission occurs through droplet spread; incubation period varies from 2 to 14 days (Peiris et al. 2003).

Typical symptoms are fever with myalgia and cough. Characteristic early CT findings include focal ground-glass opacities and crazy-paving pattern which are scattered in distribution. Subsequent development of consolidations may be seen. Air leak syndromes with development of spontaneous mediastinum or pneumothorax have also been reported. Residual fibrosis and scarring may also be seen (Chan et al. 2004).

2.5.5 Hantavirus

Hantaviruses are a group of RNA viruses belonging to the family *Bunyaviridae* (Mattar et al. 2015). Unlike other infections of *Bunyaviridae*, infection with hantaviruses is a rodent-borne zoonosis that spreads through inhalation of rodent secretions (feces, urine, or saliva), and humans are accidental hosts (Manigold and Vial 2014). Each species of hantavirus is associated with a unique rodent host, and thus the epidemiology of hantavirus infections correlates closely with the geographical distribution of the respective rodents (Manigold and Vial 2014).

Infection with hantaviruses causes two distinct clinical pictures: hemorrhagic fever with renal syndrome (HFRS) which is more common in Europe and Asia, caused by the "old world" hantaviruses, and hantavirus cardiopulmonary syndrome (HCPS) which is more common in the Americas, caused by the "new world" hantaviruses (Mattar et al. 2015; Manigold and Vial 2014). Close to 150,000–200,000 cases occur every year, commonly in Asia (Manigold and Vial 2014). In Germany, a peak in 2012 with more than 2800 new cases was reported (Kruger et al. 2013).

Pathologically both these infections are characterized by breakdown of the endothelial barrier in blood vessels and marked vasodilatation.

HFRS is characterized by fever followed by hypotension and petechial hemorrhages due to vascular leakage, oliguric phase, polyuric phase, and convalescence. Oliguric phase is the most critical phase characterized by renal failure and pulmonary edema, and most of the case fatalities occur in this stage.

After an incubation period of 9–35 days, HCPS is characterized by abrupt onset of fever and other constitutional symptoms. In the next cardiopulmonary phase, cough, dyspnea, tachycardia, and hypotension occur due to extravasation of fluids as a result of increased capillary leakage. Rapidly progressive noncardiogenic pulmonary edema and cardiogenic shock may be seen with respiratory failure and need for ventilator support. Case fatality rate is high (Manigold and Vial 2014).

Chest radiography shows features of permeability edema: in mild cases, pleural effusions and interstitial infiltrates are seen (Fig. 23). In severe cases, marked alveolar edema with predominance in the perihilar and basal regions and sparing of the periphery is typical (Boroja et al. 2002). CT shows extensive GGO in middle and lower zones with thickening of the septa (Gasparetto et al. 2007).

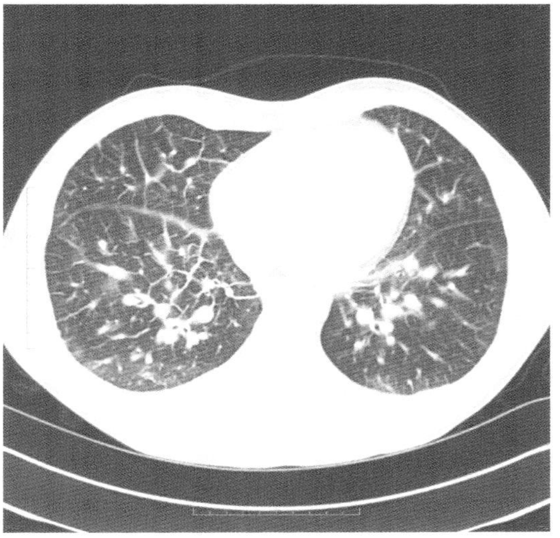

Fig. 23 A 32-year-old man with hantavirus infection: CT showing extensive thickening of the septa, areas of ground-glass, and minor pleural effusions

2.5.6 Adenovirus

They are DNA viruses belonging to *Adenoviridae* family. Many serotypes exist.

Adenovirus is a common cause of upper respiratory tract infection in children. Severe infection is seen in immunocompromised patients. It causes sequelae such as bronchiectasis, obliterative bronchiolitis, and Swyer-James syndrome (unilateral hyperlucent lung).

Pathologically, severe adenovirus pneumonia is characterized by areas of hemorrhagic consolidation, interspersed with air-trapping, atelectasis, and diffuse alveolar damage (Becroft 1967). In mild cases, inflammatory cell infiltrate in the alveoli and interstitium is seen (Chong et al. 2006).

Radiographs show unilateral or bilateral parenchymal opacities. Especially in children, areas of overinflation and atelectasis may be seen (Kim et al. 2002). On CT, extensive GGO with or without consolidations are noted. GGO correlates with areas of diffuse alveolar damage. In a study by Chong et al. in five adults with adenovirus pneumonia, one patient had shown crazy-paving appearance (Chong et al. 2006).

2.5.7 Herpes Simplex Type 1

Herpes simplex type 1 is a DNA virus of the *Herpesviridae*, along with CMV and varicella zoster virus. Primary infection is usually asymptomatic, but can manifest as pharyngitis or gingivostomatitis. Following initial infection, it remains latent and can undergo reactivation at a later stage and manifest as esophagitis or tracheobronchitis.

Pneumonia due to HSV-1 occurs commonly due to contiguous spread from upper respiratory tract or aspiration and less commonly due to hematogenous spread (Graham and Snell 1983; Ramsey et al. 1982). HSV-1 pneumonia is almost exclusively seen in immunosuppressed individuals or in patients with squamous metaplasia of the airways due to intubation, burns, or chronic smoking (Ramsey et al. 1982).

Fever, dyspnea, chest pain, and productive cough are usual clinical features. Herpes labialis and extensive oropharyngeal lesions may also be seen (Simoons-Smit et al. 2006).

The epithelial lesions are characterized by ulceration and necrosis. Pneumonia shows alveolar necrosis and exudate with inflammation (Kim et al. 2002).

On radiography, patchy segmental or lobar consolidation is usually seen, and pleural effusions are common (Aquino et al. 1998). On CT multifocal areas of GGO and consolidation are seen (Kim et al. 2002).

2.5.8 Cytomegalovirus

Cytomegalovirus (CMV) is a member of herpes family and is a DNA virus. It is well known to cause opportunistic infections in immunosuppressed individuals especially in bone marrow or solid organ transplant recipients and AIDS patients.

Clinical features include fever, cough, and dyspnea.

The pathological features of CMV infection in transplant recipients are reported to be different from those seen in AIDS patients. In transplant recipients, predominant necrotizing pneumonia is seen due to immune-mediated mechanisms, and CMV pneumonia is seen in the first few months after transplantation. AIDS patients, on the other hand, have insufficient immune response and show effects primarily due to the cytopathic effect of the virus with diffuse alveolar damage (Kim et al. 2002).

Radiographic manifestations are nonspecific and consist of reticulonodular pattern and/or airspace consolidations. CT features consist of diffuse or focal ground-glass opacities (GGO), multiple nodules, and lobar consolidation. Nodular lesions with surrounding GGO (halo sign) may be occasionally seen, GGO representing hemorrhage or inflammation (Franquet et al. 2003). Dense consolidation or mass-like opacities may be seen in AIDS patients especially with Kaposi's sarcoma (McGuinness et al. 1994).

2.5.9 Varicella Zoster

Varicella zoster is another virus belonging to *Herpesviridae* group. It causes two major manifestations: chickenpox (varicella) and herpes zoster. Pneumonia occurs most commonly in patients with chicken pox, although it may be seen in both forms (Müller et al. 2007).

Chickenpox is usually seen in children 2–8 years old; however, in recent times, the incidence in adults is increasing due to various factors (Mohsen and McKendrick 2003). While the common varicella infection in children is usually benign, infection in adults has a more fulminant course with a 25 times increased risk of pneumonia and consequent high mortality (Mohsen and McKendrick 2003).

Predisposing factors for the development of varicella pneumonia are immunosuppression, chronic lung diseases, pregnancy, or underlying malignancy like leukemia or lymphoma (Müller et al. 2007). Varicella pneumonia presents about 1–6 days after the onset of rash with cough, dyspnea, fever, and sometimes chest pain and hemoptysis (Mohsen and McKendrick 2003).

The pulmonary lesions in varicella seem to be due to hematogenous spread rather than airborne entry. The lesions are characterized by endothelial damage in pulmonary vessels with focal hemorrhagic necrosis, mononuclear infiltrates in the alveolar walls, and exudates in the alveoli (Mohsen and McKendrick 2003). Later small nodules are seen which are characterized by outer lamellated fibrous capsule and inner necrotic or hyalinized collagen with varying degrees of calcification (Kim et al. 1999).

On radiographs multiple, fleeting 5–10 mm miliary nodules are seen with a tendency to coalesce (Fig. 24). These resolve usually in a

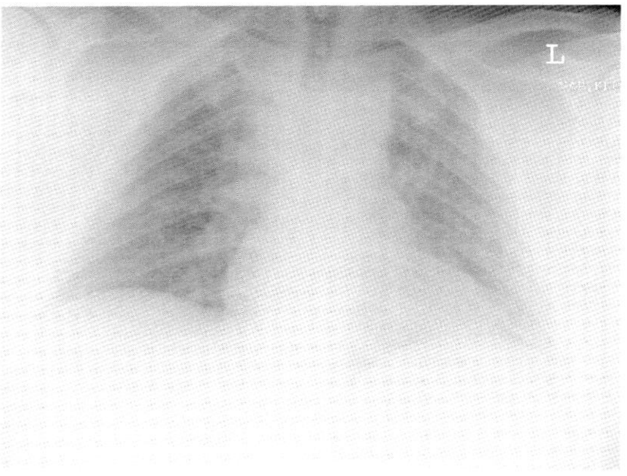

Fig. 24 A 35-year-old man with varicella virus infection: chest radiograph showing multiple fleeting 5–10 mm miliary nodules in both lungs

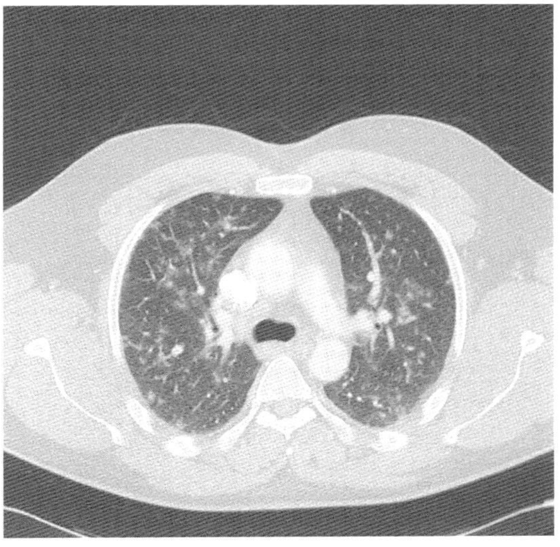

Fig. 25 Same patient as in Fig. 24: CT showing bilateral 5–10 mm nodules of soft tissue density and a ground-glass halo

week after the regression of the skin lesions, but may also be persistent for months in some patients (Sargent et al. 1966). On CT bilateral nodules of soft tissue density measuring 5–10 mm are seen (Fig. 25). Some nodules show GGO around them, while some may coalesce with adjacent nodules (Kim et al. 1999). Hilar lymph nodes and pleural effusions are less commonly seen. Dense, calcified random dense nodules measuring 2–3 mm in size may persist in some cases.

2.6 Conclusion

Although radiography and CT can be helpful in excluding a CAP, they may not be accurate in suggesting an etiological diagnosis. In every case, careful attention to the clinical history and radiological findings may help to narrow down the etiology and suggest the diagnosis.

3 Tuberculosis

3.1 Introduction

Tuberculosis is often a challenge to the clinicians and radiologists alike, particularly in areas where it is not endemic. As the clinical signs and symptoms are often nonspecific, extra attention and a high degree of suspicion are required to make the right diagnosis.

As the manifestations of tuberculosis are a result of the interaction between the offending bacteria and the host immune system, there is no definite radiological picture that defines or is typical for tuberculosis and a wide range of differential diagnoses exist. However, some features, particularly when seen in typical distributions and typical combinations, can be very helpful in suggesting the right diagnosis, as discussed below.

3.2 Background

Tuberculosis (TB) or *captain of all these men of death* is one of the oldest diseases known to mankind. It is still a disease of global concern, affecting millions of people worldwide every year. It is a leading cause of death among infectious diseases. Together with HIV, TB accounted for a staggering 1.5 million deaths in 2014 (World Health Organization 2015). Ninety-five percent of these deaths were reported in low- to middle-income countries, where tuberculosis is highly prevalent (World Health Organization 2015).

Although the incidence of TB globally has been showing a declining trend for several years, still an estimated 9.6 million new cases were reported by WHO in 2014. Majority of these cases were reported in Southeast Asia, Western Pacific, and Africa with highest number of incident cases seen in India, Indonesia, and Nigeria. 12 % of these patients were HIV positive, and notably 75 % of HIV-positive people with tuberculosis lived in Africa (World Health Organization 2015).

Europe accounts for 4 % of TB burden in the world with close to 1000 new cases per day (European Centre for Disease Prevention and Control 2015). Within the EU/EEA (European Union/European economic area), an overall declining trend in TB reporting in the last 10 years has been observed. It is noteworthy that a significant 28 % of cases were of foreign origin. In some countries like Luxemburg, Malta, Norway, Sweden, and Switzerland, the TB cases of foreign origin accounted for >70 % cases, highlighting the increased prevalence in migrants, with an increased prevalence of MDR-TB in these groups of patients (European Centre for Disease Prevention and Control 2015; Odone et al. 2015).

The early diagnosis and treatment are further challenged by the development of multidrug-resistant and extensively drug-resistant tuberculosis. Multidrug-resistant tuberculosis (MDR-TB) is defined by resistance to the two most powerful first-line drugs, isoniazid and rifampin. WHO reported that in 2014, around 3.3 % of new cases and 20 % of previously treated cases had MDR-TB. Extensively drug-resistant tuberculosis (XDR-TB) is defined as MDR-TB with additional resistance to at least one fluoroquinolone and one of the second-line injectable drugs (World Health Organization 2015). It is estimated that around 9.7 % people with MDR-TB have XDR-TB (World Health Organization 2015).

These large numbers of TB prevalence and drug resistance signify the importance of early diagnosis and treatment. To understand imaging features in tuberculosis, an understanding of the epidemiology and pathophysiology is an important prerequisite so that a high index of suspicion in appropriate clinical settings can favor a timely diagnosis, avoid life-threatening complications, and prevent further spread of this dangerous disease.

3.3 Etiology

TB is caused by bacteria of the group *Mycobacterium tuberculosis* complex. It comprises of various bacteria; common ones causing infection in humans are *Mycobacterium tuberculosis and M. bovis. M. tuberculosis* accounts for the majority of tuberculosis cases, whereas *M. bovis* is less commonly implicated due to routine pasteurization of milk.

M. tuberculosis is an obligate aerobic, nonsporing, nonmotile bacillus. Its cell wall is rich in mycolic acid, accounting for its staining properties. It resists staining by the usual Gram method, being neither Gram negative or positive. When stained with dyes such as Ziehl-Neelsen, it resists decolorization by the acid alcohol and is therefore called acid fast. It is a facultative intracellular parasite, which preferentially resides in the human macrophages. Many of these properties explain its pathogenicity and virulence.

3.3.1 Transmission

Person-to-person transmission of infection occurs through inhalation of droplet nuclei which are expelled/discharged into the air when a patient with active pulmonary or laryngeal TB coughs, talks, or sings (Leung 1999). Patients with cavitation in the lungs, sputum culture-positive TB, and sputum smear-positive pulmonary TB who expectorate around 10^6–10^7 acid fast bacillus (AFB) per mL of sputum are more contagious than sputum-negative patients (as they expectorate usually less than 10^3 AFB per ml) (Sepkowitz 1996). Additional factors that favor the spread are an improper ventilation which promotes prolonged suspension of the droplet nuclei, crowded living conditions, and prolonged contact with an "open" case.

Open tuberculosis: Not all patients with pulmonary tuberculosis are infectious to others. Those patients who show sputum positivity for the acid fast bacilli are notably more contagious than sputum-negative cases (see above). The presence of cavitation and evidence of endobronchial spread (tree-in-bud) on radiological examination serves as an indication that there is a communication between the lung lesions and the airways, thereby increasing the risk of infectivity. These "open" cases must be isolated from others.

3.4 Pathogenesis, Clinical, and Radiological Features

Classical teaching explains the lesions of pulmonary tuberculosis based on the time since infection. It states that primary disease after a recent infection manifests itself in lower lobes, lymph nodes, or as pleural effusion, whereas reactivation of latent tuberculosis causes an upper lobe predominant disease with cavitation. Although this classical "dogma" of tuberculosis which classifies the lesions based on the time since infection is widely accepted since time immemorial, it has been challenged in the recent past (Rozenshtein et al. 2015).

Recent studies based on molecular epidemiology using restriction fragment length polymorphism suggest that radiological features of pulmonary tuberculosis do not depend on time since infection (Jones et al. 1997; Glynn et al. 1999). Rather, the lesion manifestations depend on the immune status of the host. Infected persons who are immunocompetent develop apical disease with cavitation. Patients who are immunodeficient, on the other hand, develop lower lobe predominant disease with consolidation and lymphadenopathy without evidence of cavitation. This group includes HIV-positive adults with low CD4 counts and also children, as their cellular immunity is relatively weak.

This concept is further supported by the fact that HIV-positive patients with TB who have CD4 counts $>200/mm^3$ are more likely to develop apical predominant disease with cavitation (positive predictive value >78 %) and those patients with CD4 cell counts $<200/mm^3$ are more likely to have a predominantly lower lobe disease (positive predictive value 84 %), irrespective of the time since infection (Post et al. 1995).

Further studies in the coming future can make this distinction clear. Though the ongoing debate about the pathophysiology of TB has been discussed above, the terms from classical teaching, i.e., primary and reactivation tuberculosis, will be used here for the sake of simplicity as most of the literature is based on this terminology.

3.4.1 Pathogenesis

Primary Tuberculosis

Tuberculosis in a previously unexposed individual is described as primary tuberculosis. Once inhaled, the bacilli traverse the upper airways and reach the alveoli where they are phagocytosed by the pulmonary macrophages.

The subsequent outcome of infection depends on the interaction between the microbicidal capacity of the macrophage and the virulence of *Mycobacterium tuberculosis* bacillus (MTB). If the MTB are destroyed at this stage, no disease develops. But if the macrophage is not able to contain the infection or the bacillus is highly virulent, MTB multiplies multifold before the macrophage bursts. Release of various cytokines by the macrophages attracts further macrophages which phagocytose the released MTB (Knechel 2009). In the first 2–3 weeks, development of T cell-mediated immunity causes activation of macrophages which then destroy the MTB within them (van Crevel et al. 2002). This causes the formation of a typical granuloma with a caseation necrosis in the lungs and the draining lymph nodes. This attributes to the typical imaging features in primary TB. Thus, in tuberculosis destruction of the host tissue occurs as a part of the host immune response.

Once the infection is successfully brought under control, the patient becomes asymptomatic, although MTB may still lie inactive within the macrophages. Healing of the lesions occurs with fibrosis, and dystrophic calcification may also be seen (Pratt 1979).

In immunosuppressed hosts, extensive hematogenous spread of infection can manifest as a miliary TB, with multi-organ involvement.

Reactivation/*Post*primary TB

Many years, typically 3–5 years later, commonly due to reactivation and less commonly due to reinfection, there is a resurgence of the disease (Leung 1999). This stage, in previously sensitized individuals, is known as postprimary TB.

The disease is typically seen in apical and posterior segments of the upper lobes and apical segments of the lower lobes, probably due high oxygen tension and impaired lymphatic drainage in these areas which favor the growth of this obligate aerobe (Leung 1999). As the infection proceeds, the area of necrosis increases in this area, under liquefaction, and then decompresses itself into an adjacent bronchus. As a result of the formation of this communication with airways, air enters the lung parenchyma in this area of consolidation, forming what is a typical lesion of the secondary TB, that is, a cavity. As the contents of the cavity are discharged into the bronchus, the patient develops cough with expectoration. Spread of these discharges into the airways may also give rise to typical imaging appearance of endobronchial spread. When there is no cavity, endobronchial spread of Tb may still be seen due to endobronchial rupture of a lymph node, hematogenous spread of infection (Leung 1999).

3.4.2 Clinical Features

Majority of the TB cases are pulmonary with around 1/3 cases being extrapulmonary.

The clinical symptoms of tuberculosis are to an extent dependent on patient's age and immune status. At extremes of age, in children and elderly, the symptoms tend to be nonspecific and cause a delay in the diagnosis. Primary TB is most commonly seen in children, particularly in endemic areas. However, it is increasingly being seen in adults too.

The usual symptoms in pulmonary TB are cough with expectoration, low-grade fever with evening rise of temperature, malaise, and loss of weight (American Thoracic Society 1990). Hemoptysis and chest pain may also be seen.

Radiological Features

Primary pulmonary tuberculosis manifests itself radiologically variably as parenchymal opacities, lymphadenopathy, and/or pleural effusion. Chest radiography is usually the first imaging modality to suspect primary TB; however, the lesions are better appreciated on CT.

The granulomatous lesion in the pulmonary parenchyma is seen radiologically as an area of consolidation. It tends to be unilateral, in the middle or lower lobe, and is commonly observed on the right side (Leung et al. 1992). Multifocal involvement may also be seen in 12–24 % (Woodring et al. 1986). It is usually homogenous and dense, segmental, or lobar in distribution. The lesion can also be nodular or linear in appearance.

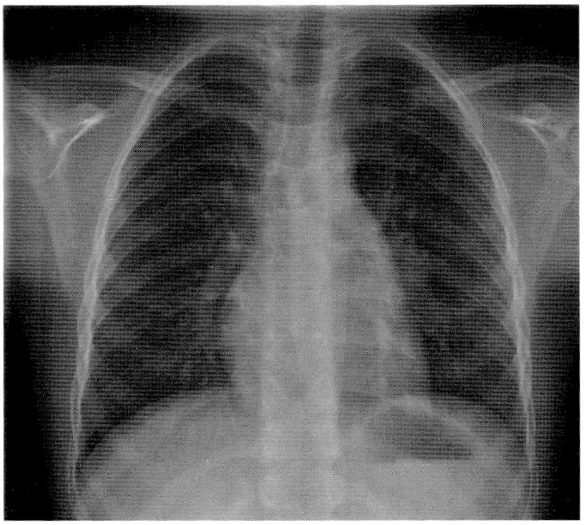

Fig. 26 A 7-year-old boy with primary TB: chest radiograph showing enlarged left hilar shadow

In two-thirds of the cases, the consolidation resolves without any sequelae (Leung 1999). In the remaining one-third cases, it heals with the formation of a linear scar or fibrosis, with calcification. This focus is called as Ghon's focus (Leung 1999). Tuberculomas which are mass-like opacities and satellite calcifications may be also seen in 9 % of the cases.

Lymphadenopathy is the most characteristic feature of primary TB. It is seen in 90–95 % of the children with primary TB. As the age increases, the prevalence of lymphadenopathy decreases in older children and adults (Leung et al. 1992). Tuberculous lymphadenopathy tends to be typically unilateral with frequent involvement of the right paratracheal and right hilar groups. This can be visualized on radiographs with the widening of the right paratracheal stripe and enlarged hilum, respectively (Fig. 26). On CT, the presence of enlarged lymph nodes, more than 2 cm with peripheral rim enhancement, is characteristic (Fig. 27). This is due to central caseous necrosis with peripheral vascular granulation tissue (Leung et al. 1992).

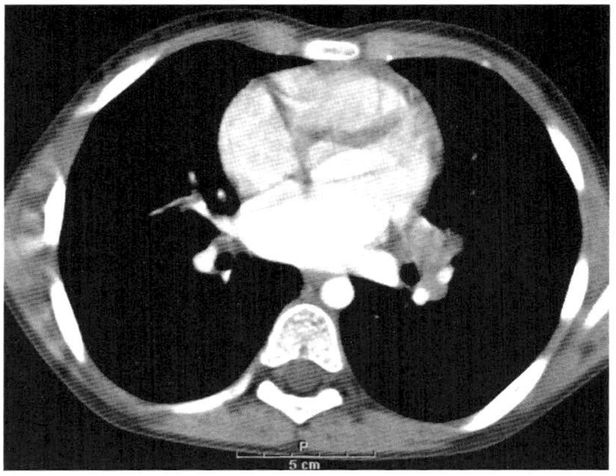

Fig. 27 A 7-year-old boy with primary TB: axial CT thorax in the same patient with mediastinal window showing enlarged left hilar lymph nodes with peripheral contrast enhancement

The enlarged lymph nodes can cause extrinsic compression of the airways. Complete obstruction of the lumen manifests as segmental or lobar collapse of the distal lung (Andreu et al. 2004). Partial obstruction, on the other hand, can present with air-trapping and hyperinflation of the involved lobe due to ball-valve-like effect and subsequent trapping of air (Arora et al. 2013).

Healing of the granulomatous lesions with dystrophic calcification leads to the formation of calcified hilar lymph node with a calcified pulmonary Ghon's lesion, also known as Ranke's complex. It serves as a telltale sign of previous TB infection in the past.

Reactivation tuberculosis is characterized by parenchymal opacifications, predominantly in the posterior and apical segments of upper lobes and apical segment of lower lobes. Multisegmental involvement is often seen. Atypical distribution involving *exclusively* other segments is rare and is seen in approximately 5 % of the cases of postprimary TB (Woodring et al. 1986). Cavities are seen in 40–45 % of cases of postprimary disease. They may be single or multiple and have varied appearances ranging from thick walled to thin walled. Cavities usually occur in areas of consolidation. Cavities may mimic carcinoma; however, careful attention to adjacent bronchogenic spread with tree-in-bud lesions and satellite nodules may aid in the diagnosis.

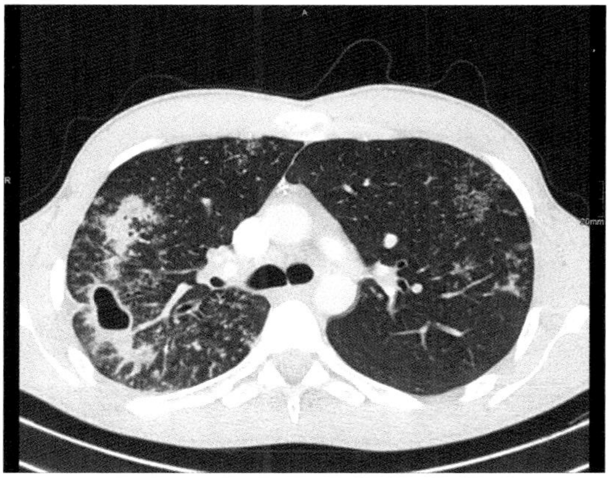

Fig. 28 A 27-year-old patient with reactivation tuberculosis: axial CT showing a thin-walled cavitary lesion in the posterior segment of the right upper lobe. Florid areas of centrilobular nodules with tree-in-bud appearance are noted on both sides. This combination is highly suggestive of reactive tuberculosis

When an area of caseous necrosis erodes into adjacent airways, bronchogenic spread is seen. It is an important hallmark of the activity of the disease. CT is more sensitive in demonstrating bronchogenic spread: in one study by Im et al., bronchogenic spread was notably seen in 95 % of patients with postprimary TB, while radiography showed these findings reliably only in 20 % patients (Im et al. 1993). Earliest markers of bronchogenic spread are sharp centrilobular nodules or linear branching opacities 2–4 mm in diameter. In extensive bronchogenic spread, a typical tree-in-bud appearance is described, the stalk represents the distal airways, and the bud represents alveolar ducts and bronchioles, which are filled with caseous material. Other signs of bronchogenic spread are bronchial wall thickening with or without bronchiectasis, poorly defined nodules 5–8 mm in diameter. Interlobular septal thickening may also be seen. These changes signify an active underlying disease and regress with effective treatment in 5–9 months (Im et al. 1993).

Tree-in-bud nodules are not specific for tuberculosis. However, presence of cavitary or nodular lesions in the typical distribution along with tree-in-bud lesions makes the diagnosis of tuberculosis highly probable and should always be considered in suitable clinical settings (Fig. 28) (Andreu et al. 2004).

Complete regression of the parenchymal lesions may be seen when healing occurs before the development of caseous necrosis, which is however rare (Pratt 1979). In posttreatment changes with development of distortion of bronchovascular structure, fibrotic bands in areas of caseous necrosis are well established. Areas of paracicatricial emphysema may develop due to bronchostenosis and traction (Im et al. 1993). Marked fibrotic reaction with upward hilar retraction is typical and may be seen in one-third of the cases. Apical pleural thickening, usually less than 1 cm, may also be occasionally seen (Woodring et al. 1986).

When to Think of TB?

Patient features: Migratory background, poor immune status

Radiological features: Primary TB: Unilateral dense segmental or lobar consolidation in lower or middle lobes, lymphadenopathy with central hypodensity on CECT

Reactivation TB: Cavitation in apical segments, centrilobular tree-in-bud nodules, with or without sequelae of primary TB infection

Hilar and mediastinal lymphadenopathy is less likely in postprimary tuberculosis. Spontaneous pneumothorax may be seen in extensive cavitary disease, although rare.

Miliary TB

At any stage, either after primary or postprimary, a fulminant infection can give rise to disseminated infection with multiple granulomas seen in various organs. These granulomas resemble millet seeds, and thus the term "miliary" tuberculosis was used to describe them. Various conditions that predispose to the development of miliary TB are HIV/AIDS, malnutrition, diabetes mellitus, underlying malignancy, immunosuppression, treatment with corticosteroids, and immunomodulators (anti-TNF alpha agents) (Sharma et al. 2012).

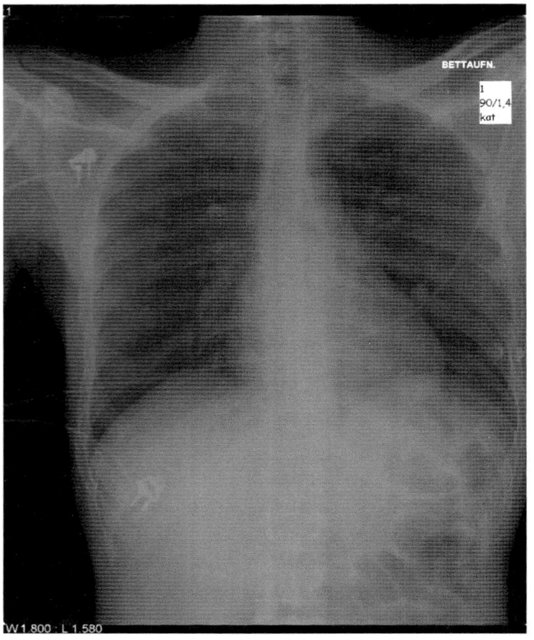

Fig. 29 A 52-year-old HIV-positive male with miliary tuberculosis: frontal radiograph showing multiple vague nodular lesions in both the lungs

Early radiographs may be normal. Evenly distributed nodules roughly 1–3 mm in size may be seen (Fig. 29). CT demonstrates these changes more clearly with sharply and poorly defined nodules seen in random distribution with respect to the secondary pulmonary lobule (Figs. 30 and 31). Smooth thickening of the interlobular septa is commonly seen (McGuinness et al. 1992). Ground-glass opacities may be seen for abnormalities that are below the resolution of CT (Hong et al. 1998). On adequate treatment, these nodules resolve usually without any residual fibrosis.

In some cases, military tuberculosis can progress to adult respiratory distress syndrome. Spontaneous pneumothorax due to rupture of subpleural nodules has also been reported (Sharma and Kumar 2002).

3.5 Pleural Involvement

Pleural effusion can be seen not only as a part of primary TB but also in patients with reactivation TB and is thus not specific for any stage of TB.

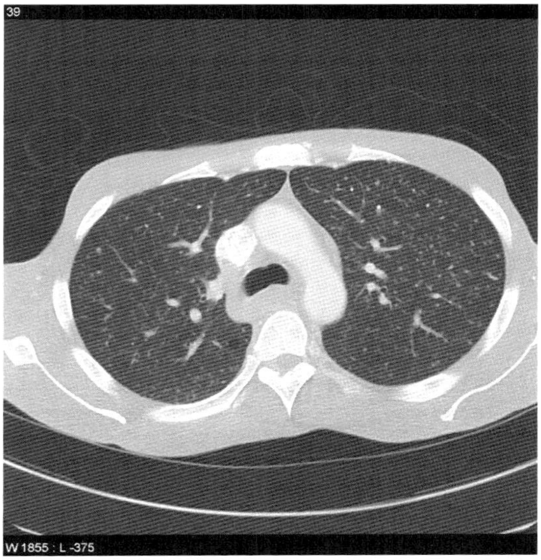

Fig. 30 A 52-year-old HIV-positive male with miliary tuberculosis: axial CT showing multiple well-defined nodules in a random distribution much better

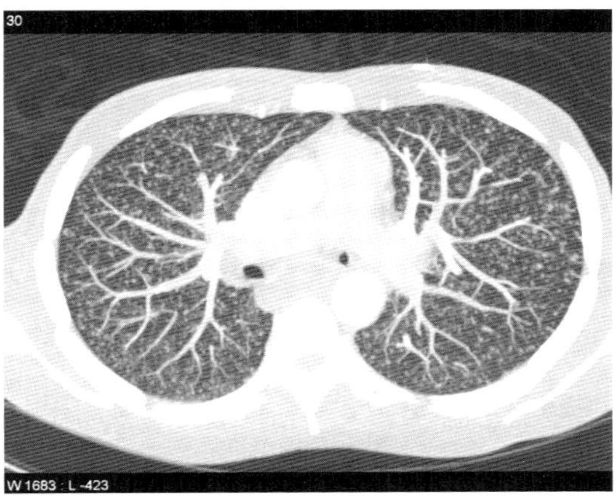

Fig. 31 A 52-year-old HIV-positive male with miliary tuberculosis: axial MiP image showing multiple miliary nodules in a random distribution better

It occurs supposedly due to a delayed hypersensitivity reaction as a result of rupture of a caseating subpleural focus into the pleural cavity. The release of inflammatory mediators causes accumulation fluid in the pleural space, which is an exudate.

Tuberculous pleuritis often presents acutely with rapid onset of pleuritic chest pain that is worsened by deep breathing, fever, and cough. In HIV-positive patients, a more subacute course is described. It is usually unilateral, often seen on the same side of the parenchymal lesion. Isolated pleural effusions without any parenchymal lesion are not rare.

On ultrasound examination, it often shows septations which are usually not appreciated on CT (Cardinale et al. 2015). On contrast-enhanced CT, pleural fluid of fluid density with smooth peripheral pleural enhancement, "split pleura" is typical (Yilmaz et al. 1998). Presence of a changing air-fluid level in the pleural space mandates ruling out a bronchopleural fistula (Johnson et al. 1973).

3.6 Airway Involvement

The involvement of airways in tuberculosis is seen in 10–20 % of patients with pulmonary tuberculosis (Moon et al. 1997). Various mechanisms responsible for the involvement of airways are spread of infection from the parenchymal lesion along the peribronchial lymphatic channels, implantation from infected sputum, erosion of an adjacent lymph node, or hematogenous spread (Moon et al. 1997; Kim et al. 1997).

Acute tracheobronchitis with involvement of the distal trachea and the proximal bronchi may be seen (Kim et al. 1997). Tracheobronchial TB is characterized commonly by a long-segment thickening (>3 cm) (smooth or irregular), causing circumferential narrowing of the airways. Less common appearances are that of a granulomatous, polypoid ulcerated mass (Andreu et al. 2004).

Chronic inflammation of the airways may cause tracheal or bronchial stenosis. Traction bronchiectasis due to fibrosis is often seen as sequel of infection.

A calcified peribronchial node that usually erodes into the adjacent bronchus is a common cause of broncholithiasis. Common sites are the proximal right middle lobar bronchus and anterior segmental bronchus of the right upper lobe.

3.7 Pericardial Involvement

Tuberculous pericarditis is seen in around 1 % pulmonary TB patients; the incidence is rising due to HIV-TB coinfection (Mayosi et al. 2005). In HIV-infected groups, 85 % of the cases of pericardial effusion are due to TB (Ntsekhe and Hakim 2005). It may present as pericardial effusion, constrictive pericarditis, or a combination of both.

The spread of infection to the pericardium occurs chiefly through the following routes:

Via infected mediastinal lymph nodes: predominant in immunocompetent individuals, it is largely a hypersensitivity reaction with paucibacillary status.

Via hematogenous route: more often encountered in HIV-positive and other immunosuppressed individuals, where is it often a more florid infection with a multibacillary status (Ntsekhe and Mayosi 2013).

Less common mode of spread is via direct spread from an adjoining pulmonary infection.

Clinical Features Typically, an insidious onset, with complaints of fever, dyspnea, chest pain, and malaise, is described. Cardiac tamponade may be frequently seen and is a late feature. Acute presentation with dyspnea, fever, and retrosternal chest pain is also possible.

Imaging On routine chest radiography, enlarged cardiac silhouette is seen in tuberculous effusion. Concomitant evidence of active pulmonary tuberculosis may be seen in 30 % of the individuals, and 30–50 % may show pleural effusions (Reuter et al. 2005). Another interesting feature to note is that the hilar lymph nodes are not usually involved; mediastinal nodes not detected with PA radiographs and therefore the lymphadenopathy in tuberculous pericarditis are not seen on routine frontal radiographs (Reuter et al. 2005). On echocardiography, pericardial thickening with evidence of strands in the fluid is commonly seen in around 60 % cases and is not specific for TB pericarditis (Mayosi et al. 2005).

Imaging features on CT may point to the tuberculous origin of the effusion. Thickened enhancing pericardium is seen; however, it may be difficult to distinguish between small effusions and thickening on CT, where ultrasound may prove more helpful. In one study, enlarged mediastinal lymph nodes were described in all patients with tuberculous pericarditis (Cherian 2004). These lymph nodes usually regress with treatment. On the contrary, other causes of effusion with mediastinal lymphadenopathy, like lymphoma, malignancy, or sarcoidosis, show hilar lymphadenopathy in addition

In constrictive pericarditis, fibrous or calcific thickening of the pericardium is seen, with or without effusion. Pericardial thickening of more than 3 mm with supporting findings of dilated inferior vena cava and deviated interventricular septum can help in accurate diagnosis, in appropriate clinical settings. Calcification of the visceral pericardium in the atrioventricular groove, interventricular groove, and crux of the heart is uncommon but may be seen (Suchet and Horwitz 1992).

3.8 Acute Complications: Tuberculosis in the Emergency Room

Tuberculosis, although as described above, has an insidious onset and progress, can also present acutely, in a previously healthy person. Common symptoms with which the patients present to the emergency room are dyspnea, fever, hemoptysis, or chest pain. It may be a challenge to diagnose tuberculosis in acute settings, especially in countries where it is less endemic and a wide other close differential diagnoses exist. However, an awareness of the migratory background and immune and HIV status of the patient, compounded by a high index of suspicion of the treating physician and the radiologist, may expedite the diagnostic process.

3.8.1 Hemoptysis

Hemoptysis, or expectoration of blood, is an acute life-threatening complication of tuberculosis. Incidence of hemoptysis in TB may be up to 7 %, depending upon the regional prevalence of tuberculosis, with a high mortality rate ranging from 9 to 18 % (Krishnan et al. 2009; Johnston and Reisz 1989; Alkhuja and Miller 2001). Hemoptysis in TB does not always signify an underlying active disease (Prasad et al. 2009).

Massive hemoptysis is defined variably in the literature, with the volume of blood ranging from 100 to 1000 mL in 24 h, although any amount of bleeding that causes hemodynamic instability should be considered significant (Corder 2003; Jean-Baptiste 2000). Almost 90% of causes of massive hemoptysis in general originate from bronchial vessels, while 10% originate from pulmonary vessels, understandably because the bronchial vessels are at systemic pressure (Yoon et al. 2002). Notable among the common causes are chronic inflammatory conditions like bronchiectasis, tuberculosis, and lung abscess and malignancies like bronchogenic carcinoma, which account for a vast majority of cases of massive hemoptysis.

The first step in managing any patient with massive hemoptysis is stabilization of the patient, resuscitation, and protection of the lower airways, as the risk of death due to asphyxiation overweighs that due to exsanguination (Marshall and Jackson 1997).

The next step is to identify the site and cause of bleeding and treat it accordingly. Various procedures form a part of the diagnostic algorithm for further evaluation, with MDCT angiography followed by bronchoscopy standing at the forefront. If the patient is clinically stable, the first logical step will be a MDCT angiography to locate the site of bleeding. CT has many advantages as it enables not only the identification of the site of bleeding but also facilitates the evaluation of the lungs to recognize the underlying cause of bleeding (Yoon et al. 2002).

On the other hand, patients who are not stable are taken up directly for rigid/flexible fiber-optic bronchoscopy. Many studies nevertheless recommend using CT angiography prior to bronchoscopy routinely in all patients with hemoptysis, as CT aids in a comprehensive evaluation with a better diagnosis of the cause of hemoptysis compared to bronchoscopy (Revel et al. 2002; Bruzzi et al. 2006).

Causes of Hemoptysis in Tuberculosis

Several underlying pathologies in tuberculosis can cause hemoptysis. Bronchial vessels are a more common source than pulmonary vessels and, when involved, tend to cause severe hemoptysis which is difficult to control.

Tuberculous bronchitis and bronchiectasis tend to cause bronchial arterial bleeding. Tuberculosis cavities can erode into adjacent structures, for example, into pleura and chest wall, and cause hemoptysis due to the involvement of intercostal, internal mammary, or subclavian vessels. Furthermore, colonization of preexisting cavities with fungus – aspergilloma – can also present as hemoptysis. Inflammation of pulmonary artery branches adjoining the cavities of TB, with consequent formation of "Rasmussen" aneurysm, can precipitate fatal hemoptysis. Erosion of the involved lymph nodes into adjacent tracheobronchial tree or vessels may also cause hemoptysis (Chatterjee et al. 2015; Halezeroglu and Okur 2014).

Bronchiectasis and Dilatation of Bronchial Arteries

Bronchial arteries are the primary source of nourishment to the bronchial tree and have microvascular connections with pulmonary circulation. These connections become functional in patients with bronchiectasis and chronic inflammation like TB.

In various chronic inflammatory conditions like tuberculosis and bronchiectasis (which can itself be as a result of tuberculosis), there is associated vasculitis and thrombosis of pulmonary vessels that cause local hypoxia. This stimulates the release of angiogenetic growth factors such as vascular endothelial growth factor, thereby promoting neovascularity, collateral formation, and enlarged bronchial arteries. This accounts for flow of blood from bronchial arteries at systemic pressure into the pulmonary vessels and hemoptysis (Bruzzi et al. 2006).

Special attention should be given to CT appearances in these patients. Presence of nodular or tubular soft tissue attenuation structures in the mediastinum, particularly around the airways, which are atypical for lymph nodes, should be viewed with suspicion. These structures may point toward hypertrophied bronchial arteries (Song et al. 1998).

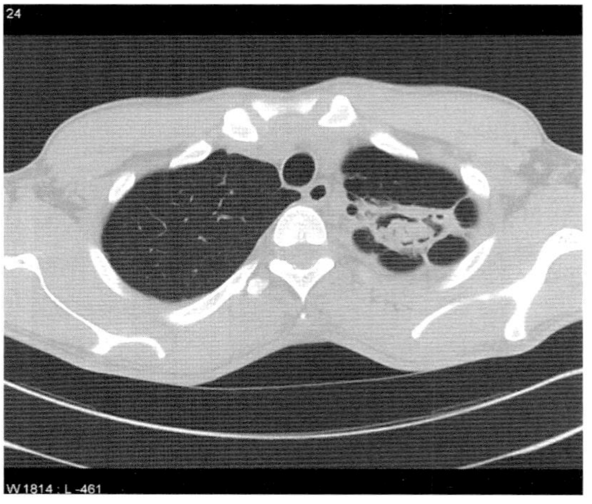

Fig. 32 A 52-year-old patient with cavitary lesion in left upper lobe. Intracavitary body with "air-crescent" sign, suggestive of aspergilloma, is seen in the left upper lobe

Aspergilloma

Aspergilloma is a fungal infection, caused commonly due to the fungus *A. fumigatus* that saprophytically colonizes preexisting cavities, and dilated bronchi, without invading them. It is commonly asymptomatic, hemoptysis being the most common symptom. On radiography, a round or oval intracavitary mass lesion is typically described, the lesion being dependent in location and surrounded by a crescent of air (air-crescent sign). Decubitus views to demonstrate the mobility of the intracavitary mass are helpful in doubtful cases. Pathologically, the lesion comprises of fungal hyphae intermixed with varying amounts of mucous and cellular debris. On CT, a soft tissue attenuation lesion located within a cavity is typical (Fig. 32). Thickening of the walls of the cavity and that of the adjacent pleura is described. This thickening may be the earliest sign of aspergillosis, even before any visible changes in the cavity are seen. It represents a hypersensitivity reaction rather than a fibrosis and is reversible with treatment (Franquet et al. 2000).

Hemoptysis in aspergilloma is often associated with vasculitis in the cavity wall and extensive collateral formation from axillary and subclavian vessels (Uflacker et al. 1983; Remy et al. 1977). Hypertrophied bronchial arteries may also be seen as the cause of hemoptysis, and these should be actively searched for on CT.

The diagnosis can be challenging when the air crescent is not clearly appreciated due to obliteration of the cavity. Other differential diagnoses for intracavitary lesions are angioinvasive aspergillosis, echinococcal cysts, Rasmussen aneurysm in a cavity, lung abscess, bronchogenic carcinoma, intracavitary clot or hematoma, and *P. carinii* pneumonia (Franquet et al. 2001)

Treatment: Spontaneous resolution may be seen in 10 % of the patients (Hammerman et al. 1973). Palliative bronchial artery embolization is undertaken for acute management of hemoptysis, although a significantly high rate of recurrent hemoptysis in aspergillosis has been reported (Uflacker et al. 1983; Remy et al. 1977). Definitive treatment is thus surgical resection with perioperative antifungal treatment.

Rasmussen's Aneurysm

Rasmussen's aneurysm is another rare cause of life-threatening hemorrhage in tuberculosis. A prevalence of 4 % in autopsy studies in patients who died of tuberculosis has been described.

Rasmussen's aneurysm is a pseudoaneurysm which arises due to erosion of a cavity into an adjacent pulmonary artery. As the inflammation of the cavity involves an adjoining pulmonary artery branch, there is progressive weakening and thinning of the arterial wall as a result of necrotizing granulomatous inflammation, giving rise to a pseudoaneurysm months or years later (Santelli et al. 1994; Kim et al. 2001). Eventual rupture can cause fatal hemoptysis.

MDCT angiography plays an important role in not only identifying the aneurysm but also in correctly characterizing it as arising from pulmonary artery, distinguishing it from bronchial artery aneurysms which are more frequent. Careful attention to the cavity on post-contrast images may exhibit a focal enhancing lesion, thereby clinching the diagnosis.

Emergency endovascular management technique like percutaneous catheter embolization of the aneurysm is the treatment of choice (Remy et al. 1980).

Hemoptysis Due to Lymph Nodes

Although extremely rare, reports of tuberculous lymph nodes causing erosion of mediastinal vessels like aorta or pulmonary artery with subsequent formation of trachea/bronchovascular fistula and fatal hemorrhage do exist (Krishnan et al. 2009; Fatimi et al. 2006).

3.8.2 Chest Pain/Dyspnea

Acute onset chest pain and difficulty in breathing in tuberculosis can be due to a variety of underlying causes: acute respiratory distress syndrome (ARDS), pleuritis, pneumothorax, pericarditis, chest wall abscess to name a few.

Pneumothorax: Secondary Spontaneous Pneumothorax

Pneumothorax can complicate the course of roughly 1 % of tuberculosis, more often in severe cavitary tuberculosis. Underlying pathology is rupture of pleural caseous nodules which undergo necrosis. It must be suspected when apical abnormality is seen after re-expansion of the lung (Kim et al. 2001).

Pneumothorax, which may also be bilateral, has been reported in patients with miliary tuberculosis, who present with acute onset of breathlessness during the course of treatment with antituberculous drugs (Sharma and Kumar 2002; Arya et al. 2011; Khan et al. 2011; Singh et al. 2014). Caseation of the subpleural miliary nodules with subsequent rupture into the pleural space has been attributed as the triggering factor. On imaging, miliary shadows may not be discernible initially and may be evident only when the lung re-expands.

4 Hematogenous Spread of Pulmonary Infection

4.1 Introduction

Hematogenous origin of pulmonary infection depends on septic pulmonary embolism (SPE). This is an uncommon syndrome characterized by pulmonary embolization of infected thrombi containing microorganisms admixed with fibrin. It depends on a primary infectious site spread out into the venous circulation, with implantation into peripheral pulmonary arterial vessels, resulting in alveolar infective infiltrates.

The most common causative Gram-positive bacteria are *Staphylococcus aureus* and *Streptococcus pneumoniae*, whereas the most frequent Gram-negative bacterium is *Pseudomonas aeruginosa* (Angus and van der Poll 2013).

Historically SPE was most commonly associated with Lemierre's syndrome, postpartum septic pelvic thrombophlebitis, and right-sided infective endocarditis (Mac Millan et al. 1978; Goldenberg et al. 2005).

In the last decade, attention has been made to changes in the epidemiology, including thrombophlebitis due to contiguous deep soft tissue or bone infection or for infected endovascular catheters and implantable devices (Brenes et al. 2012a; Cook et al. 2005a).

In fact, like all foreign bodies, venous catheters, cardiac pacemaker, implantable cardioverter defibrillator, and joint prosthesis could carry a risk of infection. Due to increase in the number of that devices, the risk of infections have become a common problem in clinical practice (Baddour et al. 2003).

The incidence of infections is 1.9 per 1000 devices per year, and the cumulative probability of device infections is higher among patients with defibrillators compared with those with pacemaker and central venous catheters or joint prosthesis (Uslan et al. 2007).

Approximately 25 % of acute cardiac pacemaker infections occur as an acute event, in a period of device to be installed in the first 1–2 months (Cook et al. 2005b) (Fig. 33). There is a high mortality (27–65 %) associated with infections of these devices (Klug et al. 1997).

Septic embolism also occurs in 22–50 % of patients with infective endocarditis. The predictors of embolism are vegetation size greater than 10 mm, mitral location, and infection of *S. aureus*.

The brain, the spleen, and lungs are the most frequent sites of embolism in left- and right-sided infective endocarditis (Takin et al. 2012).

4.1.1 Clinical Characteristics

Main risk factors for SPE are intravenous drug abuse, alcoholism, hemodialysis, diabetes, and venous catheters (Cassling et al. 1985) (Fig. 34).

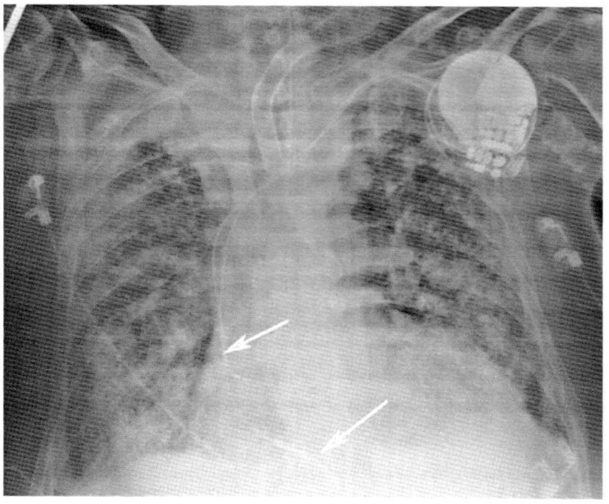

Fig. 33 Chest radiograph shows the presence of a pacemaker (*arrows*) associated with multiple lobular, patchy, pulmonary infiltrates

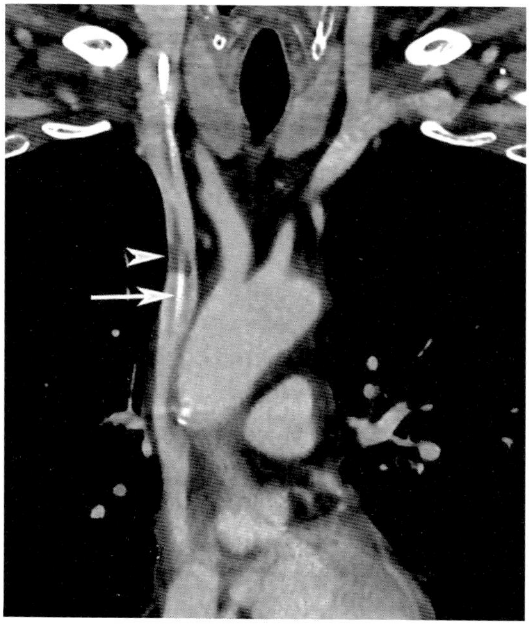

Fig. 34 Post-contrast CT coronary image of the mediastinum demonstrates a defect filling corresponding to a thrombus (*arrowhead*) that surrounds a central venous catheters (*arrow*) inside the lumen of superior vena cava

SPE diagnosis is based on the following criteria: acute clinical presentation with fever, chills, chest pain, dyspnea, hemoptysis, cough, presence of an extrapulmonary infectious site (such as pyelonephritis (Fig. 35) with or without hydronephrosis,

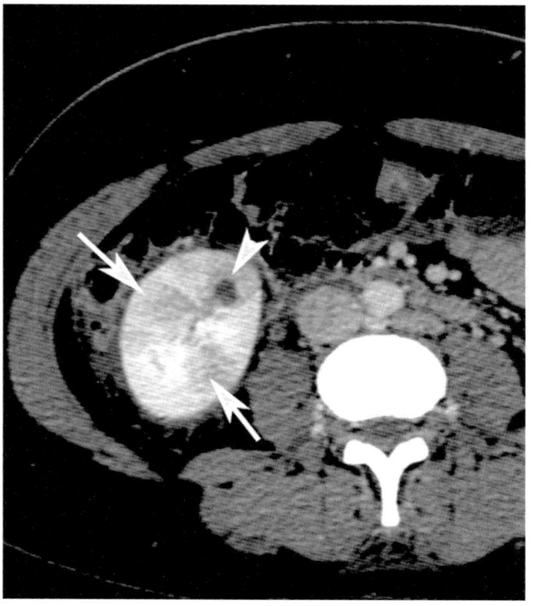

Fig. 35 Post-contrast CT axial scan of the abdomen shows multiple hypodense focal areas (*arrows*) of the right kidney, corresponding to pyelonephritis associated with a small abscess (*arrowhead*)

osteomyelitis with multiple small paraspinal abscesses, osteoarthritis (Fig. 36), liver abscesses (Fig. 37), muscle abscesses (Fig. 38), neck or oral infection (Fig. 39), etc.), frequent acute venous thrombosis that can affect any vein in the body evidenced by color Doppler-ultrasound and/or CT scan (Fig. 40), bacteremia evidenced by laboratory tests, multifocal pulmonary peripheral nodules, or infiltrates demonstrated by chest x-ray film and CT scan.

Frequently the patients with SPE have an infective endocarditis (IE) that primarily involves the cardiac valve leaflets and can spread septic emboli into the pulmonary arterial circulation. Patients with large cardiac valve-infective vegetations (>10 mm) are at high risk of pulmonary embolism. The mitral valve is the most frequent infected valve (50 %) followed by the aortic valve (40 %) and tricuspid valve (10 %). Multiple valves, usually the mitral and aortic valves, are involved in 20 % of cases (Moriera et al. 2012; Nucifora et al. 2007).

The mortality of IE is about 30–60 % and is due to septic embolism involving mitral valve, lungs, and cerebrovascular sites (Nucifora et al. 2007).

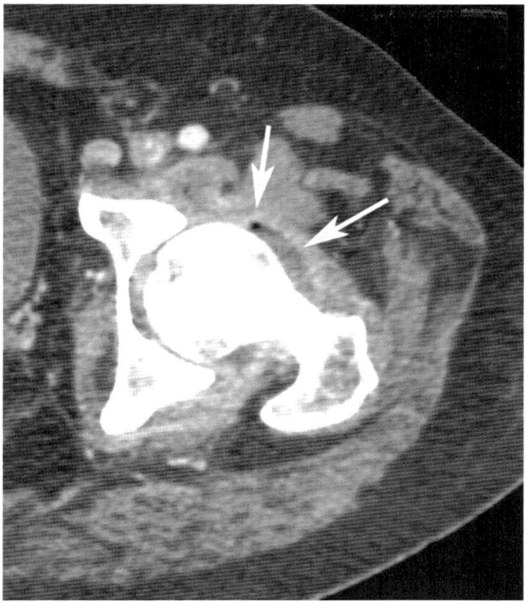

Fig. 36 Post-contrast CT axial scan of the pelvis demonstrates a thin fluid collection with air bubbles (*arrows*) inside the left hip capsule, due to osteoarthritis

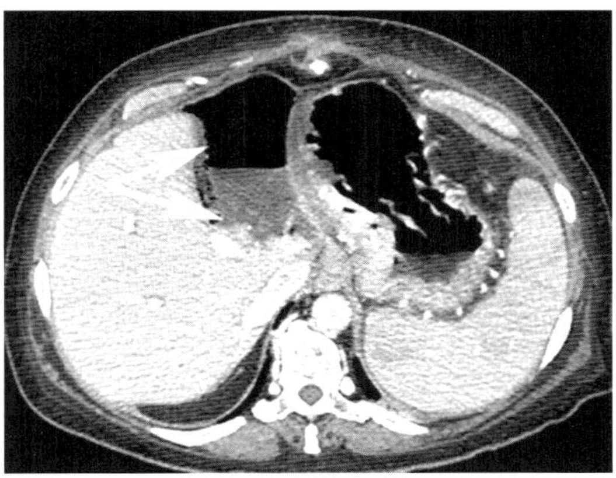

Fig. 37 Post-contrast CT axial scan of the abdomen demonstrates a large liver abscess with a typical air-fluid level (*arrow*)

4.2 Pathophysiologic Sequence

A local infection can cause extravasation of microorganisms into the venous system. Depending on the extent of the infection, edema could result in venous compression and stasis (Nourse et al. 2007) (Fig. 40).

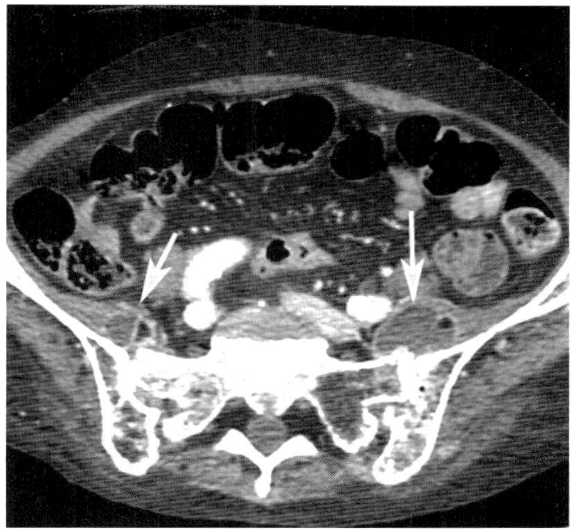

Fig. 38 Post-contrast CT axial scan of the pelvis shows bilateral iliopsoas muscle small fluid collections surrounded by a thin hyperdense capsule (*arrows*) corresponding to abscesses

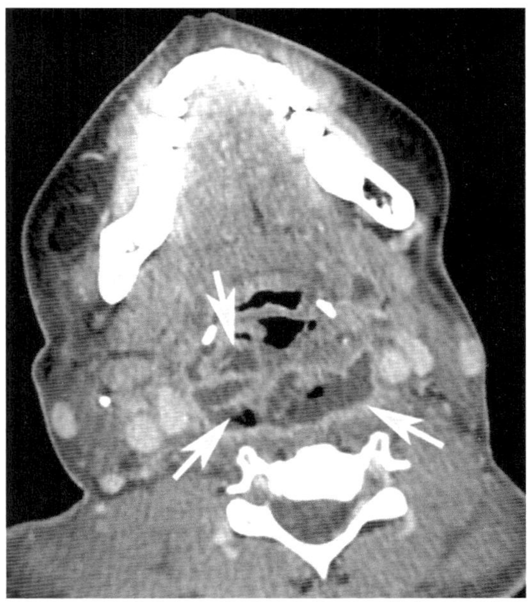

Fig. 39 Post-contrast CT axial of the neck demonstrates a pharyngeal multiloculated collection surrounded by a thin hyperdense tissue (*arrows*) corresponding to abscess

The venous endothelium could be damaged by inflammatory mediators and production of thrombogenic toxins by the microorganism, leading to venous thrombosis. The fibrin and platelet

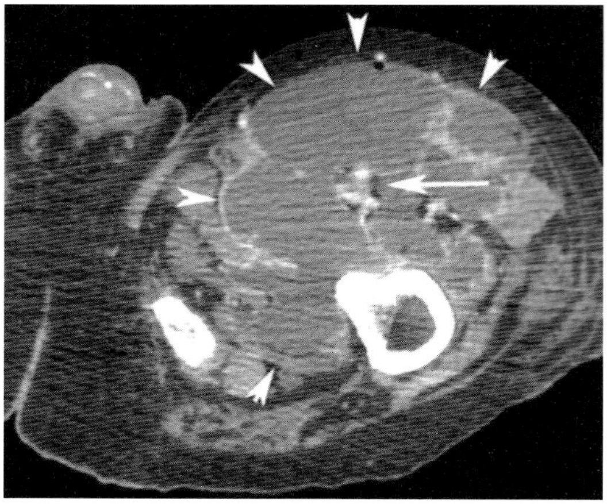

Fig. 40 Post-contrast CT axial scan of the left lower limb shows quadricipite muscle large multiloculated collection corresponding to abscess (*arrowheads*), surrounding the femoral venam that contains a thrombus (*arrow*)

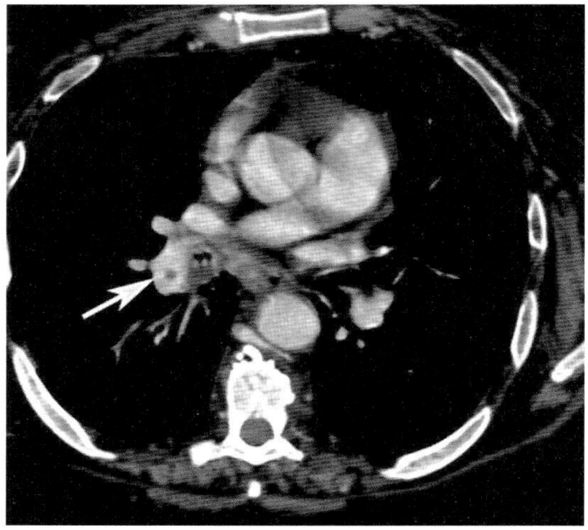

Fig. 41 Post-contrast CT axial scan of the chest shows a small defect filling corresponding to an embolus (*arrowhead*) inside the lumen of the right lower interlobar pulmonary artery

matrix serves as an ideal nidus for proliferation of the microorganism with potential for propagation and allows for distant metastatic infection as its contents are drained into the pulmonary circulation through the venous system.

Special attention should be given to *S. aureus* which can determine a severe inflammatory reaction, with direct endothelial damage through CI toxins and enzymatic mechanism, determining septic pulmonary emboli (Brenes et al. 2012b) (Fig. 41).

Specifically, it is known that *S. aureus* has a tendency to promote venous thrombosis. The bacterium produces an extracellular heat stable leukocidin that exhibits thrombogenic effects, through indirect inflammatory mechanism, including the development of reactive oxygen species and release of secondary inflammatory mediators from dying granulocytes, causing intense endothelial dysfunction (Boyle-Vavra and Daum 2007). *S. aureus* produces coagulase too, which specifically interacts with fibrinogen and causes coagulation (Gorenstem et al. 2000).

The predominance of *S. aureus* as the causative agent is related to its intrinsic thrombogenic and pro-inflammatory potential, rather than just its expected relation to the type of primary focus (Vinder Have et al. 2009; Hota et al. 2001). Once in the blood flow, the bacterium can damage directly the pulmonary parenchyma through the toxins (Boyle-Vavra and Daum 2006) and indirectly through inflammatory mediators (Holm et al. 2011) that may occasionally promote local thrombosis which serves as an additional nidus for proliferation of the bacterium. Embolization of these thrombi, inside the pulmonary arterial circulation (Fig. 41), allows for multiple infection infiltrates of the lungs, even in the absence of heart valvular involvement.

The endothelial cells of the capillaries and arterioles as well as the venules of the lungs are highly susceptible to hypoxia. Therefore, mild transient ischemia of lung tissue may result in marked vessel dilatation as well as increased vascular permeability with fluid and erythrocyte leakage inside the alveolar sacs (Wagenwoort 1995).

4.3 Radiographic Features

Chest x-ray film is low sensitive, but can help to provide important information to suggest the diagnosis of SPE. Radiological findings are based on the evidence of multiple small diffuse lung opacities (Fig. 42), look like that of a bronco-pneumonia, and/or wedge-shaped opacities in the

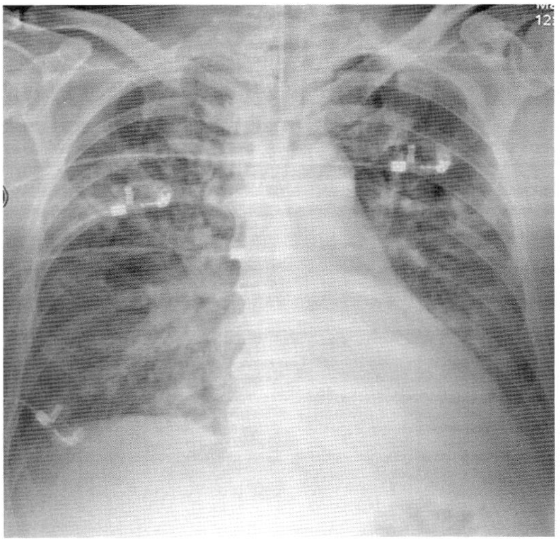

Fig. 42 Chest radiograph shows multiple bilateral lobular areas of consolidation of pulmonary parenchyma that coalescence in the right paracardiac region

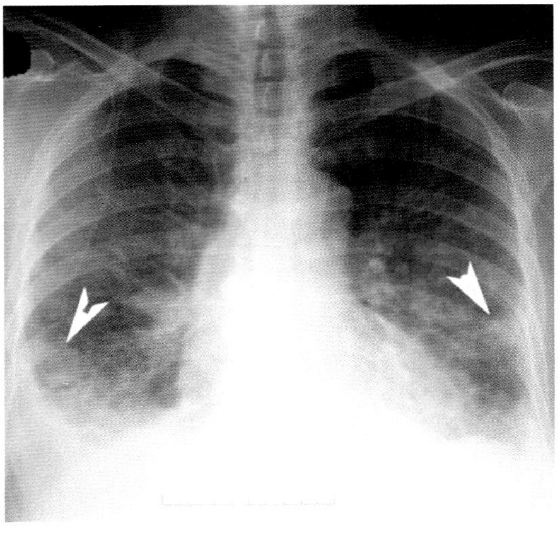

Fig. 43 Chest radiograph shows peripheral pulmonary infiltrates (*arrows*) associated with pleural effusion

periphery of lung (Fig. 43) and nodules with or without cavitations.

The gold standard to investigate the cause of acute respiratory symptoms is chest computed tomography (Farahmand et al. 2011; Cook et al. 2005c).

The typical CT findings that indicate SPE include peripheral nodules with or without

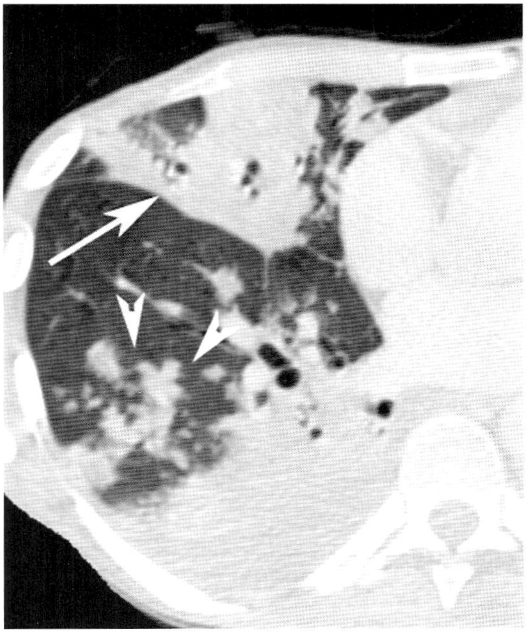

Fig. 44 CT axial scan of the chest shows a peripheral wedge-shaped opacity (*arrow*) of the medium pulmonary lobe associated with multiple patchy opacities of the lower right pulmonary lobe

cavitations, some of them showing evidence of breakdown suggestive of septic emboli, wedge-shaped peripheral lesions abutting the pleura (Fig. 44), and patchy ground-glass opacities (Fig. 45) and feeding vessel signs (Fig. 46). Other CT findings include air bronchogram within nodules (Fig. 47), focal consolidations, lung abscesses (Fig. 48), and halo signs. About 70 % of the lesions are generally located just beneath the pleura (Fig. 49) and about feeding vessels (Fig. 50). It was reported that radiographic evidence of a nodular density suspended in a thinly walled hyperlucent cavity is characteristic of septic pulmonary emboli (Yoong and Cheong 1997; Iwasaki et al. 2001).

There is also a tendency for the septic nodules to change appearance over time. Feeding vessels are observed in nodules in 60–70 % of patients (Rossi et al. 2000; Habib et al. 2010).

The microembolism is not generally observed directly on CT scan. Indirect findings of microembolism are pulmonary edema, pulmonary infarctions, and pulmonary hypertension findings with enlargement of arterial vessels.

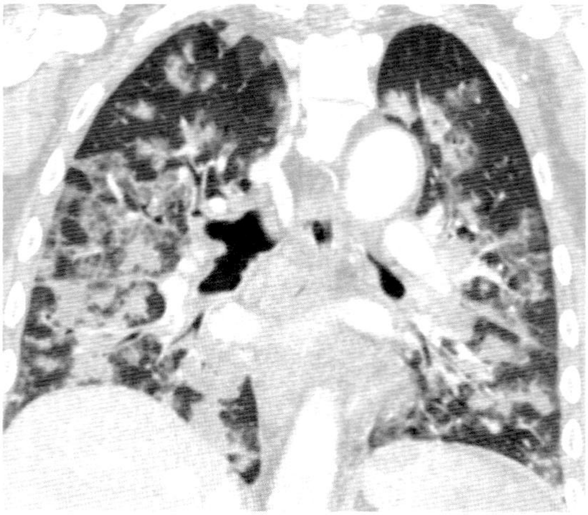

Fig. 45 CT coronal image of the chest demonstrates multiple patchy ground-glass opacities of the lungs

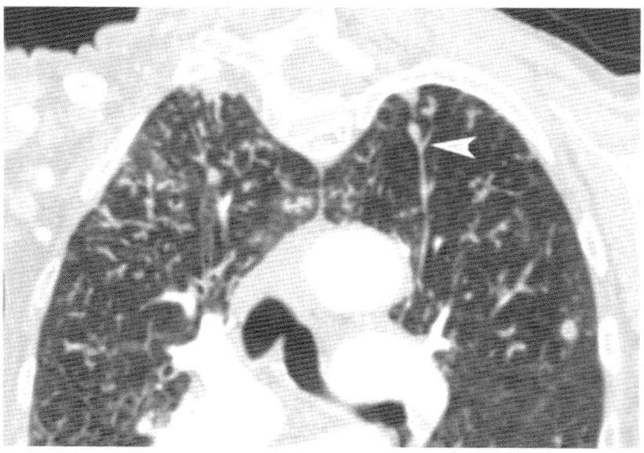

Fig. 46 CT coronal image of the chest demonstrates the feeding vessel sign (*arrow*)

The presence of parenchymal consolidation in pulmonary infarction is mainly caused by pulmonary hemorrhage (Balakrishnan et al. 1989).

Unusual presentations of SPE include pneumomediastinum and subcutaneous emphysema (Wang et al. 2004) as well as the evidence of septic emboli in the subsegmental pulmonary arteries. Pleural effusion is also observed in 70 % of patients (Fig. 42).

The chest CT findings typically lead to cardiac imaging because of the association with right-sided infective endocarditis. The absence of obvious cardiac valvular lesions should prompt careful consideration of other potential sources of infections, including venous devices

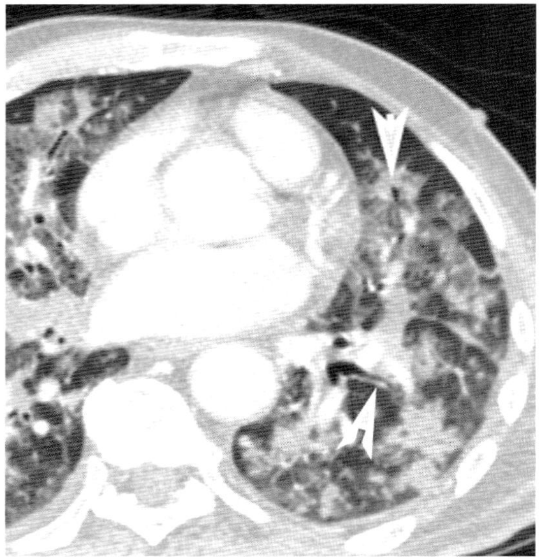

Fig. 47 CT axial scan of the chest demonstrates air bronchogram (*arrowheads*) within patchy ground-glass pulmonary opacities

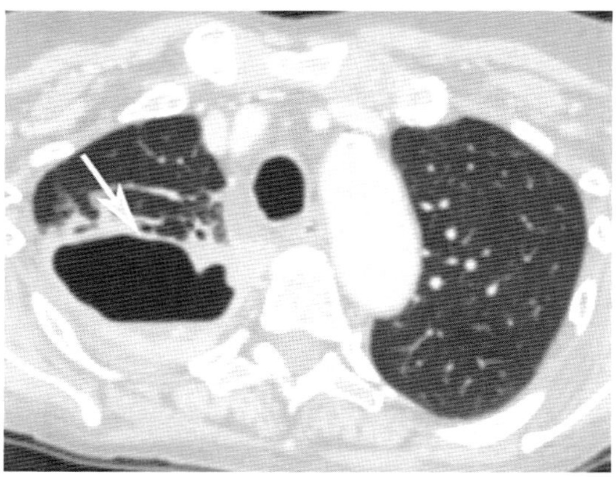

Fig. 48 CT axial scan of the chest demonstrates a large right upper pulmonary lobe abscess with a typical air-fluid level (*arrow*)

(Fig. 51), or thrombophlebitis due to soft tissue infections (Fig. 40). Additional imaging modalities including ultrasound help in delineating the root cause of infection (Gadcowski and Stout 2008).

Echocardiographic examination of all cardiac valves, including right-sided valves, should be carried out in all patients with suspecting infective endocarditis, especially when the patient has a risk factor (Chua et al. 2000). In the absence of

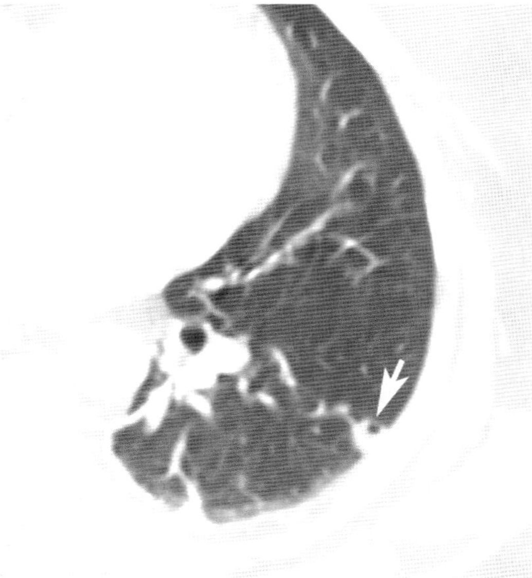

Fig. 49 CT axial scan of the chest demonstrates a small peripheral abscess with a typical air-bubble inclusion (*arrow*) localized in the left lower pulmonary lobe

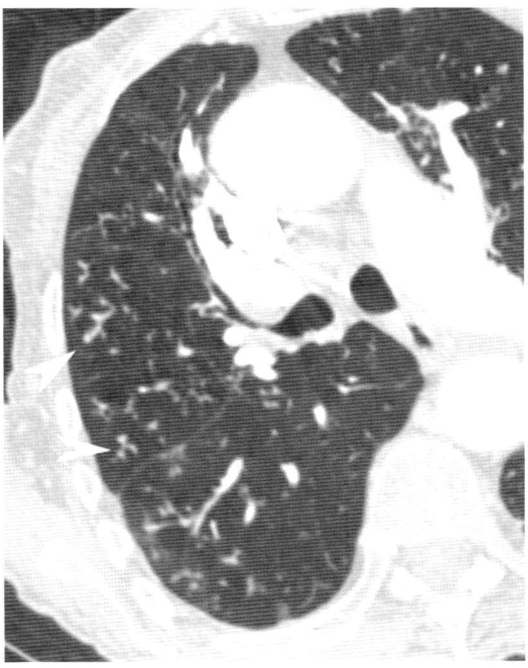

Fig. 50 CT axial scan of the chest demonstrates the feeding vessel signs (*arrowheads*)

signs of endocarditis, further evaluation to identify the infectious source is indicated (Vos et al. 2012).

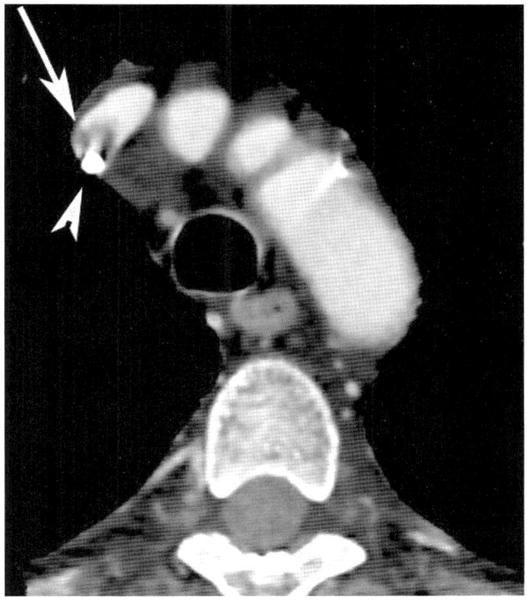

Fig. 51 Post-contrast CT axial scan of the mediastinum demonstrates a defect filling corresponding to a thrombus (*arrowhead*) that surrounds a central venous catheters (*arrow*) inside the lumen of the left brachiocephalic vein

4.4 Conclusion

Sepsis is a syndrome caused by the inefficiency of the mechanism of control and containment of the infection. It is characterized by symptoms and signs of systemic inflammatory reaction to infection and manifestations of organ dysfunction, resulting from alterations in the microcirculation. It is the second common cause of death with a mortality rate between 15 and 50% (Ferrari and Barletta 2012).

SPE has manifestations ranging from an insidious illness with fever and respiratory symptoms to acute generalized sepsis with disseminated intravascular coagulopathy or acute renal failure.

The diagnosis of SPE is based on clinical manifestations, culture data, and radiographic evidence of peripheral thrombosis and pulmonary infection. Respiratory impairment with high grade fever and marked increase of serum inflammatory markers differentiate septic pulmonary embolism from nonseptic pulmonary embolism (Melina et al. 2010).

The concurrence of an extrapulmonary source of infection with contiguous septic thrombophlebitis complicated by septic pulmonary embolism seems to affect particularly the adult populations. A high index suspicion of thrombosis is present in patients where the manifestations of the soft tissue infection (erythema, pain, and swelling) can overlap those of SPE (Fred and Harle 1969).

Chest x-ray film could be rather nonspecific, whereas chest CT scan provides the earliest and most easily identifiable indication of SPE and systemic embolization of infection.

Bibliography

Community-Acquired Pneumonia

American Thoracic Society (1995) Hospital-acquired pneumonia in adults: diagnosis, assessment of severity, initial antimicrobial therapy and preventive strategies. Am J Respir Crit Care Med 153:1711–1719

Aquino SL, Gamsu G, Webb WR et al (1996) Tree-in-bud pattern. Frequency and significance on thin section CT. J Comput Assist Tomogr 20:594–599

Austin JH, Muller NL, Friedman PJ et al (1996) Glossary of terms for CT of the lungs: recommendations of the Nomenclature Committee of the Fleishner Society. Radiology 200:327–331

Barlett JG, Finegold SM (1974) Anaerobic infections of the lung and pleural space. Am Rev Respir Dis 110:56–77

Bhalla M, Mc Loud TC (1998) Pulmonary infections in the normal host. In: Mc Loud TC (ed) Thoracic radiology, the requisites. Mosby, Philadelphia

Chastre J, Trouillet H, Vuagnat A et al (1998) Nosocomial pneumonia in patient with acute distress respiratory syndrome. Am J Respir Crit Care Med 157:1165–1172

De Paso WJ (1991) Aspiration pneumonia. Clin Chest Med 12:269–284

Franquet T (2001) Imaging of pneumonia: trends and algorithms. Eur Respir J 18:196–208

Hansell DM, Bankier AA, MacMahon H et al (2008) Fleischner Society: glossary of terms for thoracic imaging. Radiology 246:697–722

Heussel CP, Kauczor HU, Heussel G et al (1997) Early detection of pneumonia in febrile neutropenic patients. Use of thin section CT. AJR Am J Roentgenol 169:1347–1353

Ito I, Ishida T, Togashi K et al (2009) Differentiation of bacterial and non bacterial community-acquired pneumonia by thin-section computed tomography. Eur J Radiol 72(3):388–395

Kofteridis D, Samonis G, Mantadakis E et al (2009) Respiratory tract infections caused by Haemophilus influenzae: clinical features and predictors of outcome. Med Sci Monit 15:135–139

Marom EM, McAdams HP, Erasmus JJ et al (1999) The many faces of pulmonary aspiration. AJR Am J Roentgenol 172:121–128

Muller NL, Franquet T, Lee KS (2007) Bacterial pneumonia. In: Imaging of pulmonary infections. Lippincott Williams and Wilkins, Philadelphia, pp 20–28

Musher DM, Dowell ME, Shortridge VD (2002) Emergence of macrolide resistance during treatment of pneumococcal pneumonia. N Engl J Med 346:630–631

Naidich DP, McCauley DI, Khouri NF et al (1983) Computed tomography of lobar collapse. J Comput Assist Tomogr 7:745–757

Okada F, Ando Y, Tanque S et al (2012) Radiological findings in acute Haemophilus influenzae pulmonary infection. Br J Radiol 85:121–126

Primack SL, Hartman TE, Lee KS et al (1994) Pulmonary nodules and the CT halo sign. Radiology 190:513–515

Reittner P, Muller NL, Heyneman L (2000a) Mycoplasma pneumoniae pneumonia: radiographic and high resolution CT features in 28 patients. AJR Am J Roentgenol 174:37–41

Shiley KT, Van Deerlin VM, Miller WT (2010) Chest CT features of community-acquired respiratory viral infections in adult patients with lower respiratory tract infections. J Thorac Imaging 25(1):68–75

Thurlbeck WM, Miller RR, Muller NL, Rose S III (1991) Diffuse diseases of the lung: a team approach. BC Decker/Mosby Year Book, Philadelphia, pp 65–92

Vilar J, Domingo ML, Soto C et al (2004a) Radiology of bacterial pneumonia. Eur J Radiol 51:102–113

Vincent JL, Bihari DJ, Suter PM et al; EPIC International Advisory Committee (1995) The prevalence of nosocomial infection in intensive-care Units in Europe. Results of the European prevalence of infections in intensive care (EPIC) study. JAMA 274:639–644

Winer-Muram HT, Rubin SA, Ellis JV et al (1993) Pneumonia and ARDS in patients receiving mechanical ventilation: diagnostic accuracy of chest radiography. Radiology 188:479–485

Atypical Infections

Aquino SL, Dunagan DP, Chiles C, Haponik EF (1998) Herpes simplex virus 1 pneumonia: patterns on CT scans and conventional chest radiographs. J Comput Assist Tomogr 22(5):795–800

Arnold FW, Summersgill JT, Lajoie AS, Peyrani P, Marrie TJ, Rossi P et al (2007) A worldwide perspective of atypical pathogens in community-acquired pneumonia. Am J Respir Crit Care Med 175(10):1086–1093

Becroft DM (1967) Histopathology of fatal adenovirus infection of the respiratory tract in young children. J Clin Pathol 20(4):561–569

Boroja M, Barrie JR, Raymond GS (2002) Radiographic findings in 20 patients with Hantavirus pulmonary syndrome correlated with clinical outcome. AJR Am J Roentgenol 178(1):159–163

Chan MS, Chan IY, Fung KH, Poon E, Yam LY, Lau KY (2004) High-resolution CT findings in patients with severe acute respiratory syndrome: a pattern-based approach. AJR Am J Roentgenol 182(1):49–56

Chong S, Lee KS, Kim TS, Chung MJ, Chung MP, Han J (2006) Adenovirus pneumonia in adults: radiographic and high-resolution CT findings in five patients. AJR Am J Roentgenol 186(5):1288–1293

Cunha CB (2010) The first atypical pneumonia: the history of the discovery of Mycoplasma pneumoniae. Infect Dis Clin North Am 24(1):1–5

Drysdale SB, Green CA, Sande CJ (2016) Best practice in the prevention and management of paediatric respiratory syncytial virus infection. Ther Adv Infect Dis 3(2):63–71

Eaton MD, Meiklejohn G, van Herick W (1944) Studies on the etiology of primary atypical pneumonia : a filterable agent transmissible to cotton rats, hamsters, and chick embryos. J Exp Med 79(6):649–668

Fairbank JT, Patel MM, Dietrich PA (1991) Legionnaires' disease. J Thorac Imaging 6(3):6–13

Fields BS, Benson RF, Besser RE (2002) Legionella and Legionnaires' disease: 25 years of investigation. Clin Microbiol Rev 15(3):506–526

Franquet T (2011) Imaging of pulmonary viral pneumonia. Radiology 260(1):18–39

Franquet T, Lee KS, Muller NL (2003) Thin-section CT findings in 32 immunocompromised patients with cytomegalovirus pneumonia who do not have AIDS. AJR Am J Roentgenol 181(4):1059–1063

Fraser DW, Tsai TR, Orenstein W, Parkin WE, Beecham HJ, Sharrar RG et al (1977) Legionnaires' disease: description of an epidemic of pneumonia. N Engl J Med 297(22):1189–1197

Gasparetto EL, Davaus T, Escuissato DL, Marchiori E (2007) Hantavirus pulmonary syndrome: high-resolution CT findings in one patient. Br J Radiol 80(949):e21–e23

Graham BS, Snell JD Jr (1983) Herpes simplex virus infection of the adult lower respiratory tract. Medicine (Baltimore) 62(6):384–393

Guckel C, Benz-Bohm G, Widemann B (1989) Mycoplasmal pneumonias in childhood. Roentgen features, differential diagnosis and review of literature. Pediatr Radiol 19(8):499–503

Hahn DL (1999) Chlamydia pneumoniae, asthma, and COPD: what is the evidence? Ann Allergy Asthma Immunol 83(4):271–288, 91; quiz 91–92

Hsieh SC, Kuo YT, Chern MS, Chen CY, Chan WP, Yu C (2007) Mycoplasma pneumonia: clinical and radiographic features in 39 children. Pediatr Int 49(3):363–367

John SD, Ramanathan J, Swischuk LE (2001) Spectrum of clinical and radiographic findings in pediatric mycoplasma pneumonia. Radiographics 21(1):121–131

Karnak D, Beng-sun S, Beder S, Kayacan O (2001) Chlamydia pneumoniae infection and acute exacerbation of chronic obstructive pulmonary disease (COPD). Respir Med 95(10):811–816

Kim JS, Ryu CW, Lee SI, Sung DW, Park CK (1999) High-resolution CT findings of varicella-zoster pneumonia. AJR Am J Roentgenol 172(1):113–116

Kim EA, Lee KS, Primack SL, Yoon HK, Byun HS, Kim TS et al (2002) Viral pneumonias in adults: radiologic and pathologic findings. Radiographics 22(Spec No):S137–S149

Kim KW, Goo JM, Lee HJ, Lee HY, Park CM, Lee CH et al (2007) Chest computed tomographic findings and clinical features of legionella pneumonia. J Comput Assist Tomogr 31(6):950–955

Knittler MR, Sachse K (2015) Chlamydia psittaci: update on an underestimated zoonotic agent. Pathog Dis 73(1):1–15

Kruger DH, Ulrich RG, Hofmann J (2013) Hantaviruses as zoonotic pathogens in Germany. Dtsch Arztebl Int 110(27–28):461–467

Kuo CC, Jackson LA, Campbell LA, Grayston JT (1995) Chlamydia pneumoniae (TWAR). Clin Microbiol Rev 8(4):451–461

Manigold T, Vial P (2014) Human hantavirus infections: epidemiology, clinical features, pathogenesis and immunology. Swiss Med Wkly 144:w13937

Marrie TJ, Haldane EV, Noble MA, Faulkner RS, Martin RS, Lee SH (1981) Etiology of atypical pneumonias – a one year prospective study. CMAJ 125:1118–1123

Marrie TJ, Costain N, La Scola B, Patrick W, Forgie S, Xu Z et al (2012) The role of atypical pathogens in community-acquired pneumonia. Semin Respir Crit Care Med 33(3):244–256

Mattar S, Guzman C, Figueiredo LT (2015) Diagnosis of hantavirus infection in humans. Expert Rev Anti Infect Ther 13(8):939–946

Mayer JL, Lehners N, Egerer G, Kauczor HU, Heussel CP (2014) CT-morphological characterization of respiratory syncytial virus (RSV) pneumonia in immune-compromised adults. Rofo 186(7):686–692

McGuinness G, Scholes JV, Garay SM, Leitman BS, McCauley DI, Naidich DP (1994) Cytomegalovirus pneumonitis: spectrum of parenchymal CT findings with pathologic correlation in 21 AIDS patients. Radiology 192(2):451–459

Meyer Sauteur PM, Unger WW, Nadal D, Berger C, Vink C, van Rossum AM (2016) Infection with and carriage of mycoplasma pneumoniae in children. Front Microbiol 7:329

Mohsen AH, McKendrick M (2003) Varicella pneumonia in adults. Eur Respir J 21(5):886–891

Müller NL (2003) Diseases of the lung: radiologic and pathologic correlations. Lippincott Williams & Wilkins, Philadelphia, p 387

Muller NL, Miller RR (1995) Diseases of the bronchioles: CT and histopathologic findings. Radiology 196(1):3–12

Müller NL, Franquet T, Lee KS, Silva CIS (2007) Imaging of pulmonary infections. Lippincott Williams & Wilkins, Philadelphia, p vii,184 p

Murray JF, Mason RJ (2010) Murray and Nadel's textbook of respiratory medicine. Saunders Elsevier, Philadelphia. Available from: http://www.clinicalkey.com/dura/browse/bookChapter/3-s2.0-C20090378058

Oikonomou A, Muller NL, Nantel S (2003) Radiographic and high-resolution CT findings of influenza virus

pneumonia in patients with hematologic malignancies. AJR Am J Roentgenol 181(2):507–511
Okada F, Ando Y, Wakisaka M, Matsumoto S, Mori H (2005) Chlamydia pneumoniae pneumonia and Mycoplasma pneumoniae pneumonia: comparison of clinical findings and CT findings. J Comput Assist Tomogr 29(5):626–632
Peiris JS, Yuen KY, Osterhaus AD, Stohr K (2003) The severe acute respiratory syndrome. N Engl J Med 349(25):2431–2441
Pipavath SJ, Lynch DA, Cool C, Brown KK, Newell JD (2005) Radiologic and pathologic features of bronchiolitis. AJR Am J Roentgenol 185(2):354–363
Ramsey PG, Fife KH, Hackman RC, Meyers JD, Corey L (1982) Herpes simplex virus pneumonia: clinical, virologic, and pathologic features in 20 patients. Ann Intern Med 97(6):813–820
Reimann HA (1938) An acute infection of the respiratory tract with atypical pneumonia. JAMA 111:2377–2384
Reittner P, Muller NL, Heyneman L, Johkoh T, Park JS, Lee KS et al (2000b) Mycoplasma pneumoniae pneumonia: radiographic and high-resolution CT features in 28 patients. AJR Am J Roentgenol 174(1):37–41
Sargent EN, Carson MJ, Reilly ED (1966) Roentgenographic manifestations of varicella pneumonia with postmortem correlation. Am J Roentgenol Radium Ther Nucl Med 98(2):305–317
Simoons-Smit AM, Kraan EM, Beishuizen A, Strack van Schijndel RJ, Vandenbroucke-Grauls CM (2006) Herpes simplex virus type 1 and respiratory disease in critically-ill patients: real pathogen or innocent bystander? Clin Microbiol Infect 12(11):1050–1059
Tsai TF, Finn DR, Plikaytis BD, McCauley W, Martin SM, Fraser DW (1979) Legionnaires' disease: clinical features of the epidemic in Philadelphia. Ann Intern Med 90(4):509–517
Vilar J, Domingo ML, Soto C, Cogollos J (2004b) Radiology of bacterial pneumonia. Eur J Radiol 51(2):102–113
Webb WR, Higgins CB; Ovid Technologies Inc (2011) Thoracic imaging pulmonary and cardiovascular radiology. Wolters Kluwer/Lippincott Williams & Wilkins Health, Philadelphia. Available from: http://ovidsp.ovid.com/ovidweb.cgi?T=JS&PAGE=booktext&NEWS=N&DF=bookdb&AN=01437581/1st_Edition&XPATH=/PG(0)
Yagyu H, Nakamura H, Tsuchida F, Sudou A, Kishi K, Oh-ishi S et al (2003) Chest CT findings and clinical features in mild Legionella pneumonia. Intern Med 42(6):477–482

Tuberculosis

Alkhuja S, Miller A (2001) Tuberculosis and sudden death: a case report and review. Heart Lung 30(5):388–391
American Thoracic Society (1990) Diagnostic standards and classification of tuberculosis. Am Rev Respir Dis 142(3):725–735
Andreu J, Caceres J, Pallisa E, Martinez-Rodriguez M (2004) Radiological manifestations of pulmonary tuberculosis. Eur J Radiol 51(2):139–149
Arora A, Bhalla AS, Jana M, Sharma R (2013) Overview of airway involvement in tuberculosis. J Med Imaging Radiat Oncol 57(5):576–581
Arya M, George J, Dixit R, Gupta RC, Gupta N (2011) Bilateral spontaneous pneumothorax in miliary tuberculosis. Indian J Tuberc 58(3):125–128
Bruzzi JF, Remy-Jardin M, Delhaye D, Teisseire A, Khalil C, Remy J (2006) Multi-detector row CT of hemoptysis. Radiographics 26(1):3–22
Cardinale L, Parlatano D, Boccuzzi F, Onoscuri M, Volpicelli G, Veltri A (2015) The imaging spectrum of pulmonary tuberculosis. Acta Radiol 56(5):557–564
Chatterjee K, Colaco B, Colaco C, Hellman M, Meena N (2015) Rasmussen's aneurysm: a forgotten scourge. Respir Med Case Rep 16:74–76
Cherian G (2004) Diagnosis of tuberculous aetiology in pericardial effusions. Postgrad Med J 80(943):262–266
Corder R (2003) Hemoptysis. Emerg Med Clin North Am 21(2):421–435
European Centre for Disease Prevention and Control (2015) Tuberculosis surveillance and monitoring in Europe 2015 [cited 2016 20.4.2016]. Available from: http://ecdc.europa.eu/en/publications/_layouts/forms/Publication_DispForm.aspx?List=4f55ad51-4aed-4d32-b960-af70113dbb90&ID=1278
Fatimi SH, Javed MA, Ahmad U, Siddiqi BI, Salahuddin N (2006) Tuberculous hilar lymph nodes leading to tracheopulmonary artery fistula and pseudoaneurysm of pulmonary artery. Ann Thorac Surg 82(5):e35–e36
Franquet T, Gimenez A, Cremades R, Domingo P, Plaza V (2000) Spontaneous reversibility of "pleural thickening" in a patient with semi-invasive pulmonary aspergillosis: radiographic and CT findings. Eur Radiol 10(5):722–724
Franquet T, Muller NL, Gimenez A, Guembe P, de La Torre J, Bague S (2001) Spectrum of pulmonary aspergillosis: histologic, clinical, and radiologic findings. Radiographics 21(4):825–837
Glynn JR, Bauer J, de Boer AS, Borgdorff MW, Fine PE, Godfrey-Faussett P et al (1999) Interpreting DNA fingerprint clusters of Mycobacterium tuberculosis. European Concerted Action on Molecular Epidemiology and Control of Tuberculosis. Int J Tuberc Lung Dis 3(12):1055–1060
Halezeroglu S, Okur E (2014) Thoracic surgery for haemoptysis in the context of tuberculosis: what is the best management approach? J Thorac Dis 6(3):182–185
Hammerman KJ, Christianson CS, Huntington I, Hurst GA, Zelman M, Tosh FE (1973) Spontaneous lysis of aspergillomata. Chest 64(6):679–679
Hong SH, Im JG, Lee JS, Song JW, Lee HJ, Yeon KM (1998) High resolution CT findings of miliary tuberculosis. J Comput Assist Tomogr 22(2):220–224
Im JG, Itoh H, Shim YS, Lee JH, Ahn J, Han MC et al (1993) Pulmonary tuberculosis: CT findings – early active disease and sequential change with antituberculous therapy. Radiology 186(3):653–660

Jean-Baptiste E (2000) Clinical assessment and management of massive hemoptysis. Crit Care Med 28(5):1642–1647

Johnson TM, McCann W, Davey WN (1973) Tuberculous bronchopleural fistula. Am Rev Respir Dis 107(1):30–41

Johnston H, Reisz G (1989) Changing spectrum of hemoptysis. Underlying causes in 148 patients undergoing diagnostic flexible fiberoptic bronchoscopy. Arch Intern Med 149(7):1666–1668

Jones BE, Ryu R, Yang Z, Cave MD, Pogoda JM, Otaya M et al (1997) Chest radiographic findings in patients with tuberculosis with recent or remote infection. Am J Respir Crit Care Med 156(4 Pt 1):1270–1273

Khan NA, Akhtar J, Baneen U, Shameem M, Ahmed Z, Bhargava R (2011) Recurrent pneumothorax: a rare complication of miliary tuberculosis. N Am J Med Sci 3(9):428–430

Kim Y, Lee KS, Yoon JH, Chung MP, Kim H, Kwon OJ et al (1997) Tuberculosis of the trachea and main bronchi: CT findings in 17 patients. AJR Am J Roentgenol 168(4):1051–1056

Kim HY, Song KS, Goo JM, Lee JS, Lee KS, Lim TH (2001) Thoracic sequelae and complications of tuberculosis. Radiographics 21(4):839–858; discussion 59–60

Knechel NA (2009) Tuberculosis: pathophysiology, clinical features, and diagnosis. Crit Care Nurse 29(2):34–43; quiz 4

Krishnan B, Shaukat A, Chakravorty I (2009) Fatal haemoptysis in a young man with tuberculous mediastinal lymphadenitis. A case report and review of the literature. Respiration 77(3):333–336

Leung AN (1999) Pulmonary tuberculosis: the essentials. Radiology 210(2):307–322

Leung AN, Muller NL, Pineda PR, FitzGerald JM (1992) Primary tuberculosis in childhood: radiographic manifestations. Radiology 182(1):87–91

Marshall TJ, Jackson JE (1997) Vascular intervention in the thorax: bronchial artery embolization for haemoptysis. Eur Radiol 7(8):1221–1227

Mayosi BM, Burgess LJ, Doubell AF (2005) Tuberculous pericarditis. Circulation 112(23):3608–3616

McGuinness G, Naidich DP, Jagirdar J, Leitman B, McCauley DI (1992) High resolution CT findings in miliary lung disease. J Comput Assist Tomogr 16(3):384–390

Moon WK, Im JG, Yeon KM, Han MC (1997) Tuberculosis of the central airways: CT findings of active and fibrotic disease. AJR Am J Roentgenol 169(3):649–653

Ntsekhe M, Hakim J (2005) Impact of human immunodeficiency virus infection on cardiovascular disease in Africa. Circulation 112(23):3602–3607

Ntsekhe M, Mayosi BM (2013) Tuberculous pericarditis with and without HIV. Heart Fail Rev 18(3):367–373

Odone A, Tillmann T, Sandgren A, Williams G, Rechel B, Ingleby D et al (2015) Tuberculosis among migrant populations in the European Union and the European Economic Area. Eur J Public Health 25(3):506–512

Post FA, Wood R, Pillay GP (1995) Pulmonary tuberculosis in HIV infection: radiographic appearance is related to CD4+ T-lymphocyte count. Tuber Lung Dis 76(6):518–521

Prasad R, Garg R, Singhal S, Srivastava P (2009) Lessons from patients with hemoptysis attending a chest clinic in India. Ann Thorac Med 4(1):10–12

Pratt PC (1979) Pathology of tuberculosis. Semin Roentgenol 14(3):196–203

Remy J, Arnaud A, Fardou H, Giraud R, Voisin C (1977) Treatment of hemoptysis by embolization of bronchial arteries. Radiology 122(1):33–37

Remy J, Smith M, Lemaitre L, Marache P, Fournier E (1980) Treatment of massive hemoptysis by occlusion of a Rasmussen aneurysm. AJR Am J Roentgenol 135(3):605–606

Reuter H, Burgess LJ, Doubell AF (2005) Role of chest radiography in diagnosing patients with tuberculous pericarditis. Cardiovasc J S Afr 16(2):108–111

Revel MP, Fournier LS, Hennebicque AS, Cuenod CA, Meyer G, Reynaud P et al (2002) Can CT replace bronchoscopy in the detection of the site and cause of bleeding in patients with large or massive hemoptysis? AJR Am J Roentgenol 179(5):1217–1224

Rozenshtein A, Hao F, Starc MT, Pearson GD (2015) Radiographic appearance of pulmonary tuberculosis: dogma disproved. AJR Am J Roentgenol 204(5):974–978

Santelli ED, Katz DS, Goldschmidt AM, Thomas HA (1994) Embolization of multiple Rasmussen aneurysms as a treatment of hemoptysis. Radiology 193(2):396–398

Sepkowitz KA (1996) How contagious is tuberculosis? Clin Infect Dis 23(5):954–962

Sharma N, Kumar P (2002) Miliary tuberculosis with bilateral pneumothorax: a rare complication. Indian J Chest Dis Allied Sci 44(2):125–127

Sharma SK, Mohan A, Sharma A (2012) Challenges in the diagnosis & treatment of miliary tuberculosis. Indian J Med Res 135(5):703–730

Singh AS, Atam V, Das L (2014) Secondary spontaneous pneumothorax complicating miliary tuberculosis in a young woman. BMJ Case Rep 2014

Song JW, Im JG, Shim YS, Park JH, Yeon KM, Han MC (1998) Hypertrophied bronchial artery at thin-section CT in patients with bronchiectasis: correlation with CT angiographic findings. Radiology 208(1):187–191

Suchet IB, Horwitz TA (1992) CT in tuberculous constrictive pericarditis. J Comput Assist Tomogr 16(3):391–400

Uflacker R, Kaemmerer A, Neves C, Picon PD (1983) Management of massive hemoptysis by bronchial artery embolization. Radiology 146(3):627–634

van Crevel R, Ottenhoff TH, van der Meer JW (2002) Innate immunity to Mycobacterium tuberculosis. Clin Microbiol Rev 15(2):294–309

Woodring JH, Vandiviere HM, Fried AM, Dillon ML, Williams TD, Melvin IG (1986) Update: the radiographic features of pulmonary tuberculosis. AJR Am J Roentgenol 146(3):497–506

World Health Organization (2015) 20th edition of WHO global TB report. [updated 20.4.2016]. Available from: http://www.who.int/tb/publications/global_report/en/
Yilmaz MU, Kumcuoglu Z, Utkaner G, Yalniz O, Erkmen G (1998) Computed tomography findings of tuberculous pleurisy. Int J Tuberc Lung Dis 2(2):164–167
Yoon W, Kim JK, Kim YH, Chung TW, Kang HK (2002) Bronchial and nonbronchial systemic artery embolization for life-threatening hemoptysis: a comprehensive review. Radiographics 22(6):1395–1409

Hematogenous Spread of Pulmonary Infection

Angus DC, van der Poll T (2013) Severe Sepsis and septic shock. N Engl J Med 369:840–841
Baddour LM, Betmann MA, Bolger AF et al (2003) Non valvular-cardiovascular device-related infections. Circulation 108:2015–2031
Balakrishnan J, Meziane MA, Siegelman SS et al (1989) CT appearance with pathological correlation. J Comput Assist Tomogr 13(6):941–945
Boyle-Vavra S, Daum RS (2006) Community-acquired methicillin-resistant Staphylococcus aureus: the role of Panton-Valentine leukocidin. Lab Invest 87(1):3–9
Boyle-Vavra S, Daum RS (2007) Community-acquired methicillin-resistant S. aureus: the role of Panthon-Valentine leucocidin. Lab Invest 87:3–9
Brenes JA, Goswami U, Williams DN (2012a) The association of septic pulmonary embolism in adults. Oper Respir Med J 6:14–19
Brenes JA, Goswami U, Williams DN (2012b) The association of septic thrombophlebitis with septic pulmonary embolism in adults. Open Respir Med J 6:14–19
Cassling RS, Rogler WC, McManus BM (1985) Isolated pulmonic valve infective endocarditis a diagnostically elusive entity. Am Heart J 109(3):558–567
Chua JD, Wilkoff BL, Lee I et al (2000) Diagnosis and management of infections involving implantable electrophysiologic cardiac devices. Ann Intern Med 133:604–608
Cook RJ, Ashton RW, Aughenbaugh GL et al (2005a) Septic pulmonary embolism: presenting features and clinical course of 14 patients. Chest 128(1):162–166
Cook RJ, Ashton RW, Aughen GL et al (2005b) Septic pulmonary embolism presenting features and clinical course of 14 patients. Chest 128:162–166
Cook RJ, Aschton RW, Aughenbaugh GL (2005c) Septic pulmonary embolism presenting features and clinical course of 14 patients. Chest 128(1):162–166
Farahmand P, Redheuil A, Chauvaud S et al (2011) Images in endovascular medicine: septic pulmonary thromboemboli in an adolescent with Tetralogy of Fallot. Circulation 123:2164–2166
Ferrari AM, Barletta C (2012) Medicina di emergenza urgenza. Il sapere ed il saper fare del medico di emergenza tra linee guida, percorsi clinico assistenziali e rete dell'emergenza. Elsevier, Milano, pp 318–324
Fred HL, Harle TS (1969) Septic pulmonary embolism. Chest 55:483–486
Gadcowski LB, Stout JE (2008) Cavitary pulmonary disease. Clin Microbiol Rev 21(2):305–333
Goldenberg NA, Knapp-Clevenger R, Hays T et al (2005) Lemierre's and Lemierre's-like syndromes in children: survival and thromboembolic outcomes. Pediatrics 116(4):e543–e548
Gorenstem A, Gross E, Houn S et al (2000) The pivotal role of deep vein thrombophlebitis in the development of acute disseminated staphylococcal disease in children. Pediatrics 106, E87
Habib G, Badano L, Tribouilloy C et al (2010) Recommendations for the practise of echocardiography in infective endocarditis. Eur J Echocardiogr 11(2):202–219
Holm K, Frick IM, Bjork L et al (2011) Activation of the contact system at the surface of Fusobacterium necrophorum represents a possible virulence mechanism in Lemierre's syndrome. Infect Immun 79(8):3284–3290
Hota B, Lyles R, Rim J et al (2001) Predictors of clinical virulence in community onset methicillin-resistant S. aureus infections; the importance of USA 300 and pneumonia. Clin Infect Dis 53:766–771
Iwasaki Y, Nagata K, Nakanischi M et al (2001) Spiral CT findings in septic pulmonary emboli. Eur J Radiol 37(3):190–194
Klug D, Lacroix D, Savoye C et al (1997) Systemic infection related to endocarditis on pacemaker leads: clinical presentation and management. Circulation 95:2098–2107
Mac Millan JC, Milstein SH, Samson PC (1978) Clinical spectrum of septic pulmonary embolism and infarction. J Thorac Cardiovasc Surg 75(5):670–679
Melina G, El-Hamamsy I, Sinatra R et al (2010) Late fulminant pulmonary valve endocarditis after the Ross operation. J Thorac Cardiovasc Surg 139(5):e99–e100
Moriera D, Correia E, Rodrigues B (2012) Isolated pulmonary valve endocarditis in an normal hearth. Rev Port Cardiol 31(9):615–617
Nourse C, Starr M, Munckhof W (2007) Community acquired methicillin resistant S. Aureus causes severe disseminated infection and deep venous thrombosis in children: literature review and recommendations for management. J Pediatr Child Health 43:656–661
Nucifora G, Badano L, Hysko F et al (2007) Pulmonary embolism and fever: when should right-sided infective endocarditis be considered? Circulation 115(6):e173–e176
Rossi SE, Goodman PC, Franquet T (2000) Non thrombotic pulmonary embolism. AJR Am J Roentgenol 174(6):1499–1508

Takin R, Acet H, Ertas F (2012) An unusual case of endocarditis: isolated pulmonary valve in patient with patent ductus arteriosus. J Med Cases 3(6):340–343

Uslan DZ, Sohail MR, StSauver JL et al (2007) Permanent pacemaker and implantable cardioverter defibrillator infection: a population-based study. Arch Intern Med 167:669–675

Vinder Have KL, Karmazyn B, Verma M et al (2009) Community acquired methicillin resistant S. aureus in acute musculoskeletal infection in children: a game changer. J Pediatr Orthop 29(8):827–831

Vos FJ, Kullberg BJ, Sturm PD et al (2012) Metastatic infectious disease and clinical outcome in Staphylococcus aureus and Streptococcus species bacteremia. Medicine (Baltimore) 91(2):86–94

Wagenwoort CA (1995) Pathology of pulmonary thromboembolism. Chest 107(1 Suppl):10S–17S

Wang YC, Wang JM, Chow YC et al (2004) Pneumomediastinum and subcutaneous emphysema as the manifestation of emphysematous pyelonephritis. Int J Urol 11:909–911

Yoong KY, Cheong I (1997) A study of Malaysian drug addicts with human immunodeficiency virus infection. Int J STD AIDS 8:118–123

Non-infectious Parenchymal Lung Disease

G. Dalpiaz and M. Piolanti

Contents

Abstract

Acute dyspnea is a common presenting complaint in the emergency room, emergency medicine and intensive care. It may have a cardiovascular or a non-cardiovascular origin, the latter including pulmonary parenchymal diseases. Depending on the cause, it may be associated with fever, cough, hemoptysis, and/or chest pain, with a duration of symptoms that can range from hours to days.

Prompt identification of the underlying cause of acute dyspnea is essential in guiding appropriate therapy and management, as patients may rapidly progress to acute respiratory failure. Evaluation with chest radiography is vital for initial assessment and may

G. Dalpiaz, MD
Radiologia Ospedale Bellaria, AUSL Bologna, Italy
e-mail: giorgia.dalpiaz@ausl.bologna.it

M. Piolanti, MD (✉)
Radiologia Ospedale Maggiore, AUSL Bologna, Italy
e-mail: marco.piolanti@ausl.bo.it

Med Radiol Diagn Imaging (2016)
DOI 10.1007/174_2016_30, © Springer International Publishing Switzerland

reveal diffuse parenchymal abnormalities, which may require further assessment with computed tomography (HRCT).

Acute non-infectious parenchymal lung diseases are often overlooked and may be under-diagnosed. Their diagnosis requires the evaluation, along with the HRCT pattern, of the clinical and laboratory features and of the bronchoalveolar lavage. Biopsy may be necessary in more complex cases.

Although the most frequent cause of diffuse non-infectious parenchymal lung involvement is acute hydrostatic pulmonary edema, there is a wide variety of diseases that may be encountered, including acute drug toxicity, hypersensitivity pneumonitis (HP), acute respiratory distress syndrome (ARDS) and diffuse alveolar hemorrhage (DAH). In trauma patients, fat embolism syndrome (FES) must be taken into account. Acute respiratory failure is an eventuality that can occur during the course of chronic lung diseases (UIP for example), which may have been unknown until then.

1 Acute Drug Toxicity

1.1 Introduction

Drug toxicity is a common condition, often underdiagnosed. As a result, the incidence and the prevalence are underestimated. There are numerous agents with potential toxic effects on the lungs including cytotoxic and noncytotoxic drugs. Common causes of drug-induced lung disease include chemotherapeutic agents, amiodarone, antibiotics, and nonsteroidal anti-inflammatory drugs. There are a number of recognized cofactors that may enhance the likelihood of a pulmonary drug reaction, particularly reactions associated with chemotherapeutic agents. These include advanced age, prior radiotherapy, and elevated inspired oxygen levels; the presence of any or all of these factors increases the likelihood of developing a pulmonary drug reaction. Surgery may even be a precipitating event (Camus et al. 2004a).

1.2 Mechanisms of Injury

Generally, pulmonary drug reactions are the result of either direct or indirect effects of the drug. Reactions due to direct effects can be broadly divided into those that are toxic reactions (which to some extent are dose-related, such as reactions to chemotherapeutic agents) and those that are idiosyncratic reactions (which tend not to show a consistent dose-response relationship). This division is artificial and the distinction between toxic reactions and idiosyncratic reactions is not always clear cut. Several risk and exacerbating factors for diffuse lung disease have been identified. Some of them include advanced age (60 years or older) and existing pulmonary lesions (Kubo et al. 2013).

1.3 Terminology and Clinical Issues

The symptoms may be acute/subacute/chronic and are nonspecific and therefore the diagnosis requires a high index of suspicion by clinician and the radiologist. Acute respiratory failure due to drug-associated ILD generally has an unpredictable onset and rapid time course (onset of clinical manifestations within minutes to hours of taking the drug). Patients with acute drug toxicity present with the progressive or rapid onset of dry cough, high fever, and dyspnea. These patients often require admission to the intensive care unit and mechanical ventilation (Prasad et al. 2014; Camus et al. 2004b).

The identification of drug-induced lung disease requires an active consideration of any change in the patient's clinical course as a possible response to medications. There are no pathognomonic signs, symptoms, laboratory tests, or pathologic features that identify a drug as the cause of the illness. Further, drug-induced lung disease must be distinguished from more common illnesses or causes of acute exacerbation of an ongoing illness such as asthma, infection, congestive heart failure, and pulmonary thromboembolism. A history of drug exposure and a consistent radiological pattern may be diagnostic tools.

Bronchoalveolar lavage (BAL) is particularly helpful in ruling out infectious mostly before

Table 1 Acute drug toxicity: main clinical-histopathologic patterns

Acute clinical-histopathologic patterns	Typical drugs
Diffuse alveolar damage (DAD/ARDS)	Bleomycin, busulfan, cyclophosphamide, mitomycin, amiodarone
Diffuse alveolar hemorrhage (DAH)	Anticoagulants, amphotericin B, cytarabine (ara-C), penicillamine, cyclophosphamide
Pulmonary edema (PE)	Blood transfusions, tricyclic antidepressants, illicit drugs
Hypersensitivity pneumonia (HP)	Methotrexate, cyclophosphamide, nitrofurantoin

corticosteroid therapy. Biopsy can generally be avoided, as it does not always provide a specific diagnosis. Open lung biopsy is rarely performed (Müller et al. 2004).

1.4 Imaging

Several clinical-histopathologic patterns of drug toxicity with acute respiratory failure have been observed (Table 1). The HRCT features of drug-induced lung disease often reflect the histopathologic patterns of reaction (Rossi et al. 2000; Cleverley et al. 2002; Erasmus et al. 2002; Torrisi et al. 2011). For the clinical aspects and imaging of each acute clinical-histopathologic pattern listed in Table 1, we suggest to refer to the other diseases covered in this chapter. A new and continuously updated website is available for information on drug-induced pulmonary reactions: http://www.pneumotox.com.

1.5 Management and Treatment

Disease types such as pulmonary edema and hypersensitivity pneumonia generally have a favorable clinical course and most patients resolve following drug discontinuation or treatment with corticosteroids. In contrast, DAD rarely responds to treatment and has a poor prognosis, and even if it resolves, fibrosis may remain as a sequela.

2 Hypersensitivity Pneumonitis (HP)

2.1 Introduction

Hypersensitivity pneumonitis (HP), also known as extrinsic allergic alveolitis, is a syndrome that results from repeated inhalation and subsequent sensitization to a wide variety of airborne organic particles. The presentation and clinical course are highly variable and depend from intensity and duration of exposure to the antigen and the nature of the antigen and specific factors of the host, such as an individual predisposition probably genetically determined (Spagnolo et al. 2015). According to data from registries of interstitial lung diseases (ILDs) in three European countries, HP accounts for 4–15% of all ILD cases (Thomeer et al. 2001). However, the incidence and prevalence of HP are difficult to estimate with precision, mainly because of the number of cases that are misdiagnosed or not recognized and a lack of uniform diagnostic criteria.

The disease is diagnosed on the basis of a history of exposure to an offending antigen with onset of compatible clinical, HRCT, or physiological findings within 4–12 h. Other diagnostic criteria include clinical improvement after removal from exposure and recurrence on reexposure. In cases where the inciting antigen cannot be identified or in the presence of conflicting clinical, radiological, and functional findings, fiberoptic bronchoscopy with bronchoalveolar lavage (BAL) and transbronchial lung biopsy are indicated. Surgical lung biopsy is only required if these prove inconclusive (Elicker et al. 2016).

2.2 Mechanisms of Injury and Causes

HP comes from an immune-mediated inflammatory process involving the lung parenchyma (terminal bronchioles, alveoli, and interstitium), based on mechanisms likely independent from single causative agent, mediated by immune complexes in the acute phases of the disease and an altered response of T lymphocytes in the early stages subacute and

Table 2 Major classes of antigens and corresponding types of hypersensitivity pneumonitis

Class of antigens	Specific antigens	Disease prototypes
Fungi	*Aspergillus*	Farmer's lung Mushrooms worker's lung
Mycobacteria	*Mycobacterium avium-intracellulare*	Hot tub lung Swimming pool lung
Bacteria	*Saccharopolyspora rectivirgula*	Farmer's lung
Animal proteins	*Avian proteins*	Bird fancier's lung
	Silkworm proteins	Silk production HP
Chemicals	*Diisocyanates, trimellitic anhydride*	Chemical worker's lung

chronic (Vogelmeier et al. 1993; Barrera et al. 2008). HP seems that cigarette smoking can play a protective effect by reducing the intensity of hyperimmune response. The immune pathogenesis, not yet fully clarified, is linked to hyperactivity of T cells and the action of immune complexes.

In every living environment, antigens potentially causative of the disease may be present. The reported culprits have included microbes, animal and plant proteins, and low-molecular-weight chemicals that combine with host proteins to form haptens. HP-inducing antigens may be classified in broad categories represented by disease prototypes (Table 2) (Hanak et al. 2007; Spagnolo et al. 2015; Selman 2011). In the table is a selected list of the possible innumerable agents and disease.

2.3 Terminology and Clinical Issues

HP has been conventionally classified as acute, subacute, and chronic (Richerson et al. 1989), although a significant overlap exists and there are no widely accepted criteria to distinguish the various forms. In this regard, (Selman et al. 2012) proposed an alternative classification scheme based primarily on disease behavior, distinguishing between acute nonprogressive and intermittent disease, acute progressive/subacute disease, chronic nonprogressive disease, and chronic progressive disease. Which pattern of illness occurs presumably depends upon the intensity and duration of contact, the nature of the antigen, and host factors.

Acute HP is characterized by an influenza-like syndrome occurring a few hours after a substantial exposure. Symptoms gradually decrease over hours/days but often recur with reexposure. Acute episodes can be indistinguishable from an acute respiratory infection caused by viral or mycoplasmal agents. Attacks often follow exposure to the allergen within enclosed spaces with poor ventilation. Patients typically have a restrictive ventilatory defect with reduced DLCO or, in rare cases, an obstructive pattern. Mild hypoxemia at rest is common. In general, the acute form is nonprogressive and intermittent, with spontaneous improvement after antigen avoidance (Selman et al. 2012).

2.4 Imaging

2.4.1 Radiological Signs

Chest radiograph may be normal. Abnormal radiographic findings observed in some patients include a variable combination of fine nodular opacities and widespread ground-glass opacity or, more rarely, as consolidation. The zonal distribution varies from patient to patient and may vary over time in the same patient (Unger et al. 1973; Mönkäre et al. 1985).

2.4.2 CT Signs

High-resolution CT has greatly improved the radiological diagnosis of hypersensitivity pneumonitis because it is more sensitive and specific than chest X-ray. HRCT may either show typical findings, which may be virtually diagnostic of HP in the appropriate clinical setting, or provide important clues that may suggest a correct diagnosis.

HRCT findings vary widely based on the stages of the disease. Only a few reports have described HRCT abnormalities in acute HP, as HRCT is seldom performed at this stage due to the rapid resolution of symptoms. However, in cases with severe clinical manifestations

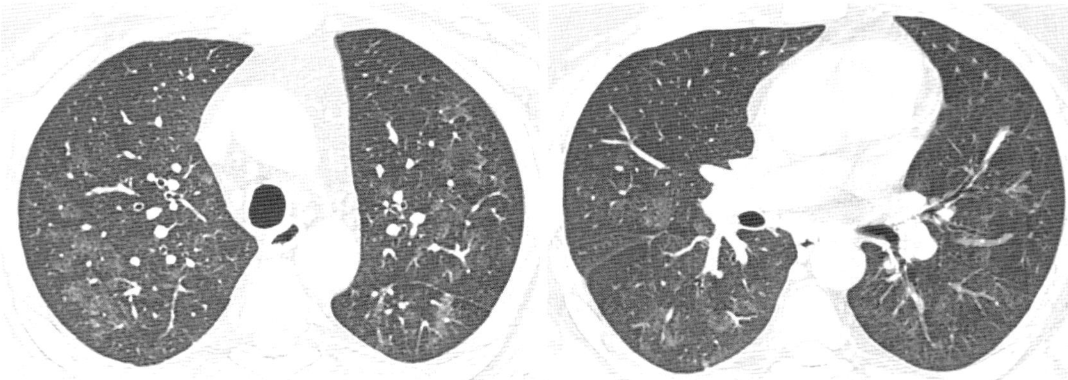

Fig. 1 Hypersensitivity pneumonitis with acute onset. High-resolution computed tomography showing diffuse ground-glass opacity, which is bilateral and symmetric

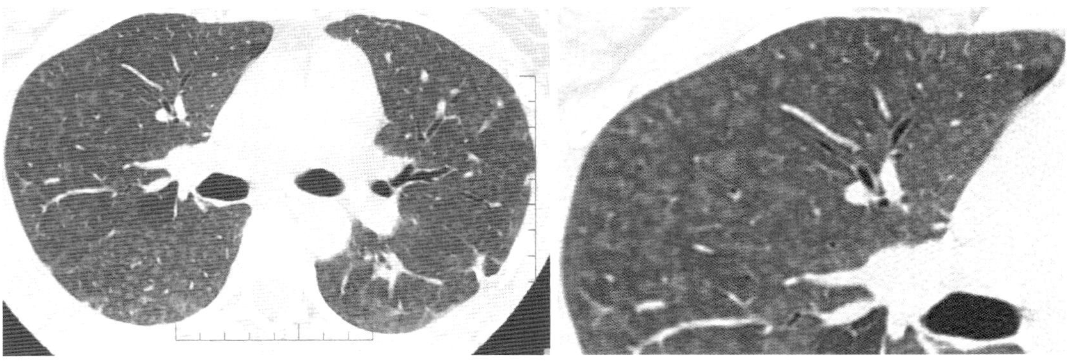

Fig. 2 Hypersensitivity pneumonitis. Axial high-resolution CT images depict bilateral and numerous centrilobular nodules with low-density and ill-defined margins. In terms of their aspect, the nodules are similar to snowflakes. The nodules are diffuse with uniform distribution. *Dark areas* of lobular size due to air trapping are also visible

(e.g., acute respiratory failure), acute HP on HRCT scans may resemble the exudative phase of diffuse alveolar damage (DAD) (Schwarz and Albert 2004). Diffuse ground-glass opacity is usually bilateral and symmetric but sometimes patchy and concentrated in the middle part and base of the lungs (Cormier et al. 2000; Zompatori et al. 2003) (Fig. 1). Furthermore, ground-glass opacity (GGO) superimposed on a background of chronic changes may be observed in acute exacerbation of chronic HP or in chronic cases following intense exposure to antigens.

HRCT abnormalities observed in the subacute phase of the disease may be more specific and include numerous poorly defined nodules, GGO, and areas of decreased attenuation. The nodules with low-density and ill-defined margins usually present less than 5 mm in diameter (also defined centrilobular ground-glass opacities). In terms of their aspect, the nodules are similar to snowflakes. Poorly defined nodules may be the predominant (Fig. 2) or only associated abnormality in patients with subacute HP. These abnormalities represent cellular bronchiolitis, peribronchiolar interstitial inflammation, or, less frequently, focal organizing pneumonia (Maffessanti and Dalpaz 2011).

The key sign to the diagnosis is the coexistence of sporadic lobular areas of air trapping appearing as patches of black lung (Fig. 3). These regions of lobular air trapping are caused by concomitant bronchiolar inflammation and obstruction.

Thus, the combination of a ground-glass opacification, lobular air trapping, and centrilobular

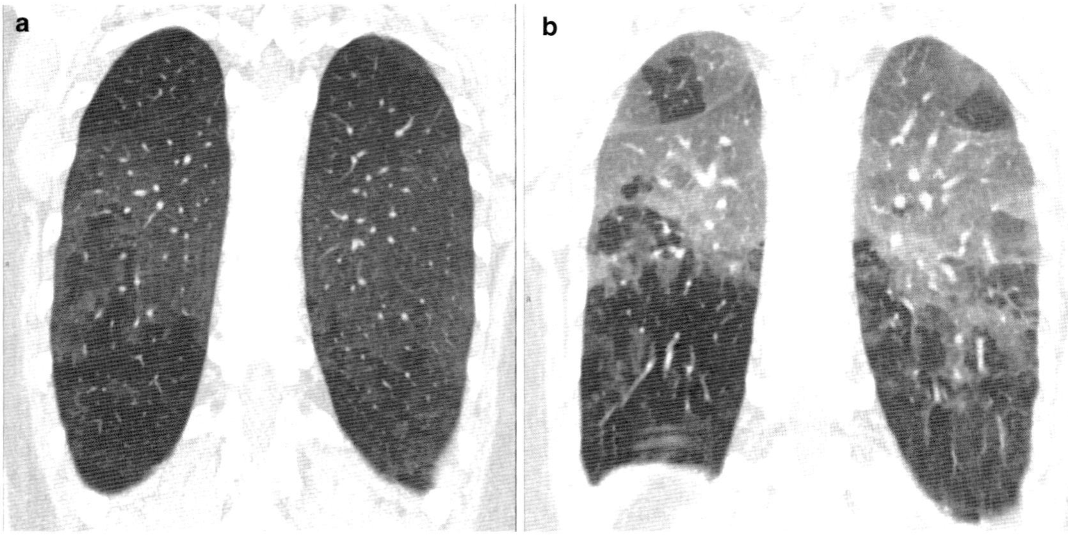

Fig. 3 Recurrent bird fancier's disease. (**a**) Coronal reformatted computed tomography (CT) image obtained at suspended inspiration demonstrates patchy ground glass involving the medium-upper zones combined with areas of decreased attenuation. (**b**) The intensity of the areas of decreased attenuation increases on expiratory CT indicating small airway involvement, an almost invariable finding in hypersensitivity pneumonitis. A few *dark areas* of lobular size due to air trapping are visible in the upper lobes

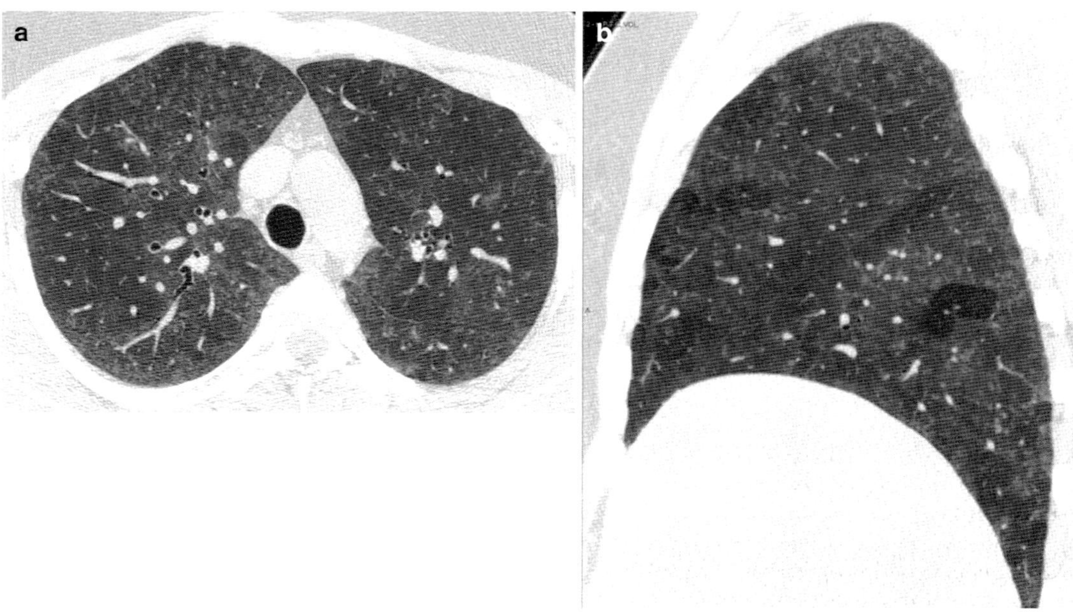

Fig. 4 (**a**, **b**) Typical high-resolution CT abnormalities in patients with hypersensitivity pneumonitis with insidious course and recurrent acute exacerbation include ground-glass opacity, air trapping, and centrilobular ground-glass opacities

nodules is particularly suggestive of acute and insidious onset without fibrosis (Fig. 4) (Silva et al. 2007).

The variable combination of areas of decreased attenuation, ground-glass opacities, and normal lung may produce the so-called head-cheese pattern, which is highly suggestive of HP (Chong et al. 2014). Coexisting thin-walled lung cysts have been reported in 13 % of patients with subacute HP (Franquet et al. 2003) and are believed to be caused by partial bronchiolar obstruction by peribronchiolar lymphocytic infiltration. These cysts are usually few in number and range in size from 3 to 25 mm. Occasionally in patients with an insidious onset of disease, focal consolidation is present, presumably representing organizing pneumonia. Mediastinal lymph node enlargement has been described in approximately 30 % of patients.

2.5 Differential Diagnosis

The differential diagnosis with other disorders manifesting with acute/subacute diffuse GGO e.g., opportunistic infections, pulmonary edema, and cellular nonspecific interstitial pneumonia (NSIP) may be difficult. However in HP the frequent association of lobular air trapping and centrilobular snowflake nodules is crucial for the diagnosis.

The so-called head-cheese pattern may also be observed in respiratory bronchiolitis-associated ILD (RB-ILD). Integrating nicotine poisoning and laboratory findings may indicate the most likely diagnosis (Chong et al. 2014).

GGO combined with cysts resemble those seen in lymphocytic interstitial pneumonia (LIP). However, LIP is often associated with other conditions, such as connective tissue diseases or lymphatic disorders (e.g., human immunodeficiency virus infection, lymphoma) (Ichikawa et al. 1994).

2.6 Management and Treatment

Patients with acute/subacute HP, if correctly and timely diagnosed and treated, generally have an excellent prognosis. The most important recommended therapy is inhibiting exposure to the causal agent by eliminating it from the environment, avoiding settings where it is present, or using a respirator in those settings. Systemic corticosteroids for a few days to weeks may improve symptoms. Indications for the use of such drugs include acute, severe, or progressive disease (Kokkarinen et al. 1992).

3 ARDS

3.1 Introduction

Acute respiratory distress syndrome (ARDS) is a condition characterized by sudden onset of severe hypoxemia and diffuse pulmonary infiltrates.

The syndrome was firstly introduced by Ashbaugh and colleagues in 1967 (Ashbaugh et al. 1967), while the criteria for the diagnosis of ARDS were first established in 1994 by the American-European Consensus Conference (AECC) (Bernard et al. 1994).

In 2012 the "Berlin definition," the new updated consensus definition of ARDS, has been published in a high-impact journal. ARDS is defined as: "[…] type of acute diffuse, inflammatory lung injury, leading to increased pulmonary vascular permeability, increased lung weight, and loss of aerated lung tissue. The clinical hallmarks are hypoxemia and bilateral radiographic opacities […]" (ARDS Definition Task Force 2012).

3.2 Mechanisms of Injury

ARDS may follow several different types of lung injury that ultimately determine the same monomorphic pulmonary response, characterized histopathologically by the presence of diffuse alveolar damage (DAD).

There are many triggering events that have been classically classified as pulmonary or extrapulmonary. Pulmonary or direct injuries are processes determining direct injury to lungs, like infection, gastric aspiration, or toxic inhalation. Extrapulmonary or indirect injuries may be systemic processes like polytrauma, drug toxicity, sepsis, transfusions, or extra-thoracic diseases like acute pancreatitis.

From a histopathologic point of view, "diffuse" refers to the involvement of the whole alveolar structure: endothelium, basal membrane, and epithelium. The process is widespread throughout the lungs, but not always in a homogeneous manner: frequently there is presence of spared areas (Kligerman et al. 2013).

The process is characterized by a sequence of phases. Not necessarily the process develops through all the phases: it can stop and reverse anytime (Castro 2006).

The early or exudative phase lasts up to 7 days and is characterized by the presence of hyaline membranes. The alveolar epithelium is damaged and the basal membrane is exposed.

The next stage is the organizing, or proliferative, phase, characterized by the presence of organizing tissue and fibrosis. If this phase does not resolve favorably, there is progression to the last phase, the fibrotic phase.

The pattern of fibrosis is atypical and usually with predilection of the anterior segments (anti-gravitational distribution). Some patients may show areas of "honeycombing," more frequently encountered following acute interstitial pneumonia (AIP), which is the "idiopathic" form ARDS (Tomiyama et al. 2001).

3.3 Terminology and Clinical Issues

The term ARDS should not be confused with the term permeability edema and it is not interchangeable with the term noncardiogenic edema. ARDS is the most severe form of permeability edema, but there are other forms of permeability edema without DAD (Ketai and Godwin 1998). Classification of pulmonary edema is discussed in the "Acute pulmonary edema" section.

ARDS, which is a life-threatening condition, is associated histopathologically to DAD.

In the AECC definition, ARDS was defined as an acute onset of hypoxemia, without specifying a timeframe to define acute; the PaO_2/FiO_2 (ratio of partial pressure of arterial oxygen to fraction of inspired oxygen) must be under <200 mmHg, with presence of bilateral infiltrates on frontal chest X-ray. Presence of left atrial hypertension must be ruled out. PaO_2/FiO_2 between 200 and 300 is termed acute lung injury (ALI).

When idiopathic, the process is termed acute interstitial pneumonia (AIP), also known as Hamman-Rich syndrome (Kliegerman et al. 2013). AIP may sometimes present with a more subacute course, and as a result, it does not always fulfill the criteria of ARDS (Janz et al. 2000).

The new definition of Berlin introduces several important changes to the old criteria (ARDS Definition Task Force 2012). The timeframe for define acute onset is specified within a week from a determinate event. A minimum level of positive end-expiratory pressure (PEEP) is established to evaluate the severity of the respiratory failure. The need to measure pulmonary wedge pressure is removed and the term ALI is suppressed. ARDS is now classified in three grades: mild ($200< PaO_2/FiO_2 <300$ with PEEP or C-PAP >5 cm H_2O), moderate ($100< PaO_2/FiO_2 <200$ with PEEP >5 cm H_2O), and severe (PaO_2/FiO_2 <100 with PEEP >5 cmH_2O). Finally, it is stated that the pathologic correlate of ARDS is DAD.

A set of training radiograph is attached to improve interobserver reliability (Ferguson et al. 2012). Opacities seen on CT scan may substitute chest X-ray evaluation for the diagnosis of diffuse pulmonary infiltrates (Table 3).

3.4 Imaging

3.4.1 Radiological Signs

The chest X-ray picture of ARDS varies depending on the phase of the process (Sheard et al. 2012).

In the early or exudative phase, there is some degree of clinical-radiological dissociation, with a latent period after the injury of about 24 h, when the radiograph results normal (Fig. 5a).

Subsequently the appearance of radiographic changes is rapid. The opacification is diffuse and symmetric, peripheral, and with presence of air-bronchograms. The heart and the vascular pedicle are not enlarged; pleural effusion is absent or limited (Fig. 5b). Septal thickening and peribronchial cuffing are less common than in HPE.

The picture remains stable for some days, or longer, during the proliferative phase. In more severe cases, the opacification is complete and

Table 3 Diagnostic criteria for ARDS according to the American-European Consensus Conference (AECC) (Bernard et al. 1994) and to the Berlin definition (ARDS Definition Task Force 2012)

	AECC 1994	Berlin 2012
Onset	"Acute" (no specific timeframe)	Acute "within 7 days of a known clinical insult"
Radiological criteria	Bilateral infiltrates on frontal CXR	"Bilateral infiltrates on frontal CXR not fully explained by effusions, lobar/lung collapse, or nodules /masses" (chest X-ray interpretation set available online)
CT	Not included	Bilateral opacities on CT
Pulmonary artery wedge pressure (PAWP)	PAWP <18 mmHg	Removed
Severity	Acute lung injury (ALI) if PaO_2/FiO_2 <300 (regardless of PEEP level) ARDS $PaO_2/FiO_2 < 200$ (regardless of PEEP level)	ALI removed Mild/moderate/severe ARDS Minimum C-PAP/PEEP level 5 cmH_2O
Pathologic correlate	Injury to both the epithelium and the endothelium	DAD (diffuse alveolar damage)

the picture is that of the so-called "white lungs" (Fig. 5d, e).

In the late phase the alterations begin to reverse. In patients who heal, the lungs return normal (Fig. 5f), while in patients who develop fibrosis, there is evidence of coarse reticular opacities.

3.4.2 HRCT Signs

The HRCT pattern of ARDS depends on the phase of the process, even if we cannot clearly distinguish the phases. In particular, the exudative phase and the early organizing phase of ARDS overlap, as well as the late proliferative phase overlap with the fibrotic phase (Ichikado 2014).

In the very beginning (early exudative phase), HRCT shows patchy ground-glass opacities (GGO) and consolidations, with geographic distribution (Figs. 5c and 6b). Small pleural effusions (missed by chest X-ray), septal pattern, and crazy paving can also be seen.

Afterward, the process quickly progress to a more homogeneous opacification of the lungs, which persists for the exudative phase and the organizing phase. At this stage ARDS may show two patterns, named typical and atypical. Originally the typical pattern has been associated with extrapulmonary ARDS, while the atypical was associated with pulmonary ARDS (Goodman et al. 1999). This has not been confirmed by a following study (Desai et al. 2001), and in any case, it is not always possible to attribute a single cause to the insurgence of this syndrome (Desai 2002).

The HRCT pattern of typical ARDS is characterized by the presence of a bilateral symmetric anterior-posterior density gradient (Fig. 6c). The density is lower anteriorly (or may be normal or hyperventilated), while posteriorly the density increases progressively, from a ground-glass opacification to a frank consolidation, in the more dependent regions.

In atypical ARDS there are patchy GGO or consolidations, randomly distributed in dependent and nondependent regions of the lungs, without the symmetric density gradient (Fig. 5c).

In the late proliferative and fibrotic phase, from 38 to 85 % of the patients show fibrotic changes in the parenchyma, characterized by an atypical coarse reticular pattern, with traction bronchiectasis and bronchiolectasis (Fig. 7). Fibrotic alterations are more frequently distributed in the ventral portions of the lungs (Fig. 6e, f). This is considered to be the consequence of the barotrauma caused by prolonged ventilation (Nöbauer-Huhman et al. 2001).

CT predictors of mortality in ARDS are signs of right heart failure, involvement of more than 80 % of the lung parenchyma, and presence of varicoid traction bronchiectasis (Chung et al. 2011).

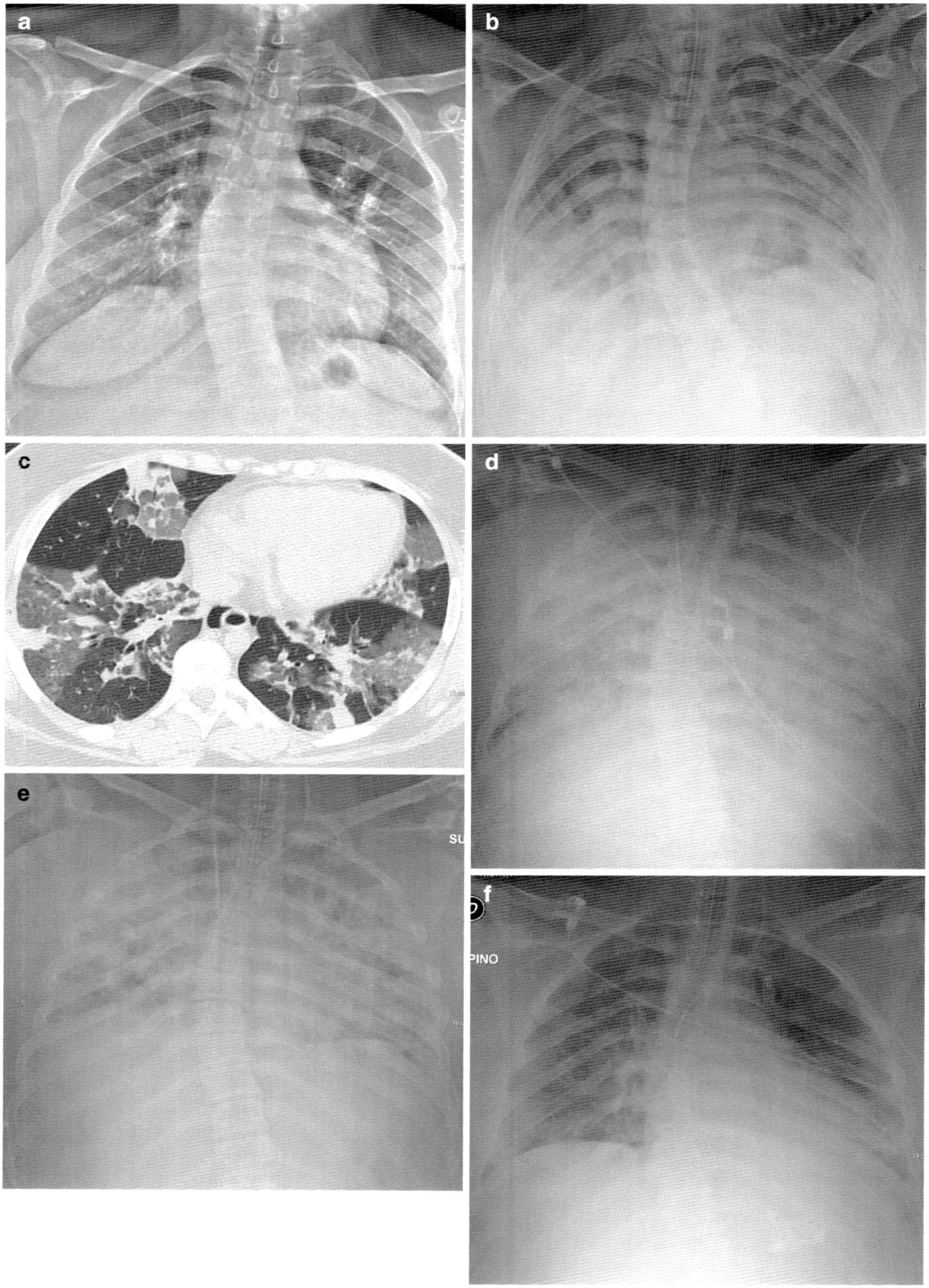
a
b
c
d
e
f
SU
PINO

3.5 Differential Diagnosis

Historically, the radiographic differentiation of hydrostatic and permeability edema has always been a big radiological challenge (Milne et al. 1985; Aberle et al. 1988).

Criteria for the radiographic differentiation of permeability edema from hydrostatic pulmonary edema (HPE) have been discussed in the acute pulmonary edema paragraph. Although there are several signs that can help the diagnosis, the distinction is frequently impossible. Moreover, chest radiograph interpretation shows poor interobserver reliability (Rubenfeld et al. 1999; Meade et al. 2000).

Likely HRCT may improve the diagnostic accuracy, but at present there is a scarcity of literature in regard. HRCT findings that suggest presence of HPE are perihilar and upper lobar distribution of GGOs, central predominant distribution of consolidations, dilatation of the pulmonary veins and of the superior cava vein, thickening of the bronchial walls (peribronchovascular thickening), and right pleural effusion. Even distribution of the GGOs and of the consolidations is found more often in ARDS. Gravity-dependent opacities, septal pattern, air bronchograms, and traction bronchiectasis did not show significant difference in prevalence between HPE and ARDS (Komiya et al. 2013).

This difficulty in the differential diagnosis of the nature of the edema is implicitly recognized by the definition of Berlin. In the Berlin definition, a differential diagnosis between cardiogenic and noncardiogenic edema on chest radiograph is not required, nor it is considered relevant: it is now recognized that hydrostatic edema and ARDS may coexist. The diagnosis of ARDS requires that the respiratory failure is not fully explained by cardiac failure, or fluid overload, using all available data (Ferguson et al. 2012). Therefore, radiologically, the focus is on the generic diagnosis of bilateral edema that must not be confused with pleural effusions, lobar/lung collapse, or nodules/masses. In fact, HPE is not the only condition with which the ARDS goes in differential diagnosis: bioptic and autoptic studies have demonstrated only moderate agreement between the clinical diagnosis of ARDS and presence of DAD. Specificity of the various criteria for presence of DAD is variable in literature, but always quite poor (Lorente et al. 2015).

There is no pathognomonic laboratory test or radiological sign to establish the diagnosis of ARDS, which is generally clinical. Apart from HPE, the most common conditions that share a similar clinical presentation are atelectasis, pneumonia, and pulmonary embolism (Murray 1975). In reality there are many more and encountered less frequently: miliary tuberculosis, CMV pneumonia, invasive aspergillosis, hantavirus pneumonia, herpes simplex pneumonia, bronchoalveolar cell carcinoma, drug toxicity, lymphangitis, acute leukemia, lymphoma, veno-occlusive disease, sickle lung, acute eosinophilic pneumonia, acute cryptogenic organizing pneumonia (COP), acute fibrinous organizing pneumonia (AFOP), diffuse alveolar hemorrhage, and acute hypersensitivity pneumonia (Dakin and Griffiths 2002; Schwarz and Albert 2004).

Some of the abovementioned conditions may show peculiar HRCT findings (many are discussed elsewhere in this book). For example, presence of subpleural peripheral distribution of the consolidations is suggestive of acute eosinophilic pneumonia, while peribronchial distribution is suggestive of COP or AFOP (Obadina et al. 2013).

Most of those mimickers (or imitators) of ARDS require a different and specific therapy. Therefore, when performing a HRCT examination in patients with clinical diagnosis of ARDS, maximum attention is required to highlight any

Fig. 5 Evolution of ARDS at chest X-ray (post-infective ARDS). Latent period: no pathologic findings (**a**). The following day appearance of bilateral patchy consolidations, with bilateral pleural effusion (**b**). HRCT, performed on the same day, shows bilateral patchy and lobular GGOs and consolidations, randomly distributed (atypical ARDS) (**c**). The day after, chest X-ray shows bilateral extensive opacification ("lung white-out") (**d**). Parenchymal opacification remains stable: chest X-ray 2 days later (**e**). The patient survived and improved quickly: marked radiographic improvement 7 days later (**f**)

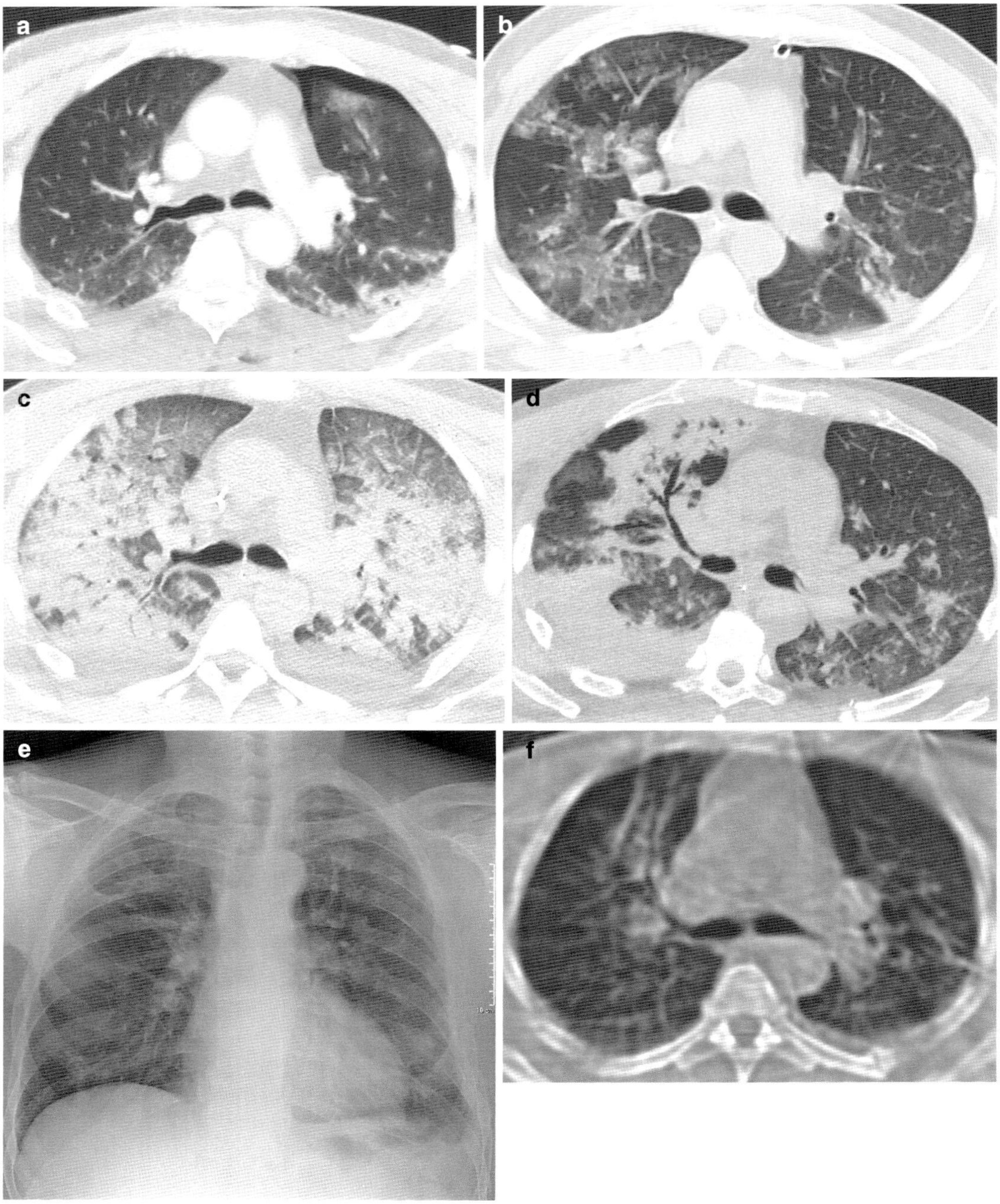

Fig. 6 Evolution of ARDS at CT (posttraumatic ARDS). At admission, left thoracic trauma with pneumothorax and lung contusion (**a**). Respiratory deterioration 7 days later: at CT appearance of bilateral patchy GGO, corresponding to the early exudative phase (**b**). Two days later, extensive lung opacification with extensive dorsal consolidation and ventral GGO: typical ARDS pattern (proliferative or organizative phase). Note presence of smooth septal thickening ("crazy-paving appearance") (**c**). Nine days later advanced regression of the lung opacities: on the right side presence of bronchiectasis and bronchocentric consolidation, located anteriorly (fibro-proliferative phase) (**d**). The patient survived and recovered well, although chest X-ray performed 2 months later demonstrates persistence of coarse fibrosis in the upper right lobe (**e**), confirmed at CT (**f**)

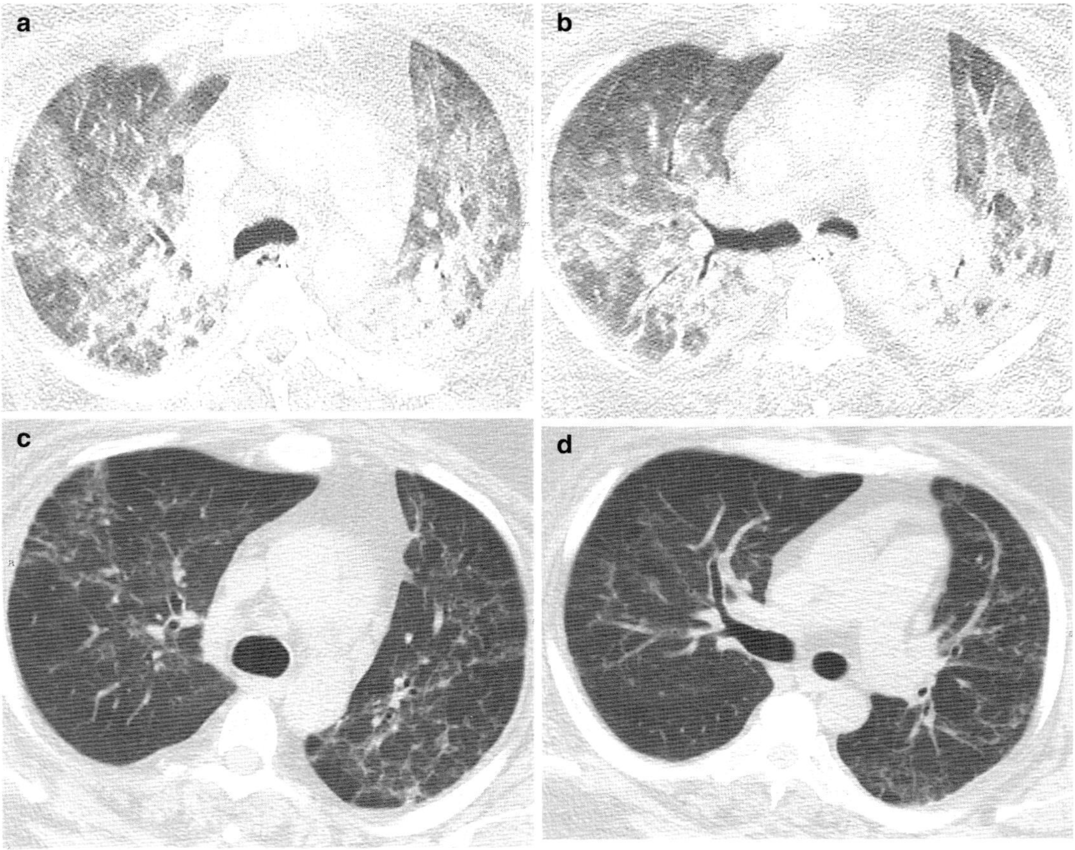

Fig. 7 Severe ARDS followed by fibrotic outcome, caused by viral H1N1 infection. Extensive bilateral consolidations and GGO (**a**, **b**). Two months later, persistence of a reticular pattern bilaterally ("atypical" fibrosis) (**c**, **d**)

sign, or pattern, that may suggest an alternative diagnosis to the complex ARDS/DAD.

3.6 Management and Treatment

No pharmacologic therapy has proved effective in the prevention or management of ARDS.

The only specific therapy for ARDS is ventilation (noninvasive or mechanical) using low tidal volumes (lung-protective strategy), to improve blood oxygen levels, and providing supportive care.

Great deal of attention must be placed to not miss a treatable cause of ARDS and to early diagnose the complications (barotrauma, ventilator-associated pneumonia, and fluid overload, among others).

4 Diffuse Alveolar Hemorrhage (DAH)

4.1 Introduction

Diffuse alveolar hemorrhage (DAH) is not a specific disorder, but a syndrome that suggests a differential diagnosis and a specific sequence of testing. DAH may be a life-threatening condition characterized clinically by the presence of hemoptysis, falling hematocrit, diffuse pulmonary infiltrates, and hypoxemic respiratory failure, which can be severe. However, chest radiographic and CT findings may be nonspecific (the alveolar infiltrates can even sometimes be unilateral), and hemoptysis may be lacking. DAH should be considered a medical emergency due to the morbidity and mortality associated with failure to treat the disorder promptly (Collard and Schwarz 2004; Lara and Schwarz 2010).

The diagnosis of diffuse alveolar hemorrhage is made on the basis of the clinical and radiological pattern and may be confirmed by bronchoalveolar lavage (BAL). In acute and severe forms, the BAL findings include bright red blood from multiple sites in different bronchi and, microscopically, hemosiderin-laden macrophages. BAL is also useful for excluding other differential diagnoses, such as infections or other endobronchial sources of bleeding (Park 2013). Once the diagnosis is established, the underlying cause must be established in order to initiate treatment.

4.2 Mechanisms of Injury and Causes

DAH is a life-threatening condition which refers to hemorrhage originating in the pulmonary microvasculature, rather than from the bronchial circulation or parenchymal abnormalities. All causes of DAH have the common denominator of an injury to the alveolar microcirculation. Pulmonary small vessel vasculitides, connective tissue disorders, and drugs make up the majority of the cases of DAH (Table 4).

DAH includes diseases associated with pulmonary capillaritis (cellular infiltrate of neutrophils in the capillaries and venules) and those associated with normal vessels (Colby et al. 2001). A pulmonary capillaritis is considered the most common underlying lesion associated with diffuse alveolar hemorrhage.

4.3 Terminology and Clinical Issues

The cardinal sign of DAH, hemoptysis, may be a dramatic event or evolve over days to weeks; however, it may be initially absent in up to 33 % of DAH cases. The other symptoms of DAH are nonspecific and include fever, cough, and dyspnea. Nonpulmonary signs and symptoms are those that accompany the underlying systemic disease. A possible association of hematuria and renal failure due to concomitant glomerulonephritis may be present (Dalpiaz et al. 2003).

The causes of diffuse alveolar hemorrhage are many, but the association with primary renal involvement (pulmonary-renal syndrome) reduces the range of diagnostic possibilities to a handful of diseases: Goodpasture's syndrome, systemic lupus erythematosus (SLE), ANCA-associated vasculitis (antineutrophil cytoplasmic antibodies), particularly micropolyangiitis (MPA), granulomatosis with polyangiitis (Wegener granulomatosis), and, more rarely, eosinophilic granulomatosis with polyangiitis (Churg-Strauss) (Jennette 2013; Chung et al. 2010; Marten et al. 2005; Mayberry et al. 2000). Knowledge of the patient's clinical data and laboratory tests may be sufficient to guide toward the possible cause of this group of patients (Table 5).

Table 4 Causes of diffuse alveolar hemorrhage (DAH)

Main causes of diffuse alveolar hemorrhage
Pulmonary small vessel vasculitides:
ANCA-associated pulmonary vasculitides:
Granulomatosis with polyangiitis (formerly Wegener's granulomatosis)
Microscopic polyangiitis (MPA)
Churg-Strauss vasculitis
Non-ANCA-associated pulmonary vasculitides:
Goodpasture's syndrome
Connective tissue disorders (SLE, mixed connective tissue disease, RA)
Drugs
Other causes of diffuse alveolar hemorrhage
Coagulative disorders
Inhaled toxins
Mitral valve disease
Pulmonary veno-occlusive disease (PVOD)
Infection
Diffuse alveolar damage
Malignancy
Autologous bone marrow transplantation
Acute lung transplant rejection
Pulmonary hemosiderosis
Antiphospholipid syndrome

Table 5 Causes of combination of DAH and glomerulonephritis (primary pulmonary-renal syndrome)

	Clinical features	Laboratory tests
Goodpasture's syndrome	Young man	Anti-GBM
Granulomatosis with polyangiitis (Wegener granulomatosis)	Upper airway disease (nasal, oral, or sinus inflammation)	c-ANCA
Microscopic polyangiitis (MPA)	Systemic symptoms	p-ANCA
Systemic lupus erythematosus (SLE)	Systemic symptoms	ANA
Eosinophilic granulomatosis with polyangiitis (Churg-Strauss)	Asthma	Peripheral eosinophilia p-ANCA

Anti-GBM anti-glomerular basement membrane antibodies, ANCA antineutrophil cytoplasmic autoantibody, *ANA* antinuclear antibodies

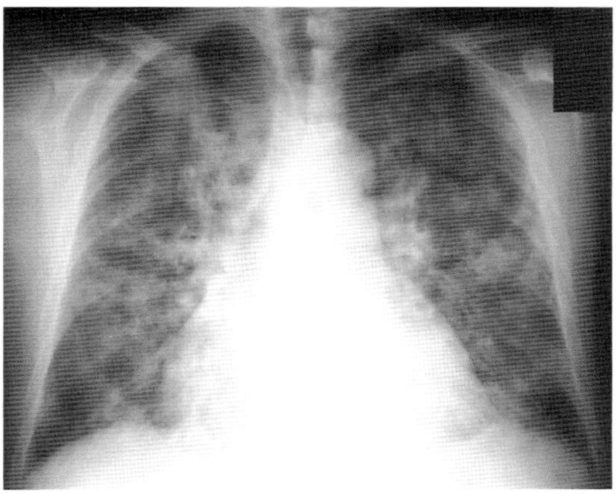

Fig. 8 Diffuse alveolar hemorrhage (DAH) in systemic lupus erythematosus (SLE). Chest radiograph shows extensive and patchy parenchymal opacities in both lungs. Both apices and subpleural lungs are relatively spared (bat's wing or butterfly pulmonary opacities)

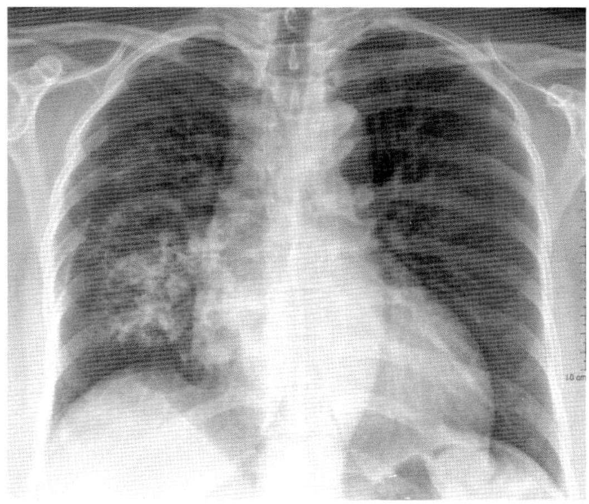

Fig. 9 Diffuse alveolar hemorrhage (DAH) and alveolar edema in mitral regurgitation resulting from myocardial infarction and papillary muscle rupture. Chest radiograph reveals asymmetrical consolidations predominantly in the right parahilar region

4.4 Imaging

4.4.1 Radiological Signs

The characteristic radiological picture of DAH often shows bilateral parenchymal consolidation or ground-gross opacities, sometimes predominant in the perihilar region ("butterfly wings" or "bat wings" opacities, Fig. 8); occasionally it is prevalently unilateral (Fig. 9) (Primack et al. 1995). The chest radiograph findings are nonspecific and the diagnosis relies combination with clinical and laboratory findings.

4.4.2 CT Signs

High-resolution CT often yields no additional diagnostic information, merely confirming the presence of infiltrates. The HRCT pattern can vary with time of onset of the hemorrhage and the clinical context is crucial in image interpretation.

Acute phase can range from lobular or lobar areas of ground-glass opacities or consolidation or extensive, perihilar (bat's wing or butterfly), or diffuse involvement (Fig. 10a, b) (Cortese et al. 2008; Castañer et al. 2010).

Within days of an acute episode of hemorrhage, interlobular septal thickening may be seen in association with ground-glass opacity (crazy-paving pattern) as hemosiderin-laden macrophages accumulate in the interstitium (Fig. 10c) (Rossi et al. 2003; De Wever et al. 2011).

CT may be useful in the follow-up period, given its ability to demonstrate even the mildest relapse arising after reduction or discontinuation

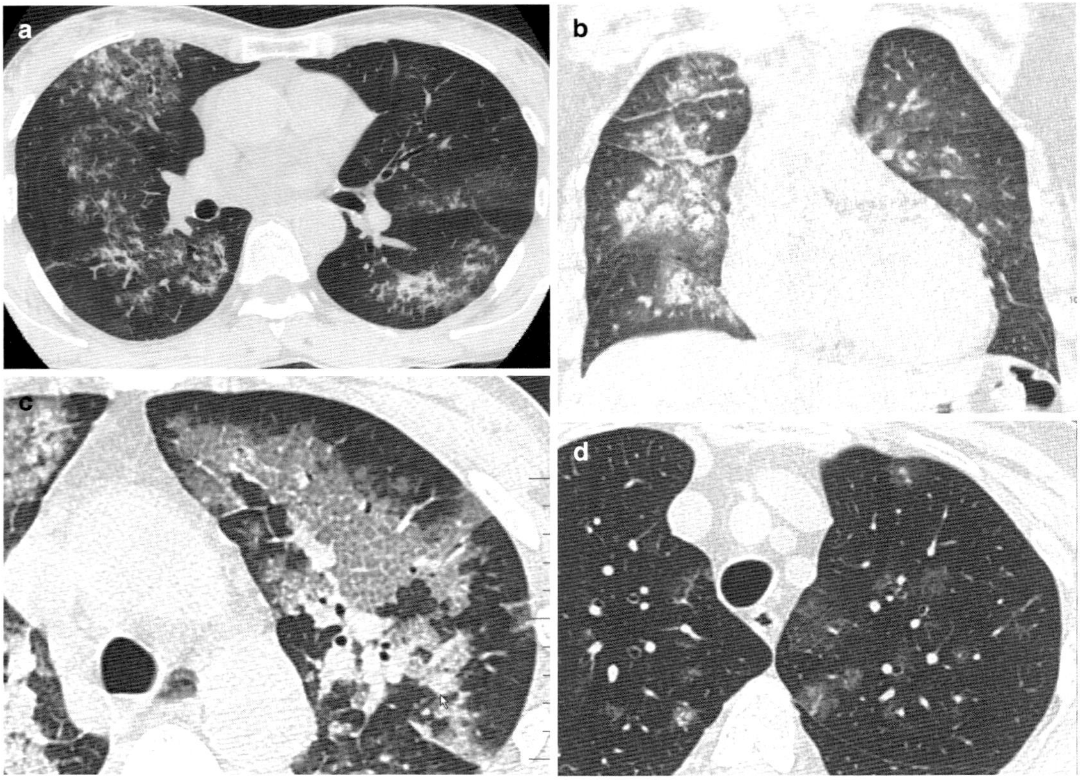

Fig. 10 Variety of high-resolution CT patterns that can be found in DAH. (**a**) Wegener granulomatosis. CT image shows extensive areas of ground-glass opacity in a predominantly perihilar distribution (bat's wing or butterfly pulmonary opacities). (**b**) Mitral regurgitation resulting from myocardial infarction and papillary muscle rupture (same patient as in Fig. 9). CT reveals asymmetrical consolidations and ground-glass opacities predominantly in the right parahilar region. Coexist interstitial edema and enlarged vessels due to concomitant interstitial edema. (**c**) Systemic lupus erythematosus (same patient as in Fig. 8). Within days of an acute episode of hemorrhage, interlobular septal thickening may be seen in association with ground-glass opacity (crazy-paving pattern). (**d**) Microscopic polyangiitis (MPA). CT image shows patchy areas of ground-glass opacity and some low-density nodules (snowflake-like nodules), some of them rounded and feeding-vessels

of cortisone and immunosuppressant therapy. Some faint scattered nodules or small areas of ground glass and some low-density nodules (snowflake-like nodules) may be seen, sometimes around the smaller vessels, which are not detected by chest radiography (Fig. 10d) (Maffessanti et al. 2005).

After repeated episodes of pulmonary hemorrhage, a persistent reticular pattern may be seen, with areas of peripheral traction bronchiectasis and distortion of the lung architecture; this pattern reflects interstitial hemosiderin deposition and mild lung fibrosis and has been termed pulmonary hemosiderosis.

4.5 Differential Diagnosis

Radiological pattern of DHA is not pathognomonic, but diffuse alveolar hemorrhage is the second cause of acute perihilar alveolar lung disease after pulmonary edema (Ribeiro et al. 2006; Dalpiaz and Maffessanti 2013). Differentiation is usually straightforward based on the clinical data and the frequent co-existence, in hydrostatic edema, of pleural effusion, enlarged vessels, and sometimes cardiomegaly. In all these cases, the differential diagnosis with other acute forms of diffuse lung disease—particularly inhalation and infectious pneumonia—based on radiological data alone becomes impossible. Hemorrhagic alveolar infiltration resolves rapidly (especially after corticosteroid therapy) but slower than pulmonary edema.

4.6 Management and Treatment

The treatment of DAH depends on the underlying cause of hemorrhage and ranges from supportive care and withdrawal of offending drugs to high-dose steroids, immunosuppressants, and plasmapheresis. Massive pulmonary hemorrhage is a life-threatening manifestation and requires aggressive immunosuppressive therapy as soon as possible.

5 Fat Embolism Syndrome (FES)

5.1 Introduction

Fat embolism syndrome (FES) is a rare complication of the fractures, mainly of the long bones. Its importance lies in the fact that it is in the differential diagnosis with other more frequent respiratory complications of trauma and polytrauma, which require a different therapy (such as pulmonary edema or bilateral bronchopneumonia). Also, more rarely, FES can occur in more severe forms such as the acute respiratory distress syndrome (ARDS) or in a fulminant form. While the radiographic findings may be mistaken for other conditions, the CT pattern may be more specific and suggest the diagnosis.

5.2 Mechanisms of Injury

The exact injury mechanism in FES has not been completely explained, nor has the histopathologic picture been completely clarified. The symptomatology has been put in relation to the release of fat particles in the venous blood flow, followed by pulmonary and systemic embolization. At present, it is thought that there are two pathogenic stages that follow one another: the mechanical phase and the biochemical phase (Akhtar 2009). The mechanical phase occurs after release of fat droplets into the venous blood, which determine mechanical obstruction of the pulmonary and systemic capillary bed. The following biochemical phase is due to the toxic effects of free fat acids (FFA) on the endothelia. It is unclear how fat droplets reach systemic circulation: likely they pass through a patent foramen oval or through the pulmonary capillary bed.

Only few studies describe the histopathologic alteration in human FES: in the majority of cases, a toxic vasculitis with alveolar hemorrhage and edema is reported, but also presence of hyaline membranes, the hallmark of diffuse alveolar damage (DAD) and ARDS, has been demonstrated (Berrigan et al. 1966; Dines et al. 1975; Curtis et al. 1979).

Usually fat embolism (FE) is caused by bone fractures, typically by long bone fractures in young patients. Rarely, FE may be due to traumatic subcutaneous fat crushing without fractures (Bolliger et al. 2011) or to nontraumatic causes (Mellor and Soni 2001).

5.3 Terminology and Clinical Issues

Fat embolism (FE) refers to the emergence of fat particles within the venous circulation with the consequent pulmonary embolization. This occurrence is practically constant after fracture, but only a small minority of patients develop clinical symptoms. In those, the resulting syndrome is called fat embolism syndrome (FES) and is characterized by the combination of acute respiratory failure, nervous system impairment, and cutaneous manifestations. The typical petechial rash, that affects the neck, trunk and armpits, characterizes cutaneous manifestations. Petechiae may be evident also in the conjunctiva, retina, or mucosae.

The incidence of posttraumatic FES varies considerably in literature (range from 0.25 % up to 35 %) (Akhtar 2009).

There is no investigation 100% specific for FES and the syndrome is diagnosed on a clinical base (Mellor and Soni 2001). The most widely accepted diagnostic criteria are those from Gurd and Wilson (Table 6) (Gurd and Wilson 1974).

Table 6 Diagnostic criteria from Gurd and Wilson

Major criteria	Minor criteria
Respiratory insufficiency	Pyrexia
Cerebral involvement	Tachycardia
Petechial rush	Retinal changes
	Anemia
	Thrombocytopenia
	High erythrocyte sedimentation rate
	Fat macroglobulinemia
	Jaundice
	Renal changes

Diagnosis of FES is established when 2 major criteria, or 1 major criterion plus 4 minor criteria, are fulfilled

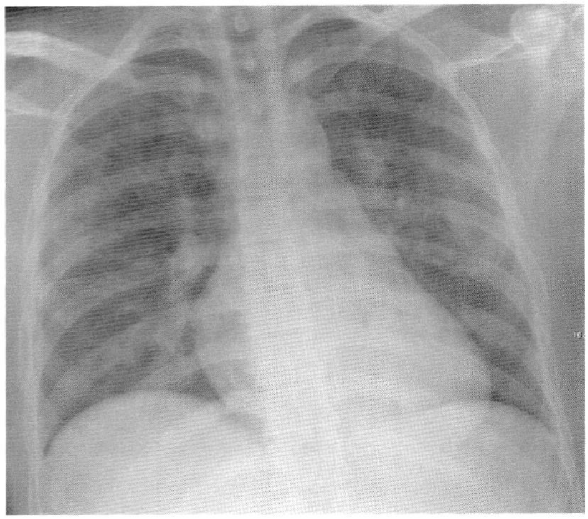

Fig. 11 Early FES. Chest X-ray performed after the onset of the respiratory failure shows poor radiographic alterations

There are three possible clinical presentation of the fat embolism syndrome. The first is classical response, characterized by transient respiratory failure. It can occur after the trauma or after fixation of the fracture.

The second presentation is with the adult respiratory distress syndrome (ARDS). The third is the so-called hyperacute syndrome: it is extremely rare, is characterized by cardiovascular collapse, and quickly leads to death.

5.4 Imaging

5.4.1 Radiological Signs

Usually the appearance of the radiographic alterations lags behind clinical symptoms, even in already, considerably, symptomatic patients (Fig. 11) (Han et al. 2003).

After an interval (up to 72 h, or even longer), radiographic alterations begin to appear in the perihilar and basal regions. Finally appears the full-blown radiographic picture, which consists of a diffuse interstitio-alveolar involvement, with widespread opacities (Fig. 12). The alterations may be patchy and show relative sparing of the apices (Feldman et al. 1975).

The radiological picture at conventional chest X-ray is considered nonspecific and of little help in the differential from other forms of diffuse airspace disease, like ARDS.

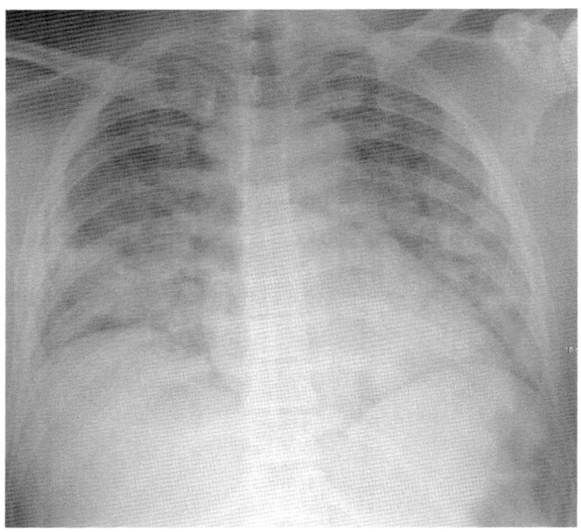

Fig. 12 Full-blown FES. Chest X-ray shows bilateral widespread opacities, with relative sparing of the upper lungs

Sometimes it is possible to identify bilateral focal lesions, described as nodular infiltrates, "rounded densities," or nodular opacities (Fig. 13) (Greenberg 1968; Heyneman and Müller 2000; Arakawa et al. 2000).

Clearing of the radiographic alterations requires a time varying from few days to more than a week (Feldman et al. 1975).

5.4.2 CT Signs

CT findings in pulmonary FES include multifocal ground-glass opacities (GGO) and consolidations, frequently in association with nodules and micronodules. The alterations tend to be bilateral and widespread, with gravitational distribution: consolidations usually have posterior-basal predominance.

The nodules have random distribution, being evident both in the central lobular region and in the subpleural region (Gallardo et al. 2006; Piolanti et al. 2016) (Fig. 14). Also they may present along the interlobular septa (Malagari et al. 2003).

GGO generally have patchy distribution, with geographic appearance (Fig. 15a), and may be frequently associated with septal thickening (Malagari et al. 2003) (Fig. 15b). Consolidations tend to have a gravity-dependent distribution and small pleural effusions are frequent (Arakawa et al. 2000). Consolidations and GGO may present as lobular or sub-lobular opacities (Fig. 14c) (Piolanti et al. 2016).

There are also some case reports of macroscopic fat embolism being detected with contrast-enhanced CT (Ravenel et al. 2002; Nucifora et al. 2007).

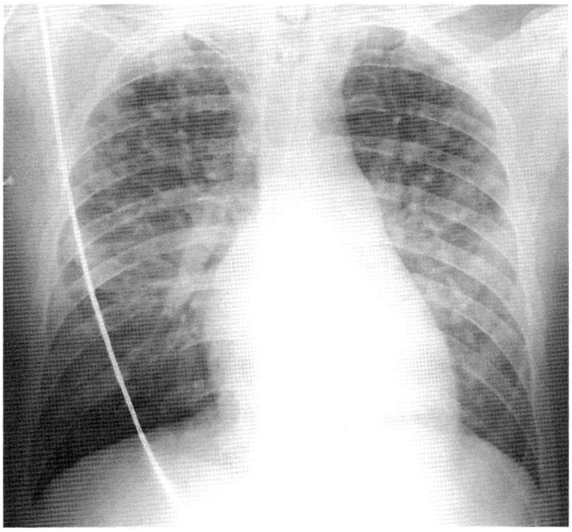

Fig. 13 Nodular pattern as presentation of pulmonary FES. Bilateral nodular and micronodular involvement

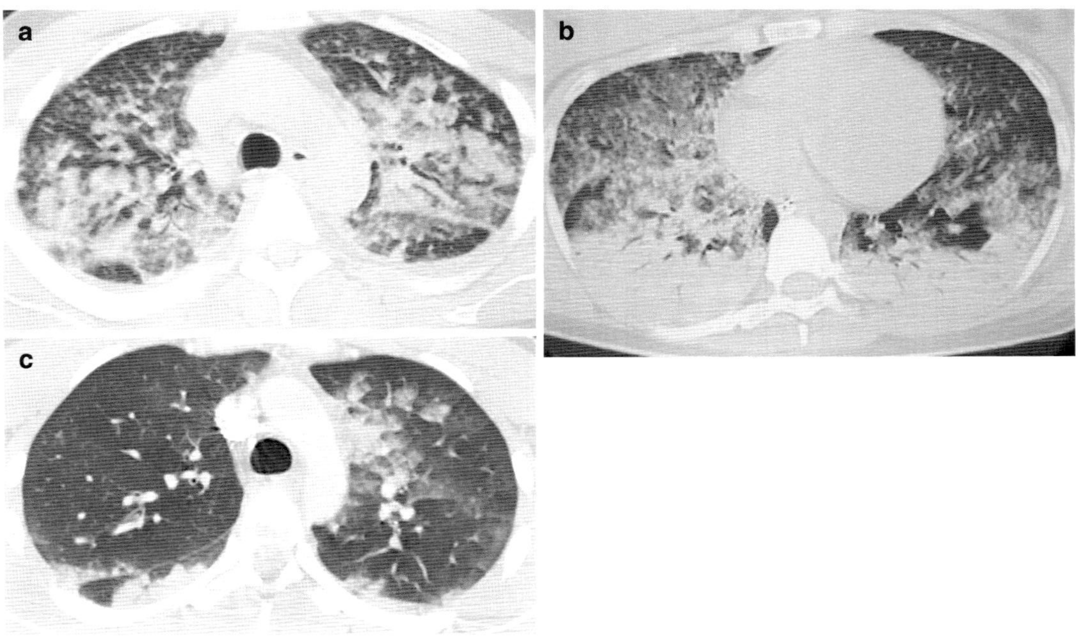

Fig. 14 Nodular pattern at lung CT. Extensive bilateral GGO and consolidations (some showing lobular shape), bilateral nodules, and micronodules: centrilobular and subpleural (randomly distributed) (**a**). Patients with FES and ARDS: anterior-posterior density gradient with dependent consolidations. Presence of an overlapping micro-nodular pattern. (**b**) Lobular and sub-lobular consolidations on the left, subpleural micronodules on the right along the superior fissure (**c**)

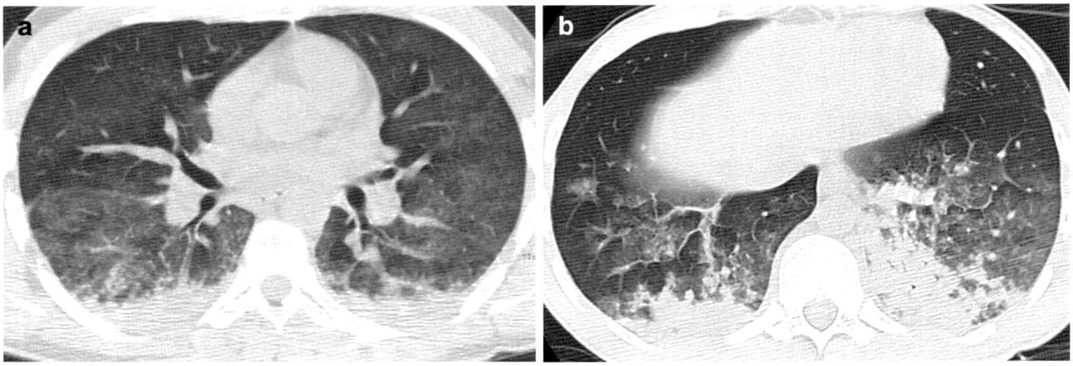

Fig. 15 GGO in acute FES. Diffuse GGO with geographic distribution (**a**). Presence of bilateral smooth interlobular septal thickening. On the right side anterior-posterior density gradient with presence of GGO anteriorly. On the left side GGO are extensive and the overlapping of septal thickening generates a crazy-paving appearance (**b**)

5.5 Differential Diagnosis

Although full-blown or severe FES is not a frequent eventuality, and its frequency is decreasing since early stabilization of the fractures was introduced, it is an important condition to be kept in mind. Its importance lies in the fact that it must be differentiated from other more common and dangerous complications of fractures and polytrauma, such as pulmonary embolism and pneumonia, requiring a specific therapy.

In fact, in the posttraumatic setting, FES has a wide range of conditions from which it must be differentiated: hydrostatic pulmonary edema, fluid overload, neurogenic pulmonary edema, pulmonary contusions, aspiration, viral pneumonia, bilateral bronchopneumonia, ventilator-associated pneumonia, sepsis, ARDS, atelectasis, pulmonary hemorrhage, pulmonary embolism, and drug reactions (Feldman et al. 1975).

Normal heart size, normal vascular distribution, and absence of signs of pulmonary hypertension (Kerley lines, peribronchial cuffing, and widening of the vascular pedicle) are considered findings helpful in differential diagnosis from HPE at chest X-ray (Han et al. 2003). In reality, septal thickening, the equivalent of the Kerley lines at HRCT, is a frequent finding in FES (Malagari et al. 2003).

Lung contusions generally appear at chest X-ray as patchy airspace opacities, unilateral and asymmetric. At HRCT they appear as GGO or consolidations, with ill-defined borders and non-segmental distribution. They may show subpleural sparing. After the trauma they may extend and reach the maximum extension in 24–48 h (Kaewlai et al. 2008; Mirka et al. 2012). This is very helpful in the differential with FES that shows up after a latent period, and its pulmonary alterations are usually bilateral and diffuse.

Viral and bacterial pneumonias may present with several different patterns at CT, with considerable overlap in the imaging appearance (Miller et al. 2011). The presence at HRCT of an "airway- centric" disease, which is characterized by bronchial wall thickening, bronco-centric nodules, lobular opacities, and tree in bud opacities, is highly suggestive of bronchopneumonia (Ketai et al. 2008). Absence of tree in bud opacities and the random distribution of the nodules in FES results to be a useful sign for the differentiation from bronchopneumonia.

Aspiration may show different HRCT patterns: obstruction of the airways by foreign body, tree in bud opacities, or segmental or lobar opacities. Aspiration tends to interest posterior segments of the upper lobes and superior segments of the lower lobes. A massive intake of gastric content causes a severe chemical pneumonia, leading to ARDS (Medelson's syndrome) (Kim et al. 2008).

5.6 Management and Treatment

The treatment of FES is essentially supportive.

Early stabilization of fractures involving the long bones decreases the incidence of FES (Talucci et al. 1983; Svenningsen et al. 1987).

However, it is still unclear what is the best surgical strategy in patients who already show signs of FES. Furthermore, effective pharmacologic therapies have not been found yet, except for steroids. However, their effectiveness has not been proven in prospective studies on a large scale (Akhtar 2009).

6 Acute Pulmonary Edema

6.1 Introduction

Pulmonary edema is defined as presence of excess extravascular fluid in the lungs. The more common type of acute pulmonary edema is hydrostatic pulmonary edema (HPE) due to acute cardiac failure or to fluid overload (overhydration or renal failure).

From a radiological point of view, HPE is the most frequent cause of acute diffuse pulmonary disease (Ketai and Washington 2002).

Chest X-ray is the classical radiological examination for the diagnosis of HPE, while lung sonography is an emerging technique (Cardinale et al. 2014).

CT is not performed for suspected HPE, but HPE is a frequent finding in CT examinations performed for different purposes (e.g., to rule out suspected pulmonary embolism).

6.2 Mechanisms of Injury

The Starling equation describes the factors determining the flow of the fluids between the pulmonary capillary circulation and the lung interstitium (Ware and Matthay 2005). Edema occurs when accumulation of extravascular fluid (transudative or exudative) exceeds the resorption mechanisms (lymphatic absorption). Factors determining the amount of capillary filtration are the transmural hydrostatic pressure, the transmural oncotic pressure, and the permeability of the capillary membrane.

Generally speaking, HPE appears when transmural hydrostatic pressure increases or intravascular oncotic pressure decreases. The fluid is a transudate with low-protein content. The excess of fluid accumulates first in the interstitium and then moves to the pleural and alveolar spaces.

Noncardiogenic edema is due to an increase in permeability of the pulmonary capillaries that allows the outflow of plasma proteins, without increase in transmural hydrostatic pressure. This protein outflow attracts fluids into the interstitial compartment generating an exudative edema, called "permeability edema." In diffuse alveolar damage (DAD), the injury to the endothelial barrier originates the increase in permeability. This is not the sole mechanism of increased capillary permeability that may also occur without DAD, like in cases of reaction to drugs (illicit drugs, interleukin-2 edema), transfusion reaction (classically defined by Milne "allergic lung"), or infection (e.g., hantavirus pulmonary syndrome) (Ketai and Godwin 1998).

6.3 Terminology and Clinical Issues

Acute pulmonary edema is classically classified into cardiogenic and noncardiogenic pulmonary edema.

Cardiogenic pulmonary edema is also referred to as hemodynamic edema or hydrostatic pulmonary edema (HPE). Elevated hydrostatic pressure follows pulmonary venous hypertension, which can be caused by left heart failure or by volume overload (Ware and Matthay 2005).

Noncardiogenic pulmonary edema is also referred to as permeability or injury edema and it is classified into two types: permeability edema with diffuse alveolar damage (DAD) and permeability edema without DAD (Ketai and Godwin 1998).

Finally, edema may be mixed hydrostatic and permeability. A cardiogenic edema may not be purely hydrostatic, since marked elevation of transmural pressure may generate some degree of epithelial damage, or a volume overload may complicate a permeability edema, generating a mixed edema.

High-altitude, re-expansion, and neurogenic pulmonary edemas are included into the mixed edema group: although their pathogenesis is still incompletely explained, in all cases a hydrostatic component is supposed to combine with some degree of increases in permeability (Ketai and Godwin 1998; Gluecker et al. 1999).

6.4 Imaging

6.4.1 Radiological Signs

Chest radiograph is routinely performed in patients with suspected HPE to confirm the diagnosis or rule out other possible causes. Radiographic findings associated with HPE are increased heart size, increased width of the vascular pedicle, balanced or inverted vascular distribution (redistribution or "cephalization" of the lung vessels), vascular haziness, central or even distribution of the opacities and presence of peribronchial cuffing, septal lines, thickening of the fissures, and pleural effusion.

Radiographically pulmonary edema is divided into three degrees: mild, moderate, and severe (Rubinowitz et al. 2007; Morgan and Goodman 1991).

Mild-degree edema or venous hypertension may show an enlarged vascular pedicle and pulmonary redistribution (cephalization or inversion), which is more frequently seen in cases of chronic heart failure (Fig. 16). Similarly, the heart does not usually enlarge at the first episode of left ventricular failure. Patients with mild edema due to volume overload or to renal failure may show balanced flow, a finding that can be evaluated only in the upright position.

Moderate or interstitial edema shows peribronchial cuffing, Kerley B-lines (septal lines), thickening of the interlobar fissures, and vascular haziness (indistinctness) (Fig. 17).

Severe or alveolar edema shows airspace opacification, prevalent in the middle and lower lung fields (perihilar or gravitational) (Figs. 18 and 19).

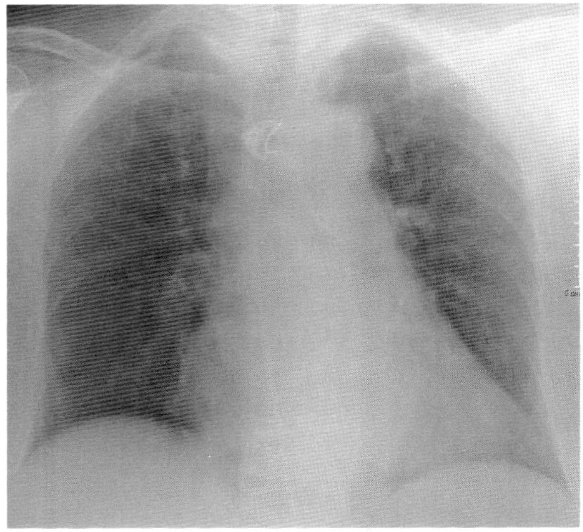

Fig. 16 Mild-degree edema or venous hypertension. Pulmonary redistribution, enlarged heart, and enlarged vascular pedicle

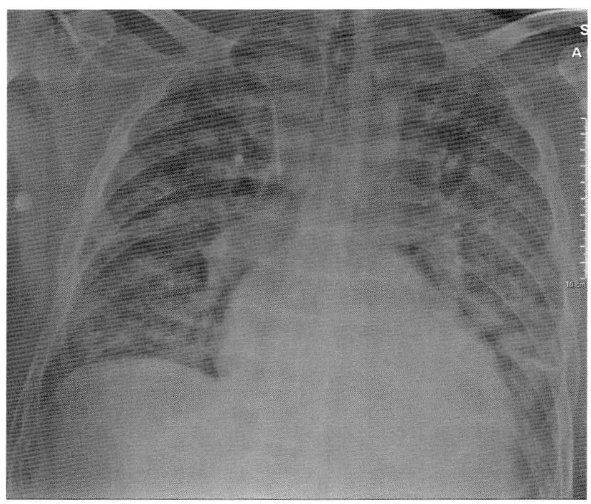

Fig. 17 Moderate or interstitial edema. Peribronchial cuffing, bilateral B Kerley lines, thickening of the interlobular fissure, and vascular haziness

The alterations typically are symmetric, but they may be asymmetric in patients with pulmonary parenchymal disease (e.g., emphysema). Unilateral edema is also possible (e.g., in case of mitral cord rupture or of lying on one side) (Fig. 20a, b).

Measurements of the vascular pedicle width can provide an estimate of the intravascular volume status, both in the upright and in the supine position. A vascular pedicle larger than 53 mm in the upright position and more than 70 mm in the supine is expression of HPE and of fluid overload (Milne and Pistolesi 1994; Ely and Haponik 2002). This measurement may provide evidence of HPE before evidence of clinical signs and help distinguish HPE from permeability edema (Milne 2010).

The radiographic picture is considered to depend from the pulmonary capillary wedge pressure (PCWP), which is an indirect measure of the left atrial pressure: however, in literature, there are great discrepancies and controversies on this topic. With PCWP under 19–25 mmHg, there is equalization or cephalization of the vasculature. Between 20 and 30 mmHg, there is a radiographic picture of interstitial edema. Alveolar flooding appears with over 25–30 mmHg, resulting in the radiological appearance of confluent acinar opacity (Morgan et al. 1991; Ketai and Godwin 1998). It is important to remember how the radiographic picture depends also from the acuteness or chronicity of

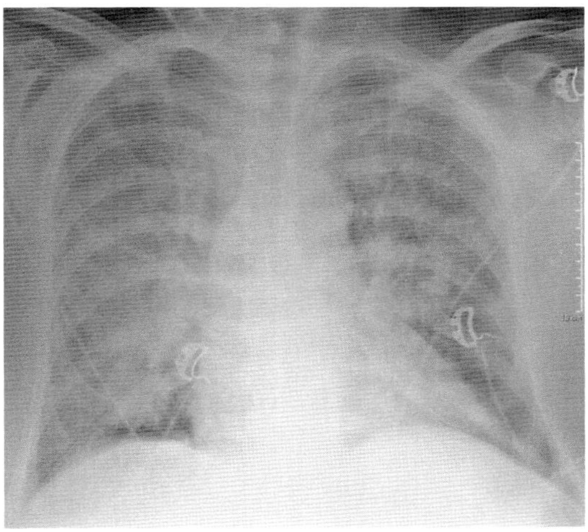

Fig. 18 Severe or alveolar edema. Bilateral airspace opacification, prevalent in the middle or lower fields

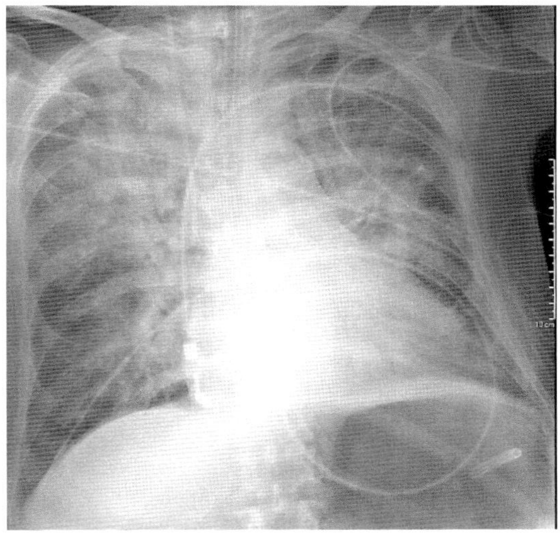

Fig. 19 Alveolar edema with the so-called "bat wings" or "butterfly wings" appearance. Non-gravitational bilateral perihilar opacities with sparing of the lung periphery

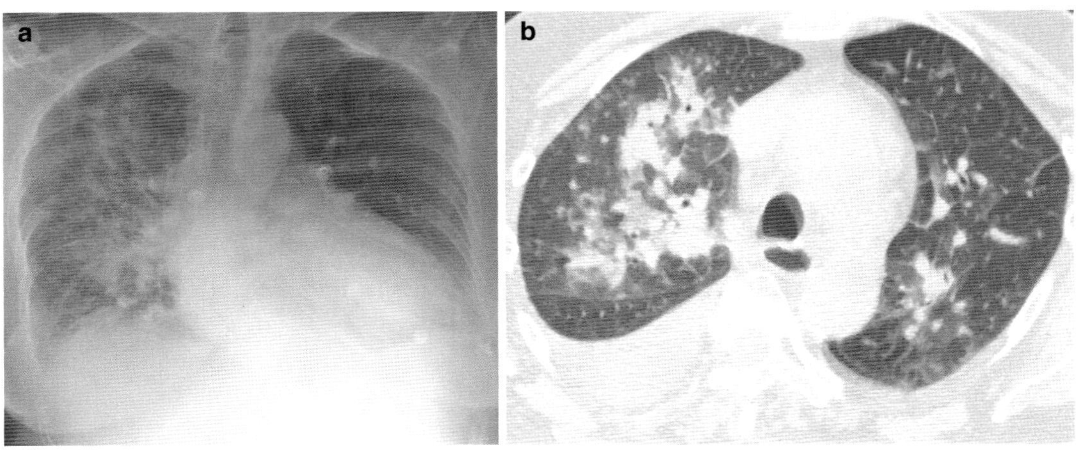

Fig. 20 Unilateral alveolar edema in a patient with acute mitral incompetence (rupture of a papillary muscle). Radiographic picture, extended right-side perihilar opacity, pulmonary redistribution, and enlarged heart (**a**); HRCT findings, presence of right lateral perihilar consolidations; bilaterally smooth septal thickening (septal pattern), bronchial wall thickening, and pleural effusion (**b**)

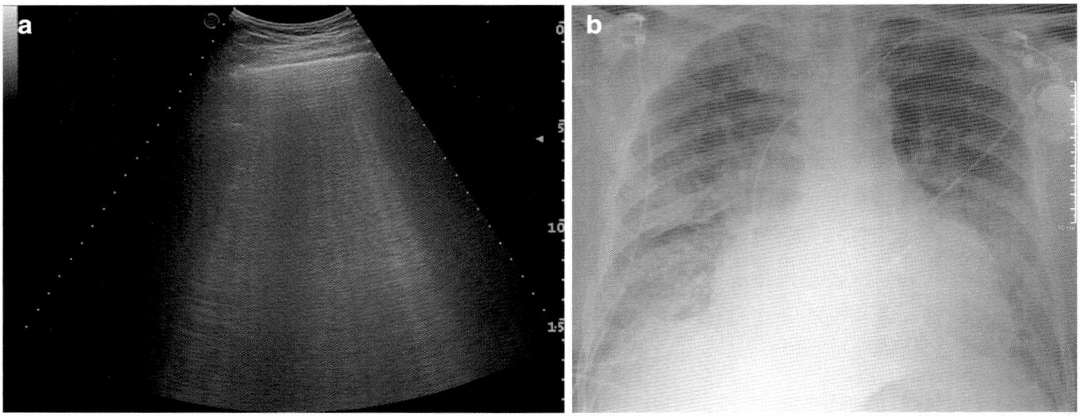

Fig. 21 Lung sonography. Interstitial syndrome characterized by presence of multiple B-lines: left-basal scan (**a**). Corresponding X-ray picture (**b**)

heart failure: edema in acute heart failure is determined by lower pressure gradients, but may not show at chest X-ray dilatation of the heart and of the vessels. On the contrary, chronic heart failure determines an increase in the compliance of the heart and of the pulmonary vessels, and higher pressures are required to determine vascular dilatation (Ketai and Godwin 1998).

Chest X-ray has some intrinsic and technical issues that limit its diagnostic accuracy (Ware and Matthay 2005; Ketai and Godwin 1998). Before radiographic changes start to appear, the water content of the lungs may have to increase up to 30 %; alterations may persist up to 24 h after regression of the edema; bedside radiograms obtained with portable X-ray equipment have intrinsically poor technical quality, and they are affected by factors related to the difficulty to optimize the technique of execution, such as positioning of the patient, patients' body weight, degree of inspiration, type of ventilation applied, and focal film distance and exposure; consolidation at chest X-ray is a nonspecific finding, reflecting loss of the air content of the alveoli, and may be subtended by processes other than HPE, such as hemorrhage, pneumonia, inflammation, or tumor.

6.4.2 Lung Sonography

Lung sonography (LUS) is a relatively new and promising technique, based on the evaluation of sonographic artifacts generated by the lungs. In particular, one of them, the so-called B-lines, underlines the so-called interstitial syndrome (Cardinale et al. 2014) (Fig. 21). LUS is highly sensitive in detecting the B-lines, which are vertical echogenic linear artifacts (reverberations).

The interstitial syndrome is a nonspecific finding, which reflects any condition of the lung where alveolar air is partially replaced with increase in interstitial fluids or cellularity. The detection of an interstitial syndrome is not an exclusive feature of HPE and does not allow differentiation of the underlying interstitial disease. Combining the distribution and the number of the B-lines, with other sonographic signs (peripheral consolidations and aspect of the pleural line) and with the physical examination, may allow to differentiate cardiogenic and noncardiogenic causes of the interstitial syndrome (Copetti et al. 2008; Gargani and Volpicelli 2014).

The advantages of ultrasound are the low cost, noninvasiveness, repeatability, the possibility to perform bedside (point-of-care sonography), and the lack of use of ionizing radiation.

This technique is meeting a great enthusiasm on the part of clinicians and researchers. Certainly, in the next few years, researchers and scientific societies will clarify the potentialities, and the role, of this innovative approach.

6.4.3 CT Signs

Lung HRCT is more sensitive in detecting edema findings compared to chest X-ray (Rubinowitz et al. 2007).

Unfortunately, it is too irradiating, and expensive, to be used routinely for the detection of HPE. For this reason, there are no studies that correlate the CT findings with the degree of HPE.

In the clinical practice, HPE is some kind of "incidentaloma," found at a CT examination performed to rule out other diseases (acute pulmonary embolism above all). It is therefore important to readily recognize HPE at CT to address properly the diagnostic and therapeutic procedures.

The main HRCT findings of HPE are septal pattern, or smooth thickening of the interlobular septa, and ground-glass opacities (GGO) (Figs. 22 and 23).

Other findings are bronchial wall thickening (or smooth peribronchovascular interstitial thickening), enlarged vessels, thickening of the fissures, and ill-defined perivascular and centrilobular opacities and consolidations (Storto et al. 1995; Ribeiro et al. 2006).

GGO are typically patchy, may be lobular, or may present as crazy paving.

At CT the distribution of the alterations tends to show parahilar and posterior distribution. HPE may also show up with a gravity-dependent density gradient (Komiya et al. 2013).

6.5 Differential Diagnosis

There are several radiographic signs that may help the differential between HPE and noncardiogenic pulmonary edema (Milne et al. 1985; Aberle et al. 1988).

Typically, cardiogenic pulmonary edema shows cardiomegaly with vascular redistribution and pleural effusions. The distribution of the opacities is typically even and perihilar (central), prevalent in the middle and lower lung fields, and the vascular pedicle may be enlarged.

Noncardiogenic edema typically shows patchy peripheral or diffuse opacification of the lung fields, with air bronchograms and without cardiomegaly and pleural effusion; vascular pedicle is not enlarged. Septal lines, or Kerley lines, are more frequent in HPE, but may be present in noncardiogenic edema as well.

Unfortunately, these two types of edema frequently do not show up with the typical picture and may share many radiological features: in reality, the distinction becomes frequently impossible, besides the fact that they may coexist in the same patient (Desai 2002).

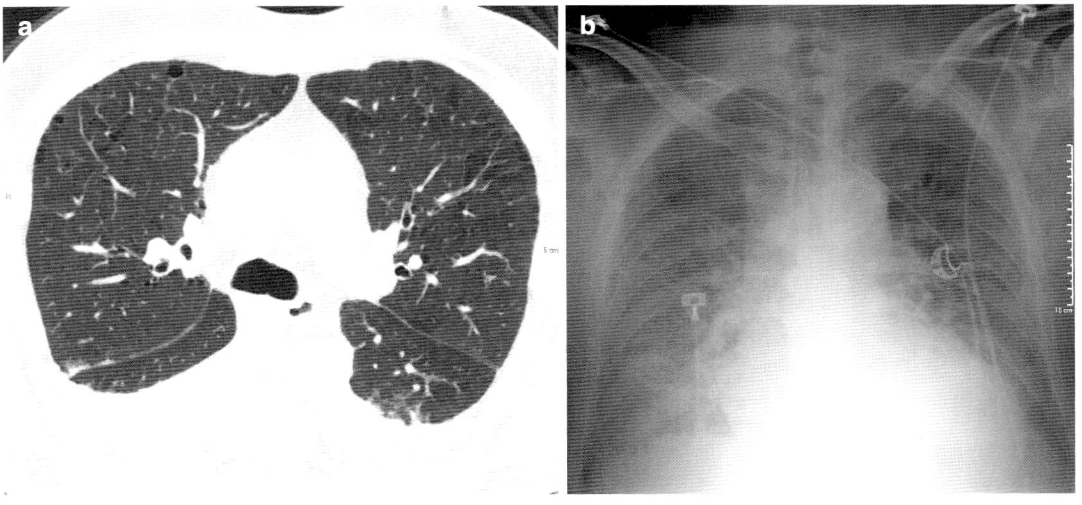

Fig. 22 Interstitial edema at HRCT. Presence of a bilateral diffuse septal pattern and mild bilateral pleural effusion (**a**). Corresponding chest X-ray picture (**b**)

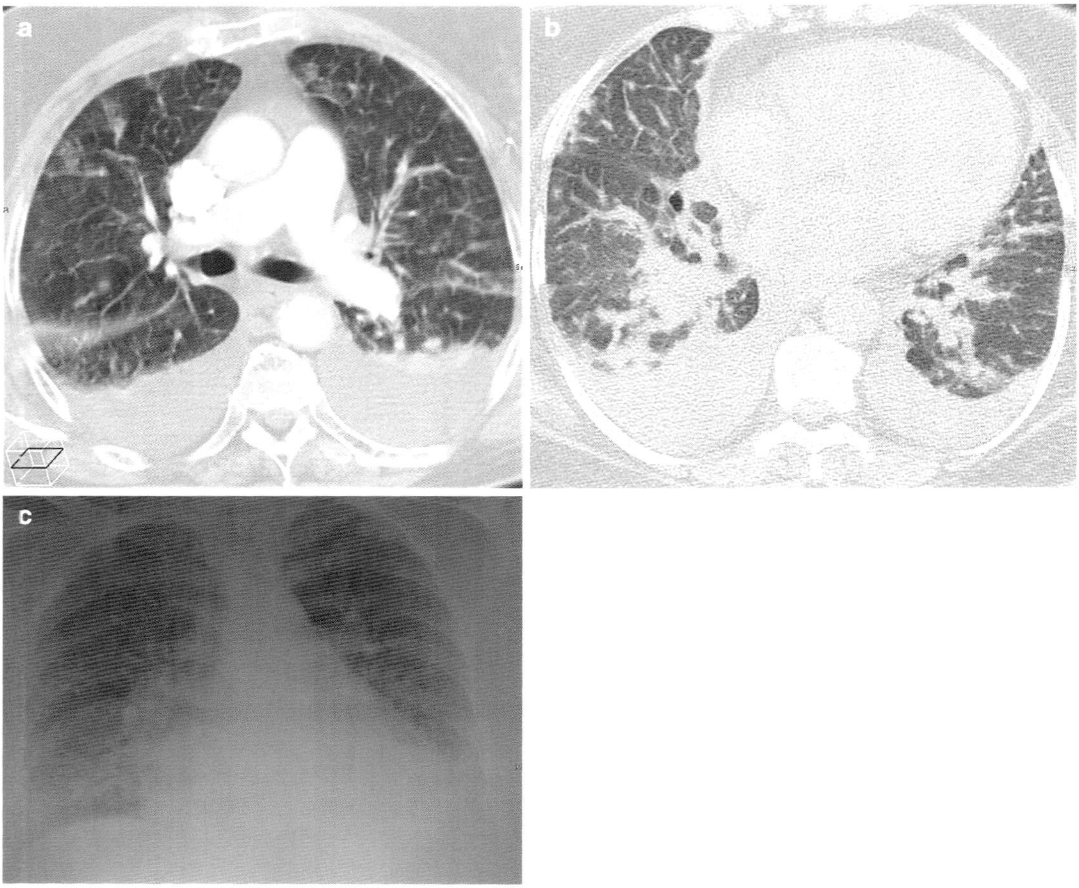

Fig. 23 HRCT findings in two cases of more advanced pulmonary edema. Extensive septal pattern, bronchial wall thickening, lobular ground-glass opacities and bilateral pleural effusion (**a**). Diffuse septal thickening, perihilar consolidations and bilateral pleural effusion (**b**); same patient of image (**b**); radiographic picture (**c**)

Furthermore, HPE has to be differentiated from several other conditions sharing a similar clinical and radiographic presentation, the so-called diffuse airspace disease. Those conditions, among others, are infective pneumonias, interstitial pneumonias, massive embolism, pulmonary hemorrhage, and aspiration (Ketai and Washington 2002).

Radiographic differentiation may be challenging and it is not always possible. HRCT may sometimes be very helpful and suggest the correct diagnosis, although in many cases it does not yield additional elements compared to chest X-ray (Ketai and Washington 2002; Rubinowitz et al. 2007).

The main HRCT finding in HPE is the septal pattern, with variable degrees of GGO. This HRCT pattern goes into differential diagnosis with several conditions, much rarer, such as pulmonary veno-occlusive disease (PVOD), lymphangitis carcinomatosis (although in this condition the septal thickening is usually nodular), sarcoidosis (which usually exhibit perilymphatic micronodules), Niemann-Pick disease, Erdheim Chester disease, cystic lymphangiectasia, lymphangiomyomatosis, and North American hantavirus infections (Oikonomou and Prassopoulos 2013).

6.6 Management and Treatment

Acute pulmonary edema is a life-threatening emergency. If necessary immediate intervention is required addressing the ABCs of resuscitation (airway, breathing, and circulation).

Subsequently, the therapy depends on the patient's condition and the cause of the pulmonary edema: measures may be aimed to preload reduction, afterload reduction, or inotropic support.

References

Aberle DR, Wiener-Kronish JP, Webb WR, Matthay MA (1988) Hydrostatic versus increased permeability pulmonary edema: diagnosis based on radiographic criteria in critically ill patients. Radiology 168(1):73–79

Akhtar S (2009) Fat embolism. Anesthesiol Clin 27(3): 533–550

Arakawa H, Kurihara Y, Nakajima Y (2000) Pulmonary fat embolism syndrome: CT findings in six patients. J Comput Assist Tomogr 24(1):24–29

ARDS Definition Task Force; Ranieri VM, Rubenfeld GD, Thompson BT, Ferguson ND, Caldwell E, Fan E, Camporota L, Slutsky AS (2012) Acute respiratory distress syndrome: the Berlin Definition. JAMA 307(23):2526–2533

Ashbaugh DG, Bigelow DB, Petty TL, Levine BE (1967) Acute respiratory distress in adults. Lancet 2(7511): 319–323

Barrera L, Mendoza F, Zuñiga J, Estrada A, Zamora AC, Melendro EI, Ramírez R, Pardo A, Selman M (2008) Functional diversity of T-cell subpopulations in subacute and chronic hypersensitivity pneumonitis. Am J Respir Crit Care Med 177:44–55

Bernard GR, Artigas A, Brigham KL et al (1994) The American-European Consensus Conference on ARDS: definitions, mechanisms, relevant outcomes, and clinical trial coordination. Am J Respir Crit Care Med 149(3 pt 1):818–824

Berrigan TJ Jr, Carsky EW, Heitzman ER (1966) Fat embolism. Roentgenographic pathologic correlation in 3 cases. Am J Roentgenol Radium Ther Nucl Med 96(4):967–971

Bolliger SA, Muehlematter K, Thali MJ, Ampanozi G (2011) Correlation of fat embolism severity and subcutaneous fatty tissue crushing and bone fractures. Int J Legal Med 125(3):453–458

Camus P, Fanton A, Bonniaud P, Camus C, Foucher P (2004a) Interstitial lung disease induced by drugs and radiation. Respiration 71(4):301–326

Camus P, Kudoh S, Ebina M (2004b) Interstitial lung disease associated with drug therapy. Br J Cancer 91(Suppl 2):S18–S23

Cardinale L, Priola AM, Moretti F, Volpicelli G (2014) Effectiveness of chest radiography, lung ultrasound and thoracic computed tomography in the diagnosis of congestive heart failure. World J Radiol 6(6):230–237

Castañer E, Alguersuari A, Gallardo X, Andreu M, Pallardó Y, Mata JM, Ramírez J (2010) When to suspect pulmonary vasculitis: radiologic and clinical clues. Radiographics 30(1):33–53

Castro CY (2006) ARDS and diffuse alveolar damage: a pathologist's perspective. Semin Thorac Cardiovasc Surg 18(1):13–19

Chong BJ, Kanne JP, Chung JH (2014) Headcheese sign. J Thorac Imaging 29(1):W13

Chung MP, Yi CA, Lee HY, Han J, Lee KS (2010) Imaging of pulmonary vasculitis. Radiology 255(2):322–341

Chung JH, Kradin RL, Greene RE, Shepard JA, Digumarthy SR (2011) CT predictors of mortality in pathology confirmed ARDS. Eur Radiol 21(4):730–737

Cleverley JR, Screaton NJ, Hiorns MP, Flint JD, Müller NL (2002) Drug-induced lung disease: high-resolution CT and histological findings. Clin Radiol 57(4):292–299

Colby TV, Fukuoka J, Ewaskow SP, Helmers R, Leslie KO (2001) Pathologic approach to pulmonary hemorrhage. Ann Diagn Pathol 5(5):309–319

Collard HR, Schwarz MI (2004) Diffuse alveolar hemorrhage. Clin Chest Med 25(3):583–592

Copetti R, Soldati G, Copetti P (2008) Chest sonography: a useful tool to differentiate acute cardiogenic pulmonary edema from acute respiratory distress syndrome. Cardiovasc Ultrasound 6:16

Cormier Y, Brown M, Worthy S, Racine G, Müller NL (2000) High-resolution computed tomographic characteristics in acute farmer's lung and in its follow-up. Eur Respir J 16(1):56–60

Cortese G, Nicali R, Placido R, Gariazzo G, Anrò P (2008) Radiological aspects of diffuse alveolar haemorrhage. Radiol Med 113(1):16–28

Curtis AM, Knowles GD, Putman CE, McLoud TC, Ravin CE, Smith GJ (1979) The three syndromes of fat embolism: pulmonary manifestations. Yale J Biol Med 52(2):149–157

Dakin J, Griffiths M (2002) The pulmonary physician in critical care 1: pulmonary investigations for acute respiratory failure. Thorax 57(1):79–85

Dalpiaz G, Maffessanti M (2013) Diffuse lung diseases. In: Geriatric imaging. Springer, Berlin/New York

Dalpiaz G, Nassetti C, Stasi G (2003) Diffuse alveolar haemorrhage from a rare primary renal-pulmonary syndrome: micropolyangiitis. Case report and differential diagnosis. Radiol Med 106(1–2):114–119

De Wever W, Meersschaert J, Coolen J, Verbeken E, Verschakelen JA (2011) The crazy-paving pattern: a radiological-pathological correlation. Insights Imaging 2(2):117–132

Desai SR (2002) Acute respiratory distress syndrome: imaging of the injured lung. Clin Radiol 57(1):8–17

Desai SR, Wells AU, Suntharalingam G et al (2001) Acute respiratory distress syndrome caused by pulmonary and extrapulmonary injury: a comparative CT study. Radiology 218:689–693

Dines DE, Burgher LW, Okakaki H (1975) The clinical and pathological correlation of fat embolism syndrome. Mayo Clin Proc 50:407–411

Elicker BM, Jones KD, Henry TS, Collard HR (2016) Multidisciplinary approach to hypersensitivity pneumonitis. J Thorac Imaging 31(2):92–103

Ely EW, Haponik EF (2002) Using the chest radiograph to determine intravascular volume status: the role of vascular pedicle width. Chest 121(3):942–950

Erasmus JJ, McAdams HP, Rossi SE (2002) High-resolution CT of drug-induced lung disease. Radiol Clin North Am 40(1):61–72
Feldman F, Ellis K, Green WM (1975) The fat embolism syndrome. Radiology 114(3):535–542
Ferguson ND, Fan E, Camporota L, Antonelli M, Anzueto A, Beale R, Brochard L, Brower R, Esteban A, Gattinoni L, Rhodes A, Slutsky AS, Vincent JL, Rubenfeld GD, Thompson BT, Ranieri VM (2012) The Berlin definition of ARDS: an expanded rationale, justification, and supplementary material. Intensive Care Med 38(10):1573–1582
Franquet T, Hansell DM, Senbanjo T, Remy-Jardin M, Müller NL (2003) Lung cysts in subacute hypersensitivity pneumonitis. J Comput Assist Tomogr 27(4): 475–478
Gallardo X, Castañer E, Mata JM, Rimola J, Branera J (2006) Nodular pattern at lung computed tomography in fat embolism syndrome: a helpful finding. J Comput Assist Tomogr 30(2):254–257
Gargani L, Volpicelli G (2014) How I do it: lung ultrasound. Cardiovasc Ultrasound 12:25
Gluecker T, Capasso P, Schnyder P, Gudinchet F, Schaller MD, Revelly JP, Chiolero R, Vock P, Wicky S (1999) Clinical and radiologic features of pulmonary edema. Radiographics 19(6):1507–1531
Goodman LR, Fumagalli R, Tagliabue P et al (1999) Adult respiratory distress syndrome due to pulmonary and extrapulmonary causes: CT, clinical, and functional correlations. Radiology 231:545–552
Greenberg HB (1968) Roentgenographic signs of post-traumatic fat embolism. JAMA 204(6):540–541
Gurd AR, Wilson RI (1974) The fat embolism syndrome. J Bone Joint Surg Br 56B(3):408–416
Han D, Lee KS, Franquet T, Müller NL, Kim TS, Kim H, Kwon OJ, Byun HS (2003) Thrombotic and non-thrombotic pulmonary arterial embolism: spectrum of imaging findings. Radiographics 23(6):1521–1539
Hanak V, Golbin JM, Ryu JH (2007) Causes and presenting features in 85 consecutive patients with hypersensitivity pneumonitis. Mayo Clin Proc 82:812–816
Heyneman LE, Müller NL (2000) Pulmonary nodules in early fat embolism syndrome: a case report. J Thorac Imaging 15(1):71–74
Ichikado K (2014) High-resolution computed tomography findings of acute respiratory distress syndrome, acute interstitial pneumonia, and acute exacerbation of idiopathic pulmonary fibrosis. Semin Ultrasound CT MR 35(1):39–46
Ichikawa Y, Kinoshita M, Koga T, Oizumi K, Fujimoto K, Hayabuchi N (1994) Lung cyst formation in lymphocytic interstitial pneumonia: CT features. J Comput Assist Tomogr 18:745–748
Janz TG, Madan R, Marini JJ, Summer WR, Meduri GU, Smith RM, Epler GR, Schnader J (2000) Clinical conference on management dilemmas: progressive infiltrates and respiratory failure. Chest 117(2):562–572
Jennette JC (2013) Overview of the 2012 revised International Chapel Hill Consensus Conference nomenclature of vasculitides. Clin Exp Nephrol 17(5):603–606
Kaewlai R, Avery LL, Asrani AV, Novelline RA (2008) Multidetector CT of blunt thoracic trauma. Radiographics 28(6):1555–1570
Ketai LH, Godwin JD (1998) A new view of pulmonary edema and acute respiratory distress syndrome. J Thorac Imaging 13(3):147–171
Ketai L, Washington L (2002) Radiology of acute diffuse lung disease in the immunocompetent host. Semin Roentgenol 37(1):25–36
Ketai L, Jordan K, Marom EM (2008) Imaging infection. Clin Chest Med 29(1):77–105
Kim M, Lee KY, Lee KW, Bae KT (2008) MDCT evaluation of foreign bodies and liquid aspiration pneumonia in adults. AJR Am J Roentgenol 190(4):907–915
Kliegerman SJ, Franks TJ, Galvin JR (2013) From the radiologic pathology archives: organization and fibrosis as a response to lung injury in diffuse alveolar damage, organizing pneumonia, and acute fibrinous and organizing pneumonia. Radiographics 33(7):1951–1975
Kokkarinen JI, Tukiainen HO, Terho EO (1992) Effect of corticosteroid treatment on the recovery of pulmonary function in farmer's lung. Am Rev Respir Dis 145:3–5
Komiya K, Ishii H, Murakami J et al (2013) Comparison of chest computed tomography features in the acute phase of cardiogenic pulmonary edema and acute respiratory distress syndrome on arrival at the emergency department. J Thorac Imaging 28(5):322–328
Kubo K, Azuma A, Kanazawa M, Kameda H, Kusumoto M, Genma A, Saijo Y, Sakai F, Sugiyama Y, Tatsumi K, Dohi M, Tokuda H, Hashimoto S, Hattori N, Hanaoka M, Fukuda Y, Japanese Respiratory Society Committee for formulation of Consensus statement for the diagnosis and treatment of drug-induced lung injuries (2013) Consensus statement for the diagnosis and treatment of drug-induced lung injuries. Respir Investig 51(4):260–277
Lara AR, Schwarz MI (2010) Diffuse alveolar hemorrhage. Chest 137(5):1164–1171
Lorente JA, Ballén-Barragán A, Herrero R, Esteban A (2015) Acute respiratory distress syndrome: does histology matter? Crit Care 19:337. doi:10.1186/s13054-015-1022-6
Maffessanti M, Dalpiaz G (2005) Diffuse lung diseases: clinical features, pathology HRCT. Springer, Milan/New York
Maffessanti M, Dalpiaz G (2011) Practical pulmonary pathology: a diagnostic approach. Elsevier, Philadelphia
Malagari K, Economopoulos N, Stoupis C et al (2003) High resolution CT findings in mild pulmonary fat embolism. Chest 123(4):1196–1201
Marten K, Schnyder P, Schirg E, Prokop M, Rummeny EJ, Engelke C (2005) Pattern-based differential diagnosis in pulmonary vasculitis using volumetric CT. AJR Am J Roentgenol 184(3):720–733
Mayberry JP, Primack SL, Müller NL (2000) Thoracic manifestations of systemic autoimmune diseases: radiographic and high-resolution CT findings. Radiographics 20(6):1623–1635
Meade MO, Cook RJ, Guyatt GH et al (2000) Interobserver variation in interpreting chest radiographs for the diag-

nosis of acute respiratory distress syndrome. Am J Respir Crit Care Med 161(1):85–90
Mellor A, Soni N (2001) Fat embolism. Anaesthesia 56(2):145–154
Miller WT Jr, Mickus TJ, Barbosa E Jr, Mullin C, Van Deerlin VM, Shiley KT (2011) CT of viral lower respiratory tract infections in adults: comparison among viral organisms and between viral and bacterial infections. AJR Am J Roentgenol 197(5):1088–1095
Milne EN (2010) Imaging expertise in critical care units. Radiology 256(3):1013
Milne EC, Pistolesi M (1994) Reading the chest radiograph: a physiologic approach. Mosby-Year Book, St Louis
Milne EN, Pistolesi M, Miniati M, Giuntini C (1985) The radiologic distinction of cardiogenic and noncardiogenic edema. AJR Am J Roentgenol 144(5):879–894
Mirka H, Ferda J, Baxa J (2012) Multidetector computed tomography of chest trauma: indications, technique and interpretation. Insights Imaging 3(5):433–449
Mönkäre S, Ikonen M, Haahtela T (1985) Radiologic findings in farmer's lung. Prognosis and correlation to lung function. Chest 87:460–466
Morgan PW, Goodman LR (1991) Pulmonary edema and adult respiratory distress syndrome. Radiol Clin North Am 29(5):943–963
Müller NL, White DA, Jiang H, Gemma A (2004) Diagnosis and management of drug-associated interstitial lung disease. Br J Cancer 91 Suppl 2:S24–S30
Murray JF (1975) Editorial: the adult respiratory distress syndrome (may it rest in peace). Am Rev Respir Dis 111(6):716–718
Nöbauer-Huhman IM, Eibenberger K, Schaefer-Prokop C et al (2001) Changes in lung parenchyma after acute respiratory distress syndrome (ARDS): assessment with high resolution computed tomography. Eur Radiol 11:2436–2443
Nucifora G, Hysko F, Vit A, Vasciaveo A (2007) Pulmonary fat embolism: common and unusual computed tomography findings. J Comput Assist Tomogr 31(5):806–807
Obadina ET, Torrealba JM, Kanne JP (2013) Acute pulmonary injury: high-resolution CT and histopathological spectrum. Br J Radiol 86(1027):20120614
Oikonomou A, Prassopoulos P (2013) Mimics in chest disease: interstitial opacities. Insights Imaging 4(1): 9–27
Park MS (2013) Diffuse alveolar hemorrhage. Tuberc Respir Dis (Seoul) 74(4):151–162
Piolanti M, Dalpiaz G, Scaglione M, Coniglio C, Miceli M, Violini S, Trisolini R, Barozzi L. Fat Embolism Syndrome: Lung Computed Tomography Findings in 18 Patients. J Comput Assist Tomogr. 2016 [Epub ahead of print] PubMed PMID: 26938691
Prasad R, Gupta P, Singh A, Goel N (2014) Drug induced pulmonary parenchymal disease. Drug Discov Ther 8(6):232–237
Primack SL, Miller RR, Müller NL (1995) Diffuse pulmonary hemorrhage: clinical, pathologic, and imaging features. AJR Am J Roentgenol 164(2):295–300
Ravenel JG, Heyneman LE, McAdams HP (2002) Computed tomography diagnosis of macroscopic pulmonary fat embolism. J Thorac Imaging 17(2): 154–156
Ribeiro CM, Marchiori E, Rodrigues R, Gasparetto E, Souza AS Jr, Escuissato D, Nobre LF, Zanetti G, de Araujo Neto C, Irion K (2006) Hydrostatic pulmonary edema: high-resolution computed tomography aspects. J Bras Pneumol 32(6):515–522
Richerson HB, Bernstein IL, Fink JN, Hunninghake GW, Novey HS, Reed CE, Salvaggio JE, Schuyler MR, Schwartz HJ, Stechschulte DJ (1989) Report of the Subcommittee on Hypersensitivity Pneumonitis. Guidelines for the clinical evaluation of hypersensitivity pneumonitis. J Allergy Clin Immunol 84:839–844
Rossi SE, Erasmus JJ, McAdams HP, Sporn TA, Goodman PC (2000) Cleverlay. Pulmonary drug toxicity: radiologic and pathologic manifestations. Radiographics 20(5):1245–1259
Rossi SE, Erasmus JJ, Volpacchio M, Franquet T, Castiglioni T, McAdams HP (2003) "Crazy-paving" pattern at thin-section CT of the lungs: radiologic-pathologic overview. Radiographics 23(6):1509–1519
Rubenfeld GD, Caldwell E, Granton JT, Hudson LD, Matthay MA (1999) Interobserver variability in applying a radiographic definition for ARDS. Chest 116(5): 1347–1353
Rubinowitz AN, Siegel MD, Tocino I (2007) Thoracic imaging in the ICU. Crit Care Clin 23(3):539–573
Schwarz MI, Albert RK (2004) "Imitators" of the ARDS: implications for diagnosis and treatment. Chest 125(4):1530–1535
Selman M (2011) Hypersensitivity pneumonitis. In: Schwarz M, King TE Jr (eds) Interstitial lung disease, 5th edn. People's Medical Publishing House-USA, Shelton, pp 597–625
Selman M, Pardo A, King TE Jr (2012) Hypersensitivity pneumonitis: insights in diagnosis and pathobiology. Am J Respir Crit Care Med 186(4):314–324
Sheard S, Rao P, Devaraj A (2012) Imaging of acute respiratory distress syndrome. Respir Care 57(4):607–612
Silva CI, Churg A, Müller NL (2007) Hypersensitivity pneumonitis: spectrum of high-resolution CT and pathologic findings. AJR Am J Roentgenol 188(2):334–344
Spagnolo P, Richeldi L, du Bois RM (2008) Environmental triggers and susceptibility factors in idiopathic granulomatous diseases. Semin Respir Crit Care Med 29:610–619
Spagnolo P, Rossi G, Cavazza A, Bonifazi M, Paladini I, Bonella F, Sverzellati N, Costabel U (2015) Hypersensitivity pneumonitis: a comprehensive review. J Investig Allergol Clin Immunol 25(4):237–250
Storto ML, Kee ST, Golden JA, Webb WR (1995) Hydrostatic pulmonary edema: high-resolution CT findings. AJR Am J Roentgenol 165(4):817–820
Svenningsen S, Nesse O, Finsen V, Hole A, Benum P (1987) Prevention of fat embolism syndrome in patients with femoral fractures – immediate or delayed operative fixation? Ann Chir Gynaecol 76(3):163–166

Talucci RC, Manning J, Lampard S, Bach A, Carrico CJ (1983) Early intramedullary nailing of femoral shaft fractures: a cause of fat embolism syndrome. Am J Surg 146(1):107–111

Thomeer MJ, Costabe U, Rizzato G, Poletti V, Demedts M (2001) Comparison of registries of interstitial lung diseases in three European countries. Eur Respir J Suppl 32:114s–118s

Tomiyama N, Müller NL, Johkoh T, Cleverley JR, Ellis SJ, Akira M, Ichikado K, Honda O, Mihara N, Kozuka T, Hamada S, Nakamura H (2001) Acute respiratory distress syndrome and acute interstitial pneumonia: comparison of thin-section CT findings. J Comput Assist Tomogr 25(1):28–33

Torrisi JM, Schwartz LH, Gollub MJ, Ginsberg MS, Bosl GJ, Hricak H (2011) CT findings of chemotherapy-induced toxicity: what radiologists need to know about the clinical and radiologic manifestations of chemotherapy toxicity. Radiology 258(1):41–56

Unger GF, Scanlon GT, Fink JN, Unger JB (1973) A radiologic approach to hypersensitivity pneumonias. Radiol Clin North Am 11(2):339–356

Vogelmeier C, Krombach F, Münzing S, König G, Mazur G, Beinert T, Fruhmann G (1993) Activation of blood neutrophils in acute episodes of farmer's lung. Am Rev Respir Dis 148:396–400

Ware LB, Matthay MA (2005) Clinical practice. Acute pulmonary edema. N Engl J Med 353(26): 2788–2796

Zompatori M, Calabrò E, Poletti V, Rabaiotti E, Piazza N, Viani S (2003) Hypersensitivity pneumonitis. High resolution CT findings with pathological correlations. A pictorial essay. Radiol Med 106(1–2):44–50

Airway Disease

Tullio Valente

Contents

T. Valente
Department of Imaging, Section of Radiology, Azienda Ospedali dei Colli, P.O. Monaldi, Naples 80100, Italy
e-mail: tullio.valente@gmail.com

Abstract

There are few conditions in emergency medicine as potentially challenging and high risk as the *acute airway obstruction*. Time is often limited, the patient's condition may be critical, and a failed airway has the potential for significant morbidity or death. Chest radiography (CXR) is useful in diagnosing and evaluating the progression of atelectasis, aspiration, pulmonary edema, pneumonia, and pleural fluid collections. Lung ultrasonography (LUS) is an excellent complementary diagnostic tool in emergency diagnosis. For patients who can tolerate lying flat for the study, thin-section multidetector computed tomography (MDCT) provides the anatomic detail that permits planning of therapy and is useful when the clinical and radiologic presentations are discrepant and the patient is not responding to therapy or in further defining a radiographic abnormality.

Imaging plays a key role in the diagnosis and monitoring of *bronchiectasis* and the management of complications. Exacerbation of bronchiectasis can confer substantial potential morbidity, usually secondary to recurrent infection. In severe cases of bronchiectasis, massive hemoptysis can lead to death. CXR is useful as an initial screening tool and during acute exacerbations, but has limited sensitivity and specificity. Thin-section MDCT is the reference standard for diagnosis and quantification of bronchiectasis, providing detailed

Med Radiol Diagn Imaging (2016)
DOI 10.1007/174_2016_39, © Springer International Publishing Switzerland

morphological informations. Radiologists must know various causes of bronchiectasis, including common causes, such as recurrent infection or aspiration, and uncommon causes, such as congenital immunodeficiencies and disorders of cartilage development.

In industrialized countries, *inhalational exposures* to various toxicants are commonplace. Most acute toxic inhalations come from industries, home, and recreational sources. In addition to individual susceptibility, the characteristics of inhaled substances such as water solubility, size of substances, and chemical properties may affect disease severity as well as its location. A detailed history becomes even more important in such a patient and may help make a difference in the often chaotic setting of the emergency department. Laboratory evaluation, arterial blood gas analysis, and supportive measures, including the ABCs (airway, breathing, and circulation), may be required. Unfortunately, the varied presentations result in a nonspecific clinical syndrome and make diagnosis somewhat difficult. Despite substantial limitations, imaging can help in showing diffuse interstitial, alveolar, or mixed infiltrates, segmental consolidation, hyperinflation, pneumothorax, and pleural effusion. Thin-section MDCT can be used to further characterize lung abnormalities and continues to demonstrate previously unidentified characteristics that shape our understanding of noxious inhaled toxicant injury.

Table 1 Main conditions associated to airway obstruction

Malignant	Nonmalignant
Primary endoluminal carcinoma	Lymphadenopathy
Bronchogenic	Sarcoidosis
Adenoid cystic	Infectious (i.e., tuberculosis)
Mucoepidermoid	Vascular
Carcinoid	Sling
Metastatic carcinoma to the airway	Cartilage
Bronchogenic	Relapsing polychondritis
Renal cell	Granulation tissue from:
Breast	Endotracheal tubes
Thyroid	Tracheostomy tubes
Colon	Airway stents
Sarcoma	Foreign bodies
Melanoma	Surgical anastomosis
Laryngeal carcinoma	Granulomatosis with polyangiitis
Esophageal carcinoma	Pseudotumor
Mediastinal tumors	Hamartomas
Thymus	Amyloid
Thyroid	Papillomatosis
Germ cell	Hyperdynamic
Lymphadenopathy	Tracheomalacia
Associated with any of the above malignancies	Bronchomalacia
Lymphoma	Webs
	Tuberculosis
	Sarcoidosis
	Goiter
	Mucus plug
	Vocal cord paralysis
	Epiglottitis
	Blood clot

1 Acute Lower Airway Obstruction and Aspiration

1.1 Introduction

Acute obstruction of the central airway is an emergent situation that results from a wide variety of malignant and benign disease processes (Table 1). Acute management involves establishing a secure and patent route for adequate gas exchange. This requires rapid determination of the location of the obstruction and nature of the obstruction followed by a thoughtful management approach based on findings. Large airway obstruction typically presents with dyspnea and wheeze (particularly during exertion and with forced exhalation maneuver), and it is commonly mistaken for refractory exacerbations of COPD; variable intrathoracic upper airway obstruction is often caused by tracheobronchomalacia, an aspirated object, or central airway tumor. Complete airway obstruction (Fig. 1) is

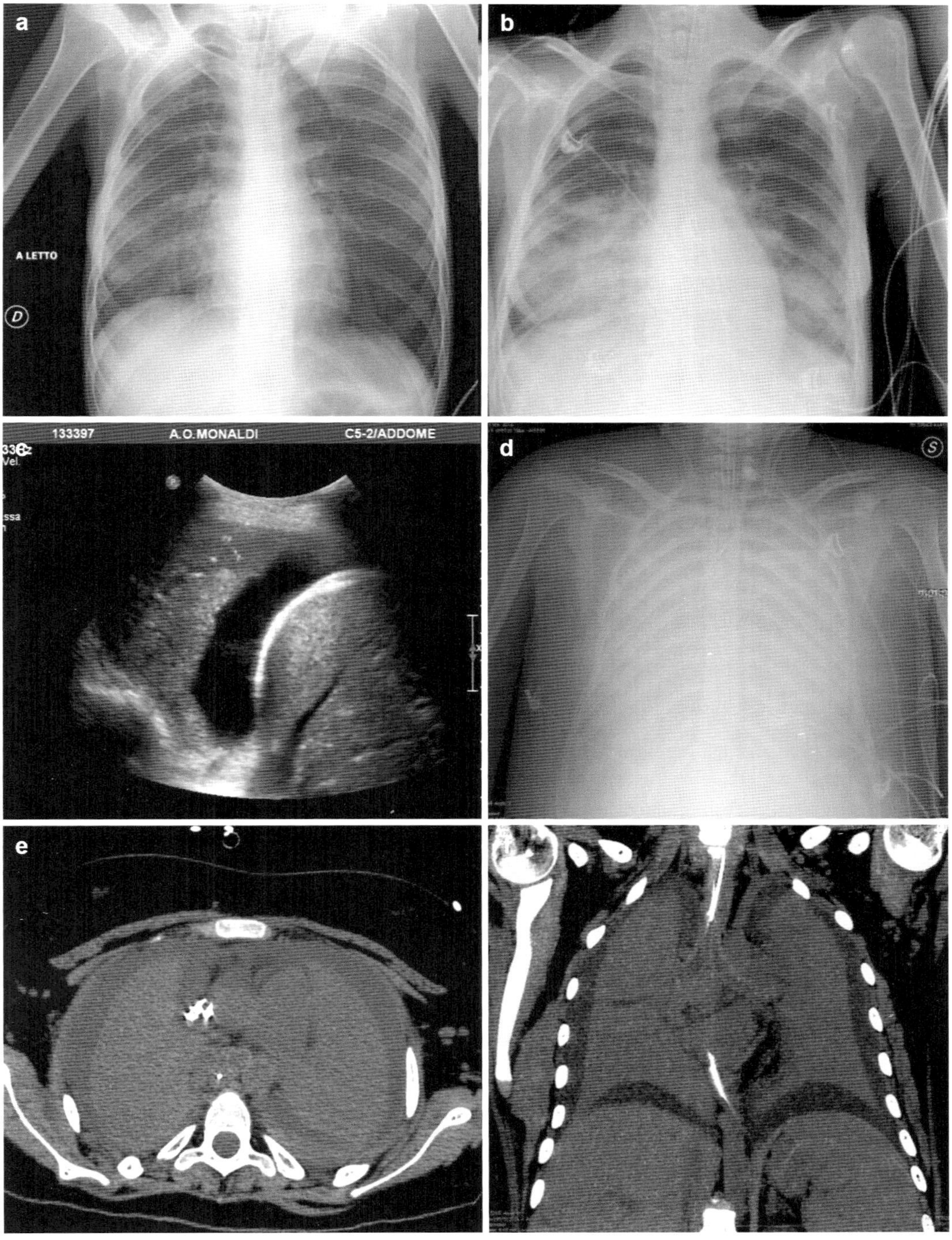

Fig. 1 Acute complete lower airway obstruction by rapid and severe course of toxic shock syndrome (TSS) in MRSA fatal progressive pneumonia. A 26-year-old menstruating woman with high fever, rash, hypotension, and rapidly evolving multiorgan failure is immediately transferred from ED into the ICU. (**a**) CXR at the admission in the ICU shows right lower lobe opacity. (**b**) Follow-up CXR 24 h later shows a new contralateral basal opacity. (**c**) Bedside longitudinal right LUS shows low right lobe complete consolidation associated to pleural effusion. (**d**) Patient in extracorporeal membrane oxygenation (ECMO). Twenty-four hours later, follow-up CXR shows completely opacified lungs. (**e**, **f**) Unenhanced MDCT axial and coronal MIP reconstructions show bilateral complete lung consolidation associated to pleural effusion. Note hypodense material that fills large airways

the worst scenario and will result in respiratory failure followed by cardiac arrest in a matter of minutes, a situation that requires an immediate, aggressive response, but it is, fortunately, very uncommon (Fig. 2).

1.2 Imaging

Patients with an acute upper airway complaint need to have their breathing issues addressed before being transferred to the radiology suite for

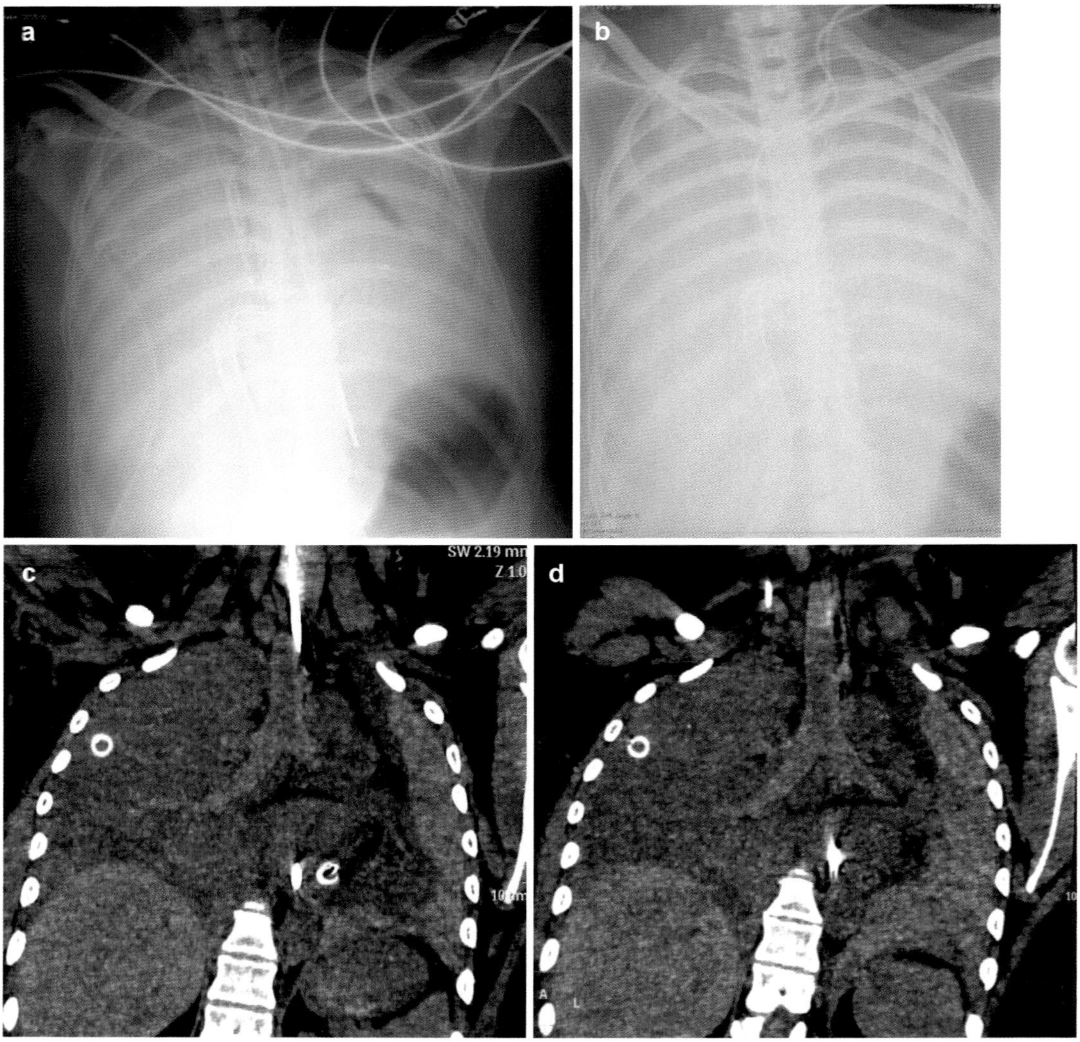

Fig. 2 Acute lower complete airway obstruction in a 16-year-old male with bleeding diathesis by treatment with anticoagulant therapy, abrupt massive postnasal bleeding, and airway hemorrhage by an highly vascularized bleeding nasopharyngeal angiofibroma.(**a**) CXR after nasogastric tube and right pleural drainages placement shows subtotal opacified lungs. (**b**) The patient was immediately transferred from ED into the ICU and CXR showed total opacified lungs.(**c**, **d**) Emergent unenhanced MDCT coronal reconstructions show hyperdense blood material that fills airways and the bloody hyperdensity mainly in the left lung (compare with Fig. 1). After nasopharyngolaryngoscopy, this patient was treated by emergent preoperative embolization. Juvenile nasopharyngeal angiofibroma is a benign, highly vascular hamartoma that arises from the nasopharynx almost exclusively in adolescent males

imaging. Intubation should be considered before any examination that requires patients to be supine (i.e., CT and MR imaging), especially if there is any suspicion of anaphylaxis or other difficulties in maintaining oxygen saturation levels. Portable anteroposterior (AP) chest radiography (CXR), complementary sonography (lung ultrasonography, LUS), and MDCT scanning of the neck and chest are the most effective initial emergent imaging studies to assess the location and extent of the airway obstruction. For patients who can tolerate lying flat for the study, MDCT provides the anatomic detail that permits planning of therapy. The study is assessed for location of primary tumor/mass, the degree of intrinsic versus extrinsic compression, and the length of the stricture. Furthermore, the relationship of the narrowing of the trachea relative to the larynx or the carina is readily assessed. For bronchial lesions, the extent of postobstructive atelectasis or infection is readily observed.

Flexible bronchoscopy provides a definitive view of the intraluminal disease but should be performed with preparation for management of the airway obstruction with laser, rigid bronchoscopy, or stent placement.

1.3 Pulmonary Parenchymal Abnormalities

Atelectasis, aspiration, airspace opacification or consolidations, air trapping and hyperinflation, hydrostatic pulmonary edema, and noncardiogenic pulmonary edema all present as pathological findings on CXR, LUS, and MDCT. Although it is often difficult, and sometimes impossible, to distinguish between these entities, certain radiographic features can aid in their diagnoses.

1.3.1 Obstructive Lung Diseases

Acute Exacerbation in Chronic Obstructive Pulmonary Disease

Chronic obstructive pulmonary disease (COPD) is defined as incompletely reversible expiratory airflow obstruction, likely caused by exposure to noxious inhaled particles (Rabe et al. 2007). The airflow limitation that underlies functional obstruction is usually progressive and associated with an abnormal inflammatory response of the lung. What is clinically called COPD reflects a complex syndrome encompassing potentially overlapping diseases such as pulmonary emphysema, chronic bronchitis, and small airway disease. Acute exacerbation of COPD is defined "as an event characterized by a change in the patient's baseline symptoms that is beyond normal day-to-day variations" is acute in onset and may warrant a change in regular medication in a patient with underlying COPD (Table 2) (Siafakas et al. 2004; Rabe et al. 2007). Three COPD phenotypes were identified based on morphologic CT changes and clinical features of COPD: phenotype A, characterized by no or minimal emphysema with or without bronchial wall thickening; phenotype E, characterized by emphysema without bronchial wall thickening; and phenotype M, characterized by emphysema with bronchial wall thickening (Fujimoto et al. 2006).

Acute Exacerbation in Asthma

Asthma is characterized by all of the following: (1) airway obstruction that is usually reversible, (2) chronic airway inflammation, and (3) nonspecific airway hyperreactivity.

The CXR features of asthma are not particularly specific, but the most common abnormality is *bronchial wall thickening*, with *hyperinflation* the second most common (identified up to 24% though less reliable) finding (Lynch 1998). In patients with asthma, CT is indicated to identify

Table 2 Summary of diseases that provoke, precipitate, or mimic an acute COPD exacerbation (Siafakas et al. 2004)

Parenchymal diseases	Pneumonia and their complications; complicated bullae
Airway diseases	Bronchial carcinoma; tracheobronchial tree infections, common pollutant
Cardiac diseases	Congestive cardiac failure, right heart failure
Lung vessels	Pulmonary hypertension, acute embolism, hemoptysis
Pleura	Pleural effusion, pneumothorax
Muscles	Muscular wasting
Mediastinum	Pneumomediastinum

suspected complications, particularly allergic bronchopulmonary aspergillosis, and mimics of asthma such as hypersensitivity pneumonitis. When it is performed, CT is helpful for evaluating the extent of airway thickening (remodeling: airway walls are thicker than healthy individuals and the degree of airway wall thickness directly correlates with the severity of airflow obstruction and clinical disease) (Aysola et al. 2008), bronchial dilation, and expiratory air trapping. Air trapping is usually defined as the percentage of the lung less than 850 HU on expiratory CT, and those individuals with an air-trapping percentage above the median value of 9.66 % defined as having an air-trapping phenotype. Bronchial dilation, or bronchiectasis (defined as a bronchus with a larger diameter than the internal diameter of the adjacent pulmonary artery), is more prevalent in asthmatic patients than in healthy subjects. Acute complications of asthma may include pneumothorax, pneumomediastinum (and rarely pneumopericardium, pneumoperitoneum, pneumoretroperitoneum, pneumorrhachis, and even subdural emphysema), mucus impaction with or without atelectasis, and pneumonia (Woods and Lynch 2009).

1.3.2 Consolidations or Airspace Opacifications or Alveolar Opacity or Alveolar Pattern

Consolidation is the most common cause of pulmonary opacities in the acute airway obstruction population. In contrast to ground-glass opacities (GGO), consolidation obscures underlying vascular structures and frequently is associated with absence of volume loss and air bronchograms by opacification of lung acini with little or no involvement of conducting airways. By definition, diseases that produce consolidation are characterized by a replacement of alveolar air by fluid, cells, tissue, or some other substances (Hansell et al. 2008). If acute, consolidation is most commonly caused by pulmonary edema (of both cardiogenic and noncardiogenic causes), pulmonary hemorrhage, acute eosinophilic pneumonia, acute extrinsic allergic alveolitis, radiation pneumonitis, pulmonary infarction, or infectious pneumonia (Table 3).

Table 3 (**a**) Diseases recognized as causing alveolar opacity or pattern

Transudate
Hemodynamic pulmonary edema[a]
Non-hemodynamic pulmonary edema
Diffuse alveolar damage (ARDS)[a]
Exudate
Infective pneumonia[a]
Eosinophilic pneumonia
Lipoid pneumonia
Hemorrhage
Diffuse alveolar hemorrhage (DAH)
Severe cardiac failure[a]
Pulmonary infarction[a]
Emboli[a]
Thromboembolism[a]
Fat embolism
Amniotic fluid embolism
Bone marrow embolism
Infiltration
Adenocarcinoma ex-bronchoalveolar cell carcinoma
Lymphoma
Miscellaneous
Pulmonary alveolar proteinosis
Acute extrinsic allergic alveolitis
Sarcoidosis
Radiation pneumonitis

[a]See other chapters of the book

Table 3 (**b**) Imaging signs of acute obstruction of airways by alveolar disease

1. Acinar or peribronchiolar nodules
2. Air alveologram and bronchiologram
3. Air bronchogram
4. Butterfly or "bat's wing" distribution
5. Coalescence (early)
6. Fluffy, ill-defined margins
7. Perihilar, diffuse, segmental, or lobar distribution
8. Present soon after onset of symptoms; rapid change

1.3.3 Thoracic Oncologic Emergencies

Oncologic patients often experience emergent complications that are either direct result of the underlying malignancy or an indirect result related to the therapy (Table 4).

Airway obstruction complicates approximately 20–30 % of patients with lung cancer, and large masses that compress the central airways may

Table 4 Thoracic oncologic direct and indirect complications

Oncologic direct complications	
Mass effect and airway compromise	Airway occlusion Tracheo- or broncho-esophageal fistula
Mass effect and vascular invasion	SVC obstruction, SVC syndrome
Mass effect and invasion of cardiac chambers	Pericardial effusion and cardiac tamponade Tumor extension into the cardiac chambers
Pleural involvement	Massive pleural effusion, hemothorax, pneumothorax Chylothorax
Neovascularity	Massive hemorrhage, pseudoaneurysm, or AV fistula
Systemic manifestations	Massive pulmonary embolism, disseminated intravascular coagulation, opportunistic infections
Oncologic indirect complications	
Postoperative or post-procedural	Pneumothorax, massive hemorrhage, hemothorax, complications of vascular injury, bronchopleural fistula
Postradiation complications	Airway edema and obstruction Radiation pneumonitis, fistula formation
Chemotherapy-related complications	Spontaneous pneumothorax, immunosuppression and opportunistic infections, fistula formation

SVC = superior vena cava; AV = arteriovenous

result in postobstructive atelectasis or pneumonia and airway compromise. Rapidly growing tracheal, mediastinal, and hilar masses are most common causes (Fig. 3) (Quint 2009; Guimaraes et al. 2014). Knowledge of airway narrowing is important before attempting percutaneous and surgical biopsy because it may lead to collapse of residual normal lung and sudden respiratory decompensation (McCurdy and Shanholtz 2012). Muscle relaxant drugs used during anesthesia may precipitate dangerous respiratory compromise in patients with pre-existing airway compression by tumor owing to loss of chest wall tone.

1.3.4 Noncardiogenic Pulmonary Edema (NCPE)

Lung edema includes (1) hydrostatic edema caused by increased capillary pressure or decreased oncotic pressure, (2) ARDS (permeability edema caused by DAD resulting in interstitial and alveolar fluid accumulation), (3) permeability edema without alveolar damage (such as heroin-induced edema, edema following cytokine administration, and high-altitude edema) primarily resulting in interstitial fluid accumulation, and (4) mixed forms of hydrostatic and permeability edema (such as neurogenic edema, reperfusion and re-expansion edema, edema following lung transplantation, etc.)

1.3.5 High-Altitude Pulmonary Edema (HAPE)

High-altitude illness includes the cerebral syndromes of acute mountain sickness (AMS), high-altitude cerebral edema (HACE), and the pulmonary syndrome of high-altitude pulmonary edema (HAPE), recognized as an alveolar fluid accumulation in unacclimatized individuals by Houston in 1960 and attributed solely to high-altitude exposure (Houston 1960); it is mainly seen in children or young adults who rapidly ascend to heights of 2000–3500 m or greater and typically occurs 3–48 h after ascent, with the hallmark symptom being dyspnea at rest, often associated to dry or with frothy pink sputum production cough and restlessness. Approximately 50 % of patients with HAPE also show symptoms of AMS/HACE, but these two forms of altitude illness can exist independently of each other (Bartsch et al. 2005). The mechanism remains unclear: HAPE is believed to be a form of noncardiogenic pulmonary edema without alveolar damage caused by exposure to the low $pO2$ found at high altitudes. Hypoxia leads to uneven areas of vasoconstriction within the pulmonary vascular bed, resulting in a pattern of patchy overperfusion (Swenson et al. 2002); these foci of high vascular pressure lead to localized violation of the capillary endothelium, causing fluid extravasation. When available, CXR features initially are heterogeneous peripheral alveolar patchy, fluffy infiltrates progressing eventually to widespread, confluent airspace involvement more severe in lung bases, but the pattern of distribution is usually unpredictable. Portable lung ultrasonography provides a more feasible imaging option in remote locations and shows progressively larger numbers of extravascular fluid

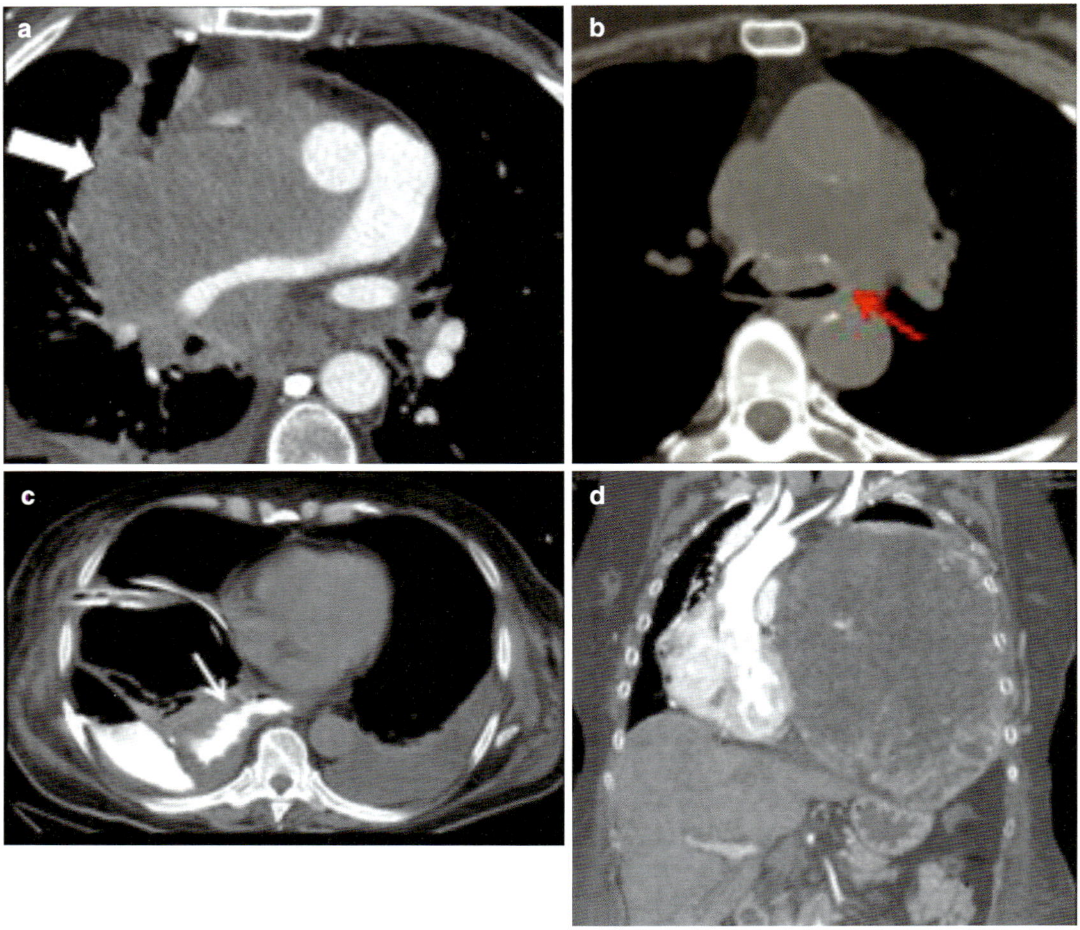

Fig. 3 MDCT of thoracic oncologic emergencies. (**a**) Lung small-cell carcinoma extending into the mediastinum with SVC syndrome (*white arrow*). (**b**) A soft tissue hilar mass with carinal and left bronchial extension (*red arrow*) in a known non-small cell carcinoma in a patient with acute breathlessness. (**c**) Esophageal carcinoma ruptured in right lung parenchyma and with esophago-pleural fistula (*white arrow*). (**d**) Mediastinal chondrosarcoma with rightward mediastinal shift and acute airway obstruction

comet tails in patients ascending to altitude and suffering from HAPE (Fagenholz et al. 2007; Pratali et al. 2010). The most modifiable risk factor for the development of HAPE is the rate of ascent to high altitude; the mainstay of therapy increases alveolar and arterial oxygen by descent or with supplemental oxygen. HAPE is a potentially life-threatening illness that is completely preventable; as the popularity of trekking and climbing grows among the general population, physicians will be increasingly relied on as a source of education, prophylaxis, and treatment, making a working familiarity with altitude-induced illnesses such as HAPE an indispensable tool for emergency physicians.

1.3.6 Neurogenic Pulmonary Edema (NPE)

A number of intracranial conditions, including head trauma, hemorrhage (usually subarachnoid), tumors, and encephalitis, can be associated with acute pulmonary edema. It can occur within a minute to hours following a neurologic insult and usually resolves within 72 h. Patients may present with varying degrees of dyspnea, tachypnea, and cyanosis shortly after suffering the brain insult. The onset of symptoms occurs in <4 h in the majority and death in 10 %. The mechanism is unclear: it has been suggested that a sudden burst of neural activity stimulates the sympathetic nervous system and an adrenergic response leading to increased extravascular lung water, increased pulmonary hydrostatic pressure, and increased lung capillary permeability (Tan and Lai 2007). The CXR picture is indistinguishable from that of cardiogenic PE (nonspecific, bilateral, rather homogeneous airspace consolidative appearances with an apical predominance are present in about half of cases) except that the heart is not enlarged and it can take up to 24 h to be apparent on imaging (Fig. 4). Radiologic findings in neurogenic pulmonary edema also disappear within 1–2 days, thereby confirming the absence of any associated DAD (Gluecker et al. 1999).

1.3.7 Re-expansion Edema (REPE)

The condition occurs often in young patients in the setting of rapid expansion of a collapsed lung, with acute-onset shortness of breath usually occurring within hours of re-expansion. The onset of pulmonary edema can be delayed by up to 24 h in some cases (Echevarria et al. 2008). It occurs following approximately 1 % of pneumothorax re-expansions or thoracentesis procedures (mostly if large-volume drainage >3 l). Although the exact mechanism of REPE has not been identified, it appears to be caused by multiple mechanisms. Increased capillary permeability due to hypoxic injury, reperfusion injury with release of toxic

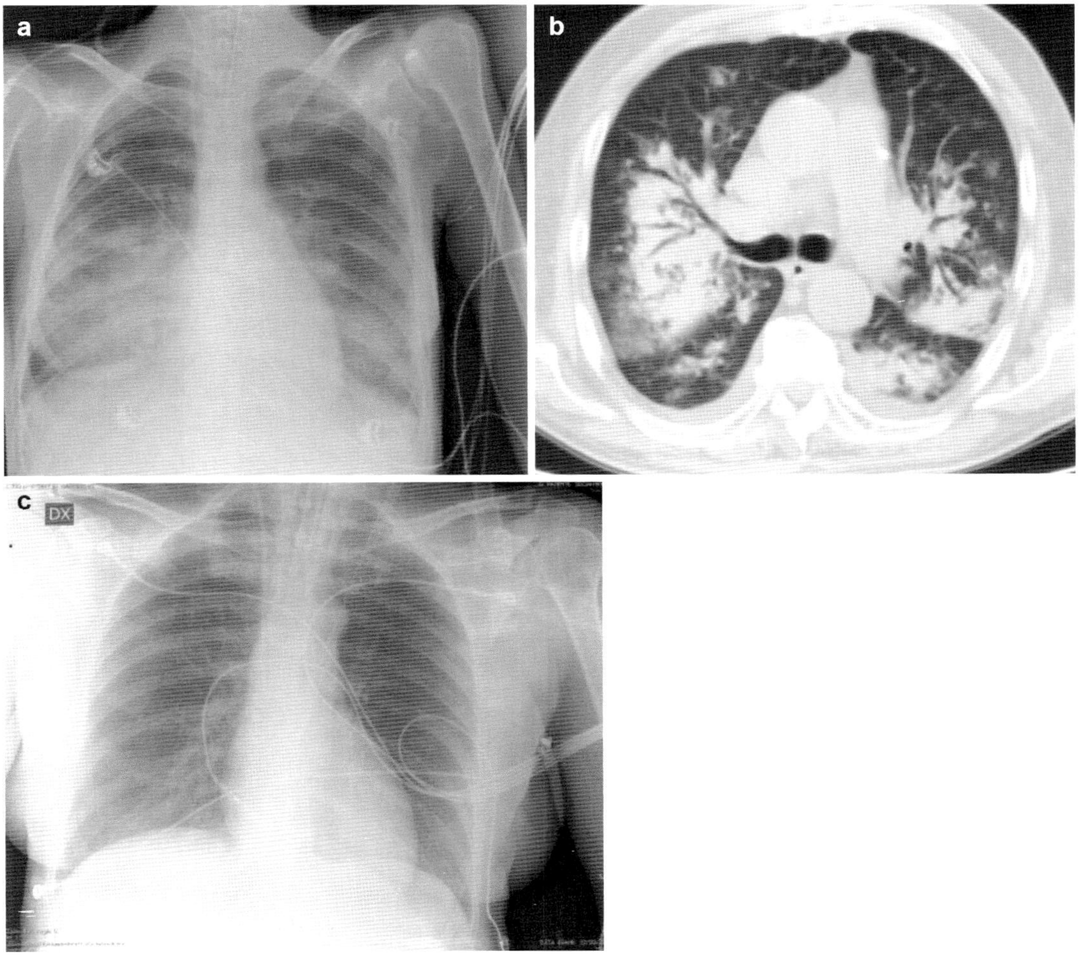

Fig. 4 Neurogenic pulmonary edema. (**a**) Anteroposterior bedside CXR view shows bilateral alveolar opacities in a 54-year-old woman with shortness of breath and subarachnoid hemorrhage, who developed neurogenic pulmonary edema. (**b**) MDCT axial scan shows diffuse bilateral and symmetric patchy ground-glass and consolidative opacities sparing the lung periphery. (**c**) Follow-up CXR 3 days later shows normal findings

oxygen free radicals, and surfactant depletion are all thought to play a major role. Furthermore, a delay in lymphatic return by stasis during prolonged collapse and bronchial occlusion may also partly account for the development of REPE. It can progress for 24–48 h and usually shows slow resolution over 5–7 days. REPE may lead to severe hypoxemia, which will increase lung damage and may result in extensive adult respiratory distress syndrome (ARDS) and multiorgan failure. CXR findings are alveolar opacities usually unilateral in those portions of the lung that were previously collapsed; rarely edema can develop in the contralateral lung (Baik et al. 2010). Thin-section MDCT findings of REPE are peripheral patchy areas of GGO frequently combined with consolidation as well as interlobular septal and intralobular interstitial thickening (Fig. 5). The British Thoracic Society guidelines suggest that less than 1.5 l of pleural fluid be drained at a time (BTS Pleural Disease Guideline 2010). Drainage catheters can be intermittently plugged to prevent rapid lung re-expansion. Rapid re-expansion of pneumothoraces is less easily controlled and caution should be taken to avoid high negative intrapleural pressures.

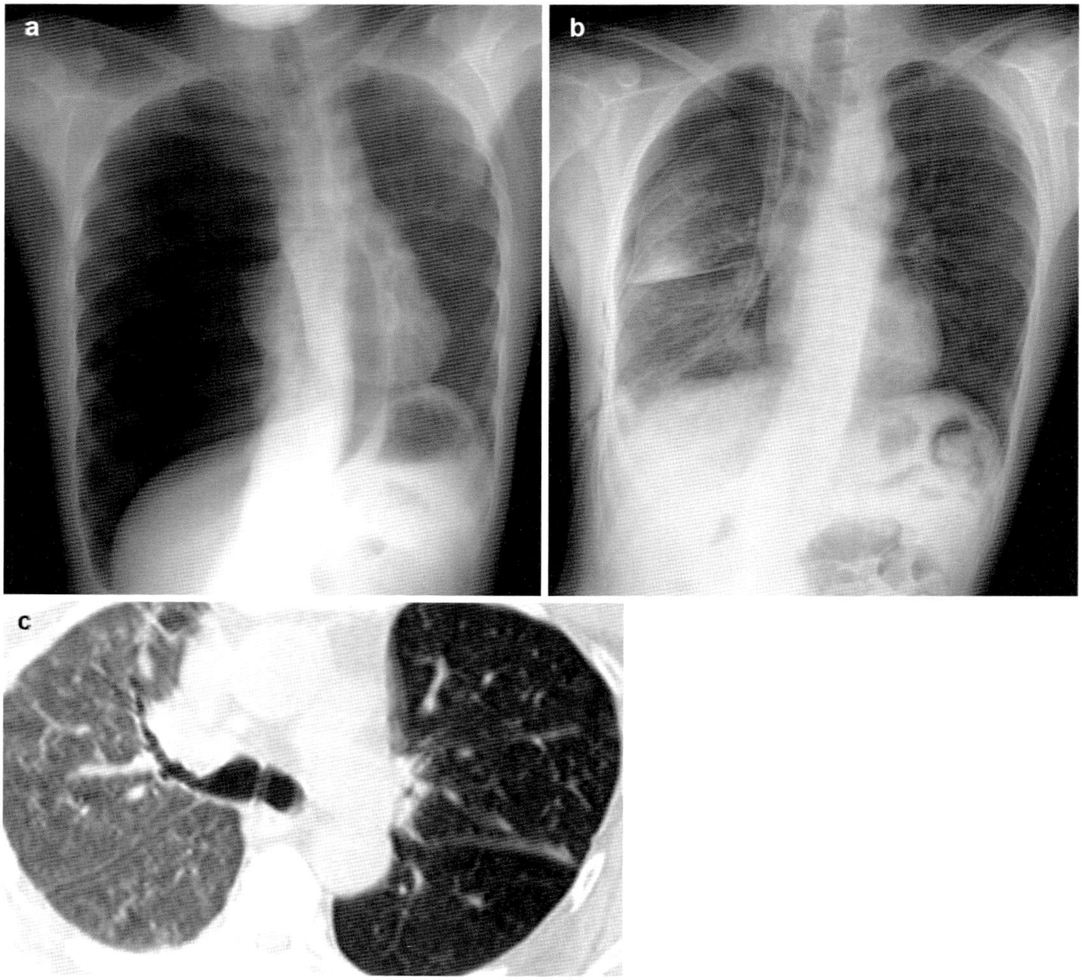

Fig. 5 Re-expansion pulmonary edema. (**a**, **b**) Standard erect PA CXR shows right lung re-expansion pulmonary edema following a spontaneous pneumothorax drainage. (**c**) Thin-section low-dose MDCT scan shows unilateral diffuse ground-glass opacity

1.3.8 Atelectasis

Atelectasis or *collapse* (Hansell et al. 2008), a decrease in lung volume accompanied by increased opacity (CXR) or attenuation (CT scan) in the affected part of the lung, is a common cause of pulmonary opacities in the acute airway obstruction population. One of the commonest mechanisms is resorption of air distal to airway obstruction (e.g., an acutely complicated endobronchial neoplasm or foreign body). Atelectasis can mimic pneumonia, particularly when signs of volume loss, such as crowding of air bronchograms, fissural deviation, mediastinal shift, and diaphragmatic elevation, are absent. Flat, platelike opacities are characteristic of discoid atelectasis. Complete lung collapse, lobar collapse, or segmental collapse can also be seen. The characteristic LUS finding is a homogenous, well-demarcated hyperechoic lung consolidation. In comparison with pneumonia, no air bronchograms are usually visible. The size of the lung consolidation may vary during the breathing cycle due to ventilation. Atelectasis is categorized according to mechanism as obstructive, compressive, cicatricial, and adhesive.

1.4 Acute Aspiration

The term *aspiration* describes a variety of situations involving the intake of solid or liquid materials into the airways and lungs (Franquet et al. 2000). The clinical and radiologic manifestations are protean, varying from asymptomatic focal inflammatory reaction with few or no radiologic abnormalities to severe life-threatening disease (Table 5).

Alcoholism is probably the most important predisposing factor for pulmonary liquid aspiration in adults, although other factors (e.g., general anesthesia, loss of consciousness, structural abnormalities of the pharynx and esophagus, neuromuscular disorders, deglutition abnormalities) may also contribute to aspiration.

Aspiration can result in airway obstruction, chemical pneumonitis, or infectious pneumonia, depending on the volume and type of aspirate. Patchy, ill-defined ground-glass, consolidative, and nodular opacities are the most frequently encountered radiographic manifestations of aspiration. Opacities typically appear rapidly and are most commonly located in the dependent regions of the lungs: the posterior segment of the upper lobes and the superior and posterior basal segments of the lower lobes (Franquet et al. 2000). Opacities may increase in conspicuity over the first 1–2 days in aspiration pneumonitis, but should resolve relatively rapidly thereafter. If opacities persist or increase over several days, aspiration pneumonia is likely present. Patchy, dependent ground-glass, and consolidative opacities are also seen on CT. "Tree-in-bud" opacities result from filling and inflammation of the distal airways (Rossi et al. 2005). When tree-in-bud opacities are present in a dependent distribution, they are highly suggestive of aspiration (Fig. 6).

Table 5 Main syndromes of acute/recurrent pulmonary aspiration

Aspirated material	Clinical effects	Imaging findings
Foreign bodies	Bronchial obstruction	Atelectasis Hyperinflation Abscess
Water	(Near) drowning	Airspace opacity
Gastric contents (Mendelson syndrome)		
Acute	Chemical pneumonitis, anaerobic infection, lung abscess	Airspace opacity Cavity
Chronic/recurrent	Recurrent aspiration Bronchiolitis Bronchiectasis	Migratory opacities Centrilobular nodules/air trapping
Acute exogenous		
Lipoid pneumonia (fire-eater hydrocarbon pneumonia)	Chemical pneumonia	Consolidations Pneumatoceles Masses

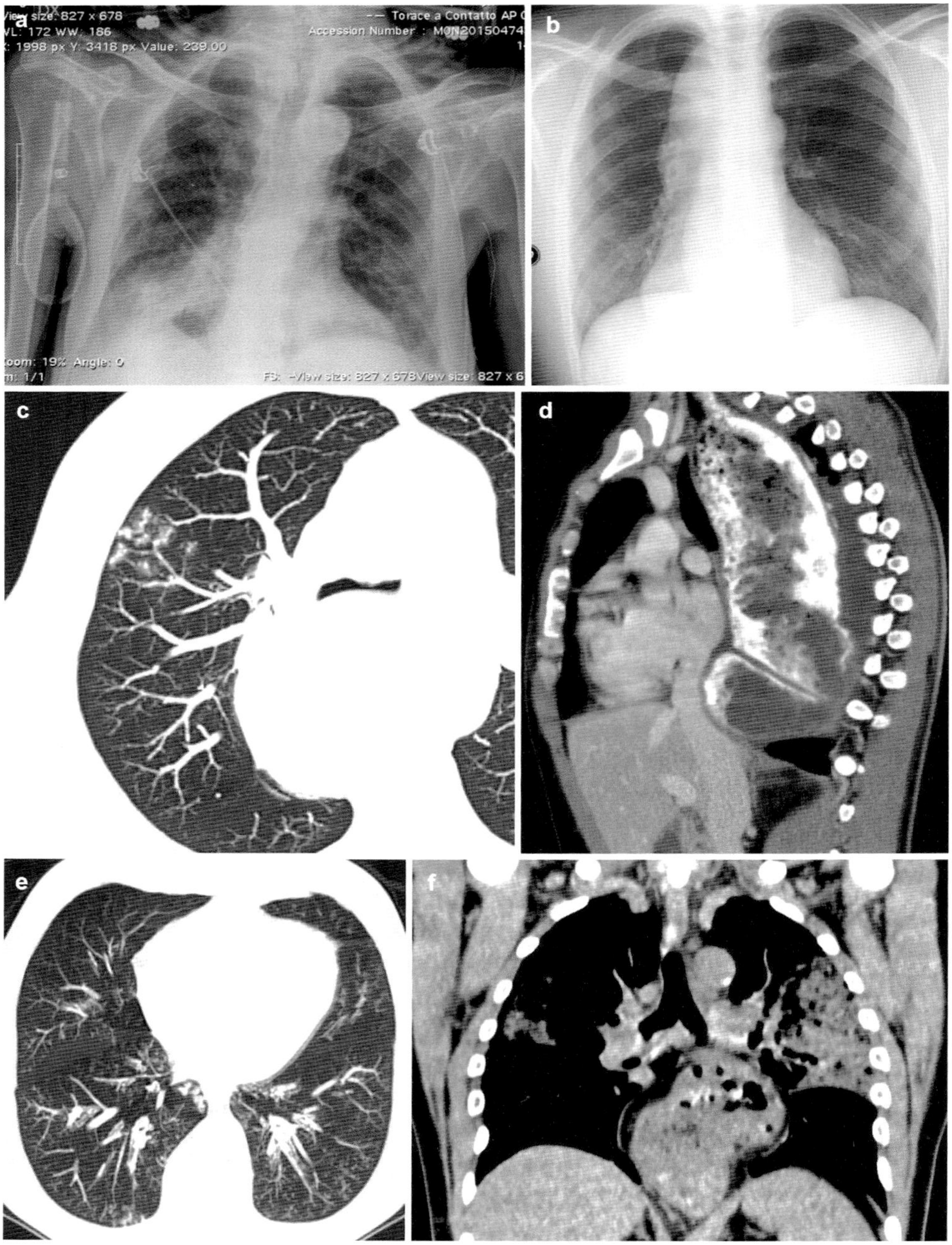

Fig. 6 Case 1. Acute aspiration pneumonia (Mendelson syndrome) in a 65-year-old man who had undergone surgery for intestinal obstruction. (**a**) Anteroposterior CXR view obtained 2 h after surgery demonstrates a focal consolidation in the right lower lobe, a finding that is consistent with aspiration pneumonia. Case 2. Aspiration bronchiolitis in a 57-year-old man with esophageal achalasia. (**b**) Frontal CXR view shows a right superior and middle paramediastinal mass. (**c**) Thin-section MDCT axial scan shows multiple diffuse centrilobular areas of increased attenuation with a characteristic tree-in-bud appearance (aspiration bronchiolitis); note that dilated esophagus displaces tracheal carina. (**d**) MDCT sagittal reconstruction shows typical findings of achalasia with contrast medium-filled esophagus, marked esophageal dilatation, and anterior bowing of the trachea. Case 3. Aspiration bronchiolitis and lung consolidations in a 46-year-old man with hiatal hernia. (**e**, **f**) Axial and coronal MDCT reconstruction shows centrilobular nodules, tree-in-bud pattern in lower lobes, consolidations in upper lobes, and large gastric hernia

1.4.1 Foreign Body Aspiration

Aspirated foreign bodies are by far the most common cause of intraluminal airway abnormalities in childhood, unusual in adults, and often overlooked as a cause of airway obstruction (Yadav et al. 2007). Up until age 15, both right and left main bronchi arise at about the same angle from the trachea so that objects may be aspirated into either side; afterward, the right main bronchus arises in a less acute, more straight path than the left (Kosucu et al. 2004). The most frequently aspirated foreign bodies are food (especially nuts), teeth, dental devices, and medical instruments, and 70 % will be nonopaque on conventional radiography (Fig. 7).

Some nuts, such as peanuts, have an oil that leads to inflammation and edema making them more difficult to expel. When a foreign body enters the lung parenchyma, prolonged irritation with intermittent infections may cause massive hemoptysis. At radiology, an aspirated foreign body may cause one lung or lobar/segmental overinflation or atelectasis (obstructive emphysema) with chronic volume loss in the affected lobe, mediastinal shift, pneumomediastinum, recurrent pneumonias, and bronchiectasis; it can occasionally mimic a congenital malformation or neoplasm (Fig. 8).

If the patient is clinically able, an expiratory CXR may demonstrate air trapping on the affected side by lack of collapse of the lung and shift of the mediastinum away from the side with the foreign body. If the patient is a child or otherwise not able to cooperate for an expiratory study, a decubitus view of the chest, with the suspected side down, may show a lack of collapse of the air-trapped lung. CT may demonstrate the foreign body and is far more sensitive than CXR in

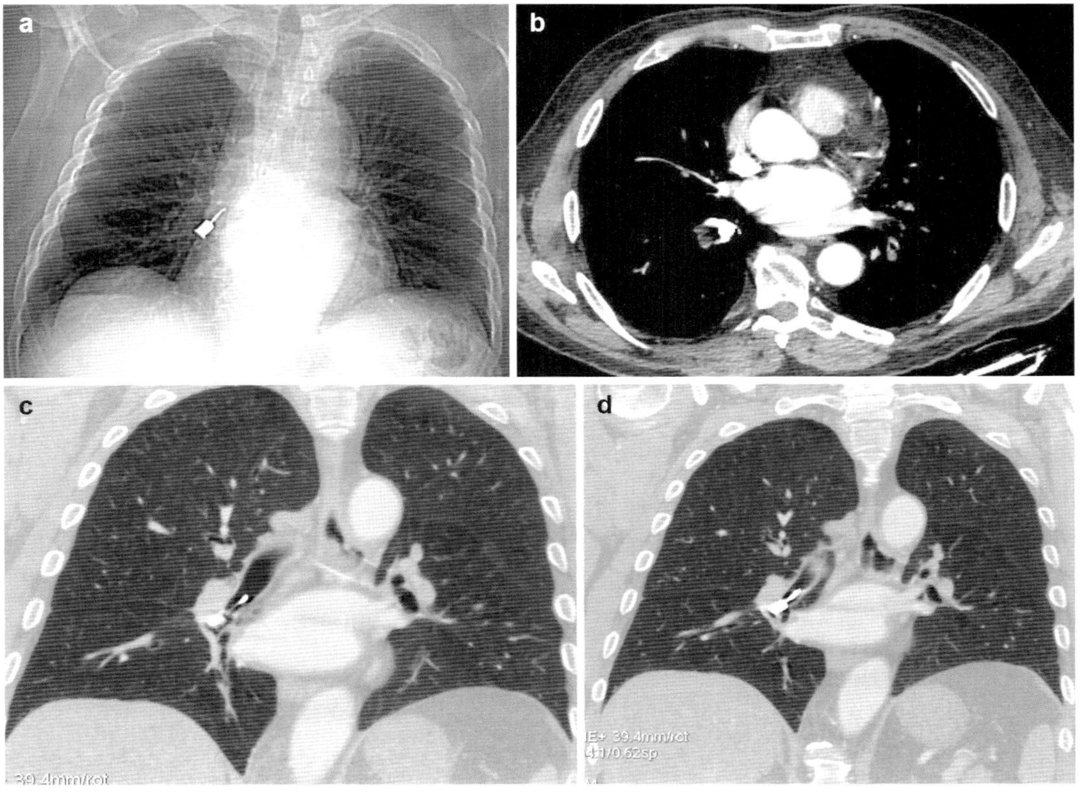

Fig. 7 Post-aspiration imaging in a 70-year-old alcoholic man. MDCT (**a**) scanogram and (**b**) axial and (**c**, **d**) coronal reconstruction images clearly show inhalation of a metallic foreign body (dental screwdriver), located in the right lower lobe bronchus

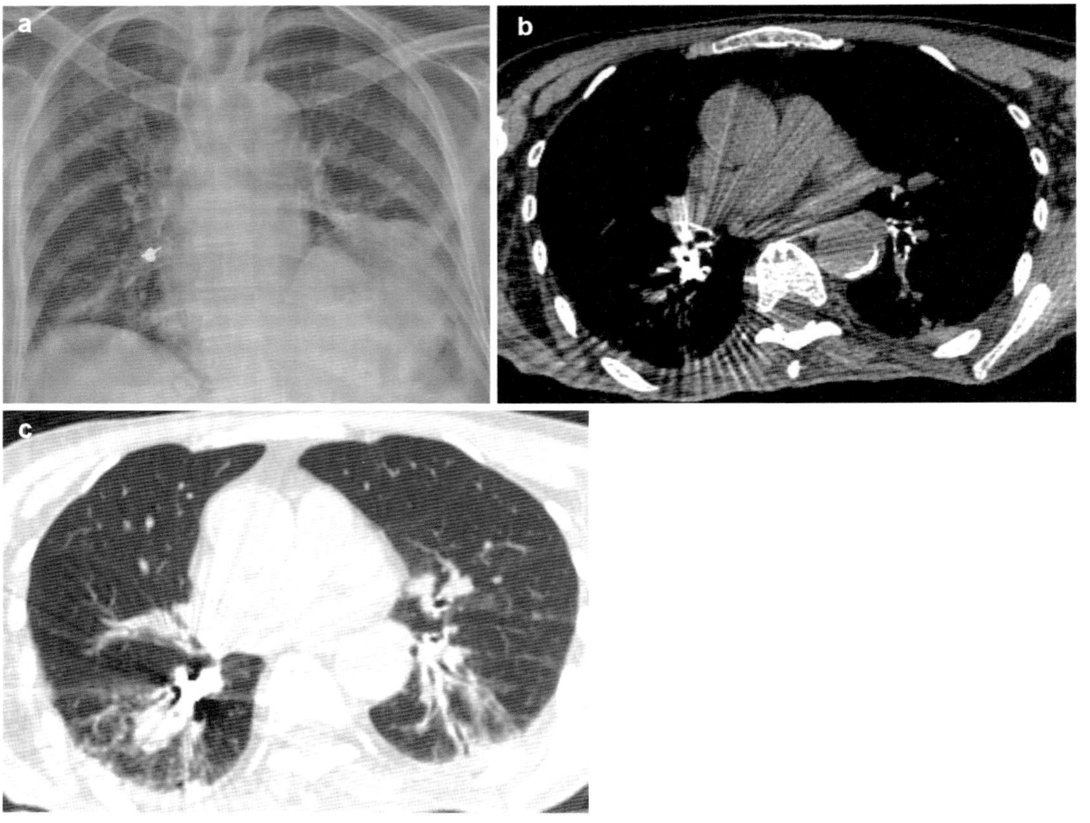

Fig. 8 Post-aspiration imaging in a 79-year-old woman. (**a**) CXR and MDCT with (**b**) mediastinal and (**c**) parenchymal windows show a foreign body inhalation, again located in the right lower lobe bronchus (earring)

demonstrating subtle low-attenuation intrabronchial material (Fig. 9) (Zissin et al. 2001).

1.4.2 Drowning or Near Nonfatal Drowning

Drowning is a process resulting in primary respiratory impairment from submersion in a liquid medium (Idris et al. 2003) and may be either a fatal or nonfatal event (Szpilman et al, 2012). Deaths because of drowning have estimated approximately 305,000 deaths in 2008 (WHO 2011). Young children are at particularly high risk of drowning, and males in general face a significantly greater risk than females. Drowning may be further classified as cold-water (<20 °C) or warm-water injury (>20 °C). The most important contributory factors to morbidity and mortality from drowning are hypoxemia and acidosis and the multiorgan effects of these processes. Central nervous system (CNS) damage may occur because of hypoxemia sustained during the drowning episode (primary injury) or may result from arrhythmias, ongoing pulmonary injury, reperfusion injury, or multiorgan dysfunction (secondary injury), particularly with prolonged tissue hypoxia. After initial breath holding, when the victim's airway lies below the liquid's surface, an involuntary period of laryngospasm is triggered by the presence of liquid in the oropharynx or larynx (stage 1, "dry drowning"). At this time, the victim is unable to breathe in air, causing oxygen depletion and carbon dioxide retention. In stage 2, the victim still usually presents with laryngospasm but may begin to swallow water into the stomach. As the oxygen tension in blood drops further, laryngospasm releases, and

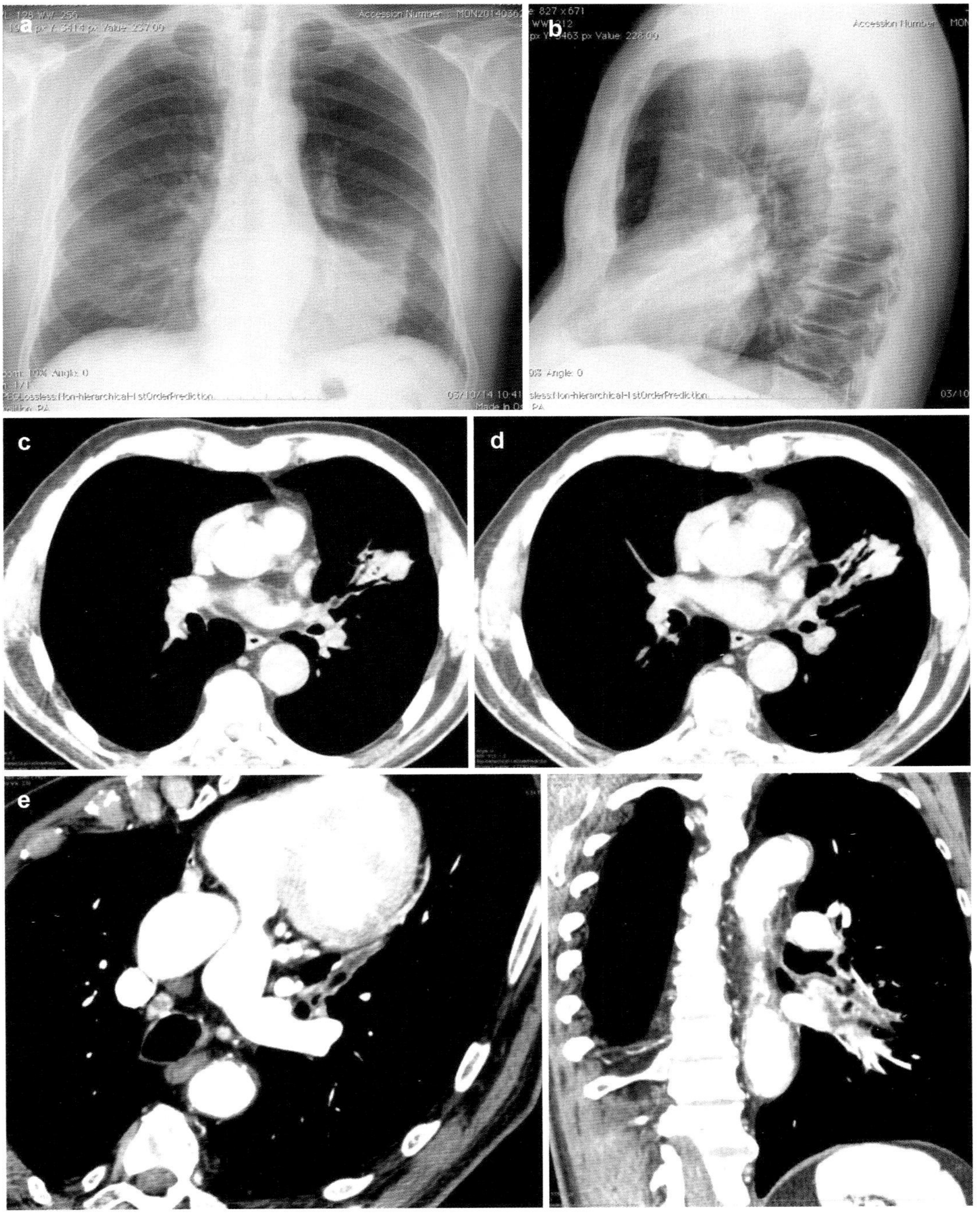

Fig. 9 Postobstructive atelectasis in a 46-year-old man who had inhaled vegetable lipid matter. (**a**) Posteroanterior and (**b**) latero-lateral CXR views show segmental lingular lung collapse, without evidence of foreign body. (**c**, **d**) Axial MDCT scans confirm lingular collapse and show possible endoluminal oval hypodensity. MDCT (**e**) oblique axial and (**f**) coronal MIP reconstructions show a lipid-density oval endobronchial mass. At bronchoscopy foreign body aspiration diagnosis was confirmed and a vegetable lipid matter was removed

the victim gasps and hyperventilates, possibly aspirating variable amounts of liquid. This leads to further hypoxemia (stage 3). Ultimately, if the process of drowning is not interrupted, hypoxia progresses to the point of complete circulatory collapse and cardiac arrest (Tourigny and Hall 2012). Pulmonary infections may occur in a delayed fashion from aspirated material, some of which may result from rare or atypical pathogens such as fungi. Patients in cardiac arrest are more likely to display a nonshockable cardiac rhythm (i.e., asystole or pulseless electrical activity). Those who survive the initial resuscitation phase are at significant risk for developing serious delayed sequelae, such as ARDS, pancreatitis, disseminated intravascular coagulation, or rhabdomyolysis during their subsequent hospital stay. The acute aspiration of massive amounts of water produces a pulmonary edema that is radiographically indistinguishable from pulmonary edema from other causes (Hunter and Whitehouse 1974; Causey et al. 2000). The clinical significance of near drowning depends more on the volume of water aspirated than on whether the aspirate is

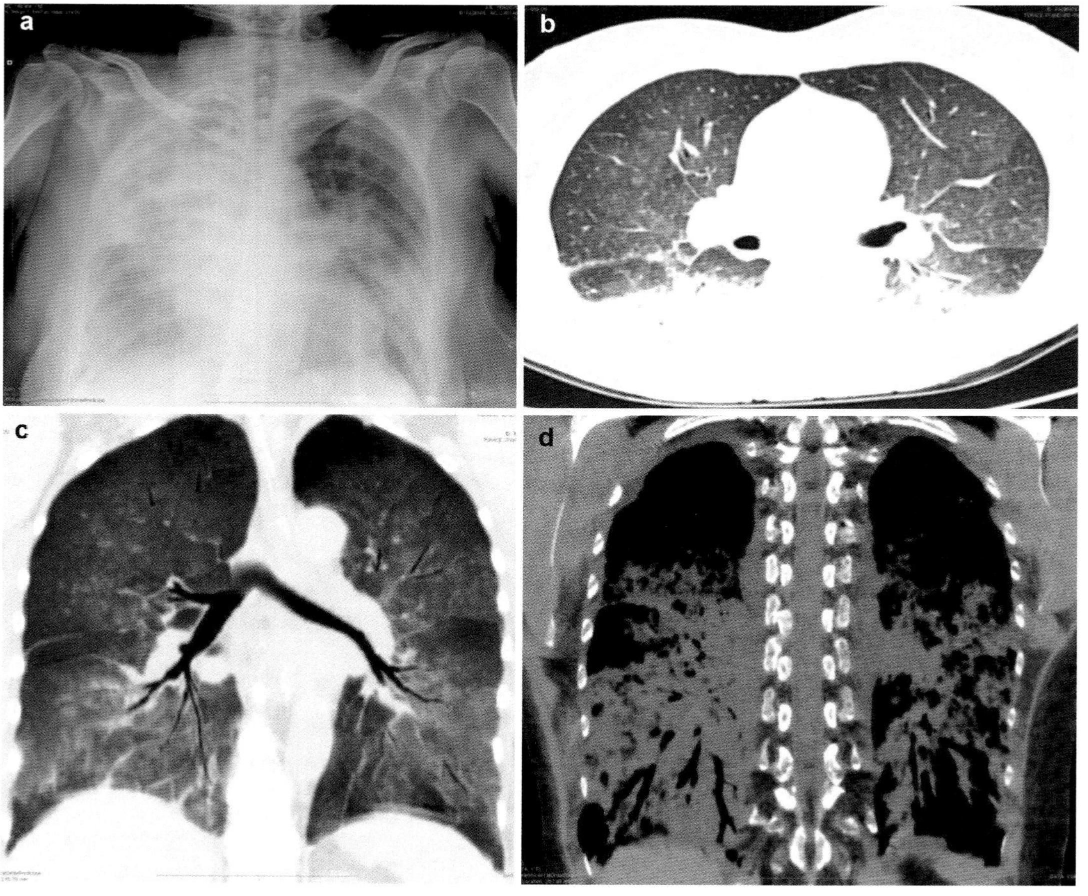

Fig. 10 Near drowning in a 67-year-old man who was admitted 3 h after nearly drowning in chlorinated water in an hotel pool. (**a**) CXR obtained at the time of admission reveals cardiac enlargement, diffuse confluent alveolar patterns of pulmonary edema, and peribronchial cuffing. Emergent MDCT (**b**) axial and (**c**, **d**) coronal reconstructions (parenchymal and mediastinal windows) show diffuse ground-glass and consolidative dependent abnormalities

freshwater or saltwater. Classic CXR findings in severe near drowning consist of alveolar edema with extensive "fluffy" areas of increased opacity that tend to coalesce throughout both lungs (Fig. 10). In mild near drowning, findings range from normal to confluent irregular peripheral areas of increased opacity in a subsegmental or segmental distribution with peripheral sparing. Pneumonia may be a complication of the aspiration of either fresh- or saltwater and, depending on the water source, may be caused by a variety of microorganisms including bacteria, fungi, and mycobacteria (Tourigny and Hall 2012).

1.4.3 Gastric Acid Aspiration (Mendelson Syndrome)

Vomiting with massive aspiration of gastric contents is a very frequent phenomenon; gastric acid with a pH <2.5 can cause pathologic reactions varying from mild bronchiolitis to hemorrhagic pulmonary edema. The posterior segments of the upper lobes and the superior segments of the lower lobes are the most frequently involved lung sites when the patient is recumbent. Acid liquid introduced into the airways is rapidly disseminated throughout the bronchial tree and lung parenchyma, producing a chemical pneumonitis within minutes. The magnitude of injury is directly related to the pH and volume of the aspirated material. The overall mortality rate associated with massive aspiration of gastric acid is approximately 30% and is greater than 50% in patients with initial shock or apnea, secondary pneumonia, or adult respiratory distress syndrome (Bynum and Pierce 1976). Classic CXR findings in acute gastric acid aspiration include bilateral perihilar, ill-defined, alveolar consolidations, multifocal patchy infiltrates, and segmental or lobar consolidation, which are usually localized to one or both lung bases (Fig. 6a).

1.4.4 Acute Exogenous Lipoid Pneumonia (Fire-Eater Pneumonia)

Exogenous lipoid pneumonia is a rare condition caused by inhalation or aspiration of plant, animal, or mineral fats and may take an acute or chronic form. Acute form is usually associated with accidental poisoning in children; in an adult population, it typically occurs in fire-eaters, who use oily substances in their shows (Betancourt et al. 2010). Clinically, acute lipoid pneumonia presents most often with cough, dyspnea, and fever. CXR pictures show consolidation, reticular and mixed alveolar-interstitial changes, as well as nodular lesions. Other rarer abnormalities, which may be noted on radiograms, are pneumatocele, pneumothorax, pneumomediastinum, and pleural effusion (Franquet et al. 2000). Most commonly, CT shows areas of a negative attenuation coefficient (between −150 and −30 HU) consolidation and ground-glass opacities as well as interstitial changes such as interlobular septal thickening and intralobular lines; fine, poorly demarcated centrilobular nodules and nodular lesions; pneumatocele; pneumothorax; pneumomediastinum; and pleural effusion (Brander et al. 1992; Laurent et al. 1999). Changes involve one or both lungs and are usually located in lower lobes or in the right middle lobe and may be multifocal or bilateral (Fig. 11).

1.5 Summary

Airway obstruction is an uncommon but potentially life-threatening condition that can be due to a number of malignant and benign processes; the diagnosis is based on the combination of characteristic findings on physical examination, as well as physiological, imaging, and endoscopic studies. Ultimately, the diagnosis is made by direct visualization of the tracheobronchial obstruction by bronchoscopy. Significant airway obstruction presenting with imminent suffocation requires immediate action to promptly and effectively reestablish and secure a patent airway and relieve the obstruction. Currently, the most comprehensive approach can be offered at centers with expertise in the management of acute complex airway disorders and availability of all endoscopic and surgical options.

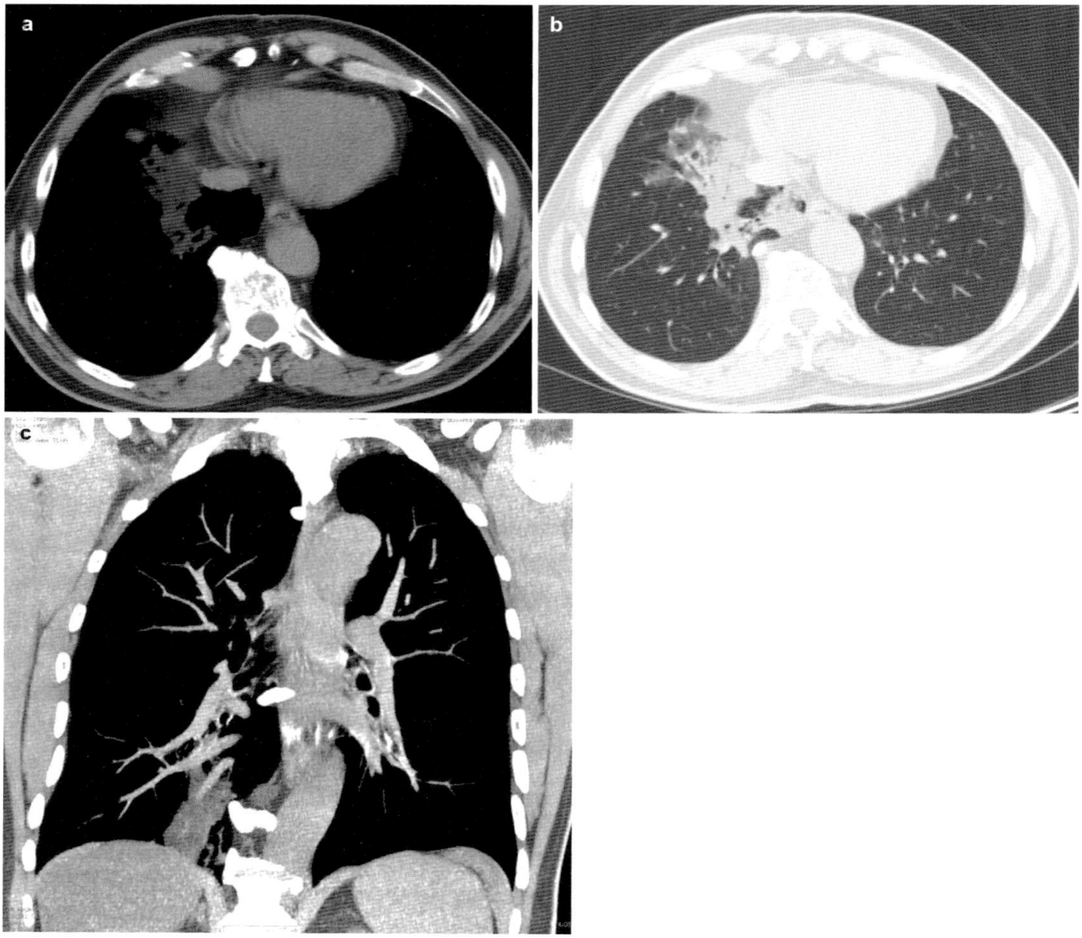

Fig. 11 Acute exogenous lipoid pneumonia. A 44-year-old actor performing in fire blowing shows who has aspirated liquid kindling for the grill 2 days before the onset of symptoms and was admitted acutely to the emergency department due to 38.8 °C fever, hemoptysis, pleuritic chest pain, and dyspnea. (**a**, **b**) Axial MDCT scans show a low-density consolidation in the middle lung lobe and scattered ground-glass opacities. (**c**) MDCT coronal MIP reconstruction better shows the low-density middle lobe consolidation. Region-of-interest measurements showed -60 to -80 Hounsfield units (HU), consistent with fat

2 Acute Exacerbation of Bronchiectasis

2.1 Introduction

The term bronchiectasis is derived from the Greek term *bronkia* (bronchial tubes), *ek* (out), and *tasis* (stretching), which together literally mean "the outstretching of the bronchi" (Feldman 2011). First described by Laennec in 1819, later detailed by Sir William Osler in the late 1800s, and further defined by Reid in the 1950s, this condition is generally defined as an abnormal and permanent focal or diffuse dilatation of the cartilage-containing airways (bronchi) caused by weakening or destruction of the muscular and elastic components of the bronchial walls (Hansell et al. 2008). Care must be taken to distinguish this large airway dilatation from dilatation of the small airways (bronchioles) that do not contain cartilage (Javidan-Nejad and Bhalla 2010). In contrast to established bronchiectasis occurring in adults, some children with bronchiectasis have been shown to have resolution or considerable improvement of the changes seen on CT scanning, suggesting the possibility that the condition may be reversible in some cases (Al Subie and Fitzgerald 2010).

Bronchiectasis results from the occurrence of one of the three main pathogenic mechanisms: bronchial wall injury, bronchial lumen obstruction, and traction from adjacent fibrosis (Shoemark et al. 2007). The latter two mechanisms are usually apparent on imaging and are suggested by an endobronchial filling defect or adjacent interstitial lung disease, while when it is met the first mechanism the radiologist is faced with a more difficult differential diagnosis (Javidan-Nejad and Bhalla 2009). The dominant feature of bronchiectasis is clearly the presence of airway inflammation, in association with bacterial infection and, in particular, nonclearing infection. An initial airway insult, such as an infection, often on the background of genetic susceptibility, compromised host clearance mechanisms and, in particular, the mucociliary escalator mechanism, which facilitated persistent bacterial colonization and infection. This damages the airway further, both directly and indirectly, as a consequence of the initiation of a secondary host inflammatory response. The three pathogenic elements in bronchiectasis—namely, airway infection, inflammation, and enzymatic activities—interact to result in progressive airway damage. Many patients eventually harbor *Pseudomonas aeruginosa* (PA) in their airway, which is associated with significant morbidity (Pappalettera et al. 2009).

The Reid morphological classification, derived from bronchographic and autopsy studies, specifies three patterns (Reid 1950):

1. *Cylindrical or tubular* bronchiectasis in which there is relatively uniform dilatation of sections of the bronchial tree, involving diffuse mucosal edema, with resultant dilated bronchi but with straight, regular outlines and that end squarely and abruptly.
2. *Varicose* bronchiectasis in which there are local constrictions superimposed on cylindrical bronchiectasis (bulbous or beaded appearance), with alternating areas of dilatation and constriction and, potentially, obstructive scarring that may subsequently result in postobstructive pneumonia and additional parenchymal damage.
3. *Saccular or cystic* bronchiectasis in which there is progressive dilatation of the airways giving a balloon-like appearance and sometimes air–fluid levels; the number of bronchial divisions is greatly reduced; it is generally acknowledged that cystic bronchiectasis represents the most advanced disease (Fig. 12).

Oftentimes, more than one type of bronchiectasis can be seen in the same patient. As the airway dilatation increases, there may be progressive collapse and fibrosis of the distal lung parenchyma. Bronchiectasis can frequently occur in parallel with more common forms of chronic lung disease including COPD (up to 50% of patients) and asthma (overlap syndromes) (Patel et al. 2004). There are many medical conditions that may lead to the development of bronchiectasis and these are detailed in Table 6.

2.2 Acute Exacerbations

The definition of an acute exacerbation is not standardized, and it has been variably defined to include some or all of the following symptoms and signs: increased cough and/or wheeze, sputum production/volume or purulence, dyspnea and lethargy, hemoptysis, or deterioration in spirometry (an unexplained significant, >10%, reduction in FEV_1 or FVC over days or weeks), chest signs, and radiographic changes; especially in the presence of severe bronchiectasis, hypoxemia may also be present (Chang et al. 2008). Impaired clearance of secretions causes colonization and infection with pathogenic organisms, contributing to the purulent expectoration commonly observed in patients with acute exacerbation of bronchiectasis. The result is further bronchial damage and a vicious cycle of bronchial damage, bronchial dilation, impaired clearance of secretions, recurrent infection, and more bronchial damage (Cole 1984). *P. aeruginosa* often causes chronic bronchial infection in

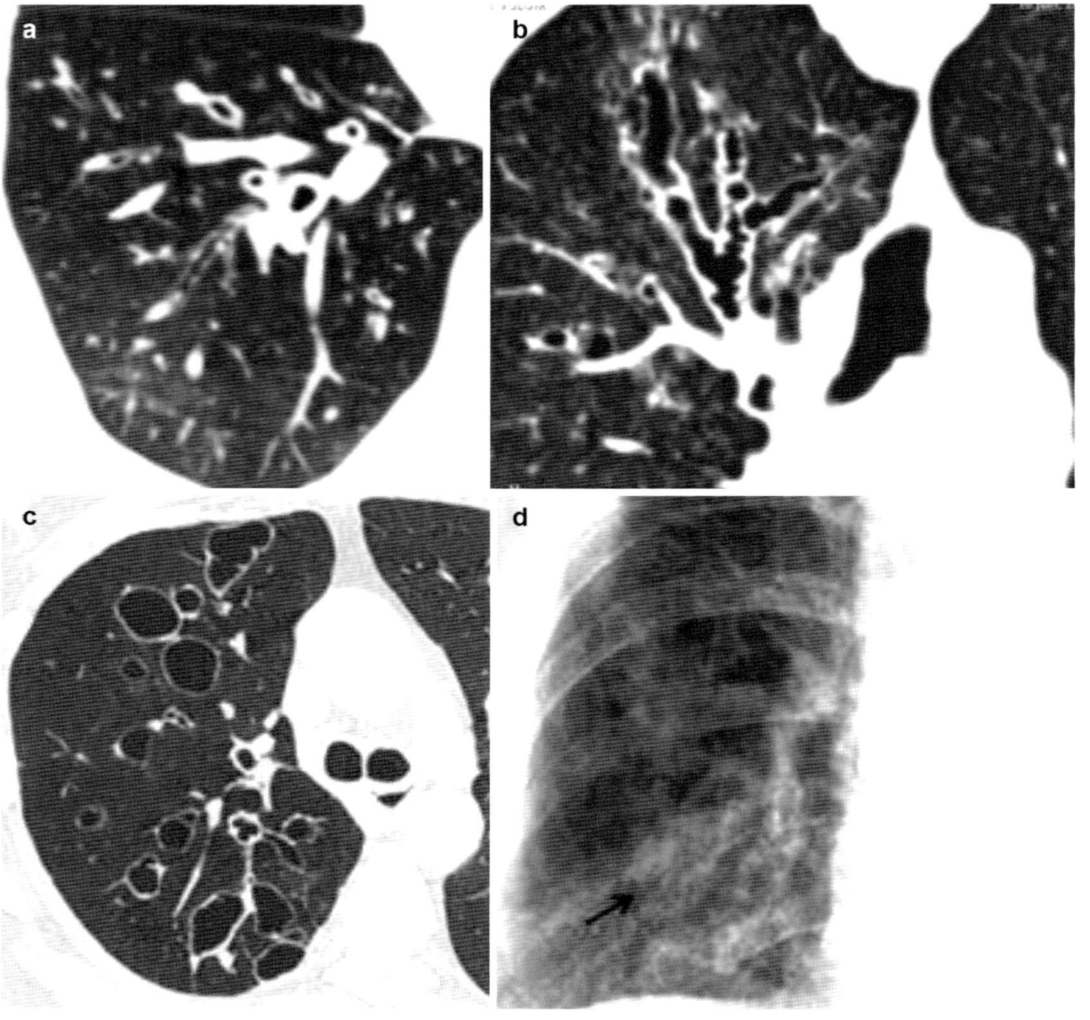

Fig. 12 The Reid morphological classification of bronchiectasis. (**a**) MDCT axial scan shows cylindrical or tubular bronchiectasis; (**b**) MDCT coronal reconstruction shows right upper lobe varicose bronchiectasis; (**c**) MDCT axial scan shows right upper lobe saccular or cystic bronchiectasis; (**d**) CXR close-up of the right lower lobe shows mucous plugging of bronchiectasis (*arrow*)

patients with non-CF bronchiectasis via a mechanism involving biofilm formation and the release of virulence factors. This suggests that *Pseudomonas* species may promote disease progression and that infection with these species may be related to worsening lung function and increased morbidity and mortality (Davies et al. 2006). Patients with chronic obstructive pulmonary disease are prone to prolonged exacerbations. Although hemoptysis is common during infective exacerbations of bronchiectasis, it may also occur in the absence of concurrent infection, so-called *dry bronchiectasis*, which is usually a sequela of tuberculosis and is found in the upper lobes. Hemoptysis, sometimes life-threatening, is caused by chronic airway inflammation and hypoxemia, which leads to bronchial arterial neovascularization (Bruzzi et al. 2006). Finally, acute exacerbations of bronchiectasis are associated with increased mortality, and the

Table 6 Causes of bronchiectasis

Causes of bronchiectasis	Imaging findings to provide clues to the diagnosis
Idiopathic (48 %)	*Often a lower lobe distribution*
Post-infective (25 %)	
Severe pneumonia	
Tuberculosis	
NTM	*Prominent nodularity in a tree-in-bud pattern or with cavitation*
Pertussis	*Lower lobe predominance*
Measles	
Impaired mucociliary clearance (9 %)	
CF	*Bilateral, proximal, parahilar, predominantly upper lobe disease*
Primary ciliary dyskinesia	*50 % associated with situs inversus, middle lobe/ lingular predominance*
Young's syndrome	*Predominantly lower lobe disease*
Chronic obstructive pulmonary disease and smoking	
Immunodeficiency (8 %)	
Common variable immunodeficiency	
Hypogammaglobulinemia	*Disproportionate bronchial wall thickening*
Specific polysaccharide antibody deficiency	
Secondary immunodeficiency, e.g., malignancy (chronic lymphocytic leukemia)	
Human immunodeficiency virus infection	
Lung and bone transplantation	
Exaggerated immune response	
Allergic bronchopulmonary aspergillosis	*Upper lobes, central bronchiectasis, prominent mucus plugging*
Graft versus host disease	
Inflammatory bowel disease (ulcerative colitis and Crohn's disease)	
c-ANCA-positive vasculitis	
Rheumatoid arthritis (3.2–35 % of patients)	
Congenital abnormalities of the bronchial wall	
Mounier-Kuhn syndrome	*(tracheobronchomegaly; enlarged tracheal diameter:>25 mm men, >23 mm women; trachea and bronchi of first to fourth order; central bronchiectasis)*
Williams-Campbell syndrome	(congenital absence of cartilage from lobar to first- to second-generation segmental airways)
Marfan syndrome	
Job syndrome (hyperimmunoglobulin E syndrome)	
Inflammatory pneumonitis	
Aspiration of gastric contents	
Inhalational exposure (smoke, ammonia, chlorine)	
Fibrosis (traction bronchiectasis)	
Sarcoidosis, radiation fibrosis, end-stage HP	*Predominantly upper lobes disease*
Idiopathic pulmonary fibrosis	*Predominantly lower lobes disease*
Mechanical obstruction (postobstructive)	*Unilateral focal bronchiectasis*
Foreign body	
Tumor	
Extrinsic compression (e.g., lymph node)	

(continued)

Table 6 (continued)

Causes of bronchiectasis	Imaging findings to provide clues to the diagnosis
Miscellaneous conditions	
Primary *Mycobacterium avium complex*	*Classic subtype: tree-in-bud opacity, patchy consolidation/cavities, upper lobes and superior segments of lower lobes*
"Lady Windermere syndrome"	*Nonclassic subtype: predominantly middle lobe and lingular disease*
Connective tissue diseases (e.g., rheumatoid arthritis, systemic lupus erythematosus, Sjogren's syndrome)	
Pulmonary sequestration	
Yellow nail syndrome	
Infertility (primary ciliary dyskinesia, cystic fibrosis, Young syndrome)	
Diffuse panbronchiolitis	
a1-Antitrypsin deficiency	
Smoke and gaseous toxins (e.g., chlorine gas and ammonia)	

majority of deaths are related to respiratory infection, with higher mortality rates associated with increasing age and number of lobes affected.

2.3 Clinical and Imaging Diagnosis

The diagnosis of bronchiectasis should be suspected in any individual presenting with persistent daily cough with mucopurulent sputum, recurrent hemoptyses, frequent infective exacerbations, and finger clubbing (Boyton 2012). The severity of airflow limitation is related to the extent and severity of the bronchiectasis (Javidan-Nejad and Bhalla 2009). In approximately 50 % of patients, a specific cause of bronchiectasis is not determined; however, in a substantial percentage of adult and children, the finding of an underlying cause results in a change in therapy and may have significant prognostic implications. The lung function studies in patients with bronchiectasis usually show an obstructive defect, and there may or may not be evidence of airway hyperreactivity. In all newly diagnosed patients with bronchiectasis, sputum should be cultured for bacteria and mycobacteria, and fungal cultures could be considered in selected cases. The main bacterial pathogens that are commonly isolated are *Haemophilus influenzae* (29–70 %) followed by *Pseudomonas aeruginosa* (12–31 %). Imaging now forms the cornerstone of diagnosis of bronchiectasis and its complications and plays an increasing role in disease monitoring and therapeutic planning.

2.3.1 Chest Radiography (CXR)

A plain chest radiography (CXR) is useful as an initial screening tool and, during acute exacerbations, may raise the initial suspicion of bronchiectasis, triggering more definitive imaging. However, it is insufficiently sensitive for the adequate diagnosis of the condition (sensitivity<50 %) (Goeminne and Dupont 2010; Currie et al. 1987), particularly in mild disease (Table 7).

Despite the obvious CXR deficiencies for the identification of bronchiectasis, an appreciation of the sometimes subtle radiographic features is necessary (Fig. 13) (Gudbjerg 1955; Woodring 1994):

(a) With more severe bronchial inflammation and fibrosis, the bronchial walls themselves become visible as parallel lines (*tram lines* or *tram tracks*) most obvious in the lower lobes on a PA view and in the middle lobe or lingula on the LL view (Westcott 1991; Feldman 2011) (Fig. 13).

Table 7 Bronchiectasis: CXR direct and indirect findings

Direct signs	Indirect signs
1. *Parallel line opacities* (*tram lines* or *tram tracks*) by dilated, thickened bronchi seen along their length	1. *Indistinct margins of vessels*
2. *Ring opacities* or *cystic* spaces (as large as 2 cm in diameter) when the bronchus is seen on end or from cystic bronchiectasis, sometimes with *air–fluid levels* (demilunes)	2. *Volume change*
3. *The signet ring sign*	(a) *Volume loss*
4. *Tubular and ovoid opacities* as *Y* or *V* shapes and sometimes the appearance of a *gloved finger* or as "finger-in-glove" opacities which radiate from the pulmonary hilum, from mucus plugging	Obscuration of the underlying hemidiaphragm
5. *Other signs:* scarring, bulla formation, pleural thickening	Crowding of pulmonary vascular markings
	Fissural displacement
	(b) Overall lung *volume increased* (compensatory hyperinflation and in generalized bronchiectasis such as in CF)
	3. Areas of *consolidation* (may be due to infection) (e.g., *Pseudomonas aeruginosa* or in ABPA)

(b) When seen end on, bronchiectatic airways appear as *ill-defined ring shadows*, ranging in size from 5 to 20 mm, notably in the mid and upper zones where the majority of airways run parallel to the radiograph beam. Signs of complications/exacerbations, such as dilated bronchi filled with pus and mucus, result in *tubular and ovoid opacities* and sometimes in the dramatic appearance of a *gloved finger*, typically seen in patients with mucoid impaction of the airways due to allergic bronchopulmonary aspergillosis (ABPA) (Fig. 14) (Martinez et al. 2008).

(c) In severe cystic disease, multiple *thin-walled ring shadows* that may contain *fluid levels* are present; the *signet ring sign* corresponds to a dilated bronchus immediately adjacent to a smaller companion pulmonary artery (Hansell 1998).

(d) Because the bronchi lie alongside the pulmonary arteries, peribronchial inflammation in early bronchiectasis makes the *margins of vessels indistinct*, particularly in the lower lobes (Hansell 1998).

(e) Associated volume loss in the lower lobes may cause *obscuration of the underlying hemidiaphragm* and *crowding of pulmonary vascular markings*, usually caused by mucous obstruction of the peripheral bronchi (Westcott 1991).

(f) Additional features of focal areas of *subsegmental collapse* and *patchy peribronchial consolidation* are nonspecific but are common in generalized disease.

(g) Signs of compensatory hyperinflation of the unaffected lung (Hansell 1998).

Extensive parenchymal consolidation is not, contrary to what might be expected, a usual feature of an infective exacerbation of bronchiectasis. Repeated infective exacerbations of subpleural bronchiectatic airways may result in a pleural reaction, although extensive pleural disease is rare unless there has been an associated empyema.

2.3.2 Thin-Section CT

Bronchography was replaced many years ago by high-resolution CT (HRCT) scanning of the chest (Young et al. 1991), which has become the gold standard (the most sensitive and specific noninvasive method, respectively, 84–97 % and 82–99 %, but higher at referral centers) for the diagnosis and that contrasts starkly with the limited ability of CXR to detect even advanced bronchiectasis (Hansell 1998). The detail afforded by 1-mm images of the peripheral airways has proved superior to virtually every other method for assessing the extent and severity of disease. Furthermore, thin-section CT features may be

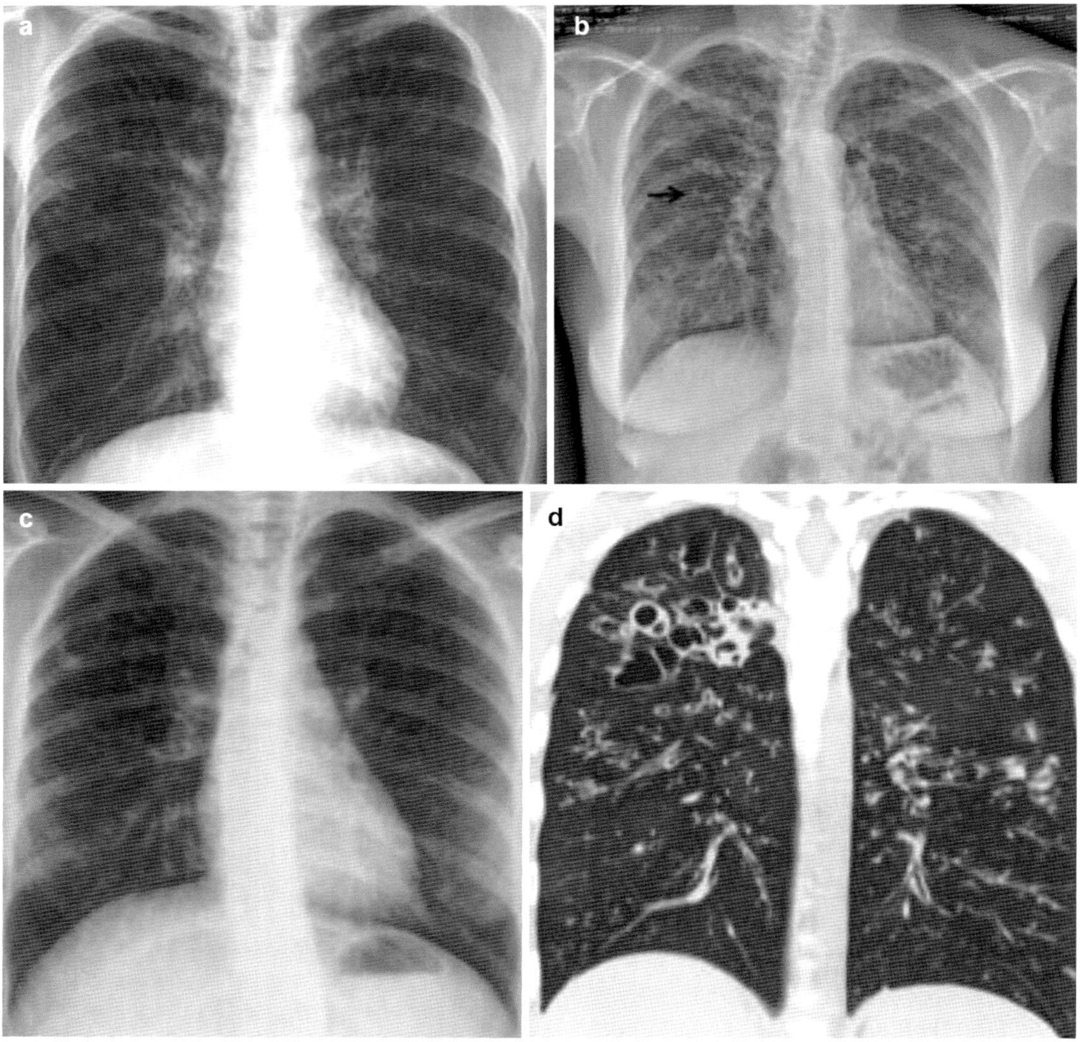

Fig. 13 Chest radiography findings in bronchiectasis. (**a**) In both upper lobes, CXR shows parallel tubular opacities due to partial fluid-filled airways. (**b**) The signet ring sign (*arrow*), a dilated bronchus immediately adjacent to a smaller companion pulmonary artery. (**c**, **d**) Integrated imaging (CXR and MDCT) shows upper right lobe ring opacities or cystic spaces, sometimes with air–fluid levels (demilunes)

suggestive of certain underlying conditions but require correlation with clinical and laboratory assessments, and images should be examined for findings suggesting ABPA, cystic fibrosis, immotile cilia, opportunist mycobacteria, and tracheobronchomegaly (Fig. 15) (Milliron et al. 2015).

Multidetector CT (MDCT) with volumetric acquisition, subsecond data acquisition, and initial thinnest possible collimation minimizes respiratory and cardiac motion, allows isotropic image reconstructions, and increases the sensitivity in detection of subtle nontapering airways, opening potentially unique automated, quantitative methods for evaluating the peripheral airways (Studler et al. 2005; Sung et al. 2003). Using MDCT as the gold standard, the sensitivity, specificity, and positive and negative predictive values of incremental HRCT in detecting bronchiectasis were 71 %, 93 %, 88 %, and 81 %, respectively (Hill et al. 2010; Dodd et al. 2006).

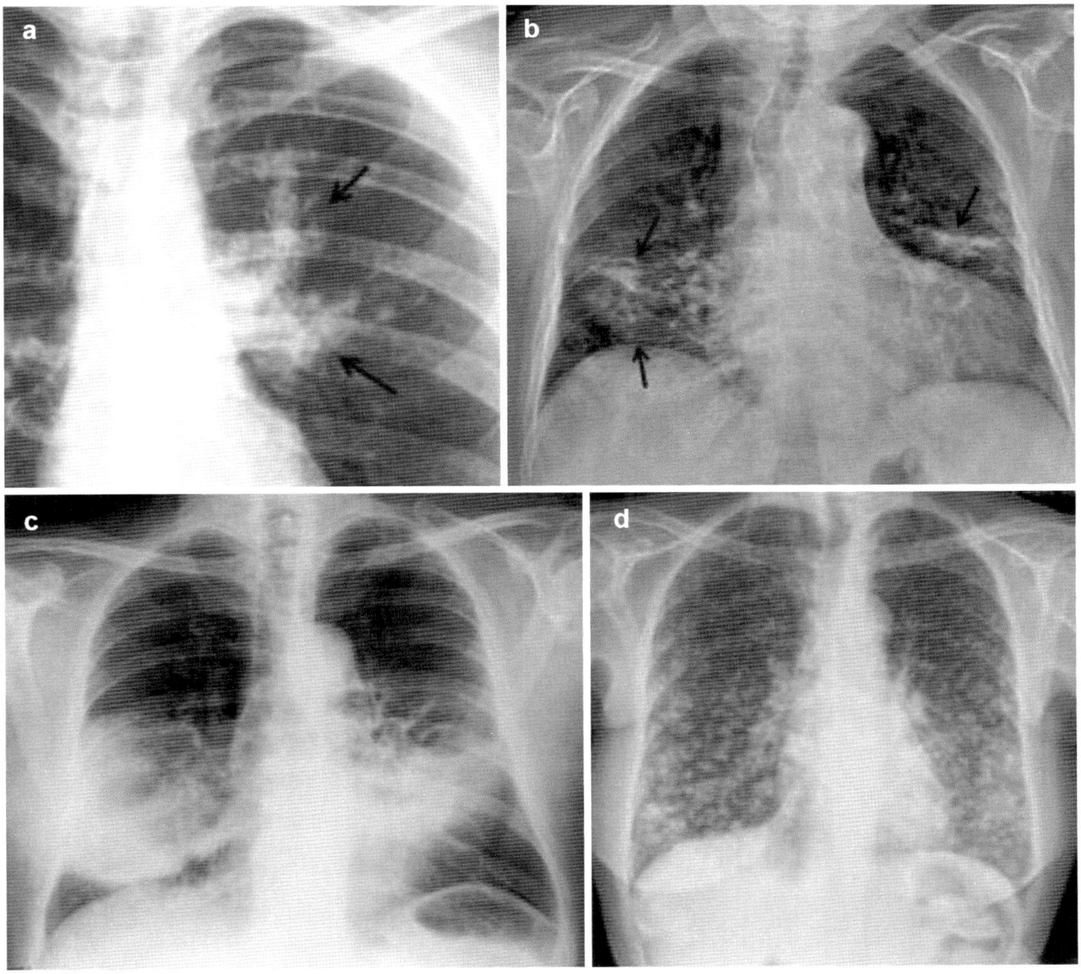

Fig. 14 Chest radiography findings in acute exacerbation of bronchiectasis. (**a**) CXR of a parahilar "gloved finger," typically seen in patients with mucoid impaction of the airways due to ABPA (*arrows*). (**b**) Bilateral focal areas of subsegmental collapse and patchy peribronchial consolidation from mucous plugging (*arrows*). (**c**) Large consolidations in both mid-lower lungs are an unusual feature of an infective exacerbation of bronchiectasis. (**d**) CXR shows diffuse lung nodular-like pattern from mucous filled airways (*P. aeruginosa*)

Interobserver agreement for the presence, extent, and severity of bronchiectasis was also better for MDCT (kappa 0.64, 0.5, and 0.48, respectively) than for incremental HRCT (kappa 0.65, 046, and 0.25, respectively) (Dodd et al. 2006). Because today most patients present with relatively mild bronchiectasis, with few (if any) physical signs, the diagnosis is usually made by *a combination of the patient's history and a thin-slice MDCT examination.* It is important to include expiratory imaging as part of the routine MDCT acquisition (Bankier et al. 1996). If it is possible, continuous acquisition of images during a forced or slow expiratory maneuver (dynamic expiratory CT) is not only more sensitive for detection of air trapping but also leads to identification of air trapping in normal individuals (Gotway et al. 2000). MinIP reconstructions are useful to demonstrate winding, interconnected tubular structures. Serious limitations for the use of quantitative airway measurements, most often including lumen diameter,

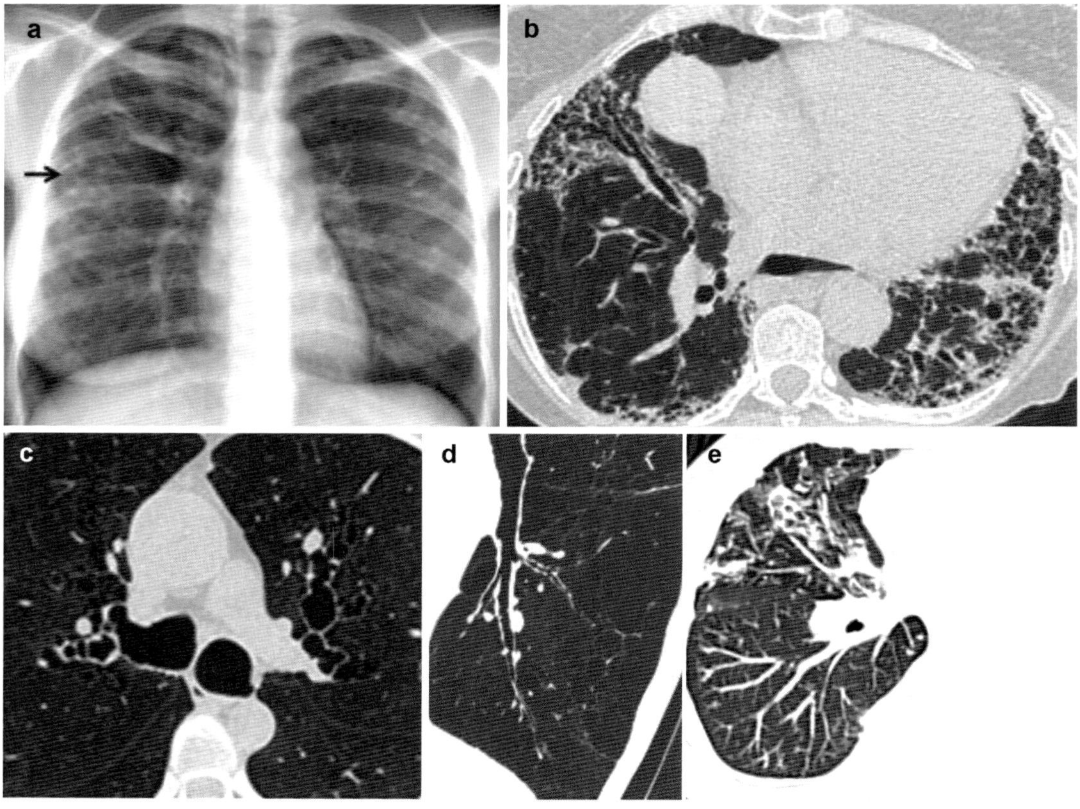

Fig. 15 Imaging findings suggestive of related diseases in bronchiectasis. (**a**) In cystic fibrosis (CF), CXR findings include hyperinflation, mucoid impactions, and bilateral parahilar mainly upper lobe bronchiectasis (*arrow*). (**b**) Traction bronchiectasis in fibrotic idiopathic interstitial pneumonia caused by peribronchial scarring. (**c**) Mounier-Kuhn syndrome is an idiopathic disease secondary to a marked atrophy of the elastic fibers and smooth muscle within the wall of the trachea and main bronchi; MDCT axial scan shows enlargement of the lumen in inspiration (>3 cm) and collapse during expiration (not shown). (**d**) Bronchiectatic airway remodeling in COPD. (**e**) ABPA bronchiectasis: ABPA is a hypersensitivity reaction to Aspergillus fumigatus antigens, affecting mostly patients with asthma and cystic fibrosis; bronchiectasis, mainly centric and in the upper lobes, is the hallmark of the disease. In ABPA retained secretions may appear sufficiently dense to mimic calcification or may calcificate

bronchoarterial ratio (BAR), lumen area (LA) and volume, wall thickness/diameter ratio (T/D ratio), and wall area percent (WA%), have been repeatedly documented, and none of these have proved of value in everyday routine clinical practice (Brillet et al. 2009; Williamson et al. 2009). As a consequence of these limitations, visual inspection remains the standard for clinical assessment of airway disorders; the potential for new methods for obtaining clinically useful automated quantitative airway evaluation remains to be evaluated. The extent of involvement of the lungs documented on HRCT scanning has been shown to correlate with both functional changes (PFT) and clinical outcomes, and HRCT score correlates significantly with exacerbation frequency (Brody et al. 2005). Although volumetric CT has numerous advantages, the radiation dose is higher and can be mitigated by several techniques (McCollough et al. 2009). Because of concerns of the level of radiation exposure with CT, particularly in children, MRI has been studied more recently for the diagnosis of bronchiectasis and been found to be a potentially suitable radiation-free alternative to CT, although the poorer spatial resolution of MRI limits the ability to visualize smaller airways and nodules (Montella et al. 2009). The most specific thin-slice CT scanning direct findings suggestive of bronchiectasis are (Table 8) (Naidich et al. 1982; Grenier et al. 1986; Hansell 1998; Javidan-Nejad and Bhalla 2009; King and Daviskas 2010; Bonavita and Naidich 2012) (Fig. 16):

1. Bronchoarterial ratio (BAR) > of 1–1.5: internal diameter of the bronchus is wider than the adjacent pulmonary artery at an equivalent branching level (i.e., a dilated bronchus cut in a horizontal section with an adjacent pulmonary artery representing the stone, signet ring formation); severity can be graded as mild, moderate, or severe (luminal diameter slightly greater, 2–3 times or >3 times than that of adjacent blood vessel in Bhalla scoring system). Care must be taken not to misinterpret bronchial dilatation as bronchiectasis in the setting of underlying acute parenchymal consolidation (so-called reversible bronchiectasis).
2. Failure of the bronchi to taper (bronchial diameter should remain unchanged for at least 2 cm distal to a branching point), a finding best appreciated toward the outer one-third of the lungs; however, this sign can be difficult to interpret in nonvolumetric CT studies (Kim et al. 1997a, b).
3. The bronchi being visualized in the outer 1–2 cm of the lung fields and visibility of airways within 1 cm of the pleural surface or abutting the mediastinal pleural surface (Kim et al. 1997a, b). Mucus plugging of dilated bronchi is readily identified, causing either complete or partial luminal filling and may be reversible. Plugging of the smaller peripheral airways and peribronchiolar inflammation are characterized by a tree-in-bud appearance, with V- and Y-shaped branching nodular opacities (Fig. 17).

Table 8 Bronchiectasis: thin-section CT direct and indirect findings

Direct signs	Indirect signs
1. *Bronchial dilatation*	1. *Bronchial wall thickening*
Increased bronchoarterial ratio (BAR)	Best assessed visually on images obtained at right angles through vertically oriented airways
Contour abnormalities (wall thickening)	2. *Mucoid impaction/ fluid-filled airways*
2. *Lack of airway tapering* >2 cm distal to point of bifurcation	Tubular or Y-shaped structures; branching or rounded opacities in cross section +/− air–fluid levels
3. *Airway visibility within 1 cm* of the costal pleura or fissures	3. *Bronchiolitis*
	Clustered ill-defined centrilobular nodules with a tree-in-bud configuration
	4. *Mosaic attenuation caused by air trapping*
	Best identified on expiratory HRCT images
	5. *Mosaic perfusion*
	Better identified on contrast-enhanced dual-energy CT of the pulmonary parenchyma
	6. *Bronchial artery hyperplasia*
	7. *Pulmonary hypertension findings*

The severity of bronchiectasis can also be assessed on the basis of the extent of disease, mucous plugging, and sacculations or abscesses and in terms of the number of bronchial divisions and lobes/segments involved, and a radiographic severity scoring system developed for use in CF has been used to assess patients with non-CF bronchiectasis (Bhalla et al. 1991). *Mosaic attenuation* is a term used to denote heterogeneous lung density, often exhibiting a distinctly geographic distribution. This nonspecific finding typically results from one of the following three causes: (1) foci of abnormally increased lung density caused by a variety of infiltrative and/or airspace filling diseases; (2) alternating low-density and high-density foci reflecting variations

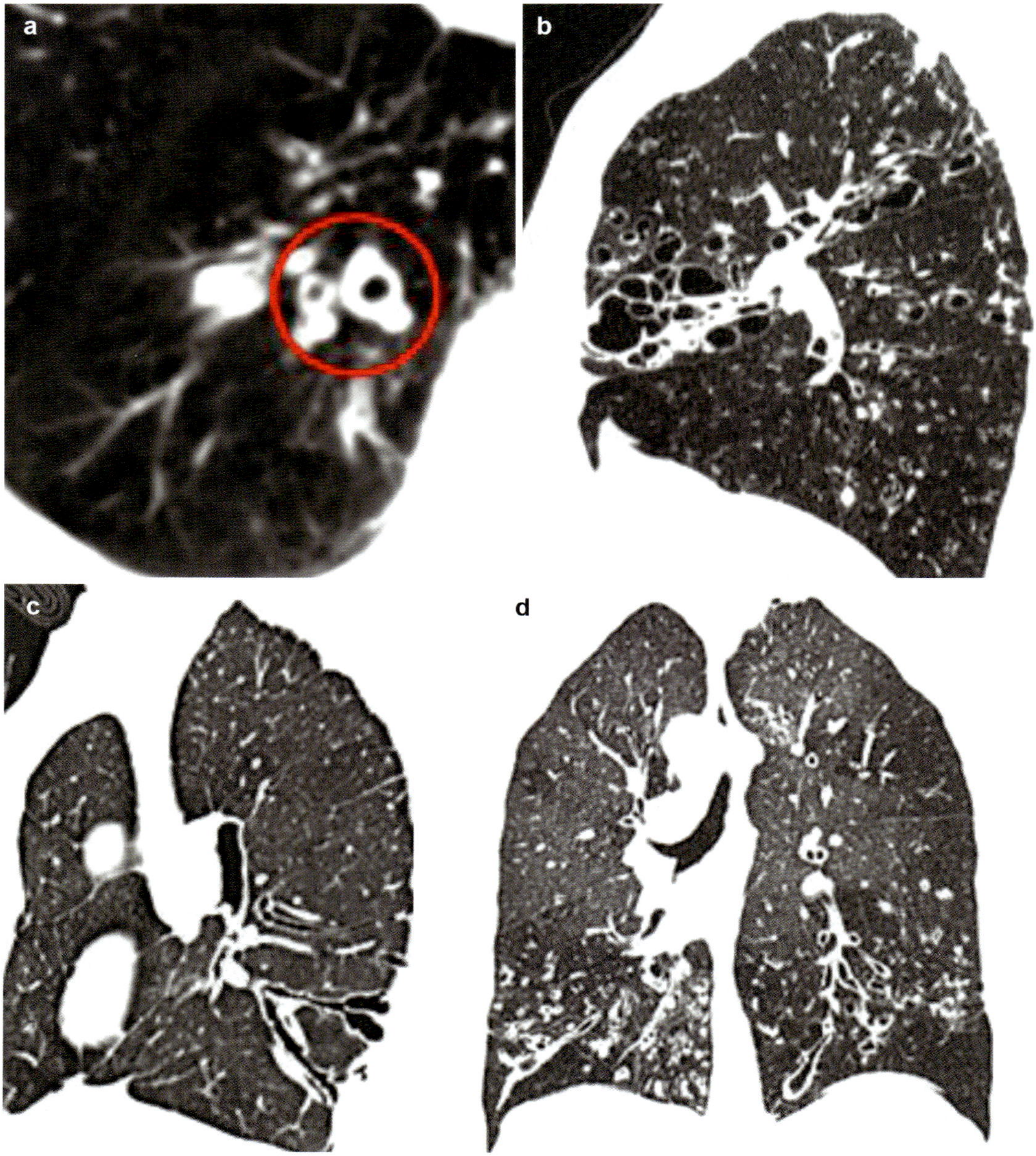

Fig. 16 Thin-section CT findings in bronchiectasis. (**a**) The so-called signet ring sign (*circle*), a bronchus with an internal diameter greater than the diameter of the adjacent pulmonary artery. (**b**) Sagittal reconstruction shows a bronchiectatic bunch of grapes in the middle lobe. (**c**) Sagittal reconstruction shows lack of airway tapering >2 cm distal to point of bifurcation, bronchial wall thickening, and bronchi abutting the pleural surface. The wall thickness evaluation varies depending on slice thickness and window levels. (**d**) Coronal reconstruction shows lack of airway tapering and mosaic attenuation pattern

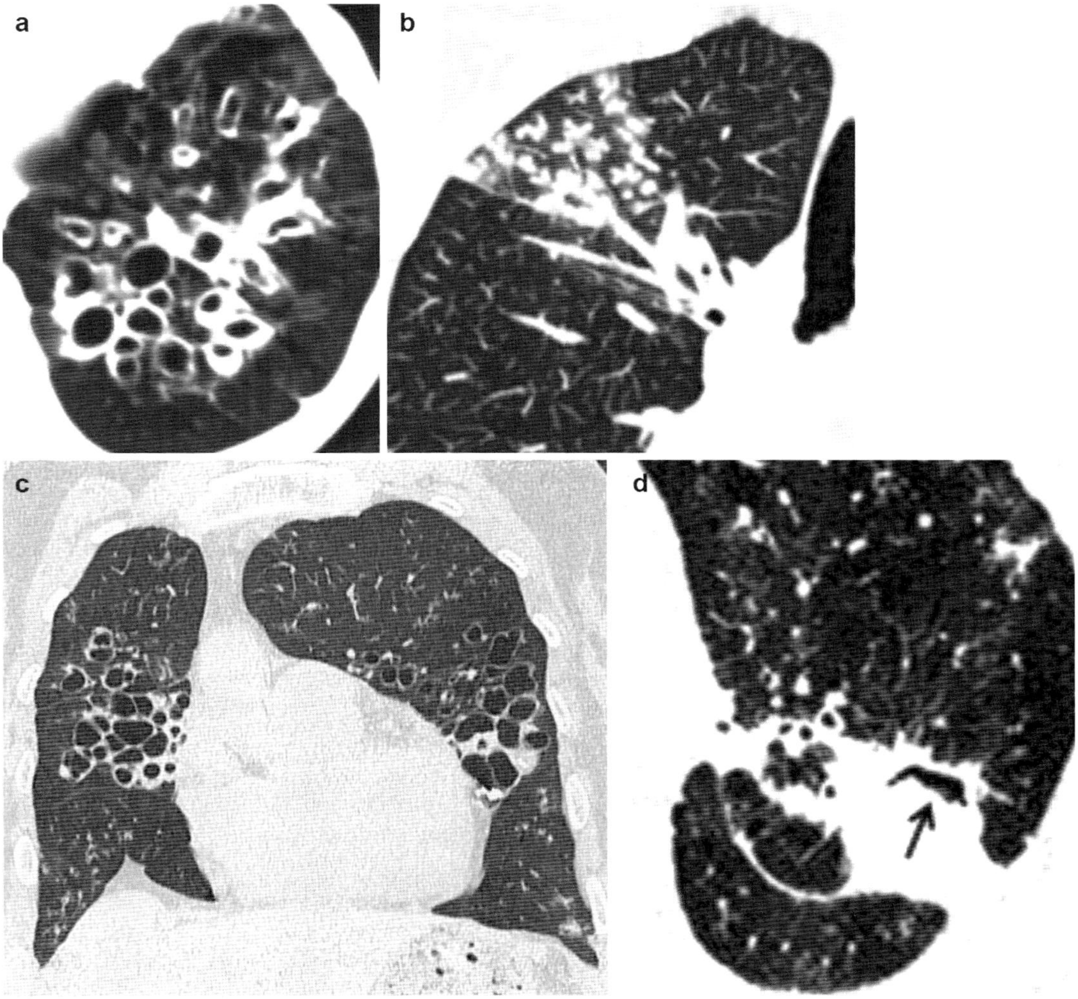

Fig. 17 Computed tomography findings in acute exacerbation of bronchiectasis. (**a**) Axial scan shows ring clustered cystic spaces in the lower right lobe with air–fluid levels (demilunes). (**b**) Coronal reconstruction shows right upper lobe clustered ill-defined centrilobular nodules with a tree-in-bud configuration by mucus-impacted small airways (bronchiolitis). (**c**) Coronal reconstruction shows bilateral cystic exacerbated bronchiectasis with air–fluid levels. (**d**) Axial closeup scan shows cystic bronchiectasis with fungal overinfection/mycetoma (*arrow*)

in lung perfusion, characteristically the result of chronic embolic pulmonary hypertension; and (3) foci of abnormally decreased lung density caused by focal air trapping in patients with underlying obstructive small airway disease (Bonavita and Naidich 2012). Differentiation between these causes is best accomplished on images acquired in deep expiration. Air trapping results either from mucous plugging and abnormal bronchial compliance or inflammation/fibrosis of the small airways, reflecting a combination of both large and small airway obstruction.

Another ancillary finding is the *presence of dilated bronchial arteries* in patients with long-standing severe bronchiectasis. This finding is easily identified following administration of intravenous contrast as irregular, tortuous vessels arising from the proximal descending thoracic aorta extending along the central airways toward the pulmonary hila. Identification of hypertrophied bronchial arteries may explain hemoptysis that is otherwise unaccounted for in select acute exacerbation cases (Fig. 18).

In acute exacerbation, more frequent imaging findings are air–fluid levels in bronchiectatic airways, mucous plugging, centrilobular nodules, and peribronchial thickening, all potentially reversible signs.

A variety of different CT-based methods for assessing the *extent and severity* of disease have been proposed (Bhalla et al. 1991; Ooi et al. 2002; de Jong et al. 2004; Oikonomou

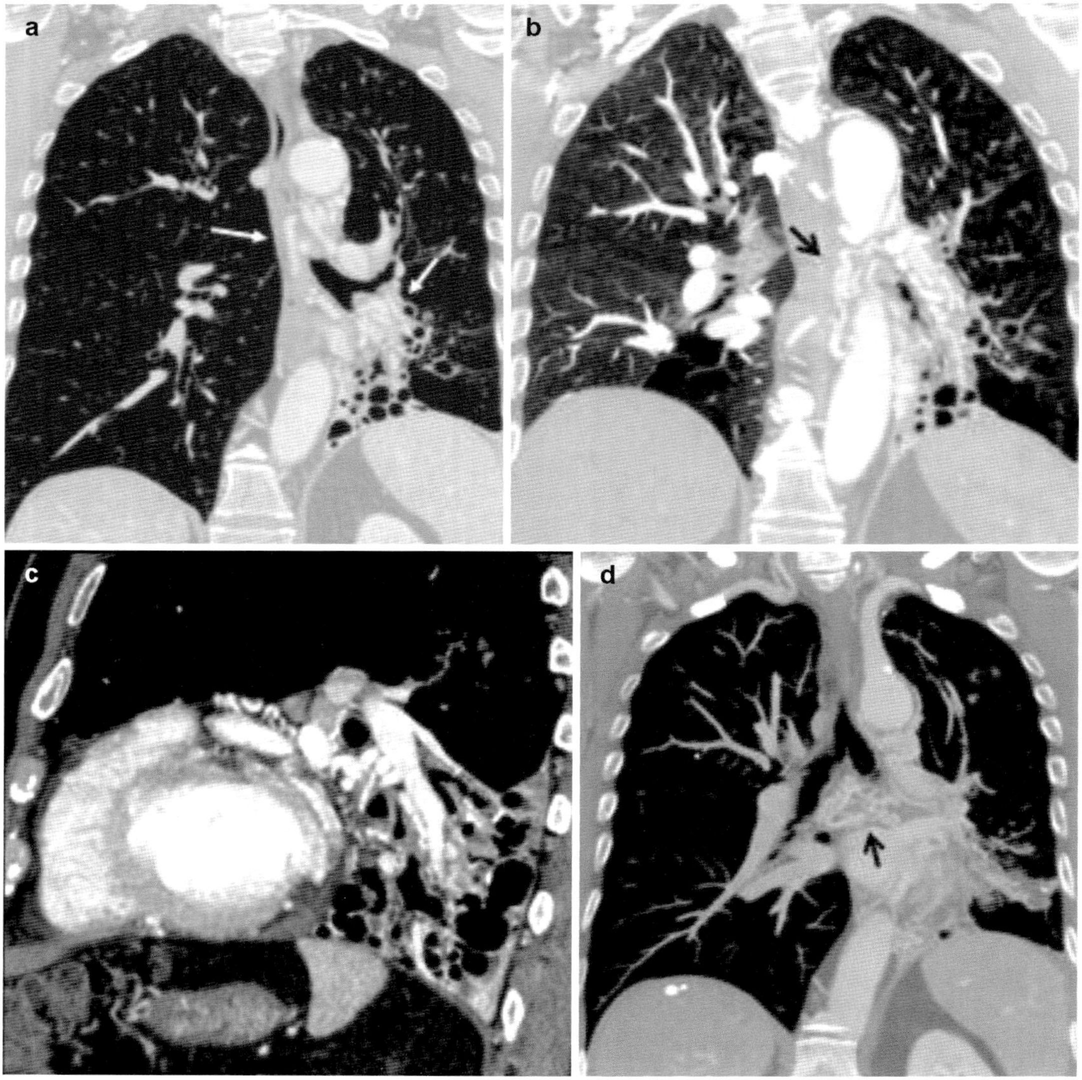

Fig. 18 Massive hemoptysis in a 41-year-old man with common variable immunodeficiency and a history of recurrent infections beginning during childhood. MDCT arterial phase (**a**, **b**, **d**) coronal and (**c**) oblique sagittal reconstructions reveal bilateral lower lobes bronchiectasis with mosaic attenuation and focal consolidation (likely hemorrhage) and tortuous hypertrophied bronchial arteries (*arrows*). The patient was treated with repeated bronchial artery embolizations

et al. 2008); they have emphasized a few or all of the following: generations of bronchial divisions (including the number of lobes/segments involved), peribronchial thickening, mucoid impaction (both large and small airway, the latter identified as resulting in a tree-in-bud pattern), signs of obstructive airway disease including CT evidence of emphysema, and mosaic attenuation (especially as documented on expiratory images). Although clearly requiring further validation, it is apparent that true routine, automated, quantitative global scoring of bronchiectasis (including color-coded 3D maps and dual-energy CT measurements of airway wall enhancement) is feasible and, if established (Bonavita and Naidich 2012), would represent an important milestone in the use of CT to assess patients with a wide variety of airway diseases.

2.4 Summary

Imaging plays a crucial role in the diagnosis and monitoring of bronchiectasis and the management of complications. CXR is useful as an initial screening tool and during acute exacerbations, but has limited sensitivity and specificity. Thin-section MDCT is the reference standard for diagnosis, quantification, and low-dose routine surveillance of bronchiectasis, providing detailed morphological and physiologic consequence evaluation; furthermore, it is valuable in diagnosing and managing complications in exacerbations and acute setting.

3 Toxic Gas Inhalation

3.1 Introduction

Acute injury to the airways and lung parenchyma may occur as a result of an industrial disaster, occupational exposure, recreational mishap, natural catastrophe, chemical warfare, and acts of terrorism (Kales and Christiani 2004). According to AEGL, acute exposures are single, non-repetitive exposures that do not exceed 8 h (Acute Exposure Guideline Levels, AEGLs).

In industrialized countries, most acute toxic inhalations come from industries, home, and recreational sources; new industrial practices and materials are increasingly recognized as causes of acute lung disease, but much of our present knowledge of inhalation injury has been gathered from burn units in smoke inhalation injury (SII), where pulmonary insufficiency is a major cause of death (Rabinowitz and Siegel 2002). In this section, we illustrate the spectrum at imaging of lung injury related to acute toxic exposures.

3.2 Definitions and Classification

Numerous classification schemes have been developed as a way to organize the enormous numbers of possible inhaled toxicants (Table 9) (Rabinowitz and Siegel 2002; Miller and Chang 2003; Nelson and Hoffman 2006; McKay 2014; Borron and Bebarta 2015; Salem and Katz 2015).

Table 9 Scheme of possible inhaled toxicants

Gases	A state of matter consisting of particles that have neither a defined volume nor a defined shape at normal temperatures and pressures and can expand to occupy an available space
Vapors	A condensable gas, that is, a state of matter that can be converted to another physical form by alterations of temperature and/or pressure, but there are no significant chemical or physical differences between a vapor and a gas
Fumes	They form when a solid, which has been volatilized by evaporation or vaporization, condenses in cool air
Particulates	Microscopic solid or liquid matter suspended in a medium, usually air in the Earth's atmosphere
Aerosols	Commonly refers to the particulate/air mixture, as opposed to the particulate matter alone
Dusts	Suspensions of solid particles in a gaseous media
Smokes	Result from the incomplete combustion of carbon-containing material including oil and coal

The severity pattern of disease is a function of the toxin or mix of toxins (*particle size*, *density*, *water solubility*, *shape*) that constituted the exposure, *duration* of *exposure*, *minute ventilation*, and the host factor status of the individual. The total inhaled dose is equal to agent concentration multiplied by time of exposure and minute ventilation (Rabinowitz and Siegel 2002; Borron and Bebarta 2015; Nelson and Hoffman 2006; McKay 2014; Salem and Katz 2015). The effects of inhalation exposure to toxicants can be thought of as follows: simple asphyxiants, tissue asphyxiants, nonrespiratory systemic toxicants with pulmonary absorption, and direct airway cellular injury. Such injuries in general occur either through localized pulmonary damage or by systemic absorption after inhalation (Miller and Chang 2003).

Those that cause localized pulmonary damage can be subdivided further into *irritant gases* (in that the chemical interaction of the agent and the water at the mucosal surface of the airways and/or other cellular components results in direct tissue injury via the generation of acids, alkali, or other reactive compounds) and those that cause *pulmonary sensitization* (associated with the late occurrence of "reactive airway dysfunction syndrome" or RADS in which subsequent exposure to small concentrations of the same agent or other potential respiratory irritants results in an asthma-like condition with bronchospasm, bronchoconstriction, and decreased airflow; RADS is not associated with immunoglobulin E-mediated histamine release) (Gorguner et al. 2004). Those that cause systemic toxicity can be subdivided into *simple asphyxiants* (displace atmospheric oxygen following Dalton's law of partial pressures but are otherwise essentially physiologically inert), *systemic asphyxiants* (usually interfere with transport or use of oxygen within tissues and organs; some chemicals exert systemic toxic effects when absorbed by way of the pulmonary circulation but cause no direct acute airway or lung injury), *organophosphates*, *hydrocarbons,* and *metal fumes* (Table 10) (Rabinowitz and Siegel 2002; Mokhlesi and Corbridge 2003; Borron and Bebarta 2015; Salem and Katz 2015).

Table 10 Pulmonary and systemic main inhalational toxicants

Pulmonary inhalational toxicants	Systemic inhalational toxicants
Irritant gases	*Asphyxiants*
Ammonia	Carbon monoxide (CO)
Chlorine	Methemoglobin inducers[a]
Formaldehyde	Hydrogen cyanide (HCN)
Nitrogen dioxide	Hydrogen sulfide (H2S)
Phosgene	Carbon dioxide (CO_2)
Hydrogen fluoride	Nitric oxide (NO)
Acrolein	Methane
Ozone	Helium, argon, krypton, xenon
Antigens/sensitizers	*Organophosphates*
Ammonia	Nerve gases (cholinesterase inhibitors)
Chlorine	Sarin (GB)
Formaldehyde	Tabun (GA)
Nitrogen dioxide	Soman (GD)
Methyl isocyanate (MIC)	Venon X
Toluene	Insecticides
Vinyl plastics	*Hydrocarbons*
Animal and plants proteins	Freon
Bacteria	Benzene
Fungi	Toluene
	Vinyl chloride
	Trichloroethylene
	Trichloroethane
	Metal fumes
	Beryllium
	Cadmium
	Mercury
	Nickel
	Zinc
	Chromium

There can be significant overlap, as many toxicants can fit in multiple categories

[a]Methemoglobinemia is a state of oxidized hemoglobin in which the hemoglobin iron is in the ferric state (Fe^{31}) and is unable to bind to or transport oxygen

3.3 Mechanisms of Toxicity

Direct airway cellular injury results from epithelial cell injury and death and from airway edema; the *nasopharynx* and *larynx* manifest these cellular injuries earliest because they are exposed to the highest concentrations of inhaled toxicants

(Garnier 1998; Mokhlesi and Corbridge 2003). Gases that are *highly water-soluble*, such as ammonia, sulfur dioxide, and hydrogen chloride, generally cause acute irritant injury to mucus membranes, including the eyes and the lining of the nose and upper airway, and spare the lower respiratory tract. This irritant injury causes unpleasant symptoms that often encourage an individual to rapidly leave an area of exposure; this prevents more severe clinical effects. *Less soluble gases*, such as phosgene, ozone, and nitrogen oxides, often cause no symptoms or ill effects in the upper airway. They penetrate into the lower airway and cause irritant effects in the bronchi, terminal bronchioles, and alveoli. Pulmonary irritants with *intermediate solubility* can produce a mixed clinical picture; whether upper or lower tract symptoms predominate depends on the duration and intensity of the exposure. Chlorine gas is a prototypical example of an intermediate solubility irritant and can produce a broad spectrum of clinical syndromes depending on the circumstances surrounding a given exposure (Rabinowitz and Siegel 2002). There is a gradual but progressive airway response to direct cellular injury. Within a few hours of postexposure, there is extensive but mild mucosal edema, no ulceration, and deceptively minimal clinical symptoms. Over the next 8–48 h, there is progressive airway edema, mucopurulent membrane production, and bronchorrhea. Within 48–72 h, there is mucosal slough and evolution of a membranous tracheobronchitis.

If toxic agents pass to the level of the *conducting airways*, damage to the epithelial cells and tight junctions can increase mucosal permeability to other substances, which increases inflammation and cellular damage. This can lead to bronchoconstriction, peribronchial edema, and bronchial mucosal slough and all can contribute to the development of atelectasis. Substances that have lower water solubility and particles less than 5 μm in diameter can penetrate into the lower respiratory tract. In the *distal airways and alveoli*, epithelial and endothelial injury results in permeability-induced edema. This can manifest anywhere from mild interstitial edema to pulmonary insufficiency. As in other forms of the acute respiratory distress syndrome (ARDS), this results in decreased lung compliance, increased alveolar-arterial oxygen gradient, and increased pulmonary vascular resistance (Ferguson et al. 2012; Fanelli et al. 2013). Pulmonary edema may be immediate in pulmonary high-concentration toxicant exposure or may be delayed 24–48 h postexposure (Miller and Chang 2003). Aggressive supportive care is often lifesaving, and treatment is usually symptomatic with the exception of organophosphates, certain chemical asphyxiants, such as cyanide and carbon monoxide, and opioid poisonings and toxicant-induced methemoglobinemia (Endorf and Gamelli 2007; Micak et al. 2007; Heitkamp et al. 2012). Airway injury is present in up to one-third of patients with major burns. Pulmonary insufficiency is a major cause of death in burn victims from residential or commercial structure fires and has been shown to result from inhalation of toxic products of combustion including the oxides of sulfur, nitrogen, aldehyde gases, and particulates, rather than from thermal injury. Carbon monoxide is rapidly transported across the alveolar membrane and binds to hemoglobin. Smoke inhalation also adds to mortality from cutaneous thermal burns and represents a combination of direct pulmonary injury and systemic and metabolic toxicities (mortality rates are approximately 5–8 %) (Table 11) (Darling et al. 1996).

Table 11 Factors of lung pathophysiologic response to smoke inhalation injury (SII)

Smoke lung injury
Patient preinjury health status (reactive airway disease or chronic lung changes)
Direct mucosal injury compromises the mucociliary escalator and particulate, mucus, and bacterial clearance Increase in bronchial blood vessel permeability
Tissue destruction and secondary inflammatory response results in mucosal slough
Systemic smoke inhalation injury
Decrease in cardiac filling pressure and cardiac index
The inflammatory effects causing capillary leak are complementary following cutaneous burns and inhalation Inflammation within the airways and lung parenchymal injury

3.4 Clinical Setting, Imaging, and Management

A detailed history becomes even more important in such a patient and may help make a difference in the often chaotic setting of the emergency department (ED). Laboratory evaluation and arterial blood gas analysis (particularly the anion, osmolal, and the oxygen saturation gaps) and supportive measures, including the ABCs (airway, breathing, and circulation), may be required (Darling et al. 1996; Mokhlesi and Corbridge 2003; Micak et al. 2007). Unfortunately, the varied presentations result in a nonspecific clinical syndrome (toxidrome) and make diagnosis somewhat difficult (Micak et al. 2007). The Abbreviated Injury Scale (AIS) criteria (0, no injury; 1, mild; 2, moderate; 3, severe; and 4, massive injury) constitute a standardized fiber-optic bronchoscopic (FOB) scoring system for the degree of burn and other inhalational injuries (Endorf and Gamelli 2007; Hassan et al. 2010; Albright et al. 2012; Mosier et al. 2012). Serial tracheobronchial washings for clinical care purposes are usually performed using an antiseptic solution (Miramistin, chlorhexidine gluconate). Blood gas analysis, functional respiratory tests, and FOB results were used to choose an appropriate respiratory support tactics in the patients with inhalation injury.

Despite substantial limitations (Putman et al. 1977), radiography of the chest (CXR) remains the most widely used method for diagnosis and monitoring of many acute inhalational lung diseases. When in admission CXR reveals recent infiltrate, this is evidence of more severe inhalation injury, thereby indicating a worse prognosis (Lee and O'Connell 1988; Wittram and Kenny 1994; DiPoce et al. 2012).

Lung ultrasound (LUS) is an excellent complementary diagnostic tool in emergency diagnosis of tracheal structures, lung consolidation, atelectasis, and pleural effusion; patient safety can be enhanced by performing procedures under US guidance, e.g., thoracentesis and vascular line access (Lichtenstein et al. 2004; Lichtenstein 2014).

Thin-section multidetector computed tomography (MDCT) of the chest is a more sensitive tool to detect inhalation injury, to value its extent, severity, and complications, and continues to demonstrate previously unidentified characteristics that shape our understanding of noxious inhaled toxicant injury (Reske et al. 2005; Koljonen et al. 2007). Since the lung has a fairly uniform response to toxicant injury, the imaging approach to burn and industrial accident victims is similar. Parameters such as estimates of the volume of infusion, as well as assessment of the need for mechanical ventilation management, the possibility of pneumonia development, and outcome are necessary.

The severity of the injury at imaging is directly related to the concentration of the toxicant and the duration of exposure. The choice of imaging studies and the information sought in the patient with a history of inhalation of a toxic gas vary according to the time elapsed since the acute event; we can distinguish:

- The *acute stage or early resuscitation phase* (the first 24–36 h postexposure, as the time the patient is managed in the ED and is usually characterized by acute pulmonary insufficiency); the goal of the radiologist is to document the extent of injury and to determine whether the toxic gas has been inhaled deeply or whether laryngospasm has confined the injury to the upper airway. A *normal CXR*, usually obtained in decubitus AP view at the often unstable patient's bedside at ED admission, may be valuable as a baseline for subsequent CXR or follow-up and does not exclude parenchymal or airway injury *which may only be evident 24–48 h after the acute event* (ARDS latent period), despite clinical evidence of lung injury (arterial hypoxemia, elevated carboxyhemoglobin levels) (Wittram and Kenny 1994). An *abnormal CXR* on admission is variable in severity and extent, indicates a worse prognosis, and may show various disease patterns:
  (a) Subglottic edema with a conical narrowing of the airway, tracheal narrowing, diffuse peribronchial infiltration, moderate venous congestion, peripherally located small round clear bubbles closely arranged to each other in a shape resembling a mulberry, and focal or diffuse patchy opacities that

usually (if not complicated by ARDS) evolve over the first few days or clear within 4–6 days, most likely due to atelectasis and consolidations (Fig. 19). Causes of atelectasis include decreased mucociliary clearance, inspissated secretions of the bronchi and bronchioles, reflex bronchoconstriction, and surfactant inactivation.

(b) Bilateral diffuse alveolar opacities more likely represent progressive noncardiogenic pulmonary edema, by increased permeability diffuse alveolar damage (DAD) with resultant transudation into the alveolar spaces (ARDS), leading to hypoxemia that is refractory to usual oxygen therapy (Ferguson et al. 2012). This can manifest anywhere from mild interstitial edema to pulmonary insufficiency (Fig. 20). ARDS is the final pathway of acute lung injury caused by a variety of agents, including inhaled toxins, aspiration, and infection (George et al. 2003). CXR may help in differentiating it from typical pulmonary edema: CXR features usually develop 12–24 h after initial lung insult, and within 1 week, alveolar pulmonary edema (hyaline membrane) occurs due to type 1 pneumocyte damage.

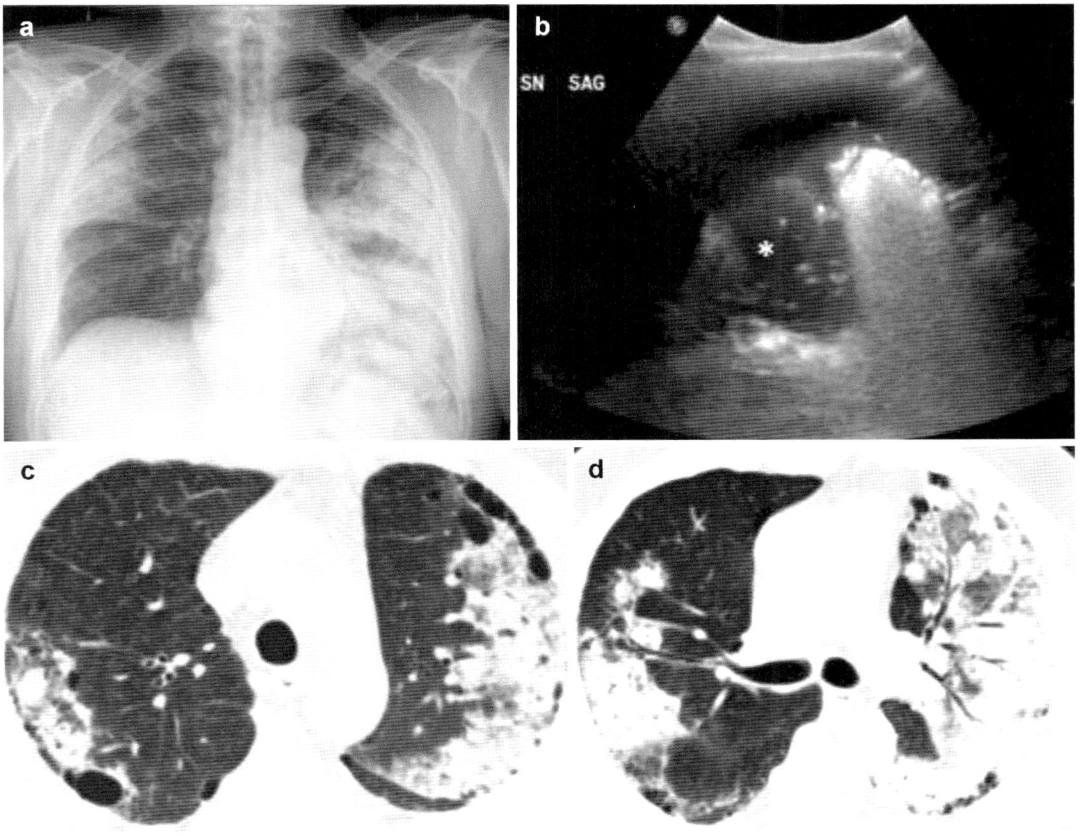

Fig. 19 Integrated imaging (CXR, US, MDCT) of asymmetrical pattern of airspace disease, greater in the left lung, in a 62-year-old man with acute presentation of shortness of breath after 24 h of smoke inhalation (SII). (**a**) CXR on admission shows bilateral consolidations. (**b**) Complementary LUS left sagittal scan shows coexistent pleural effusion and spots (air bronchogram) in consolidated lung (*). (**c**, **d**) MDCT shows airspace consolidation, air bronchograms, and pre-existing subpleural blebs; the bronchial wall thickness (BWT) was 4.2 mm on admission, 4.5 mm after 24 h, and 2.4 mm after 7 days (see text). Bronchoscopic AIS was 3 (severe injury). He developed pneumonia and remained in the ICU for 6 days

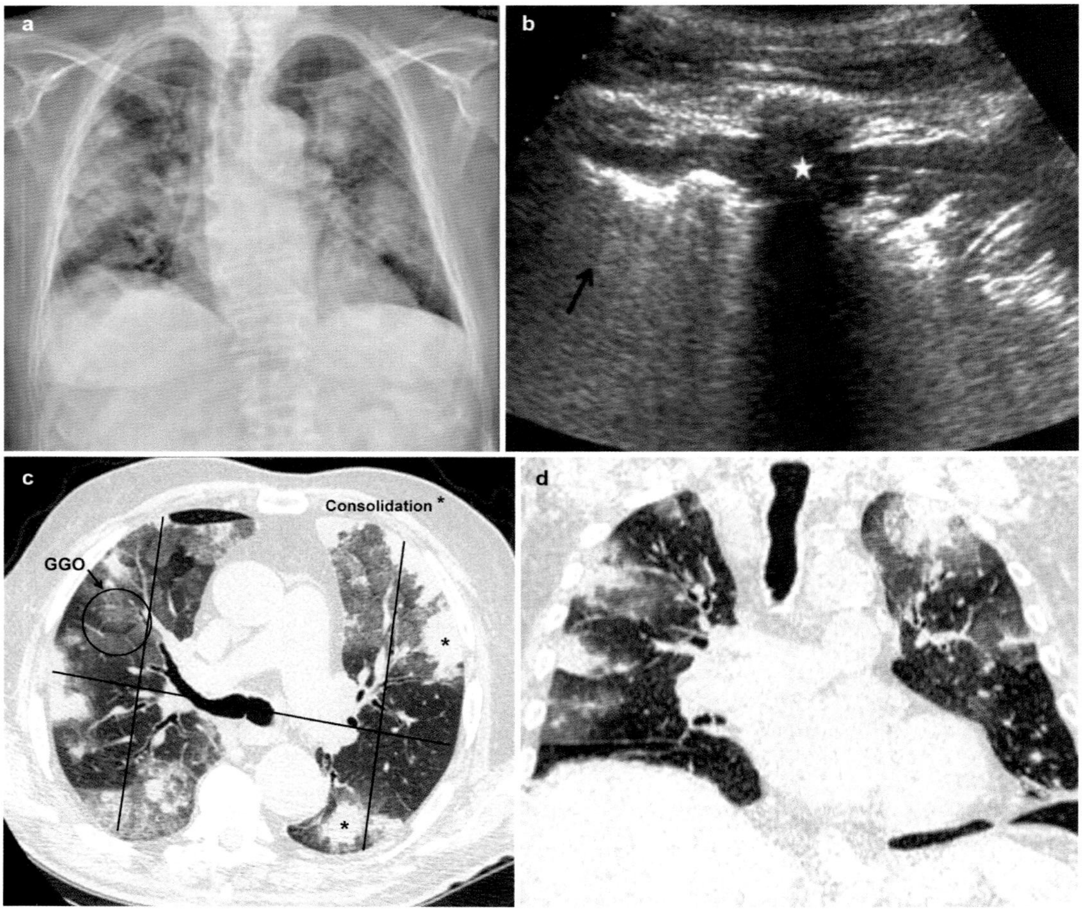

Fig. 20 Integrated imaging (CXR, US, MDCT) in a non-smoking, previously healthy 35-year-old man was presented in the emergency room after an unintentional exposure to chlorine gas at a community swimming pool. (**a**) CXR on presentation shows patchy bilateral lung consolidations. (**b**) Complementary LUS axial scan on the anterior chest at the fifth intercostal space shows focal consolidation (*star*) and aerated lung (*arrow*), without pleural effusion. MDCT (**c**) axial and (**d**) coronal reconstruction scans better demonstrate the extent of focal consolidations (*) and GGO areas; in (**c**) it has shown an example of radiologist's score (RADS) findings in chest CT axial scan (see text)

In contrast to cardiogenic pulmonary edema, which clears in response to diuretic therapy, ARDS persists for days to weeks. In addition, as the initial radiographic findings of ARDS clear, the underlying lung appears to have a reticular pattern secondary to type 2 pneumocyte proliferation and fibrosis.

In the *acute exudative phase,* pleural effusion, cardiomegaly, and septal lines are typically absent (Gluecker et al. 1999). Injury may progress to mucosal sloughing and intrapulmonary hemorrhage with mechanical obstruction of lower airways, hemoptysis, and flooding of alveoli. Rarely, early alveolar flooding may be caused by retrograde bronchorrhea.

On CXR lung opacities are bilateral, diffuse, patchy, or homogeneous, involving at least three quadrants, and cannot be fully explained by pleural effusion, atelectasis, or nodules (Fig. 21) (Lee and O'Connell 1988; Wittram and Kenny 1994; DiPoce et al. 2012; Fanelli et al. 2013). LUS is superior to auscultation and complementary to bedside CXR in the detection and follow-up of the main lung pathologic entities in ARDS (pleural

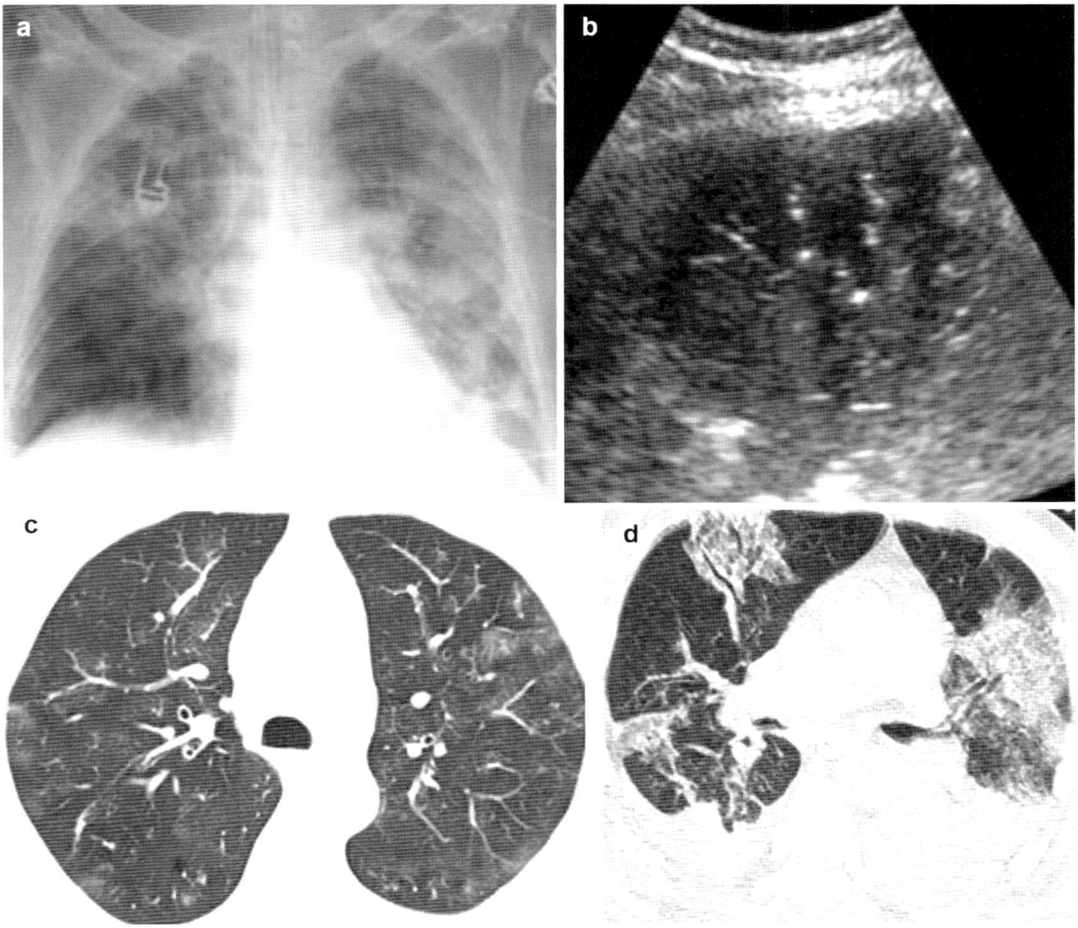

Fig. 21 Integrated imaging (CXR, US, MDCT) in a 43-year-old man working in a chemical industry who was admitted to the emergency department with a complaint of shortness of breath and hemoptysis, which began 3 h after accidental inhalation of nitric acid fumes from falling over the unlocked nitric acid container. He was urgently intubated for respiratory failure approximately 5 h after exposure, and copious serosanguinous secretion was aspirated from endotracheal tube. (**a**) CXR on admission shows bilateral ground-glass opacities. (**b**) Complementary LUS sagittal scan on the lateral chest at the seventh intercostal space shows focal consolidation in the lower left lobe. MDCT (**c**, **d**) axial scans show GGO patchy areas in the upper lobes and widespread GGO with early consolidations in both lower lobes and pleural effusion. Nitric acid is commonly used in various industries and its accidental spillage generates oxides of nitrogen, including nitrogen dioxide, a potent lung toxin when inhaled

effusion, alveolar consolidations, and alveolar-interstitial syndrome), when considering CT as the reference for a correct diagnosis (Lichtenstein et al. 2004; Lichtenstein et al. 2014).

Few hours after injury, MDCT on admission can show subtle ground-glass opacifications with mainly peribronchial distribution and patchy peribronchial consolidations centrally located (Oh et al. 2012; Yamamura et al. 2013) and can be semiquantitatively utilized as a means of stratifying inhalation injury by semiautomated measure of the abnormal lung parenchymal areas: each quadrant of each slice is scored subjectively adding the highest radiologist's score (RADS) (0 = normal, 1 = interstitial markings, 2 = ground-glass appearance, and 3 = consolidation) (Park et al. 2003; Oh et al. 2012). A high RADS score (>8 per slice) in addition to a positive bronchoscopy (high AIS score) was associated with a high probability (12.7-fold increase) of pneumonia, acute lung injury/ARDS, and death, thus showing the potential for chest CT to complement bronchoscopy in detecting clinically significant inhalation injury (Oh et al. 2012). Yamamura et al. used CT imaging to demonstrate the significant association between bronchial wall thickness (BWT) on admission and development of pneumonia; BWT, measured 2 cm distal from the tracheal bifurcation at three time points (at admission, 24 h after, and 7 days after admission), may be a predictor of the severity of SII (Yamamura et al. 2013) (Fig. 22). While the BWT of the normal volunteers is <2 mm, on admission BWT cutoff value of >3.0 mm can predict the total number of ventilator days, ICU stay days, and pneumonia development with a sensitivity of 79 %, specificity of 96 %, positive predictive value of 91 %, and a negative predictive value of 88 % (Yamamura et al. 2013).

In the acute exudative ARDS stage, MDCT shows a gravitationally dependent gradient, with more consolidation in the posterobasal regions, as a result of compressive gravitational forces (Gattinoni and Pesenti 2005). In the acute phase of ARDS, MDCT scans, notwithstanding the difficulties and risks of moving patients from and to the ICU, typically show a nonhomogeneous distribution and a ventrodorsal gradient of density, with more dense consolidations in the dependent regions, widespread ground-glass opacities, and relatively normal or hyperinflated parenchyma (in case of mechanical ventilation) in nondependent areas. Atypical ARDS, characterized by predominantly anterior consolidations in supine decubitus, can be observed in 5 % of patients during the first stage of the disease, probably due to regional differences in ventilation. MDCT predictors of mortality are >80 % of lung involvement, enlargement of the right atrium, or development of traction varicoid bronchiectasis (Chung et al. 2011; Kligerman et al. 2013).

In the *subacute stage or postresuscitation phase* (2–6 days post-injury, characterized by mucosal necrosis and slough, viscous secretions, and distal airway obstruction with atelectasis, pulmonary interstitial edema, and bronchopneumonia), imaging studies are directed toward monitoring

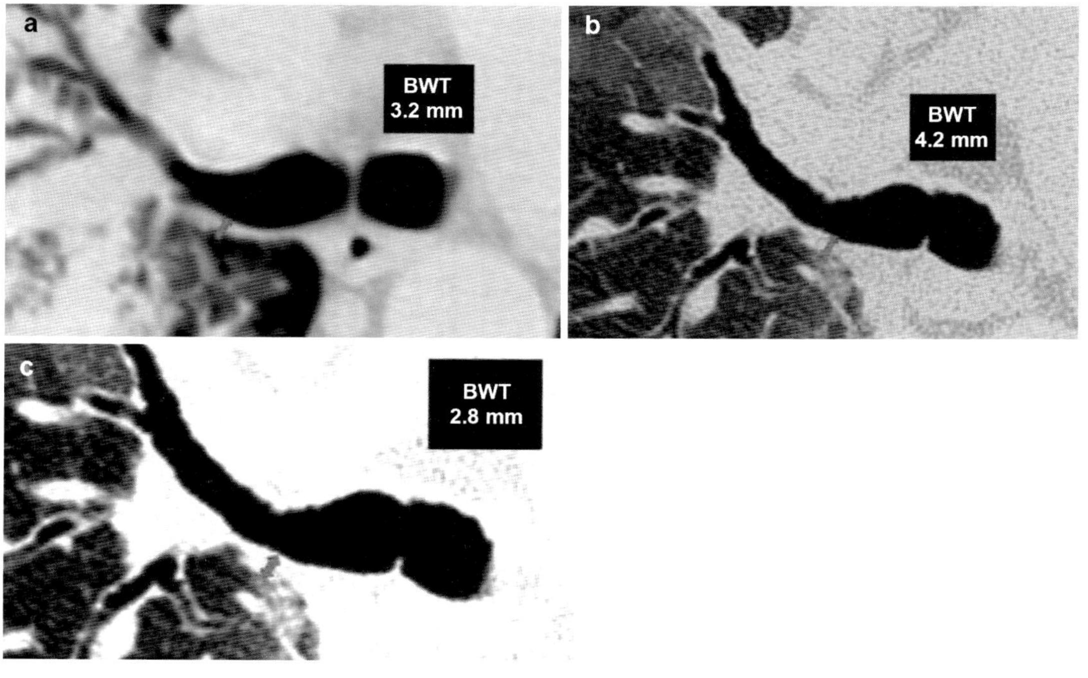

Fig. 22 Indices of bronchial wall thickness (*BWT*) on noncontrast 1 mm helical scan according Yamamura et al. (2013) in a case of smoke inhalation injury (SII). The *double headed arrows* indicate the measurement of bronchial wall thickness (*BWT*) was 3.2 mm on admission (**a**), 4.2 mm after 6 days (**b**), and 2.8 mm after 10 days (**c**). This patient had associated pneumonia and remained in the ICU for 13 days

pulmonary complications in the hospitalized patient (e.g., in burn victims, ranges are from 15 to 42 %), including infection, septicemia, ARDS, barotraumas (usually from intubation and positive pressure ventilation), multiorgan failure (MOF), and fluid overload (George et al. 2003). In severely burned patients in ICU, it may be difficult to discriminate among these various components on CXR. The most challenging differential diagnosis is still between ARDS and cardiogenic edema. Because these lung complications are associated with a significant increase in mortality, ranging from 50 to 89 %, diagnosis of pulmonary injury is important for both therapeutic and prognostic considerations and must be performed, if it is possible, by thin-slice MDCT. Early signs of barovolutrauma often correspond to interstitial emphysema and subpleural cystic airspaces. Subsequently, imaging studies can demonstrate the development of pneumomediastinum, pneumothorax (often hypertensive in mechanically ventilated patients), and subcutaneous emphysema (Gattinoni et al. 2006) (Fig. 23).

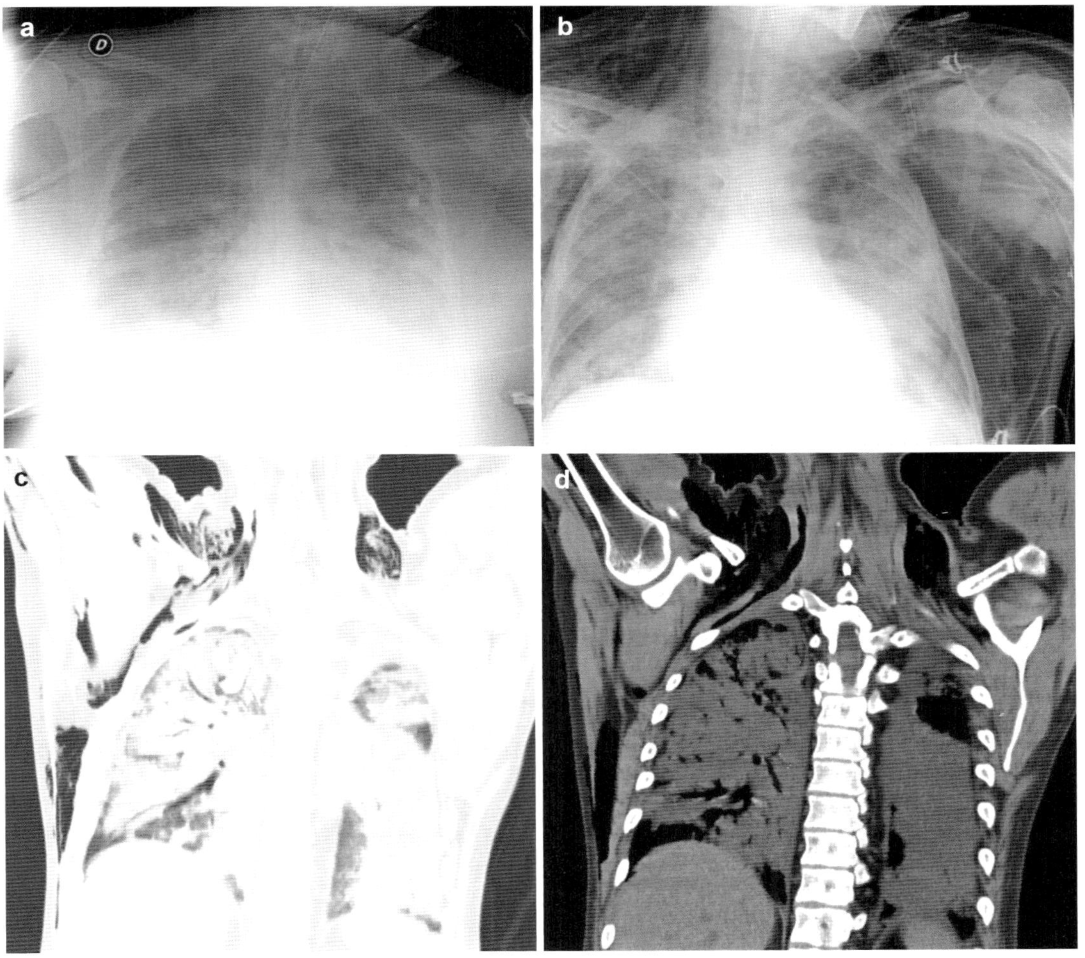

Fig. 23 A 47-year-old male, working at plating industry, was accidentally exposed to HNO3 vapor for 3–4 min. After that accident, he shows mild dyspnea. He suffered from no underlying disease. Ten hours after exposure, ICU admission (**a**) CXR shows diffuse bilateral coalescent GGO opacities in lower lobes. Next day (**b**) follow-up CXR shows extensive pulmonary consolidations appeared at the mid-lower lobes and diffuse subcutaneous emphysema. Four days later, MDCT (**c**, **d**) coronal reconstructions show bilateral progressing consolidations, pleural effusion, and a severe pneumomediastinum with subcutaneous emphysema

Extracorporeal membrane oxygenation (ECMO) is a therapy that has been used in severe cases of ARDS when patients fail to improve with traditional management (Koh 2014).

The *inflammatory–infection phase* and *chronic sequelae of acute exposures* are approximately 7 days and beyond in the post-injury period and continues until there are lung healing and burn wound closure. In intermediate or proliferative phase of ARDS, reticular opacities may appear in the diffuse and persisting background of alveolar opacities; however, unless iatrogenic complications or superimposed pneumonia develops, the radiological findings are rather stable in this phase. The extent of CT opacities (>80 % of lung volume), along with the presence of bronchiectasis, honeycombing, and signs of pulmonary hypertension (dilatation of pulmonary arteries and right ventricle), indicates early fibrosis and predicts mortality (Ichikado et al. 2006). In the later or fibrotic ARDS stage, MDCT generally demonstrates persistent ground-glass densities and reticulations, air cysts, and bullae, mainly located in the ventral regions of the lung, more often than CXR (Masclans et al. 2011). Late exposure complications such as occupational asthma, reactive airway dysfunction syndrome (RADS), increased airway responsiveness, and decreased residual volume have been described. Chronic effects of lower respiratory tract injury include bronchiolitis obliterans, bronchiolitis obliterans organizing pneumonia (BOOP), and pulmonary fibrosis. Bronchiolitis obliterans produces a pattern of fixed airway obstruction that may develop several weeks after injury, following a period in which symptoms improve. Granulation tissue plugs develop within small airways and alveolar ducts, accompanied by small airway destruction with obliterative fibrous scarring.

3.5 Some Unique Pulmonary Acute Toxins and Toxicants

3.5.1 Smoke Inhalation Injury (SII)

"Smoke inhalation" is a generic term that refers to a potential exposure to a wide variety of substances because of the complex chemistry of heat decomposition and pyrolysis (Glazer 2003; Miller and Chang 2003). Thermal airway injury is generally limited to supraglottic structures, whereas injury to the lower airway is chemical in nature. Smoke inhalation injury (SII) complicates burns in approximately 10–20 % of patients and is a major cause of mortality in burn patients because it can trigger pneumonia, acute respiratory distress syndrome (ARDS), and problems with fluid balance (El-Helbawi and Ghareeb 2011; You et al. 2014). Victims of fire accidents may be divided into three categories: those suffering only cutaneous injury, those with cutaneous and inhalational injury, and those with inhalational injury alone (Dries and Endorf 2013). Cutaneous burns are assessed in percent of total body surface area (TBSA) affected by the burn and by evaluating the burn depth. The soot present on the face, in the nose, or in the mouth of a fire victim must raise the suspicion of the inhalation injury. The injury may be limited to the upper airways and manifested by nasopharyngeal irritation, hoarseness, stridor, and dry cough or may extend deeper causing tracheobronchial and alveolar destruction with the symptoms of dyspnea, chest discomfort, bronchial breath sounds, wheezing, rales, cyanosis, and carbonaceous sputum. An abnormal CXR in the first 48 h was stated to be a poor prognostic indicator (Wittram and Kenny 1994; Miller and Chang 2003). The noxious products of combustion induce a laryngotracheobronchitis that may be severe enough to be hemorrhagic, ulcerative, or necrotizing. Surfactant and the surfactant-producing type II pneumocytes may be destroyed or damaged, leading to a DAD, loss of lung compliance, and the damaged vascular endothelium leading to an increased microvascular permeability with resultant edema (Fig. 24).

3.5.2 Paraquat (PQ)

Paraquat is a diquaternary amine aromatic nonselective herbicide whose unintentional or intentional poisoning and mucosal exposure can result in frequently fatal pulmonary toxicity, and this is why it is restricted in some countries. Although it can induce oxygen radical

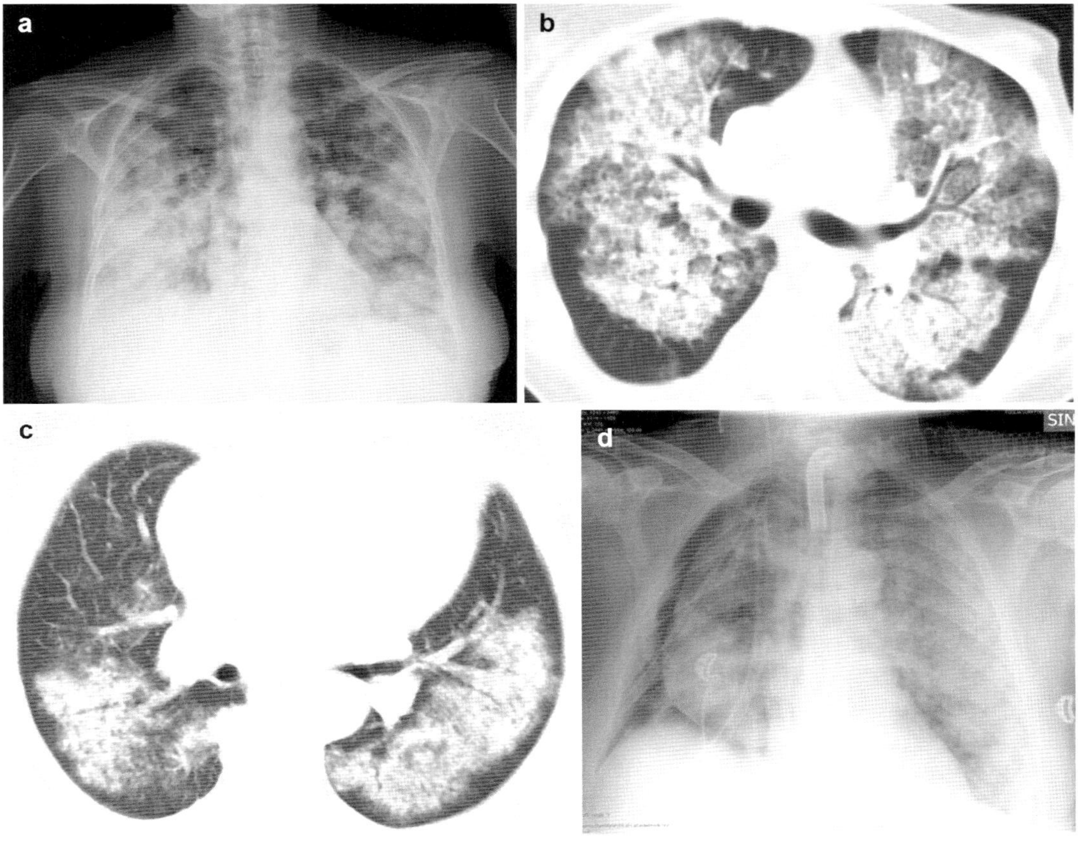

Fig. 24 A 44-year-old man with extensive burns (24% TBSA) from intentional pouring of petrol, who was then set on fire, with acute presentation and early ICU admission. On the first day, bedside ED (**a**) CXR shows bilateral consolidations. On the fourth day, (**b**, **c**) MDCT axial scans show diffuse bilateral ground-glass opacities sparing the lung periphery and the absence of pleural effusions that are typical of noncardiogenic pulmonary edema. (**d**) Follow-up CXR on the sixth day shows right pneumothorax

formation in all tissues, a structural homology results in its active uptake by pneumocytes from the circulation. The high concentration of polyamine transporters on the luminal side of the type I and type II pneumocytes and club (formerly Clara) cells results in as much as a tenfold concentration of PQ in the pneumocytes (Zhang et al. 2013). Should patients survive the initial caustic ingestion, progressive pulmonary fibrosis with death occurring up to a month later can be expected. In the shortly exposed survivor group, thin-section CT may show ground-glass opacities, consolidations, pleural effusion, and early fibrosis findings (Im et al. 1991; Lee et al. 1995; Kim et al. 2009; Zhang et al. 2013).

3.5.3 Silica

More commonly, chronic inhalation of small amounts of silica (SiO_2), 0.05 mg/m_3, results in predominantly upper lung zone deposition of silica dust that leads to the formation of 1-mm to 10-mm inflammatory nodules and results in local tissue damage. With high-intensity silica acute inhalation, as might be rarely seen in sandblasting or mining, a proliferation of type II pneumocytes can occur, with alveolar proteinosis from excessive surfactant production. This condition is known as acute silicosis also called silicoproteinosis (Dee et al. 1978; Marchiori et al. 2007). Thin-section CT scans show a diffuse GGO (ground-glass opacity) or alveolar pattern with septal thickening, similar

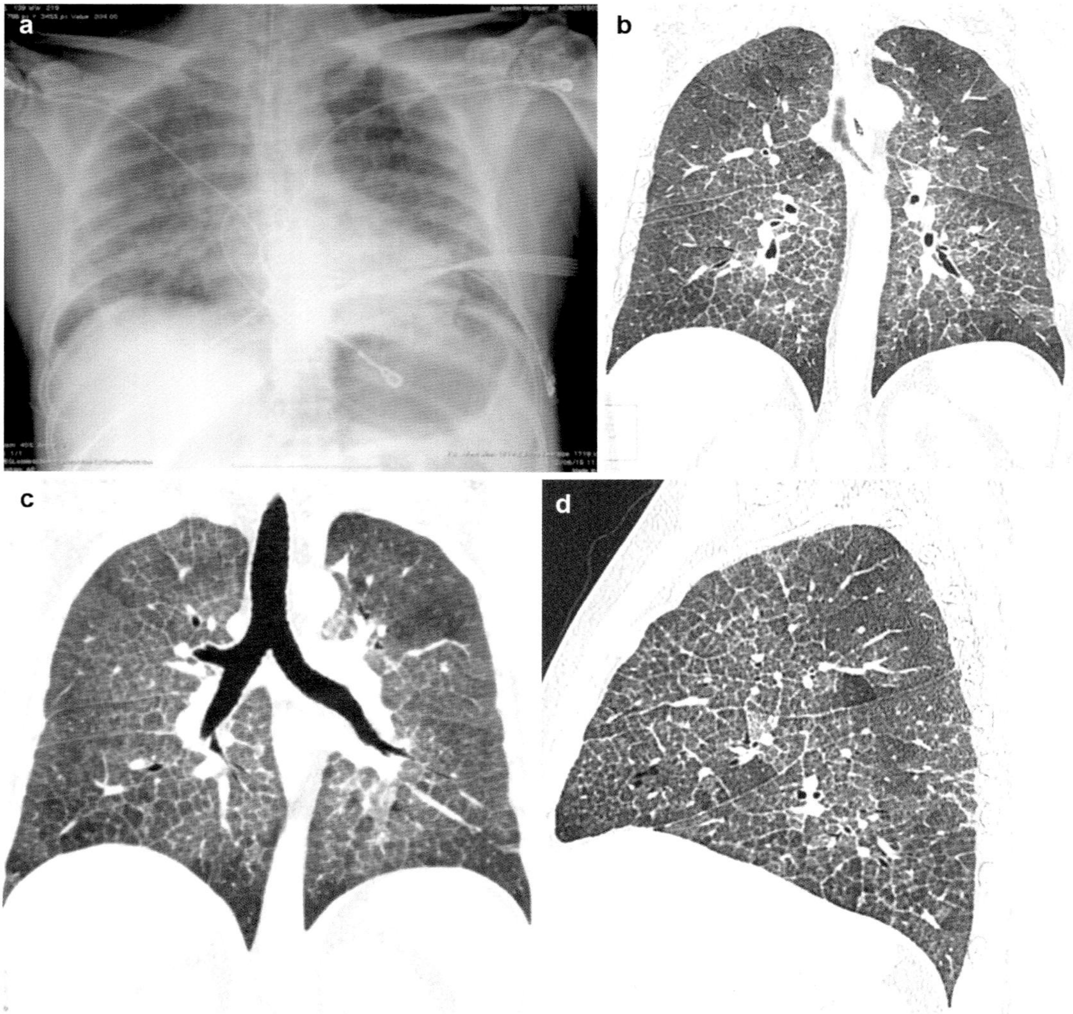

Fig. 25 A rare case of acute silicosis in a 45-year-old-man that was heavily exposed (buried for about 7 h) to very high concentrations of fine silica debris due to the outbreak of his house. He suffered from no underlying disease and had bilateral femoral necks and acetabular comminuted fractures. After about 1 week from the trauma, he presented dyspnea and dry cough. On the sixth day, (**a**) CXR showed diffuse ground-glass appearance of all lung fields. On the eighth day, chest MDCT (**b**, **c**) coronal and (**d**) sagittal reconstructions showed a "crazy-paving" pattern, highly suggestive of secondary alveolar proteinosis

to pulmonary alveolar proteinosis (Buechner and Ansari 1969) (Fig. 25).

3.6 Summary

The lungs can be an efficient means for the absorption of inhaled toxicants, resulting in airway and pulmonary injury or systemic toxicity. Although a few specific antidotes exist for inhaled toxicants, the syndrome of acute inhalation injury and clinical therapeutics are linked by common pathways of pathophysiology. Understanding and prompt diagnosis of the main imaging patterns of acute inhalation injury can simplify the decision-making process for the emergency physicians when confronted with a patient exposed to a myriad of potential inhaled toxicants.

References

Acute exposure guideline levels (AEGLs)|OPPT|US EPA. www.epa.gov/oppt/aegl/

Al Subie H, Fitzgerald DA (2010) Non-cystic fibrosis bronchiectasis. J Paediatr Child Health. doi:10.1111/j.1365-2230.2010.03857.x

Albright JM, Davis CS, Bird MD, Ramirez L, Kim H, Burnham EL et al (2012) The acute pulmonary inflammatory response to the graded severity of smoke inhalation injury. Crit Care Med 40:1113–21. doi:10.1097/CCM.0b013e3182374a67

Aysola RS, Hoffman EA, Gierada D et al (2008) Airway remodeling measured by multidetector computed tomography is increased in severe asthma and correlates with pathology. Chest 134(6):1183–91

Baik JH, Ahn MI, Park YH et al (2010) High-resolution CT findings of re-expansion pulmonary edema. Korean J Radiol 11(2):164–8. doi:10.3348/kjr.2010.11.2.164

Bankier AA, Fleischmann D, Mallek R et al (1996) Bronchial wall thickness: Appropriate window settings for thin-section CT and radiologic-anatomic correlation. Radiology 199:831–6

Bartsch P, Mairbaurl H, Maggiorini M et al (2005) Physiological aspects of high altitude pulmonary edema. J Appl Phys 98:1101–10

Betancourt SL, Martinez-Jimenez S et al (2010) Lipoid pneumonia: spectrum of clinical and radiologic manifestations. AJR Am J Roentgenol 194:103–9

Bhalla M, Turcios N, Aponte V et al (1991) Cystic fibrosis: scoring system with thin-section CT. Radiology 179:783–8

Bonavita J, Naidich PD (2012) Imaging of bronchiectasis. Clin Chest Med 33:233–248

Borron SW, Bebarta VS (2015) Asphyxiants. Emerg Med Clin North Am 33:89–115, http://dx.doi.org/10.1016/j.emc.2014.09.014

Boyton RJ (2012) Bronchiectasis. Medicine. Respir Dis 40(5):267–272

Brander PE, Taskinen E, Stenius-Aarniala B (1992) Fire-eater's lung. Eur Respir J 5:112–114

Brillet PY, Fetita CI, Capderou A et al (2009) Variability of bronchial measurements obtained by sequential CT using two computer-based methods. Eur Radiol 19:1139–47

Brody AS, Sucharew H, Campbell JD et al (2005) Computed tomography correlates with pulmonary exacerbations in children with cystic fibrosis. Am J Respir Crit Care Med 172:1128–1132

Bruzzi JF, Remy-Jardin M, Delhaye D et al (2006) Multidetector row CT of hemoptysis. Radiographics 26:3–22

Buechner HA, Ansari A (1969) Acute silico-proteinosis: a new pathologic variant of acute silicosis in sandblasters, characterized by histologic features resembling alveolar proteinosis. Dis Chest 55:274–278

Bynum LD, Pierce AK (1976) Pulmonary aspiration of gastric contents. Am Rev Respir Dis 114:1129–1136

Causey A, Tilelli J, Swanson M (2000) Predicting discharge in uncomplicated near drowning. Am J Emerg Med 18:9–11

Chang AB, Bilton D (2008) Exacerbations in cystic fibrosis: 4 – non-cystic fibrosis bronchiectasis. Thorax 63:269–76. doi:10.1136/thx.2006.060913

Chung JH, Kradin RL, Greene RE et al (2011) CT predictors of mortality in pathology confirmed ARDS. Eur Radiol 21:730–737

Cole PJ (1984) A new look at the pathogenesis, management of persistent bronchial sepsis: a 'vicious circle' hypothesis and its logical therapeutic connotations. In: Davies RJ (ed) Strategies for the management of chronic bacterial sepsis. Medicine Publishing Foundation, Oxford, pp 1–20

Currie DC, Cooke JC, Morgan AD et al (1987) Interpretation of bronchograms and chest radiographs in patients with chronic sputum production. Thorax 42:278–284

Darling GE, Keresteci MA, Ibanez D et al (1996) Pulmonary complications in inhalation injuries with associated cutaneous burn. J Trauma 40:83–89

Davies G, Wells AU, Doffman S, Watanabe S, Wilson R (2006) The effect of Pseudomonas aeruginosa on pulmonary function in patients with bronchiectasis. Eur Respir J 28:974–9

de Jong PA, Ottink MD, Robben SGF et al (2004) Pulmonary disease assessment in cystic fibrosis: comparison of CT scoring systems and value of bronchial and arterial dimension measurements. Radiology 231:434–439

Dee P, Suratt P, Winn W (1978) The radiographic findings in acute silicosis. Radiology 126:359–63

DiPoce J, Guelfguat M, DiPoce J (2012) Radiologic findings in cases of attempted suicide and other self-injurious behavior. Radiographics 32:2005–2024

Dodd JD, Souza CA, Muller NL (2006) Conventional high-resolution CT versus helical high-resolution MDCT in the detection of bronchiectasis. AJR Am J Roentgenol 187:414–420

Dries DJ, Endorf FW (2013) Inhalation injury: epidemiology, pathology, treatment strategies. Scand J Trauma Resusc Emerg Med 21:31

Du Rand I, Maskell N, Hooper C, Lee YCG et al (2010) British Thoracic Society Pleural Disease Guideline Group: a sub-group of the British Thoracic Society Standards of Care Committee. Management of spontaneous pneumothorax. Thorax 65(Suppl 2):ii18–eii31. doi:10.1136/thx.2010.136986

Echevarria C, Twomey D, Dunning J et al (2008) Does re-expansion pulmonary oedema exist? Interact Cardiovasc Thorac Surg 7:485–9

El-Helbawi RH, Ghareeb FM (2011) Inhalation injury as a prognostic factor for mortality in burn patients. Ann Burns Fire Disasters XXIV(2):82–88

Endorf FW, Gamelli RL (2007) Inhalation injury, pulmonary perturbations, and fluid resuscitation. J Burn Care Res 28:80–83

Fagenholz PJ, Gutman JA, Murray AF et al (2007) Chest ultrasonography for the diagnosis and monitoring of high-altitude pulmonary edema. Chest 131:1013–8

Fanelli V, Vlachou A, Ghannadian S et al (2013) Acute respiratory distress syndrome. New definition, current and future therapeutic options. J Thorac Dis 5:326–334
Feldman C (2011) Bronchiectasis: new approaches to diagnosis and management. Clin Chest Med 32:535–546. doi:10.1016/j.ccm.2011.05.002
Ferguson ND, Fan E, Camporota L et al (2012) The Berlin definition of ARDS: an expanded rationale, justification, and supplementary material. Intensive Care Med 38:1537–1582
Franquet T, Gimenez A, Roson N et al (2000) Aspiration diseases: findings, pitfalls, and differential diagnosis. Radiographics 20:673–85
Fujimoto K, Kitaguchi Y, Kubo K et al (2006) Clinical analysis of chronic obstructive pulmonary disease phenotypes classified using high-resolution computed tomography. Respirology 11:731–40
Garnier R (1998) Acute toxic pneumopathies. Rev Prat 48:1319–23
Gattinoni L, Pesenti A (2005) The concept of "baby lung". Intensive Care Med 31:776–784
Gattinoni L, Caironi P, Valenza F et al (2006) The role of CT-scan studies for the diagnosis and therapy of acute respiratory distress syndrome. Clin Chest Med 27:559–570
George A, Gupta R, Bang RL, Ebrahim MK (2003) Radiological manifestation of pulmonary complications in deceased intensive care burn patients. Burns 29:73–78
Glazer CS (2003) Acute inhalational injury. In: Hanley ME, Welsh CH (eds) Current diagnosis & treatment in pulmonary medicine, Internationalth edn. Mc-Graw Hill, New York, pp 354–60
Gluecker T, Capasso P, Schnyder P et al (1999) Clinical and radiologic features of pulmonary edema. Radiographics 19(6):1507–31
Goeminne P, Dupont L (2010) Non-cystic fibrosis bronchiectasis: diagnosis and management in 21st century. Postgrad Med J 86:493–501
Gorguner M, Aslan S, Inandi T, Cakir Z (2004) Reactive airways dysfunction syndrome in housewives due to a bleach-hydrochloric acid mixture. Inhal Toxicol 16:87–91
Gotway MB, Lee ES, Reddy GP et al (2000) Low-dose, dynamic, expiratory thin-section CT of the lungs using a spiral CT scanner. J Thorac Imaging 15:168–72
Grenier P, Maurice F, Musset D et al (1986) Bronchiectasis: assessment by thin-section CT. Radiology 161:95–99
Gudbjerg CE (1955) Roentgenologic diagnosis of bronchiectasis. An analysis of 112 cases. Acta Radiol 43:209–217
Guimaraes MD, Bitencourt AGV, Marchiori E, Chojniak R, Gross JL, Kundra V (2014) Imaging acute complications in cancer patients: what should be evaluated in the emergency setting? Cancer Imaging 14:18
Hansell DM (1998) Bronchiectasis. Radiol Clin North Am 36:107–28
Hansell DM, Bankier AA, MacMahon H, McLoud TC, Müller NL, Remy J (2008) Fleischner Society: glossary of terms for thoracic imaging. Radiology 246:697–722. doi:10.1148/radiol.2462070712
Hassan Z, Wong JK, Bush J, Bayat A, Dunn KW (2010) Assessing the severity of inhalation injuries in adults. Burns 36:212–6. doi:10.1016/j.burns.2009.06.205
Heitkamp DE, Mohammed TL, Kirsch J et al (2012) ACR appropriateness criteria (®)acute respiratory illness in immunocompromised patients. J Am Coll Radiol 9:164–9
Hill LE, Ritchie G, Wightman AJ, Hill AT, Murchison JT (2010) Comparison between conventional interrupted high-resolution CT and volume multidetector CT acquisition in the assessment of bronchiectasis. Br J Radiol 83:67–70
Houston CS (1960) Acute pulmonary edema of high altitude. N Engl J Med 263:478–80
Hunter TB, Whitehouse WM (1974) Fresh-water near-drowning: radiological aspects. Radiology 112:51–56
Ichikado K, Suga M, Muranaka H et al (2006) Prediction of prognosis for acute respiratory distress syndrome with thin section CT: validation in 44 cases. Radiology 238:321–329
Idris AH, Berg RA, Bierens J et al (2003) Recommended guidelines for uniform reporting of data from drowning: the "Utstein style". Circulation 108:2565–74
Im JG, Lee KS, Han MC, Kim SJ, Kim IO (1991) Paraquat poisoning: findings on chest radiography and CT in 42 patients. AJR Am J Roentgenol 157:697–701. doi:10.2214/ajr.157.4.1892020
Javidan-Nejad C, Bhalla S (2009) Bronchiectasis. Radiol Clin North Am 47:289–306. doi:10.1016/j.rcl.2008.11.006
Javidan-Nejad C, Bhalla S (2010) Bronchiectasis. Thorac Surg Clin 20:85–102
Kales SN, Christiani DC (2004) Acute chemical emergencies. N Engl J Med 350:800–8
Kim JS, Muller NL, Park CS et al (1997a) Bronchoarterial ratio on thin section CT: comparison between high altitude and sea level. J Comput Assist Tomogr 21:306–311
Kim JS, Muller NL, Park CS et al (1997b) Cylindrical bronchiectasis: diagnostic findings on thin-section CT. AJR Am J Roentgenol 168:751–754
Kim YT, Jou SS, Lee HS, Gil HW, Yang JO, Lee EY et al (2009) The area of ground glass opacities of the lungs as a predictive factor in acute paraquat intoxication. J Korean Med Sci 24:636–40. doi:10.3346/jkms.2009.24.4.636
King PT, Daviskas E (2010) Pathogenesis and diagnosis of bronchiectasis. Breathe 6:343–51
Kligerman S, Franks T, Galvin J (2013) Organization and fibrosis as a response to lung injury in diffuse alveolar damage, organizing pneumonia, and acute fibrinous and organizing pneumonia. Radiographics 33:1951–1975
Koh Y (2014) Update in acute respiratory distress syndrome. J Intensive Care 2:2. doi:10.1186/2052-0492-2-2. http://www.jintensivecare.com/content/2/1/2
Koljonen V, Maisniemi K, Virtanen K, Koivikko M (2007) Multi-detector computed tomography demonstrates smoke inhalation injury at early stage. Emerg Radiol 14:113–6
Kosucu P, Ahmetoglu A, Koramaz J et al (2004) Low-dose MDCT and virtual bronchoscopy in pediatric patients

with foreign body aspiration. AJR Am J Roentgenol 183:1771–1777
Laurent F, Philippe JC, Vergier B et al (1999) Exogenous lipoid pneumonia: HRCT, MR, and pathologic findings. Eur Radiol 9:1190–96
Lee MJ, O'Connell DJ (1988) The plain chest radiograph after acute smoke inhalation. Clin Radiol 39:33–37
Lee SH, Lee KS, Ahn JM, Kim SH, Hong SY (1995) Paraquat poisoning of the lung: thin-section CT findings. Radiology 195:271–4
Lichtenstein D, Goldstein D, Mourgeon E et al (2004) Comparative diagnostic performances of auscultation, chest radiography, and lung ultrasonography in acute respiratory distress syndrome. Anesthesiology 100:9–15
Lichtenstein D (2014) Lung ultrasound in the critically ill. Curr Opin Crit Care 20:315–22
Lichtenstein D, van Hooland S, Elbers P, Malbrain ML (2014) Ten good reasons to practice ultrasound in critical care. Anaesthesiol Intensive Ther 46:323–35. doi: 10.5603/AIT.2014.0056
Lynch DA (1998) Imaging of asthma and allergic bronchopulmonary mycosis. Radiol Clin North Am 36(1):129–42
Marchiori E, Souza CA, Barbassa TG et al (2007) Silicoproteinosis: high-resolution CT findings in 13 patients. AJR Am J Roentgenol 189:1402–6
Martinez S, Heyneman LE, McAdams HP, Rossi SE, Restrepo CS, Eraso A (2008) Mucoid impactions: finger-in-glove sign and other CT and radiographic features. Radiographics 28:1369–82
Masclans JR, Roca O, Munoz X et al (2011) Quality of life, pulmonary function, and tomographic scan abnormalities after ARDS. Chest 139:1340–1346
McCollough CH, Primak AN, Braun N, Kofler J, Yu L, Christner J (2009) Strategies for reducing radiation dose in CT. Radiol Clin North Am 47:27–40
McCurdy MT, Shanholtz CB (2012) Oncologic emergencies. Crit Care Med 40:2212–2222
McKay CA Jr (2014) Toxin-induced respiratory distress. Emerg Med Clin North Am 32:127–147, http://dx.doi.org/10.1016/j.emc.2013.09.003
Micak RP, Suman OE, Herndon DN (2007) Respiratory management of inhalation injury. Burns 33:2–13
Miller K, Chang A (2003) Acute inhalation injury. Emerg Med Clin North Am 21:533–557
Milliron B, Henry TS, Veeraraghavan S, Little BP (2015) Bronchiectasis: mechanisms and imaging clues of associated common and uncommon diseases. Radiographics 35:1011–30. doi:10.1148/rg.2015140214
Mokhlesi B, Corbridge T (2003) Toxicology in the critically ill patient. Clin Chest Med 24:689–711
Montella S, Santamaria F, Salvatore M et al (2009) Assessment of chest high-field magnetic resonance imaging in children and young adults with noncystic fibrosis chronic lung disease: comparison to high resolution computed tomography and correlation with pulmonary function. Invest Radiol 44:532–8
Mosier MJ, Pham TN, Park DR, Simmons J, Klein MB, Gibran NS (2012) Predictive value of bronchoscopy in assessing the severity of inhalation injury. J Burn Care Res 33:65–73
Naidich DP, McCauley DI, Khouri NF et al (1982) Computed tomography of bronchiectasis. J Comput Assist Tomogr 6:437–444
Nelson LS, Hoffman RS (2006) Inhaled toxins. In: Marx JA, Hockberger RS, Walls RM (eds) Rosen's emergency medicine: concepts and clinical practice, 6th edn. Mosby Elsevier, Philadelphia
Oh JS, Chung KK, Allen A, Batchinsky AI, Huzar T, King BT et al (2012) Admission chest CT complements fiberoptic bronchoscopy in prediction of adverse outcomes in thermally injured patients. J Burn Care Res 33:532–8. doi:10.1097/BCR.0b013e318237455f
Oikonomou A, Tsanakas J, Hatziagorou E et al (2008) High resolution computed tomography of the chest in cystic fibrosis (CF): is simplification of scoring systems feasible? Eur Radiol 18:538–547
Ooi GC, Khong PL, Chan-Yeung M et al (2002) High-resolution CT quantification of bronchiectasis: clinical and functional correlation. Radiology 225:663–72
Pappalettera M, Aliberti S, Castellotti P et al (2009) Bronchiectasis: an update. Clin Respir J 3:1752–6981
Park MS, Cancio LC, Batchinsky AI, McCarthy MJ, Jordan BS, Brinkley WW et al (2003) Assessment of severity of ovine smoke inhalation injury by analysis of computed tomographic scans. J Trauma 55:417–27. doi:10.1097/01.TA.0000083609.24440.7F
Patel IS, Vlahos I, Wilkinson TM et al (2004) Bronchiectasis, exacerbation indices, and inflammation in chronic obstructive pulmonary disease. Am J Respir Crit Care Med 170:400–7
Pratali L, Cavana M, Sicari R et al (2010) Frequent subclinical high-altitude pulmonary edema detected by chest sonography as ultrasound lung comets in recreational climbers. Crit Care Med 38:1818–23
Putman CE, Loke J, Matthay RA, Ravin CE (1977) Radiographic manifestations of acute smoke inhalation. AJR Am J Roentgenol 129:865–70. doi:10.2214/ajr.129.5.865
Quint LE (2009) Thoracic complications and emergencies in oncologic patients. Cancer Imaging 9:S75–S82
Rabe KF, Hurd S, Anzueto A et al (2007) Global strategy for the diagnosis, management, and prevention of chronic obstructive pulmonary disease: GOLD executive summary. Am J Respir Crit Care Med 176: 532–55
Rabinowitz PM, Siegel MD (2002) Acute inhalation injury. Clin Chest Med 23:707–715
Reid LM (1950) Reduction in bronchial subdivision in bronchiectasis. Thorax 5:233–47
Reske A, Bak Z, Samuelsson A, Morales O, Seiwerts M, Sjöberg F (2005) Computed tomography – a possible aid in the diagnosis of smoke inhalation injury? Acta Anaesthesiol Scand 49:257–60
Rossi SE, Franquet T, Volpacchio M et al (2005) Tree-in-bud pattern at thin-section CT of the lungs: radiologic-pathologic overview. Radiographics 25:789–801
Salem H, Katz SA (eds) (2015) Inhalation toxicology, 3rd edn. CRC Press/Taylor & Francis group, Boca Raton
Shoemark A, Ozerovitch L, Wilson R (2007) Aetiology in adult patients with bronchiectasis. Respir Med 191:1163–70

Siafakas NM, Anthonisen NR, Georgopoulos D (eds) (2004) Management of acute exacerbation of COPD. Marcel Dekker Inc., New York

Studler U, Gluecker T, Bongartz G, Roth J, Steinbrich W (2005) Image quality from high-resolution CT of the lung: comparison of axial scans and of sections reconstructed from volumetric data acquired using MDCT. AJR Am J Roentgenol 185:602–7

Sung YM, Lee KS, Yi CA, Yoon YC, Kim TS, Kim S (2003) Additional coronal images using low-milliamperage multidetector-row computed tomography: effectiveness in the diagnosis of bronchiectasis. J Comput Assist Tomogr 27:490–5

Swenson ER, Maggiorini M, Mongovin S et al (2002) Pathogenesis of high-altitude pulmonary edema: inflammation is not an etiologic factor. JAMA 287(17):2228–35

Szpilman D, Bierens JJLM, Handley AJ, Orlowski JP. (2012) Drowning. N Engl J Med 366:2012–10

Tan CK, Lai CC (2007) Neurogenic pulmonary edema. CMAJ 177(3):249–50

Tourigny PD, Hall C (2012) Diagnosis and management of environmental thoracic emergencies. Emerg Med Clin North Am 30:501–528. doi:10.1016/j.emc.2011.10.006

Westcott JL (1991) Bronchiectasis. Radiol Clin North Am 29:1031–42

Williamson JP, James AL, Phillips MJ et al (2009) Quantifying tracheobronchial tree dimensions: methods, limitations and emerging techniques. Eur Respir J 34:42–55

Wittram C, Kenny JB (1994) The admission chest radiograph after acute inhalation injury and burns. Br J Radiol 67:751–4

Woodring JH (1994) Improved plain film criteria for the diagnosis of bronchiectasis. J Ky Med Assoc 92:8–13

Woods AQ, Lynch DA (2009) Asthma: an imaging update. Radiol Clin North Am 47:317–329. doi:10.1016/j.rcl.2008.11.008

World Health Organization. Causes of death 2008 summary tables. Available at: http://www.who.int/evidence/bod. Accessed 14 June 2011

Yadav SP, Singh J, Aggarwall N et al (2007) Airway foreign bodies in children: experience of 132 cases. Singapore Med J 48:850–853

Yamamura H, Kaga S, Kaneda K et al (2013) Chest computed tomography performed on admission helps predict the severity of smoke-inhalation injury. Crit Care 17:R95. doi:10.1186/cc12740

You K, Yang HT, Kym D, Yoon J, Haejun Y, Cho YS et al (2014) Inhalation injury in burn patients: establishing the link between diagnosis and prognosis. Burns 40:1470–5. doi:10.1016/j.burns.2014.09.015

Young K, Aspestrand F, Kolbenstvedt A (1991) High resolution CT and bronchography in the assessment of bronchiectasis. Acta Radiol 32:439–41

Zhang H, Liu P, Qiao P, Zhou J, Zhao Y, Xing X, Li G (2013) CT imaging as a prognostic indicator for patients with pulmonary injury from acute paraquat poisoning. Br J Radiol 86(1026):20130035. doi:10.1259/bjr.20130035

Zissin R, Shapiro-Feinberg M, Rozenman J et al (2001) CT findings in the chest in adults with aspirated foreign bodies. Eur Radiol 11:606–611

Pleural Diseases

Selen Bayraktaroglu and Chiara Andreoli

Contents

Abstract

Pleurisy and Empyema

Pleural diseases are common and represent a significant contribution to the workload of emergency department.

Patients with pleural effusions may be asymptomatic; however, they generally present with symptoms such as pleuritic chest pain or dyspnea.

Imaging of Spontaneous Pneumothorax

Spontaneous pneumothorax is a relatively common cause of thoracic pain in young, thin, and tall males without preexistent lung diseases, although it is known that its occurrence is due to the rupture of underlying small subpleural bullae and blebs at the lung apices, found at thoracoscopy or detected on CT.

Signs and symptoms may be nonspecific, and often the clinical suspicion requests a diagnostic confirmation, primarily based on X-rays and, in complicated cases, on CT: in this chapter, the authors will review the radiological and CT signs of spontaneous pneumothorax and will discuss signs which can predict its recurrence and informations which strongly influence the management and the treatment choice.

S. Bayraktaroglu (✉)
Department of Radiology, Ege University Hospital, Izmir, Turkey
e-mail: selenb2000@gmail.com

C. Andreoli
Radiology, Emergency Department, La Sapienza University of Rome, Rome, Italy
e-mail: chiarandreoli@gmail.com

Med Radiol Diagn Imaging (2016)
DOI 10.1007/174_2016_43, © Springer International Publishing Switzerland

1 Pleurisy and Empyema

Selen Bayraktaroglu

1.1 Introduction

Pleural diseases are common and represent a significant contribution to the workload of emergency department.

Patients with pleural effusions may be asymptomatic; however, they generally present with symptoms such as pleuritic chest pain or dyspnea.

1.2 Terminology and Clinical Issues

The pleura is composed of visceral and parietal layers. The lungs and interlobar fissures are covered by the visceral pleura. The parietal pleura lines the mediastinum, ribs, and diaphragm. These two layers of pleura are continuous with one another. The area between the two layers is the pleural space. Normally, there is a small amount of fluid within pleural cavity (Collins and Sten 2008; White et al. 2009). Pathological processes may lead to the development of pleural effusions by causing disequilibrium between the rates of pleural fluid formation, pleural permeability, and pleural fluid absorption (Sahn 2008). The pleural fluid can originate from the pleura or may be extrapleural in origin. Pleural effusions may also be seen in the setting of infectious and inflammatory diseases, malignancies, and cardiovascular and systemic diseases (Table 1).

Table 1 Causes of pleural effusion

1. Infectious diseases (bacterial and viral pleurisy, tuberculosis)
2. Collagen vascular diseases (lupus pleuritis, rheumatoid pleurisy)
3. Neoplasm (pleural metastases, mesothelioma, leukemia, Non-Hodgkin lymphoma)
4. Pulmonary embolism
5. Cardiovascular disease (congestive heart failure, constrictive pericarditis)
6. Uremic pleuritis
7. Hypoalbuminemia
8. Chylothorax
9. Drug-induced pleural disease
10. Hypothyroidism
11. Pancreatitis
12. Subdiaphragmatic abscess
13. Hepatic hydrothorax
14. Trauma

1.3 Imaging

The chest X-ray (*CXR*) remains the initial examination of choice in the investigation of pleural disease. *Ultrasound* (*US*) is an easily applicable, cheap, and radiation-free method and is most frequently used to assess pleural disease detected on CXR. It can be performed at bedside. In addition to confirmation of pleural effusion, it may be used to guide aspiration or chest-drain insertion (Evans and Gleeson 2004). *Computed tomography* (*CT*) is a method that not only detects pleural space but also gives information about the lung parenchyma, mediastinum, and chest wall. CT has ability to determine the presence of pleural fluid loculations and pleural thickening, and it is the best method to differentiate peripheral lung abscess from empyema (King and Thomson 2002; McLoud 1998). Pleural fluid collections and pleural thickening that remain undetermined after CT may undergo *magnetic resonance imaging* (MRI) (Falaschi et al. 1996).

Positron emission tomography (*PET*) or *positron emission tomography-computed tomography* (*PET-CT*) is used in the detection of pleural malignancy and in differentiation between benign and malignant pleural disease (Duysinx et al. 2004; Goldsmith and Kostakoglu 2000).

1.4 Pleural Effusion and Emphyema

The appearance of pleural effusion depends on the patient's position at the time of the radiologic examination. Pleural fluid tends to collect along dependent surfaces. In an upright person, fluid collects mainly in the lower pleural space, and accumulation of 200 mL or

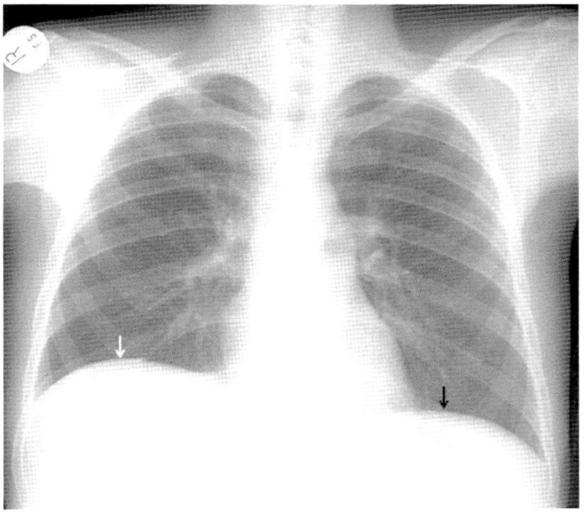

Fig. 1 Posteroanterior chest X-ray of a patient with right subpulmonic pleural effusion. Subpulmonic effusion can simulate elevated diaphragm. The peak of the elevated pseudo-diaphragm is more laterally located than normal (The *black arrow* demonstrates the peak point of left diaphragm, the *white arrow* shows the laterally located peak point of left pseudo-diaphragm)

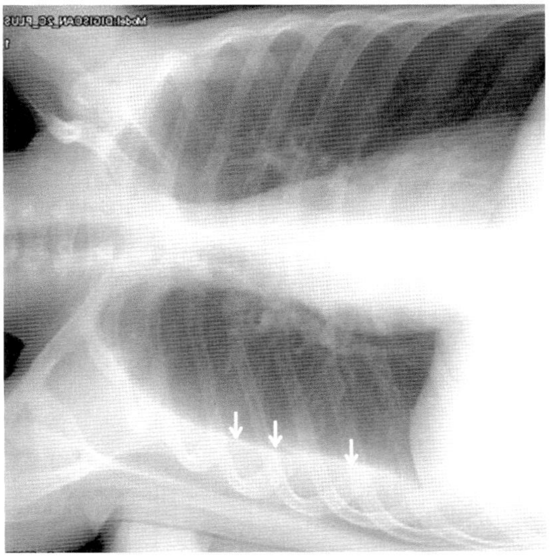

Fig. 2 Right lateral decubitis projection shows right pleural effusion by demonstrating the dependent layering of pleural fluid (*white arrows*)

more of fluid leads to blunting of the lateral costophrenic sulcus. However, it is important to note that the plain film can be normal with up to 500 mL fluid (Blackmore et al. 1996; Collins et al. 1972). As the amount of pleural fluid increases, the diaphragm appears flattened and a homogeneous lower zone opacity with a concave upward border develops. Occasionally, a large amount of pleural fluid may accumulate in the subpulmonic location and may be difficult to diagnose on erect CXR. In case of subpulmonic effusion, the upper edge of the fluid mimics the contour of the diaphragm on the chest radiograph creating an appearance similar to elevated diaphragm (pseudo-diaphragm). However, the peak of the elevated pseudo-diaphragm is more laterally located than normal (Müller 1993) (Figs. 1 and 2). The lateral decubitus view is sensitive in the detection of pleural fluid and can demonstrate as little as 5 mL of fluid. Large amounts of fluid can be missed on a supine radiograph. On a supine radiograph, as fluid accumulates on dependent surfaces, a general increased haziness over the lower pulmonary zones or a density over the apex of hemithorax develops (Fig. 3). Blunting of costophrenic angle may be seen (Müller 1993; Henschke et al. 1989).

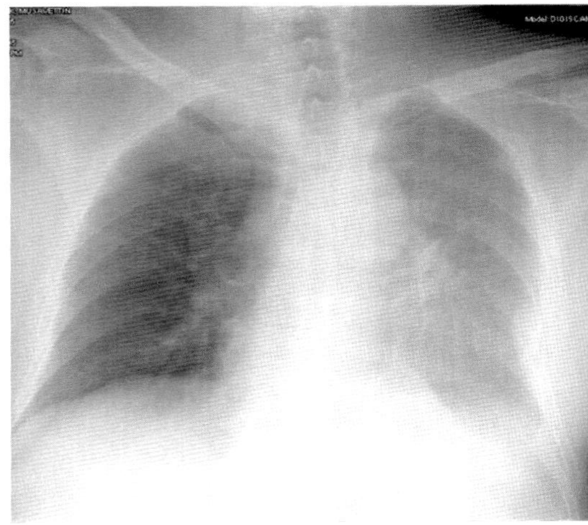

Fig. 3 Pleural effusion on left hemithorax on a supine radiograph. The pleural fluid accumulates on dependent surfaces leading to an increased haziness over the left pulmonary zones. There is blunting of left costophrenic angle

Loculated effusions can appear confusing on CXR and may be difficult to distinguish from a peripheral lung abscess. The loculated effusion is generally lenticular in shape and does not shift freely in the pleural space with changes in patient position. Incomplete layering may be detected on decubitis films (King and Thomson 2002). Infectious pleural effusions are most commonly associated with pneumonia and are defined as a parapneumonic effusion. Other mechanisms where the pleura may be contaminated by infecting organisms are the rupture of subpleural tuberculous foci or dissemination of infectious particles by the bloodstream. Intra-abdominal infections may reach the pleural space passing through the diaphragm. Penetrating injury to the chest wall or rupture of esophagus can also result in the introduction of organisms into the pleura (Rahman and Davies 2008).

Parapneumonic effusions can be separated into three stages.

1. Exudative stage
2. Fibropurulent stage
3. Organizing stage

In the *exudative stage* of parapneumonic effusion, pneumonic process causes inflammation of the visceral pleura and results in the accumulation pleural fluid. The pleural fluid in this stage is characterized by negative bacterial studies. Pleural thickening may be seen in 50 % of cases at this stage (Rahman and Davies 2008; Kienzl et al. 2012). The *fibropurulent stage* is caused by pus in the pleural space. The pleural fluid in this stage is infected and is characterized by positive bacterial studies. Progression to emphyema occurs in this stage. At this stage, the split pleura sign is seen on contrast material–enhanced CT images. There is enhancement of the thickened inner visceral and outer parietal pleura, with separation by a collection of pleural fluid (Fig. 4) (Rahman and Davies 2008; Kraus 2007). As the disease progress to *organizing stage*, fibroblasts grow into the pleural fluid from both the visceral and parietal pleura leading to pleural fibrosis. CT findings at this stage include thickened pleura with multiple loculations. The thickened pleura may calcify. Expansion of extrapleural fat and periosteal changes at adjacent ribs develops. Inability of the lung to expand after tube thoracostomy is seen at this stage (Light 2006). Extensive pleural calcifications may be associated with minimal pleural fluid. This finding is important because residual infection in pleural space may extend to adjacent chest wall and lead to empyema necessitatis or may result in bronchopulmonary fistula formation (Fig. 5a, b) (Collins and Sten 2008). On ultrasound, pleural fluid is most frequently seen as an anechoic or hypoechoic collection.

The majority of parapneumonic effusions and empyemas are associated with septations, and the pleural fluid at this stage appears hyperechoic on US examination. Pleural thickening is hard to

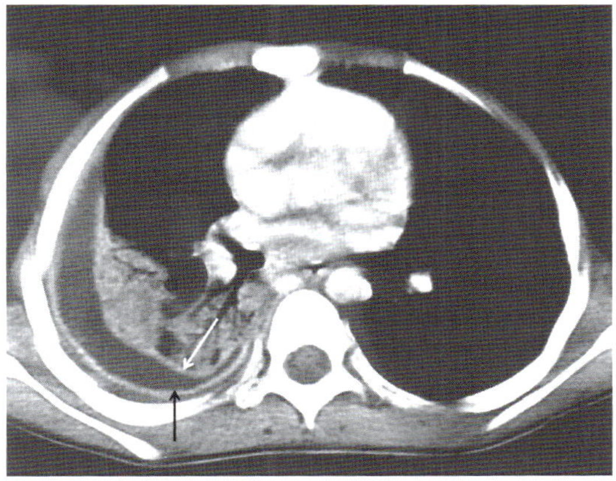

Fig. 4 The split pleura sign in emphyema. Contrast-enhanced axial CT image show enhancement of the thickened inner visceral (*white arrow*) and outer parietal pleura (*black arrow*) with separation by a collection of pleural fluid

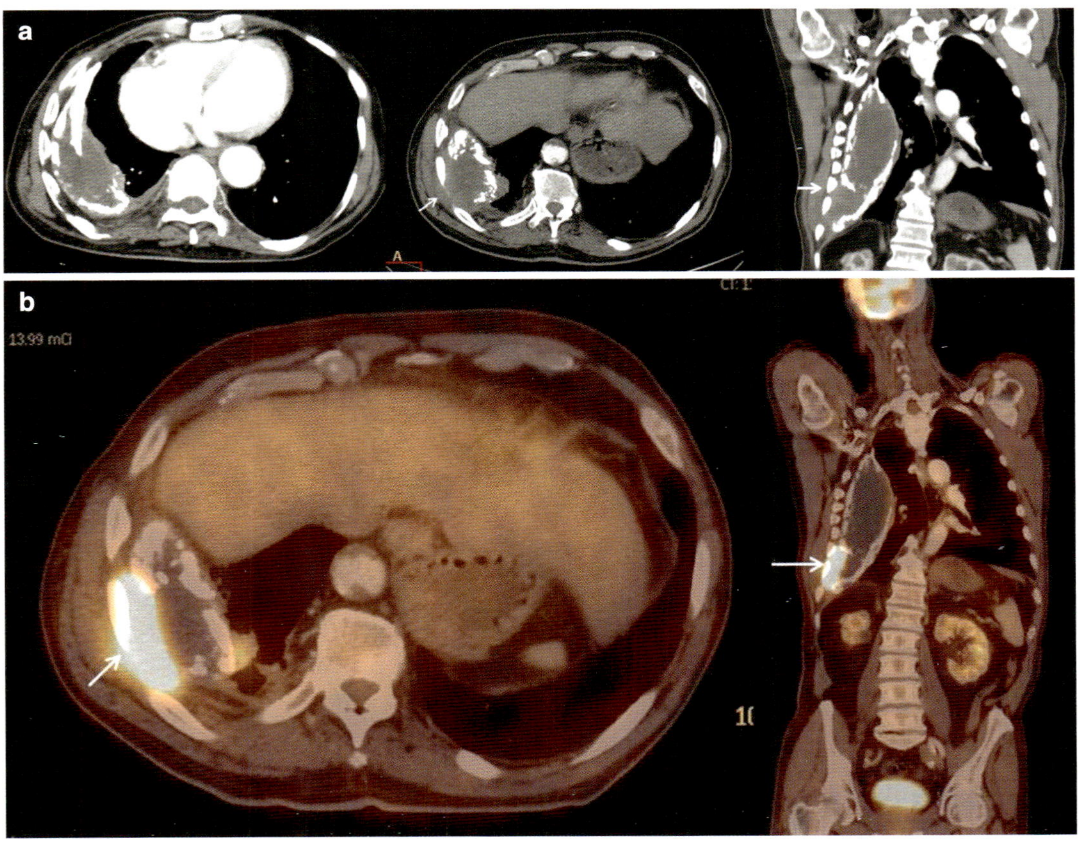

Fig. 5 (**a**) Empyema necessitatis in a patient with prior history of tuberculosis pleurisy. Contrast-enhanced axial and coronal CT images show thick and calcified pleural layers and associated pleural fluid between the pleural layers. There is extension of pleural infection to the thoracic wall (*white arrows*). (**b**). Axial and coronal fused PET-CT images show increased ^{18}F-flurodeoxyglucose (^{18}F-FDG) uptake at level of chest wall extension of pleural infection (*white arrow*)

visualize sonographically and if confirmation of this is required, contrast-enhanced CT should be performed. Apparently, there is no definitive correlation between US appearance and the stage of evolution of the effusion (Gleeson 2008).

Sometimes it may be difficult to differentiate between empyema and a pleural-based pulmonary abscess. The pulmonary abscess appears round in shape and forms an acute angle with the chest wall. However, empyemas usually form an obtuse angle with the chest wall. Pulmonary abscesses tend to have thicker walls than empyemas. The "split pleura" sign referring to the separation of enhancing parietal and visceral pleura is seen in empyema and can be used also to differentiate it from an abscess (Gleeson 2008).

1.5 Chylothorax

Chylothorax is defined as an accumulation of chyle in the pleural space most often secondary to thoracic duct injury or malignant invasion. The largest part of the thoracic duct lies in the right hemithorax, and the thoracic duct drains into the junction of the left axillary and internal jugular veins. Most chylous effusions are right sided as expected from this anatomic location. The attenuation of chylous effusions at CT may be low due to the fat content of the fluid. However because of the rich protein content of the chyle, it is generally difficult to differentiate it from other effusions (Radiographic et al. 1997).

1.6 Malignant Effusion

Metastatic seeding of the pleura is seen most commonly in lung, breast, ovarian, and gastrointestinal carcinomas. Primary pleural tumors such as mesothelioma and pleural lymphoma are rare. Certain infiltrative hematologic malignancies (e.g., acute myeloid leukemia) may also involve the pleura (Kienzl et al. 2012; Bonomo et al. 2000; Sahn 1997). Most patients with pleural metastases have large amount of effusions. However, the definitive diagnosis of malignant pleural disease generally requires pleural fluid cytologic examination, pleural biopsy, or even open chest surgery (Collins and Sten 2008; Gleeson 2008). Contrast-enhanced CT is the most commonly performed study in patients with suspected malignant pleural effusion and negative cytology on aspiration. CT signs indicating for both primary and metastatic diseases of pleura include thickening of the mediastinal pleura, parietal pleural thickening of greater than >1 cm, and focal and/or diffuse nodularity of the pleura. Using these criteria for assessment, contrast-enhanced CT has been shown to have a sensitivity of >80 %. CT examination may also give information about associated metastases (Fig. 6). Pleural or diaphragmatic nodules can be detected sonographically in cases with pleural metastases, but CT is better than US for the evaluation of pleural thickening (Evans and Gleeson 2004; Leung et al. 1990). US can be used as a tool to aid thoracentesis. MRI is superior to CT in the detection of small pleural nodules. However, the respiratory and cardiac motion artifacts are the major drawbacks of MRI examination (McLoud 1998; Gleeson 2008). PET and PET-CT have an increasing impact in the diagnosis of malignant pleural tumors. Several studies have mentioned the high accuracy of 18F-FDG PET/CT in differentiating benign and malignant pleural disease, especially in the setting of indeterminate CT findings. Increased pleural FDG uptake usually indicates the presence of pleural metastases (Fig. 7) (Schaffler et al. 2004; Kramer et al. 2004). PET/CT also plays an important role in tumor staging to detect distant metastases and to monitor therapy response. The disadvantage of PET or PET-CT is that they poorly discriminate between infective and malignant causes. Nonspecific FDG uptake can be seen in patients who have undergone prior talc pleurodesis, radiotherapy, intrapleural chemotherapy, etc. (Duysinx et al. 2004; Erasmus et al. 2000). Small volume disease or low grade malignancies such as epitheloid mesothelioma can hardly be detected with PET (Makis et al. 2012).

1.7 Management and Treatment

Interventional procedures such as thoracentesis, percutaneous drainage, and pleural biopsies are generally performed with the guidance of imaging

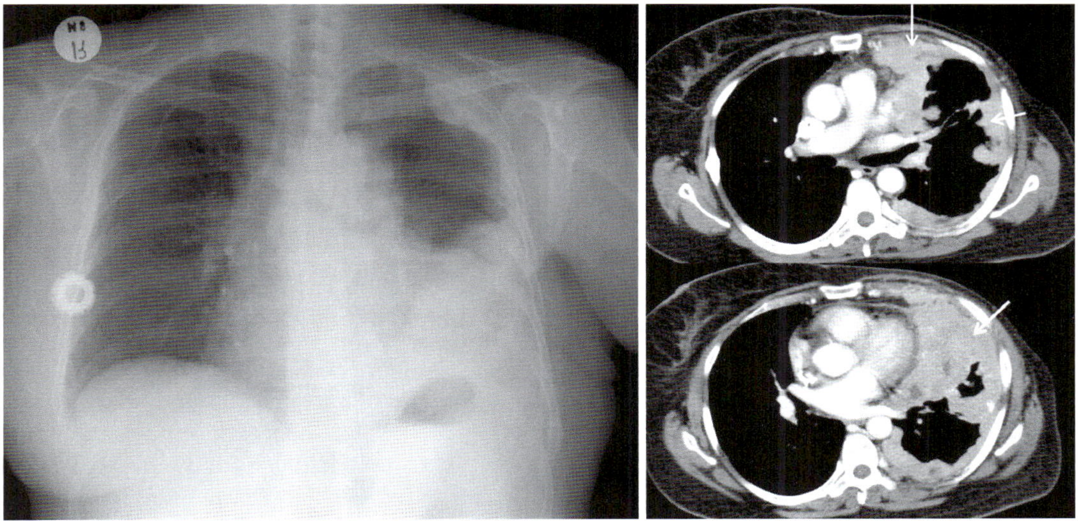

Fig. 6 Pleural metastases in a patient with breast cancer. Posteroanterior chest X-ray and axial contrast-enhanced CT images show left-sided pleural effusion, pleural thickening, and pleural mass lesions (*white arrows*). There is asymmetry at level of soft tissues due to left mastectomy

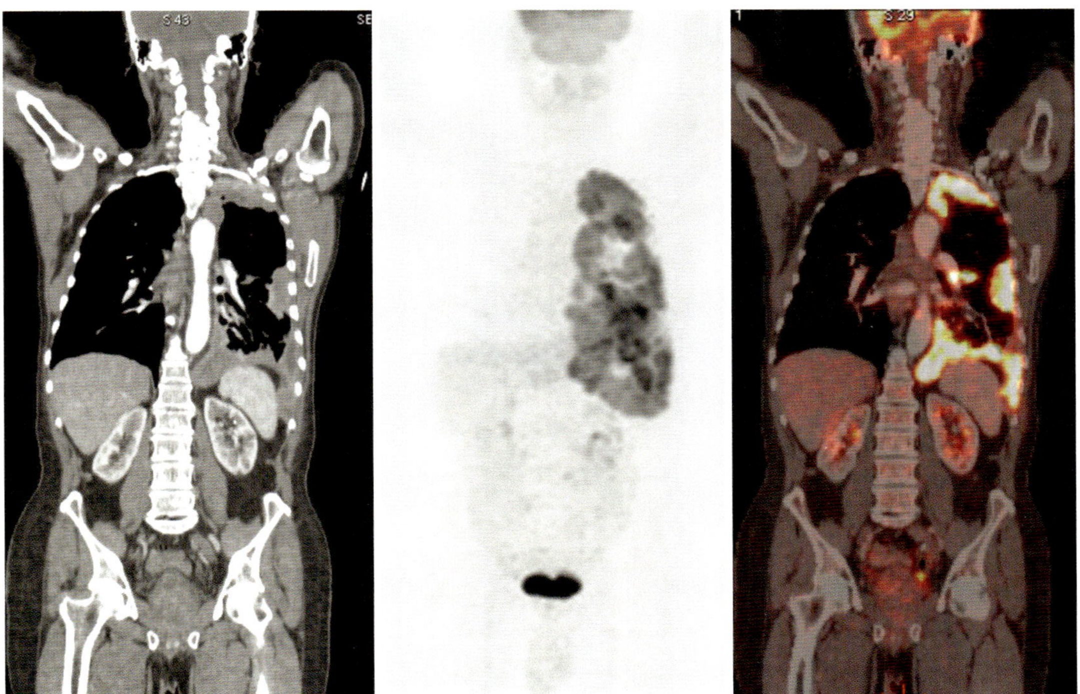

Fig. 7 Pleural carcinomatosis. Coronal CT, PET, and PET-CT fusion images show pleural thickening and increased pleural ^{18}F-flurodeoxyglucose (^{18}F-FDG) uptake

techniques. Imaging guidance helps identification of the correct placement site and proper insertion of the catheter into the pleural cavity and also helps to avoid complications that can occur during the procedure. The modality of choice depends on several factors such as the location, size, complexity of pleural fluid, local availability of the equipments, and experience of the operator. US can detect small amount of fluid in pleural cavity so it is commonly preferred in bedside percutaneous aspiration and catheter drainage of uncomplicated pleural fluid. CT is generally preferred in case of encapsulated, loculated complex pleural collections. Depending on the characteristics of the pleural fluid such as the amount, pH, glucose levels, bacteriological features, the proper therapeutic method is selected in case of parapneumonic effusion (Light and Rodriguez 1998). Therapeutic methods can vary from therapeutic thoracentesis, insertion of thoracostomy tube, administration of thrombolytics to decortication surgery. Malignant pleural effusion which cannot be controlled by systemic chemotherapy is treated interventionally. The treatment options may be repeated thoracentesis, pleural sclerosis by injection of intrapleural drugs, and long-term pleural catheters (Noukoua Tchuisse et al. 2007).

Reexpansion pulmonary edema (RPE) is a rare but important complication that may occur after treatment of lung collapse caused by pleural effusion. The rapid reexpansion of a chronically collapsed lung, after removal of a large amount of fluid from the pleural space may lead to RPE. The condition appears within 1–24 h after the evacuation. Radiologically, alveolar filling pattern is seen within a few hours of reexpansion of the lung. It is usually unilateral and is detected in those portions of lung that were previously collapsed (Fig. 8) (Tarver et al. 1996). The

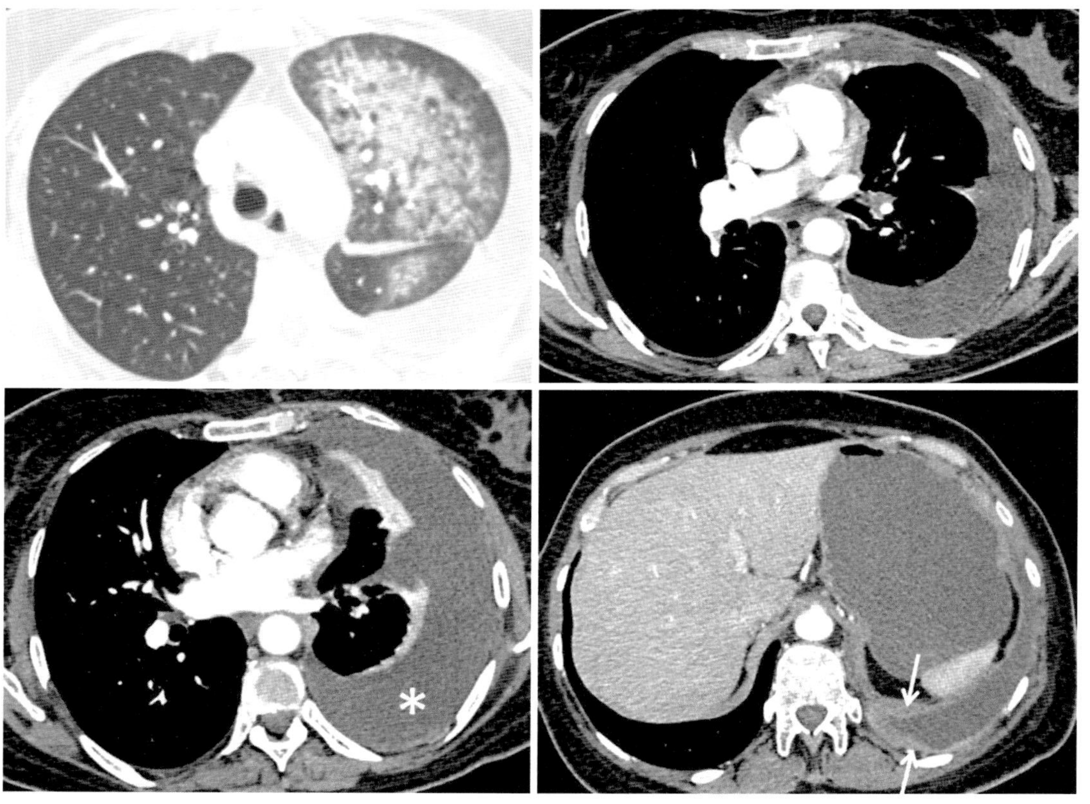

Fig. 8 Reexpansion pulmonary edema in a patient with mesothelioma. Axial chest CT image at lung window settings show ground glass areas and air space opacities in left lung after thoracentesis. CT images at mediastinal window settings shows left pleural effusion (*white asterisk*) and pleural thickening at level of left costophrenic sinus (*white arrows*)

treatment is generally supportive. As a prevention, limitation of therapeutic thoracentesis to 1000 mL is advised (Light et al. 1980).

2 Imaging of Spontaneous Pneumothorax

Chiara Andreoli

2.1 Introduction

Pneumothorax is defined as the presence of air in the pleural cavity, between the lung and the parietal pleura.

It represents a relatively common cause of admission to the emergency department, with a reported incidence of 18–28/100,000 cases per year for men and 1.2–6/100,000 cases per year for women (Noppen 2010; Bense et al. 1987; MacDuff et al. 2010).

Pneumothorax can be distinguished in "primary spontaneous pneumothorax" (PSP) that occurs in healthy patients without obvious causes and secondary spontaneous pneumothorax (SSP), due to underlying predisposing diseases, such as emphysema, tuberculosis, fibrosis, etc (MacDuff et al. 2010).

Primary pneumothorax occurs more frequently in young, thin, and tall males without predisposing lung disease, although it is known that its occurrence is due to the rupture of underlying small subpleural bullae and blebs at the lung apices, found at thoracoscopy or detected on CT: these conditions are called *emphysema-like changes* (ELCs) (Currie et al. 2007; Lesur et al. 1990; Donahue et al. 1993).

It seems that smoking increases the risk of developing primary pneumothorax nine times in young people, although the mechanism is unknown. Secondary pneumothorax (SSP) occurs when an underlying lung pathology exists: the most frequent predisposing pathological conditions are obstructive airway disease, emphysema, tuberculosis, interstitial lung disease, pulmonary fibrosis, histiocytosis X, sarcoidosis, and pulmonary infections (Currie et al. 2007).

Clinically, patients with SSP are more severe than those with PSP, because of preexisting pulmonary disease, which reduces their ventilation ability and requires several days of hospitalization and a more complex management.

Pneumothorax can be clinically silent for several days before the onset of symptoms, and often, their severity is independent from the extension of pneumothorax. The severity of symptoms is the factor that most of all influences the diagnostic-therapeutic management; the more typical symptoms are chest pain, dyspnea, and breathlessness (MacDuff and MacDuff 2009; Harcke et al. 2007). When severe symptoms and signs as cyanosis, sweating, severe tachypnea, tachycardia and hypotension, and cardiorespiratory distress appear, tension pneumothorax must be considered, which is a true medical emergency, causing mediastinal shift and cardiovascular collapse.

2.2 Diagnosis

The clinical suspicion, based on typical symptoms as abrupt onset of pleuritic pain and breathlessness and typical signs as reduced breath sounds, decreased ipsilateral chest expansion, and hyperresonant percussion at clinical examination, is usually confirmed by imaging techniques which may also yield informations about the size of the pneumothorax and the amount of air visible between the lung and chest wall: according to the British Thoracic Society guidelines, small pneumothorax is considered when the space between the lung edge and chest wall is <2 cm and large pneumothorax when this space is >2 cm at chest radiograph (MacDuff et al. 2010; Currie et al. 2007).

Chest radiography is routinely used for the diagnosis, while in complex cases, the use of CT is recommended. Chest ultrasound is used in some centers, especially in case of pediatric patients and pregnant women, in order to reduce radiation dose exposition.

2.2.1 X-ray

Usually, the standard erect posteroanterior chest radiograph is considered adequate for the diagnosis, although it is limited in accurately quantifying pneumothorax size.

The advent of digital chest imaging has implemented the visualization of pneumothorax due to the ability to change the window, allowing to better visualize the interface between the lung edge and pleural cavity.

Specific signs of pneumothorax at chest radiograph are (Figs. 9, 10, and 11):

- The visualization of the visceral pleural edge as a very thin, sharp, white, convex-shaped line which runs parallel to the chest wall
- The absence of the lung parenchyma peripheral to this line
- Radiolucency of the peripheral space compared to adjacent lung
- In up to 50 % of cases, an air-fluid level visible in the costophrenic angle (arrow in Fig. 9a)
- In severe cases, collapse of the lung
- Mediastinal shift in case of tension pneumothorax (Fig. 11a)

While the diagnosis of PSP is easier because of the normality of the adjacent parenchyma, the diagnosis of the SSP may be harder: the presence of bullous lung disease can indeed lead to the erroneous diagnosis of pneumothorax; in complex cases, the use of CT is recommended, especially if interventional treatment is the choice (MacDuff et al. 2010).

Generally there is no need to request an expiratory film in the daily practice, because it does not always provide additional benefits in the routine assessment of pneumothorax (Schramel et al. 1996; Seow et al. 1996). In expiratory phase, the lung becomes smaller and denser, and the pneumothorax is better visible, although it seems more conspicuous.

In patients who cannot stand erect, if the use of CT scan is avoided for dosimetric reasons, and it is uncertain whether a pneumothorax is present or not, the use of additional projections such as the lateral view may provide additional informations (Glazer et al. 1989), although it is not routinely used in daily clinical practice: it should be performed with the suspected affected side up, and it is based on the assumption that the lung will "fall away" from the chest wall and that

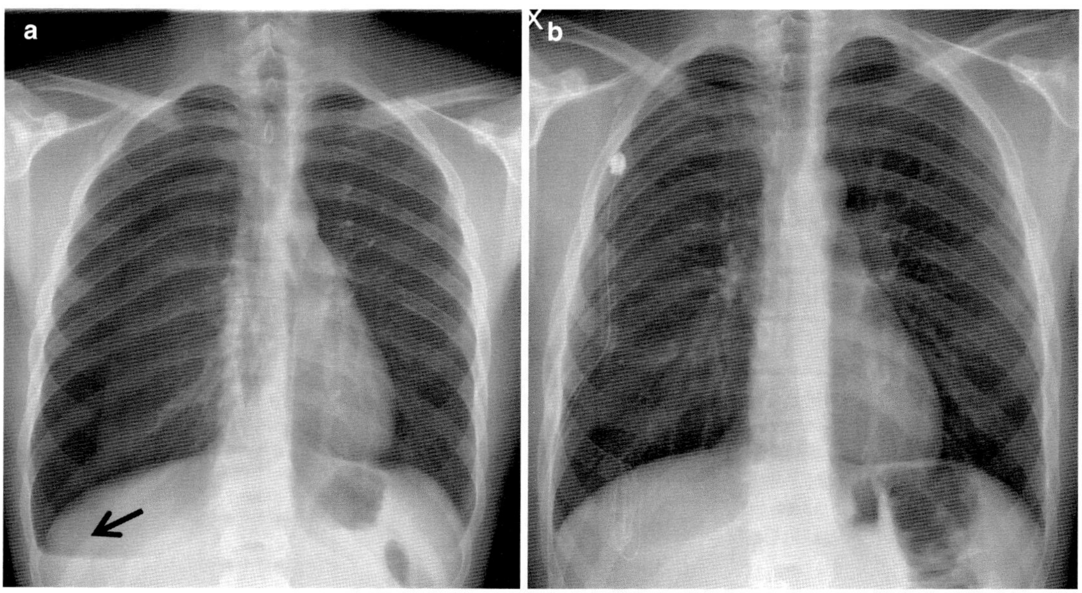

Fig. 9 In (**a**) Spontaneous pneumothorax causing partial collapse of the right lung, denser than the contralateral. The thin pleural line and the lack of the pulmonary parenchyma peripherally are clearly demonstrated. An air-fluid level is seen in the costophrenic angle (*black arrow*), due to pleural effusion. No mediastinal shift is visible. In (**b**), check after placement of drainage tube, with apex to the third intercostal space

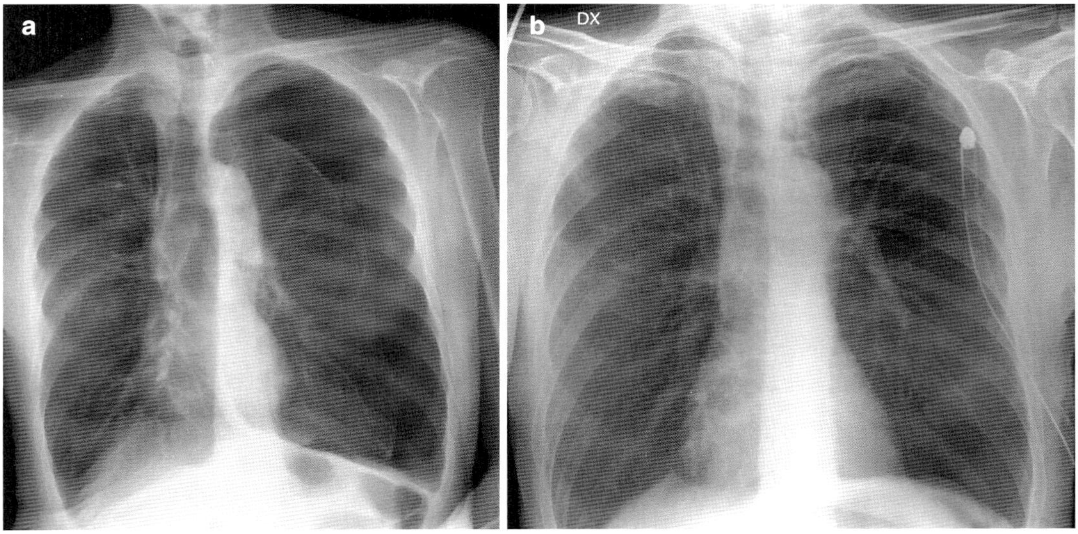

Fig. 10 In (**a**) Large pneumothorax causing compression of the left lung, depression of the hemidiaphragm and mediastinal shift. In (**b**), after placement of drainage tube, the pneumothorax is well drained

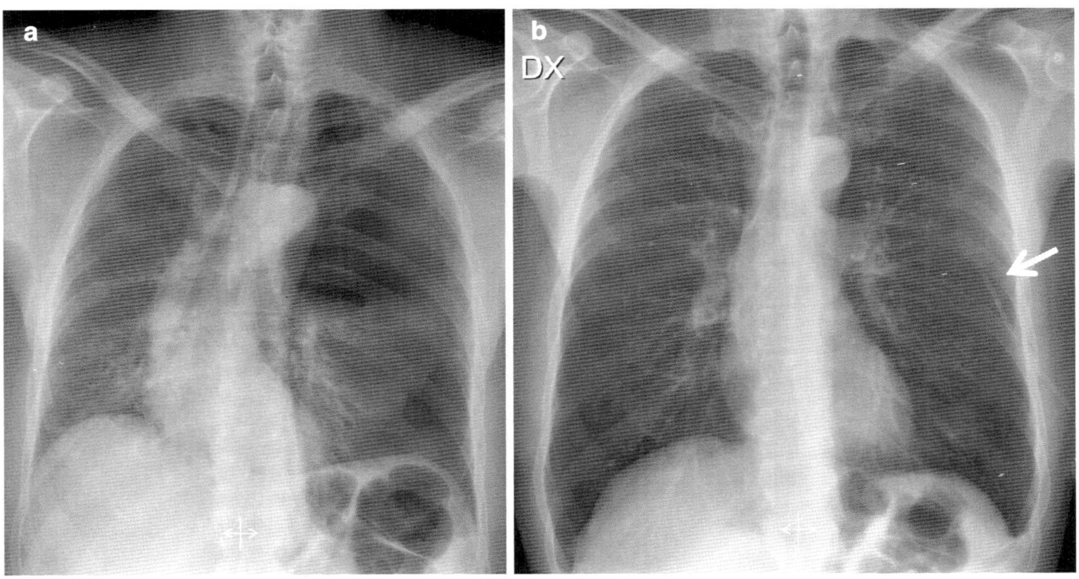

Fig. 11 Tension pneumothorax. In (**a**) a large pneumothorax causes compression of the mediastinal structures, with shift of the heart and trachea and depression of the hemidiaphragm. The left lung is collapsed. In (**b**), after positioning of a small drainage tube (*white arrow*), the pneumothorax is totally resolved

allows to better visualize the free air in the pleural space.

The tension pneumothorax represents a true thoracic emergency, due to compression of the air on mediastinal structures, and it should be promptly treated.

The compression of mediastinal structures is clearly visible on the X-rays as the shift of the heart and trachea to the contralateral side and depression of the hemidiaphragm on the affected side (Fig. 11). Often, it is clinically suspected and should be treated promptly even before performing an X-ray.

Mimics on X-radiographs

In the clinical practice, we are often facing with artifacts that can mimic the presence of a pneumothorax and that should be known to avoid mistakes, especially if the treatment is the choice: the medial border of the scapula can mimic the lung edge, and skin folds overlying the chest wall also can simulate a visceral pleural line; these mistakes are accentuated by the fact that a characteristic reduction of lung markings is often present in the upper zones of the lung, especially in children.

If the doubt persists, it is useful to repeat the radiographs removing the clothes or repositioning the arms.

Occasionally, a large bulla can mimic a pneumothorax: in that case, if there is still doubt, CT can be performed (MacDuff et al. 2010).

2.2.2 Ultrasound

Thoracic ultrasound is a promising technique, increasingly used in the shock room to quickly diagnose the presence of traumatic pneumothorax in unstable trauma patients. In B mode modality, normal lung interface with pleura shows lung sliding with vertical comet tails running down from the pleural surface. In case of pneumothorax, this sliding and the comet tail artifacts are absent. M mode can be used to confirm or to exclude movement of the lung within the rib interspace. Small air collections in the pleural space are best appreciated anteriorly in the supine position, whereas large pneumothorax is well seen laterally in the midaxillary line (Husain et al. 2012; Stone 2008; Lichtenstein et al. 2005; Ianniello et al. 2014; Zhang et al. 2006). According to the literature, in polytrauma patients, the sensitivity and specificity of US for the detection of pneumothorax ranged from 86 to 98 % and 97 to 100 %, respectively, against the supine AP chest radiographs that has a sensitivity for the detection of pneumothorax from 28 to 75 % (Wilkerson and Stone 2010).

As well as for trauma patients, in which it is impossible to perform X-rays in the upright position, thoracic ultrasound can be useful to check spontaneous pneumothorax in limited cases, such as in children and pregnant women, for dosimetric reasons.

2.2.3 Computed Tomography (CT)

As mentioned above, computed tomography is occasionally performed when the radiographic diagnosis of pneumothorax is unclear or in complex cases, for example, in order to distinguish a pneumothorax from a large emphysematous bulla, or when there is a clinical-radiological discrepancy (MacDuff et al. 2010).

CT is considered a highly reliable and decisive technique only if done with rigorous method: a high-resolution CT scan of the thorax should be performed with spiral scanner, acquiring images with slice thickness of 1 mm and section spacing of 10 mm. The lung window is used to analyze the lung parenchyma, looking for underlying pathological conditions, while the mediastinal window is useful to confirm the presence of pleural fluid or hemorrhagic collections (Shi-ping 2010).

If carried out following these parameters, CT is a method considered the "gold standard" in the detection of small pneumothorax, also called "occult pneumothorax," and in size evaluation (MacDuff et al. 2010). If the surgical procedure is the choice, it's also often used before it, in order to better study the underlying lung abnormalities, such as interstitial lung disease and enphysematic disease (Figs. 12 and 13).

Pneumothorax is very easily identified on CT and should not be a diagnostic challenge: it shows as a black band (air) around the often collapsed lung; sometimes, pleural fluid or hemorrhagic collections are present, and this condition are called hydro-/pneumothorax or hemo-/pneumothorax.

In addition to the diagnostic confirmation in emergency setting, the added value of CT scan is that CT findings can predict pneumothorax recurrence (Mitlehner et al. 1992; Warner et al. 1991), through direct visualization of invisible findings on radiographs such as little bullae and blebs located in lung apices (Fig. 14) (Ouanes-Besbes et al. 2007; Verschoof et al. 1988; Lippert et al. 1991).

Indeed, the finding of dystrophic lesions in the lung of patients affected by recurrent pneumothorax is very common: in a recent paper, Lamia

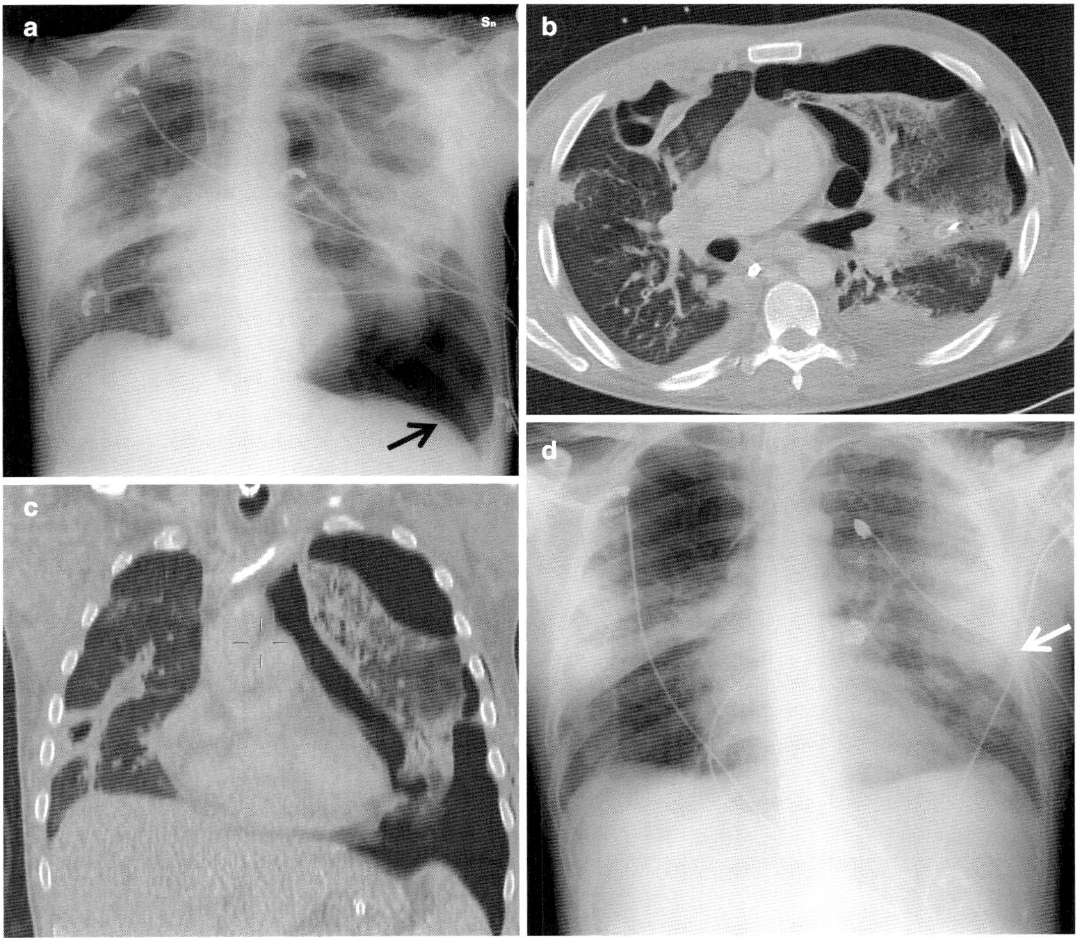

Fig. 12 In (**a**), the radiogram shows diffuse fibrosis of the lung parenchyma bilaterally and a voluminous air collection confined in the left base (*black arrow*). The CT scans (axial in **b** and coronal in **c**) confirm the severe lung fibrosis but demonstrates that the pneumothorax is more conspicuous than the amount shown at X-ray. In (**d**), it has shown the optimal positioning of the drainage tube with the resolution of pneumothorax

found dystrophic lesions in 72.5 % of cases. After that, several studies suggested that pulmonary CT scan findings, including the number and size of bullae and blebs, can predict pneumothorax recurrence, although it's known that this is not the only factor that predicts the rate of recurrence (Ouanes-Besbes et al. 2007).

The two dystrophic lesions most frequently associated with the development of recurrent pneumothorax are the pulmonary blebs and bullae, often not detected at chest X-ray: pulmonary blebs are defined as small subpleural thin-walled air spaces, not larger than 1–2 cm in diameter, with a wall thickness less than 1 mm; pulmonary bullae are cystic air spaces that have an imperceptible wall (less than 1 mm), as the blebs, but the difference between blebs and bullae is in their size, because bullae have a transverse diameter >2 cm. It should be considered that blebs can coalesce to form bullae (Lippert et al. 1991; Cantin et al. 2010; Hansell et al. 2008; Sahn and Heffner 2000; O'Connor and Morgan 2005).

There is a lot of disagreement in the literature about this topic: some studies revealed no correlation between recurrence and lung CT

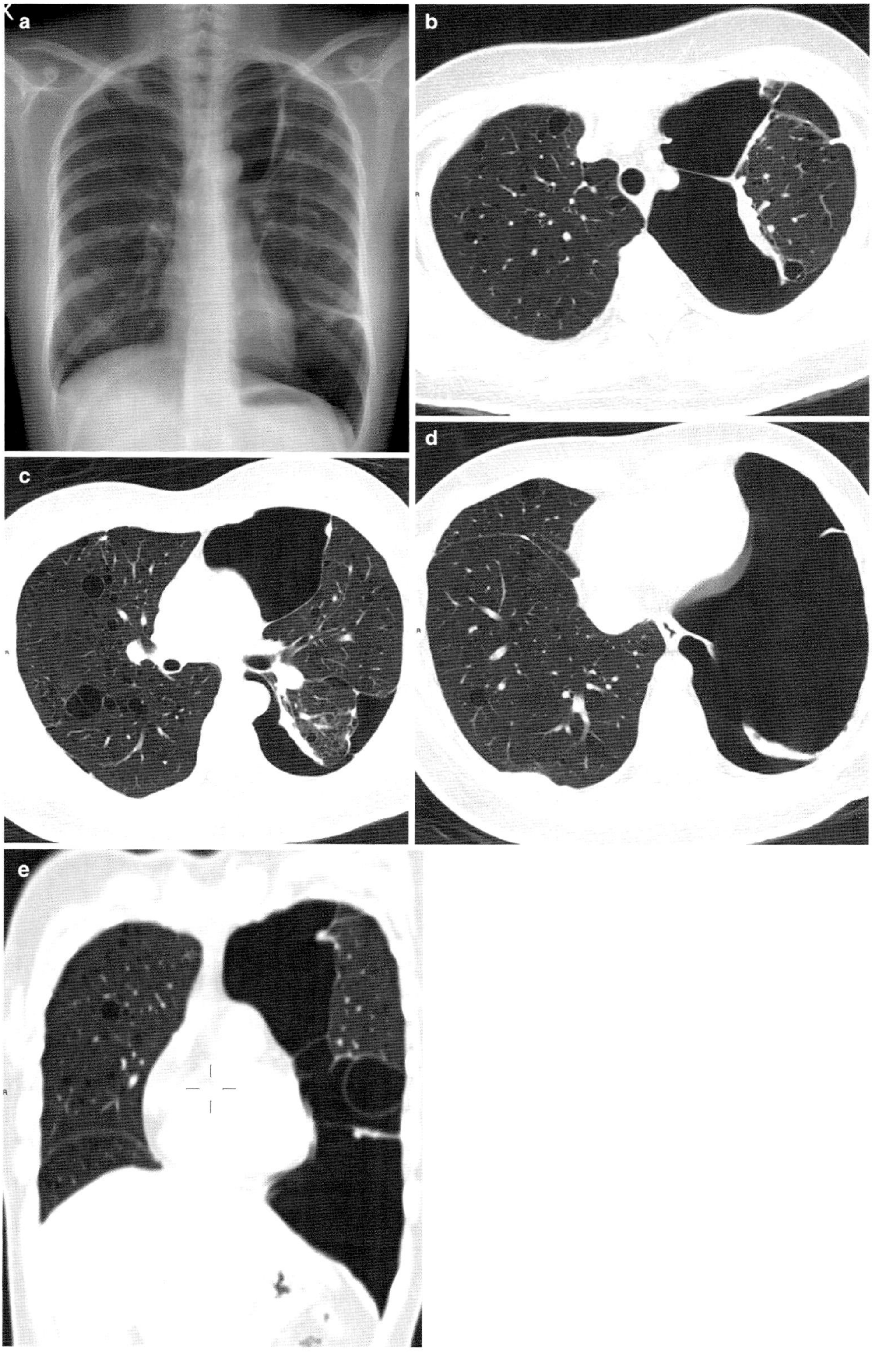
a
b
c
d
e

findings, while most of the authors agree that the incidence of recurrence derives from the therapeutic choice (as the size of the drainage tube, chemical pleurodesis rather than surgical) (Ouanes-Besbes et al. 2007).

However, in addition to assessing the need of surgical intervention, CT scan can also be used to localize the bullae/blebs at unusual sites (Shiping 2010) and to detect the presence of hemopneumothorax, which influences the treatment choice: these above informations can help in planning surgical strategies and in explaining the indication, risks, and benefits to the patients (Chen et al. 2009).

CT scans can also be used to detect the presence of bullae and blebs on the contralateral lung, which predicts the risk of contralateral spontaneous pneumothorax (Sihoe et al. 2000): one-fourth of patients with contralateral blebs developed PSP in the untreated lung.

Conclusions

Pneumothorax is a relatively common condition that needs to be promptly managed in an appropriate way. It may represent a true medical emergency, as is the case of tension pneumothorax, which requires an immediate operative treatment, while in most cases a conservative treatment is the choice.

Imaging plays a crucial role at the time of diagnosis, through the evaluation of the extent of the pneumothorax and the anatomical modifications of the lung parenchyma, which represents essential information in order to choose the best and most appropriate treatment for that patient.

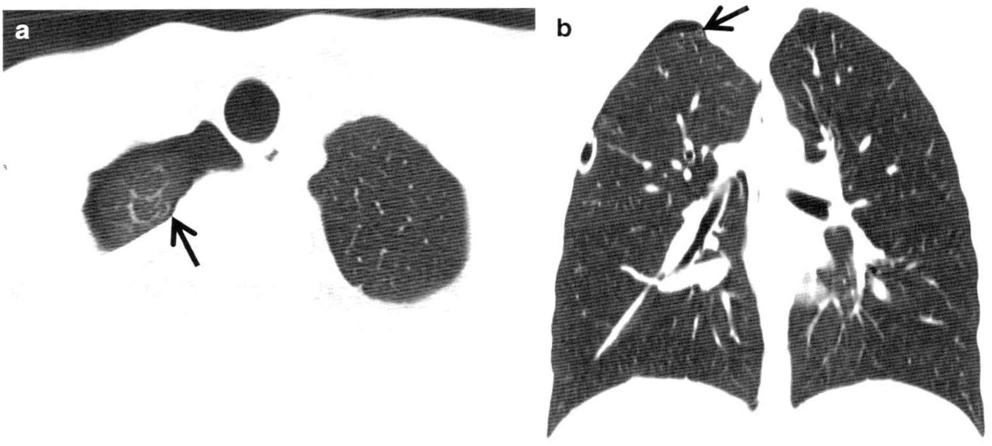

Fig. 14 The same patient of Fig. 9. Axial CT scan (**a**) and coronal reconstruction (**b**) the day after positioning of the drainage tube show the presence of some small bubbles in the right pulmonary apex (*black arrow*), clearly visible through the window of the lung parenchyma

Fig. 13 In (**a**), the radiograph shows air collection in the apical and basal zone of the left hemithorax, but no abnormalities of the parenchyma are suspected. In axial CT scans (**b–d**) and in the reformatted coronal reconstruction (**e**), centrilobular emphysema is seen, with multiple diffuse bullae spread in the parenchyma, and a conspicuous pneumothorax is well demonstrated

References

Bense L, Wiman LG, Hedenstierna G (1987) Onset of symptoms in spontaneous pneumothorax: correlations to physical activity. Eur J Respir Dis 71:181–186

Blackmore CC, Black WC, Dallas RV, Crow HC (1996) Pleural fluid volume estimation: a chest radiograph prediction rule. Acad Radiol 3:103–109

Bonomo L, Feragalli B, Sacco R, Merlino B, Storto ML (2000) Malignant pleural disease. Eur J Radiol 34: 98–118

Cantin L, Bankier AA, Eisenberg RL (2010) Multiple cystlike lung lesions in the adult. AJR Am J Roentgenol 194(1):W1–W11

Chen JS, Hsu HH, Kuo SW et al (2009) Management of recurrent primary spontaneous pneumothorax after thoracoscopic surgery: should observation, drainage, redo thoracoscopy, or thoracotomy be used? Surg Endosc 23(11):2438–2444

Collins J, Sten EJ (2008) Pleura, chest wall and diaphragm. In: Collins J, Stern EJ (eds) Chest radiology: the essentials, 2nd edn. Wolters Kluwer Health/Lippincott Williams & Wilkins, Philadelphia, pp 139–162

Collins JD, Burwell D, Furmanski S, Lorber P, Steckel RJ (1972) Minimal detectable pleural effusions. Radiology 105:51–53

Currie GP, Alluri R, Christie GL et al (2007) Pneumothorax: an update. Postgrad Med J 83:461–465

Donahue DM, Wright CD, Viale G et al (1993) Resection of pulmonary blebs and pleurodesis for spontaneous pneumothorax. Chest 104:1767e9. (2L)

Duysinx B, Nguyen D, Louis R et al (2004) Evaluation of pleural disease with 18-fluorodeoxyglucose positron emission tomography imaging. Chest 125:489–493

Erasmus JJ, McAdams HP, Rossi SE et al (2000) FDG PET of pleural effusions in patients with non-small cell lung cancer. Am J Roentgenol 175:245–249

Evans AL, Gleeson FV (2004) Radiology in pleural disease: state of the art. Respirology 9:300–312

Falaschi F, Battolla L, Mascalchi M et al (1996) Usefulness of MR signal intensity in distinguishing benign from malignant pleural disease. Am J Roentgenol 166: 963–968

Glazer H, Anderson J, Wilson BS et al (1989) Pneumothorax: appearances on lateral chest radiographs. Radiology 173:707e11

Gleeson FV (2008) Radiology: diagnostic. In: Light RW, Lee YCG (eds) Textbook of pleural diseases, 2nd edn. Hodder Arnold, London, pp 233–255

Goldsmith SJ, Kostakoglu L (2000) Nuclear medicine imaging of lung cancer. Radiol Clin North Am 38: 511–524

Hansell DM, Bankier AA, Macmahon H (2008) Fleischner Society: glossary of terms for thoracic imaging. Radiology 246(3):697–722

Harcke HT, Pearse LA, Levy AD et al (2007) Chest wall thickness in military personnel: implications for needle thoracentesis in tension pneumothorax. Mil Med 172:1260–1263

Henschke CI, Davis SD, Romano PM, Yankelevitz DF (1989) Pleural effusions: pathogenesis, radiologic evaluation, and therapy. J Thorac Imaging 4:49–60

Husain LF, Hagopian L, Wayman D et al (2012) Sonographic diagnosis of pneumothorax. J Emerg Trauma Shock 5(1):76–81

Ianniello S, Di Giacomo V, Sessa B (2014) First-line sonographic diagnosis of pneumothorax in major trauma: accuracy of e-FAST and comparison with multidetector computed tomography. Radiol Med 119(9):674–680

Kienzl D, Prosch H, Töpker M, Herold C (2012) Imaging of non-cardiac, non-traumatic causes of acute chest pain. Eur J Radiol 81:3669–3674

Kim EA, Lee KS, Shim YM et al (1997) Radiographic and CT findings in complications following pulmonary resection, chylothorax and pseudochylothorax. Eur Respir J 10:1157–1162

King S, Thomson A (2002) Radiological perspectives in empyema. Br Med Bull 61:203–214

Kramer H, Pieterman RM, Slebos DJ et al (2004) PET for the evaluation of pleural thickening observed on CT. J Nucl Med 45:995–998

Kraus GJ (2007) The split pleura sign. Radiology 243: 297–298

Lesur O, Delorme N, Fromaget JM et al (1990) Computed tomography in the etiologic assessment of idiopathic spontaneous pneumothorax. Chest 98:341–347

Leung AN, Müller NL, Miller RR (1990) CT in differential diagnosis of diffuse pleural disease. Am J Roentgenol 154:487–492

Lichtenstein DA, Mezière G, Lascols N et al (2005) Ultrasound diagnosis of occult pneumothorax. Crit Care Med 33(6):1231–1238

Light RW (2006) Parapneumonic effusions and emphyema. Proc Am Thorac Soc 3:75–80

Light RW, Rodriguez RM (1998) Management of parapneumonic effusions. Clin Chest Med 19:373–382

Light RW, Jenkinson SG, Minh VD, George RB (1980) Observations on pleural fluid pressures as fluid is withdrawn during thoracentesis. Am Rev Respir Dis 121:799–804

Lippert HL, Lund O, Blegvad S, Larsen HV (1991) Independent risk factors for cumulative recurrence rate after first spontaneous pneumothorax. Eur Respir J 4(3):324–331

MacDuff A, Arnold A, Harvey J. (2010) Management of spontaneous pneumothorax: British Society pleural disease guideline. Thorax 65(suppl 2):18–31

MacDuff A, MacDuff R (2009) Pleural depth in medical patients. Chest 136:948–949

Makis W, Ciarallo A, Hickeson M et al (2012) Spectrum of malignant pleural and pericardial disease on FDG PET/CT. Am J Roentgenol 198:678–685

McLoud TC (1998) CT and MR in pleural disease. Clin Chest Med 19:261–276

Mitlehner W, Friedrich M, Dissmann W (1992) Value of computed tomography in the detection of bullae and blebs in patients with primary spontaneous pneumothorax. Respiration 59(4):221–227

Müller NL (1993) Imaging of the pleura. Radiology 186:297–309
Noppen M (2010) Spontaneous pneumothorax: epidemiology, pathophysiology and cause. Eur Respir Rev 117:217–219
Noukoua Tchuisse C, Ghaye B, Dondelinger RF (2007) Imaging and treatment of thoracic fluid and gas collections. In: Marincek B, Dondelinger RF (eds) Emergency radiology: imaging and intervention, 1st edn. Springer, Berlin/Heidelberg, pp 391–406
O'Connor AR, Morgan WE (2005) Radiological review of pneumothorax. BMJ 330(7506):1493–1497
Ouanes-Besbes L, Mondher G, Jalel K (2007) Prediction of recurrent spontaneous pneumothorax: CT scan findings versus management features. Respir Med 101(2):230–236
Rahman NM, Davies RJ (2008) Effusions from infections: parapneumonic effusion and empyema. In: Light RW, Lee YCG (eds) Textbook of pleural diseases, 2nd edn. Hodder Arnold, London, pp 341–366
Sahn SA (1997) Pleural diseases related to metastatic malignancies. Eur Respir J 10:1907–1913
Sahn SA (2008) Approach to patients with pleural diseases. In: Light RW, Lee YCG (eds) Textbook of pleural diseases, 2nd edn. Hodder Arnold, London, pp 201–206
Sahn SA, Heffner JE (2000) Spontaneous pneumothorax. N Engl J Med 342(12):868–874
Schaffler GJ, Wolf G, Schoellnast H et al (2004) Nonsmall cell lung cancer: evaluation of pleural abnormalities on CT scans with 18F-FDG PET. Radiology 231:858–865
Schramel FM, Golding RP, Haakman CD et al (1996) Expiratory chest radiographs do not improve visibility of small apical pneumothoraces by enhanced contrast. Eur Respir J 9:406e9
Seow A, Kazerooni EA, Cascade PN et al (1996) Comparison of upright inspiratory and expiratory chest radiographs for detecting pneumothoraces. AJR Am J Roentgenol 166(2):313–316
Shi-ping LUH (2010) Diagnosis and treatment of primary spontaneous pneumothorax. J Zhejiang Univ Sci B 11:735–744
Sihoe AD, Yim AP, Lee TW et al (2000) Can CT scanning be used to select patients with unilateral primary spontaneous pneumothorax for bilateral surgery? Chest 118:380–383
Stone MB (2008) Ultrasound diagnosis of traumatic pneumothorax. J Emerg Trauma Shock 1(1):19–20
Tarver RD, Broderick LS, Conces DJ Jr (1996) Reexpansion pulmonary edema. J Thorac Imaging 11: 198–209
Verschoof AC, Ten Velde GP, Greve LH, Wouters EF (1988) Thoracoscopic pleurodesis in the management of spontaneous pneumothorax. Respiration 53(3): 197–200
Warner BW, Bailey WW, Shipley RT (1991) Value of computed tomography of the lung in the management of primary spontaneous pneumothorax. Am J Surg 162(1):39–42
White S, Duran-Mendicuti A, Sodickson A, Viscomi S, Stella M, Ledbetter S (2009) Nontraumatic emergency radiology of the thorax. In: Soto JA, Lucey BC (eds) Emergency radiology, the requisites, 1st edn. Mosby Elsevier, Maryland, pp 234–274
Wilkerson RG, Stone MB (2010) Sensitivity of bedside ultrasound and supine anteroposterior chest radiographs for the identification of pneumothorax after blunt trauma. Acad Emerg Med 17(1):11–17
Zhang H, Liu Z-H, Yang J-X et al (2006) Rapid detection of pneumothorax by ultrasonography in patients with multiple trauma. Crit Care 10:R112

Part III

Vascular Chest Emergencies

Cardiac Emergencies: Acute Chest Pain

Florian Schwarz

Contents

F. Schwarz
Institut für Klinische Radiologie, Klinikum der Universität München (LMU), Marchioninistraße 15, München 81377, Germany
e-mail: Florian.Schwarz@med.uni-muenchen.de

1 Indications for Coronary CTA in Acute Chest Pain

1.1 Introduction

Acute chest pain is one of the most common complaints in patients presenting to the emergency department (ED). In a survey of emergency room utilization in the United States in 2011, chest pain accounted for 5.2 % of all visits and was thus second only to abdominal pain as the most common presenting complaint (Anon 2014). In male patients age 65 or older, chest pain is the most common complaint accounting for 9.0 % of all visits.

Chest pain encompasses both acute life-threatening and benign diseases, and determination of the exact etiology is often difficult and time-consuming. The diagnostic strategy underlying AHA and ESC guidelines focuses on rapidly excluding diagnoses with the greatest short-term mortality risk. Acute coronary syndrome (ACS) has a prevalence of approximately 20–40 % (Roffi et al. 2015) in unselected patients presenting with acute chest pain, comprising unstable angina, ST-segment elevation myocardial infarction (STEMI), and non-ST-segment elevation myocardial infarction (NSTEMI). Pulmonary embolism (PE) and acute aortic syndromes (AASs) are other potentially life-threatening diagnoses that can manifest primarily as chest pain.

Recently, multiple professional societies, including the American College of Cardiology

Med Radiol Diagn Imaging (2016)
DOI 10.1007/174_2016_73, © Springer International Publishing Switzerland

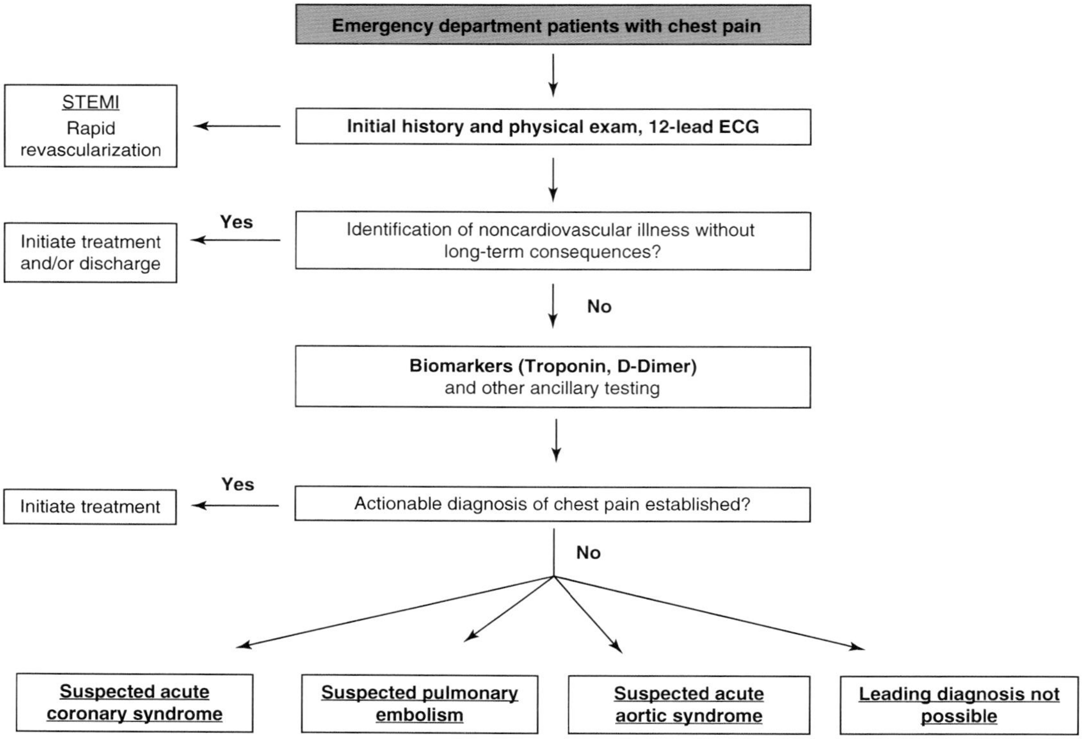

Fig. 1 Early triage of ED patients presenting with chest pain (Adapted from Rybicki et al. 2016)

(ACC) and the American College of Radiology (ACR), have published appropriate use criteria for chest pain imaging that include specific recommendations for several clinical scenarios of ACS, PE, and AAS or indeterminate chest pain (Rybicki et al. 2016). The major clinical scenarios for ACS will be discussed the following paragraphs with respect to the appropriateness of the use of coronary CT angiography (CCTA).

1.2 Early Clinical Triage of Patients with Chest Pain

On initial presentation to the ED (Fig. 1), all patients will undergo initial evaluation including history and physical examination, immediate 12-lead electrocardiography (ECG), and chest x-ray to identify or exclude STEMI and to identify noncardiovascular illnesses without long-term consequences as underlying pathology. Furthermore, immediate cardiac and pulmonary biomarker analysis is central (troponin and D-dimer). Patients in whom STEMI is established will have to undergo rapid invasive angiography for revascularization and are treated according to the guidelines. Patients with noncardiac causes of the chest pain often don't require specific CT imaging. In either of these two scenarios, coronary CT angiography (CCTA) is rarely considered appropriate (Rybicki et al. 2016).

Based on this initial evaluation, the ED physician has to risk-stratify the majority of the remaining patients into one of the three groups of diagnoses of concern (ACS, PE, or AAS) or state that the establishment of a leading diagnosis is not possible (Fig. 1). For ACS and PE, several risk scores have been thoroughly evaluated (the most common ones being the TIMI risk score (Antman et al. 2000) and the GRACE score (Fox et al. 2006) (http://www.gracescore.org/website/WebVersion.aspx) for ACS and the PE Wells score (Wells et al. 2000) and have proven to result in improved clinical decision-making, thus facilitating the classification of a patient into a particular category.

1.3 Triage Pathways in Suspected Acute Coronary Syndrome

In ACS patients, ECG findings diagnostic for myocardial ischemia or early biomarkers confirming myocyte damage are present in only a minority of patients with acute chest pain. The remaining clinically stable patients, however, still have possible myocardial ischemia and suspected NSTEMI ACS. It is in this subgroup of patients in which many are admitted and placed into chest pain units for telemetric observation – which is often referred to as "observational pathway."

However, in most of these patients, symptoms will later be ascribed to nonischemic causes – in these patients admission to an intermediate care unit could have been avoided if appropriate (imaging) test results had clearly ruled out an ischemic cause at the time of presentation. Strategies aiming at an early imaging-based exclusion of a coronary etiology of the presenting symptoms are commonly dubbed "early assessment path."

1.4 Indications for CCTA in the "Early Assessment Pathway"

Appropriateness of coronary CTA as part of the early assessment pathway will depend on the initial ECG, initial biomarker, and status of symptoms at the time of presentation. Four randomized trials have compared current standard-of-care management with early CCTA in chest pain patients presenting with a low-to-intermediate probability for ACS (Goldstein et al. 2007; Goldstein et al. 2011; Cury et al. 2013; Litt et al. 2012; Hoffmann et al. 2012). These trials have – individually and in aggregate (Hulten et al. 2013) – confirmed the safety and efficacy of an early CCTA approach in this clinical context.

Based on these trial results, in the large proportion of chest pain patients with low-to-intermediate risk for ACS, without ECG changes typical for ischemia and normal initial troponin, CCTA is considered appropriate (Rybicki et al. 2016).

In patients with initial ECG changes suggesting ischemia (other than ST-segment elevation) and positive initial biomarkers (positive initial diagnosis of NSTEMI/ACS), coronary CTA is not considered appropriate since in these patients, early revascularization may be associated with more favorable outcomes (Roffi et al. 2015).

In European countries, high-sensitivity troponin (hsTrop) assays have recently become widely available. Due to a lack of FDA approval, these are not (yet) available in the United States, however. In patients presenting with chest pain, in whom early hsTrop values are negative and who have a TIMI risk score of 0, no further testing might be considered – however, even in this extremely low-risk setting, coronary CTA is considered appropriate (Rybicki et al. 2016).

In several clinical scenarios, the diagnosis NSTEMI/ACS would be equivocal: either because clinical symptoms resolved hours before (<3 h) and the patient is asymptomatic at the time of presentation to the ED or because the initial troponin is equivocal or elevated without additional evidence of ACS. In these scenarios, coronary CTA is considered appropriate for early assessment of possible ACS (Rybicki et al. 2016).

1.5 Indications for Coronary CTA in the "Observational Pathway"

Several clinical scenarios exist after a patient is admitted in the context of an observational pathway for which recommendations for the use of coronary CTA exist. In the first scenario, any ECG and/or serial troponin unequivocally confirms NSTEMI or ACS. In this context of troponin-positive NSTEMI or ACS, several randomized trials have shown a more favorable outcome of an early invasive strategy, i.e., early revascularization. Coronary CTA is not considered appropriate in these patients unless there is significant comorbidity (particularly renal failure) which would decrease the advantage of an early invasive approach.

On the other hand, serial ECG and biomarkers might be negative or borderline for NSTEMI or ACS. In either case, the use of coronary CTA would be considered appropriate. With negative biomarkers, CTA can be performed on an outpatient basis.

2 CT Imaging and Post-processing Techniques

2.1 General Considerations

With increasing availability of state-of-the-art CT coronary angiography, the role of a calcium-scoring scan only (i.e., non-enhanced, ECG-synchronized scan of the heart) for chest pain evaluation has dwindled. While there were several studies in the late 1990s who investigated this strategy (Georgiou et al. 2001; Laudon et al. 1999; McLaughlin et al. 1999), over the years it has become apparent that the frequency of patients who present with very low calcium scores and yet show highly significant stenoses on coronary CTA or myocardial ischemia on provocative testing is too high to be negligible (Schenker et al. 2008). Furthermore, since many chest pain patients present with significant amounts of calcium, (CT) angiographic workup would be necessary in the majority of patients.

The acquisition of an unenhanced calcium-scoring scan prior to CCTA is controversial. It has been demonstrated that in patients presenting with acute chest pain, there is no incremental prognostic information gained from an independent prior calcium-scoring study (Chang et al. 2011).

At our institution, we perform an initial unenhanced CT scan for calcium scoring in all ACS patients who are over 45 years of age. To keep additional effective dose at the minimum, we choose a high-pitch acquisition protocol on a dual-source CT for this unenhanced scan regardless of the patients' heart rate and rhythm intending to scan the heart during diastole (we usually do not repeat the scan if there are motion artifacts). In our experience, this has several advantages, both regarding the diagnostic information obtained and familiarizing the patient with the breath holding and table movement procedure. It facilitates the customization of the scan range and thus contributes to dose reduction. Diagnostically, the calcium score will provide a first estimate of the amount of coronary atherosclerosis. It supports the correct interpretation of the subsequent CT angiography scan since it is unambiguous for calcification (Fig. 2). At very high calcium scores, subsequent CT angiography might be waived due to the high probability of not contributing more diagnostic information, although in appropriately selected patients, this only leads to the exclusion of very few (Chang et al. 2011). Furthermore, in patients in whom acute pathologies of the aorta also cannot be excluded, we perform an unenhanced, ECG-triggered scan of thorax covering the entire thoracic aorta intending to scan the heart at diastole. This allows for a 180-mm field-of-view (FoV) reconstruction for the coronary calcium score as well as reconstructions with full FoV for the exclusion of intramural hematoma within the aorta, hemorrhagic pericardial effusion, or hemorrhagic pleural effusions. In our experience, measurements of Hounsfield units within pericardial effusions tend to be the most accurate in unenhanced scans.

2.2 CCTA Protocol

Besides the usual relative and absolute contraindications for the administration of CT contrast material (impaired renal function, severe allergy to iodinated contrast material, manifest hyperthyroidism and pregnancy), specifically complicating factors for coronary CTA are irregular heart rhythms (atrial fibrillation, frequent extrasystoles) or contraindications to beta-blockers such as moderate-to-severe asthma. However, the vast majority of patients presenting with potential ACS will already have been administered beta-blockers to reduce myocardial oxygen demand prior to referral for coronary CTA (Roffi

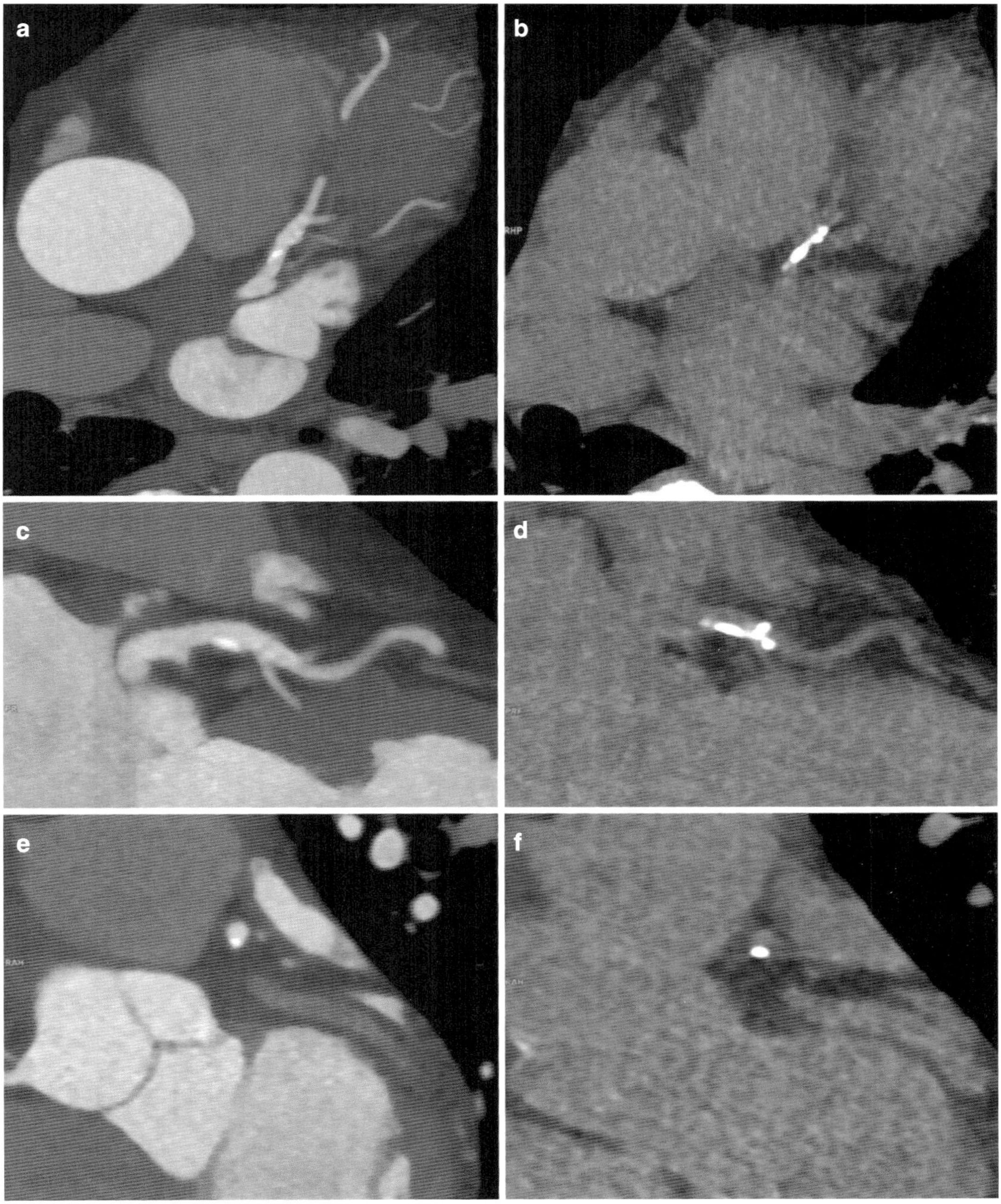

Fig. 2 Comparison of a contrast-enhanced CT-angiography series (a, c, f, 90 kVp) and non-enhanced series (b, d, f, 120 kVp) in a 52 year-old patient presenting with atypical chest pain showing a calcified plaque in the proximal LAD in corresponding 5 mm maximum intensity projection (MIP) reformations. This example illustrates how calcifications are better delineated on non-contrast series

et al. 2015). In patients with acute chest pain, we perform additional rate control in close collaboration with the treating physician in hemodynamically stable patients using intravenous metoprolol at 5 mg intervals up to a maximum total dose of 20 mg and a target heart rate of ≤70 bpm.

Prior to contrast administration and also in close collaboration with the referring physician, we also apply sublingual nitrates. Importantly, recent use of phosphodiesterase type 5 inhibitors (i.e., within 24 h for sildenafil and vardenafil and 48 h for tadalafil; used for erectile dysfunction or pulmonary hypertension, critical aortic stenosis, and hypotension) needs to be excluded prior to nitrate administration. We would also avoid nitrates in patients with a history of glaucoma. When beta-blockers have been administered previously, reactive tachycardia to nitrates is not a relevant problem in our experience. Particularly in younger patients, patient education about potentially severe headaches is mandatory.

For coronary CTA in patients with chest pain, we usually perform a test bolus acquisition first to determine optimal scan delay. In our opinion a test bolus strategy has several advantages over bolus triggering: in this patient cohort with a very wide range of ejection fractions, a test bolus approach allows for the most accurate modeling of early contrast dynamics. Furthermore, some patients (particularly with cardiac pacemakers) will suffer from chronic subclavian thrombosis which severely impairs contrast material inflow and can be detected during the test bolus. Finally, many patients will develop reactive tachycardia during contrast administration. When using bolus triggering, the heart rate can increase considerably during contrast administration, whereupon the scan protocol cannot be adjusted to the sudden change in heart rate. A scan protocol that would have been adequate for a slow steady heart rate frequently will result in nondiagnostic image quality at higher heart rates. When working with a test bolus, on the other hand, the administration of contrast material for the test bolus will often precipitate the contrast-induced tachycardia already, so the scan protocol can then be adjusted. Conversely, if the heart rate stays low during and after the test bolus, no sudden increase in heart rate during administration of the main contrast bolus is to be expected.

For optimal image quality with sound opacification of the distal coronary segments, a high iodine delivery rate is mandatory. In nonobese patients, we typically use a triphasic injection protocol with an initial bolus of 60 ml pure contrast material (350 mgI/ml or 400 mgI/ml) at 5.0 ml/s followed by a second phase of diluted contrast material (30 ml of a 50:50 mixture at 5.0 ml/s), followed by a saline chaser of 100 ml at the same injection rate.

The choice of scan protocol will be based on patient age, renal function, heart rate, and available scanner hardware. Naturally, the younger the patient, the higher the effort should be to reduce effective dose. In young patients it seems a reasonable strategy to apply an ultra low-dose (<1 mSv) scan protocol first even when there is a non-negligible risk of producing nondiagnostic image quality due to motion artifacts (Deseive et al. 2015). If image quality turns out to be nondiagnostic, the repeated contrast injection necessary for a second scan using a more complex scan protocol will usually not pose a problem to a younger patient's kidneys. All patients in whom the initial scan produced diagnostic image quality will have received a scan at extremely low effective dose. Patients who need a repeat scan with a more complex protocol (in the range 5 mSv), however, will only have a small increase in the total effective dose.

In older patients, on the other hand, who often suffer from impaired renal function, a scan repeat can be much more problematic due to the doubling of contrast material volume. In these patients, the choice would certainly be leaning toward performing the more complex scan protocol if there is any risk of producing nondiagnostic images with a low-dose scan protocol.

Applying this strategy (initial low-dose scan first) in younger patients, it is important, however, to closely surveil the frequency of scan repeats.

At our institution we use a third-generation dual-source CT to scan patients with acute chest pain. In patients with slow sinus rhythm

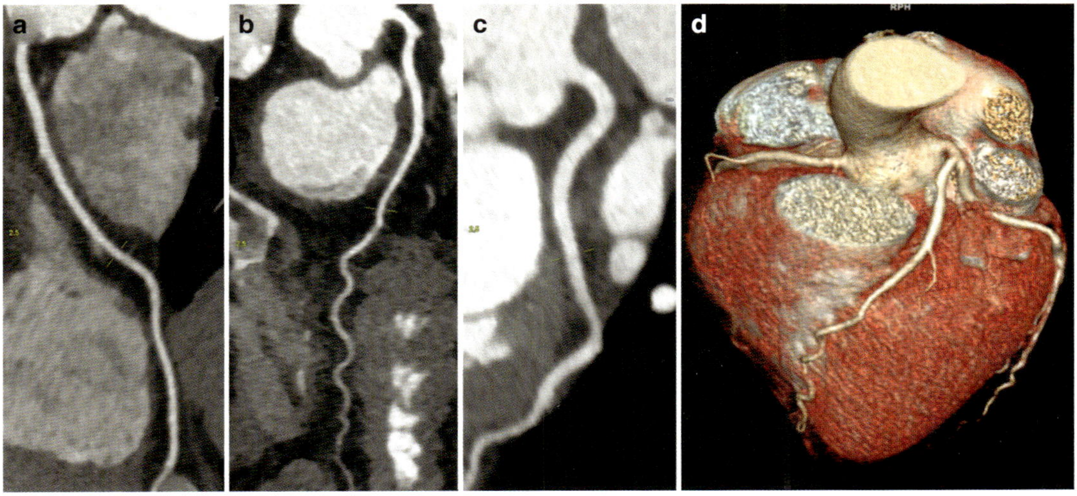

Fig. 3 45 year old female patient presenting with atypical chest pain: Coronary CTA allows the confident exclusion of coronary artery disease and thus acute coronary syndrome. (**a**) Curved Planar Reformation (CPR) of the right coronary artery (RCA); (**b**) CPR of the LAD; (**c**) CPR of the LCx; (**d**) Volume rendered image of the coronary artery system

(<70 bpm), a high-pitch CT acquisition will produce diagnostic image quality in the vast majority of patients. At higher frequencies (>70 bpm), a prospectively triggered "step-and-shoot approach" will be used with image acquisition during diastole. In very old patients or patients with very high rate retrospective, ECG gating with ECG-dependent dose modulation will be performed. Dose modulation will be switched off only in patients with severe arrhythmias.

2.3 Post-processing Techniques

Studies are reviewed by radiologists on dedicated 3D workstations or using advanced post-processing software application on a thin client-server solution. For export to PACS, thin MIPs with a slice thickness of 5 mm and 1 mm reconstruction increment are generated along the major cardiac planes (i.e., four-chamber orientation, two-chamber orientation, short axis). Likewise curved planar reformations are generated for the three major vessels and exported as rotating series in 10° intervals (i.e., 36 images per vessel) to unequivocally document correct center line positioning.

Coronary arteries are evaluated for the presence or absence of plaques and/or stenoses. Stenoses are graded according to the luminal diameter at the stenosis in relation to the luminal diameter in adjoining coronary segments as either mild (<50 %), moderate (50–69 %), or severe (≥70 % diameter stenosis) (Galperin-Aizenberg et al. 2015). In clinical routine, this measurement is usually performed by "eyeballing"; however, digital calipers are available and can be helpful in ambiguous cases.

3 Interpretation and Clinical Application of CCTA Findings

The interpretation of coronary CT angiography datasets as well as the application of findings to clinical decision-making requires considerable radiological and clinical expertise.

There is abundant data from large clinical trials that the absence of any plaque on coronary CT angiography confidently excludes ACS (Fig. 3). In ROMICAT-I, 50.3% of patients (183/368) did not exhibit any plaques in their coronary arteries (Hoffmann et al. 2009). In this subgroup no patient had a diagnosis of ACS during index hospitalization. Furthermore, in this subgroup no single patient experienced major adverse cardiac events within 2 years of follow-up. In the CTA arm of ROMICAT-II, 44.5 % of patients (210/472) did not exhibit any coronary plaques (Hoffmann et al. 2012). Among these not a single one received the diagnosis of ACS during index hospitalization either.

On the other hand, significant stenoses on coronary CTA are associated with considerable frequencies of ACS (Fig. 4). For example, in ROMICAT-I, the presence of a stenosis >50 % had a PPV for ACS of 35 % (24/68). In the CTA arm of ROMICAT-II, the presence of significant CAD (stenosis >50 %) had a PPV for ACS of 64 % (29/45).

The picture gets more complex, however, when patients do have coronary plaques or low- to intermediate-grade coronary stenoses. On the one hand, there is abundant evidence in favor of extremely low rates of ACS and MACE among patients with low-grade stenoses on CCTA:

- In a 1-year follow-up of 481 patients presenting with low-risk acute chest pain who had a maximal stenosis of less than 50 % on CCTA (Hollander et al. 2009), there was only one death (indeterminate cause). No patient sustained myocardial infarction or received coronary revascularization. Under the conservative assumption that this death was cardiac, the 1-year MACE rate was 0.2 % (1/481).
- In a registry study by Miller et al.(Miller et al. 2012) including 1419 patients presenting with low-risk acute chest pain (TIMI score≤2), 15 % (219/1419) were found to have a maximum stenosis in the 25–50 % range on coronary CTA. Among these, only a single patient (0.5 %, 1/213) developed MACE within 30 days. In this patient who experienced MI with a rise in troponin on serial evaluation, invasive angiography revealed a 99 % stenosis in an

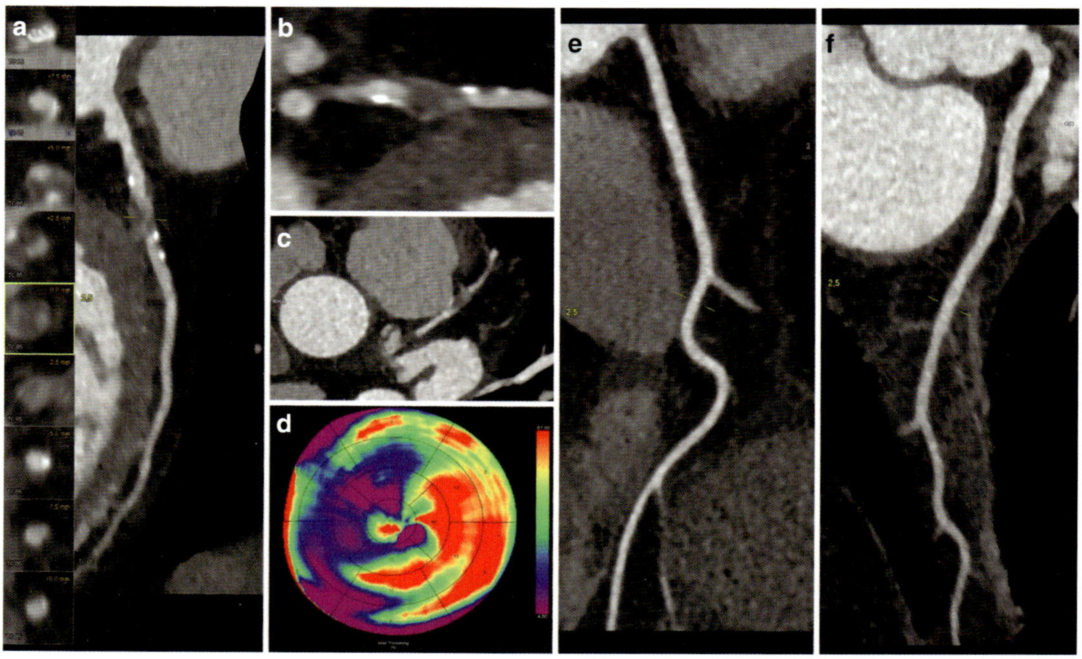

Fig. 4 55-year male patient presenting with atypical chest pain. CT-angiography shows occlusion of the mid-LAD (**a**, **b**, **c**) with corresponding hypokinesia of the anterior and septal myocardium (**d**), while no plaques were detected in the RCA (**e**) and only minimal plaques in the proximal LCx (**f**). (**a**) CPR of the LAD with yellow marker at site of occlusion; multiple small inserts on the left border displaying adjacent crosssections of the LAD; (**b**, **c**) 5 mm MIP-reformation of the site of LAD occlusion in long axis (**b**) and transverse (**c**) reformation; (**d**) 17-segment polar-map of segmental myocardial wall thickening displaying reduced contractility in the mid-ventricular anterior, anteroseptal and posteroseptal segments and the apical anterior and septal segment; (**e**) CPR of the RCA; (**f**) CPR of the LCx.

obtuse marginal branch which in retrospect could have been identified on CCTA.

- In the CTA arm of the CT-STAT trial (Goldstein et al. 2011), the 6-month MACE rate for patients who had a normal or near-normal CCTA scan (here defined as maximal stenosis < 25 %) was 0.8 % (2/268, two PCI revascularizations, 0 acute MIs, 0 deaths).
- In the CCTA arm of the ACRIN-PA trial (Litt et al. 2012), 70 % (640/908) of patients had a maximum stenosis of < 50 %. None of these patients died or had a myocardial infarction within 30 days after presentation. Within 1 year, one of these 640 experienced cardiac death (sudden cardiac death due to ventricular fibrillation arrest; the patient had reported a history of cocaine use during index visit; MACE rate 0.16 % [1/640]), and none had myocardial infarction in this period (Hollander et al. 2016).

On the other hand, data from several other studies taint this notion of an extremely low probability of ACS in patients with low- to intermediate-grade stenoses. In ROMICAT-I, 23 % of patients (7/31) who received a diagnosis of ACS during index hospitalization did show coronary plaques but no relevant stenosis at CCTA. Among patients developing NSTEMI, 38 % (3/8) did have plaques but no relevant stenosis on CCTA. In the CTA arm of ROMICAT-II, 22 % of patients (8/37) who received the diagnosis of ACS during index hospitalization only had stenoses < 50 % (i.e., nonsignificant CAD). These results appear similar to earlier invasive angiography studies which reported an absence of significant stenoses in 12–14 % of patients with ACS (Roe et al. 2000). These patients tend to present with small-vessel disease which is a known limitation of CCTA.

Several strategies have been pursued for further risk stratification of patients with low- to intermediate-grade coronary stenosis. Recent scientific efforts have been directed toward the identification of certain high-risk plaque features beyond the degree of luminal stenosis. It has been known for a long time that the culprit lesions in ACS responsible for acute coronary occlusion frequently are not associated with high-grade stenosis but rather with low- or intermediate-grade stenosis (Giroud et al. 1992). Features of high-risk plaques derived from CCTA are large plaque volume, positive coronary remodeling, spotty calcifications (Kitagawa et al. 2009), larger proportion of noncalcified plaques, low mean and minimal CT attenuation values, and the so-called napkin-ring sign (Maurovich-Horvat et al. 2012; Maurovich-Horvat et al. 2010) (defined as a ringlike peripheral higher attenuation of the noncalcified portion of the coronary plaque). The diagnostic value of high-risk plaque features had already been demonstrated for the ROMICAT-I trial (Ferencik et al. 2012). In a post hoc analysis of the ROMICAT-II trial, high-risk plaque features predicted ACS independently from high-grade stenosis (Puchner et al. 2014). Among the tested high-risk plaque features, the most extensive relative risk for ACS was conferred by the presence of spotty calcifications within coronary plaques (RR 37.2). As stated in the previous paragraph, 22 % of ACS patients in ROMICAT-II did not exhibit stenoses > 50 % on CCTA – however, all of these patients showed at least one high-risk plaque feature. Therefore, the authors suggest that patients with mild stenosis and high-risk plaque cannot be safely discharged. It is important to note, however, that these criteria have to date not been tested in a prospective study context.

References

Anon (2014) National Center for Health Statistics. National Hospital Ambulatory Medical Care Survey: 2011 emergency department summary tables

Antman EM et al (2000) The TIMI risk score for unstable angina/non-ST elevation MI: a method for prognostication and therapeutic decision making. JAMA 284(7):835–842

Chang AM et al (2011) Does coronary artery calcium scoring add to the predictive value of coronary computed tomography angiography for adverse cardiovascular events in low-risk chest pain patients? Acad Emerg Med Off J Soc Acad Emerg Med 18(10):1065–1071

Cury RC, Budoff M, Taylor AJ (2013) Coronary CT angiography versus standard of care for assessment of chest pain in the emergency department. J Cardiovasc Comput Tomogr 7(2):79–82

Deseive S et al (2015) Image quality and radiation dose of a prospectively electrocardiography-triggered high-pitch data acquisition strategy for coronary CT angiography: the multicenter, randomized PROTECTION IV study. J Cardiovasc Comput Tomogr 9(4):278–285

Ferencik M et al (2012) A computed tomography-based coronary lesion score to predict acute coronary syndrome among patients with acute chest pain and significant coronary stenosis on coronary computed tomographic angiogram. Am J Cardiol 110(2):183–189

Fox KAA et al (2006) Prediction of risk of death and myocardial infarction in the six months after presentation with acute coronary syndrome: prospective multinational observational study (GRACE). BMJ (Clin Res Ed) 333(7578):1091

Galperin-Aizenberg M et al (2015) Cardiac CT angiography in the emergency department. AJR Am J Roentgenol 204(3):463–474

Georgiou D et al (2001) Screening patients with chest pain in the emergency department using electron beam tomography: a follow-up study. J Am Coll Cardiol 38(1):105–110

Giroud D et al (1992) Relation of the site of acute myocardial infarction to the most severe coronary arterial stenosis at prior angiography. Am J Cardiol 69(8): 729–732

Goldstein JA et al (2007) A randomized controlled trial of multi-slice coronary computed tomography for evaluation of acute chest pain. J Am Coll Cardiol 49(8): 863–871

Goldstein JA et al (2011) The CT-STAT (coronary computed tomographic angiography for systematic triage of acute chest pain patients to treatment) trial. J Am Coll Cardiol 58(14):1414–1422

Hoffmann U et al (2009) Coronary computed tomography angiography for early triage of patients with acute chest pain: the ROMICAT (Rule Out Myocardial Infarction using Computer Assisted Tomography) trial. J Am Coll Cardiol 53(18):1642–1650

Hoffmann U et al (2012) Coronary CT angiography versus standard evaluation in acute chest pain. N Engl J Med 367(4):299–308

Hollander JE et al (2009) One-year outcomes following coronary computerized tomographic angiography for evaluation of emergency department patients with potential acute coronary syndrome. Acad Emerg Med Off J Soc Acad Emerg Med 16(8):693–698

Hollander JE et al (2016) Coronary computed tomography angiography versus traditional care: comparison of one-year outcomes and resource use. Ann Emerg Med 67(4):460–468.e1

Hulten E et al (2013) Outcomes after coronary computed tomography angiography in the emergency department: a systematic review and meta-analysis of randomized, controlled trials. J Am Coll Cardiol 61(8): 880–892

Kitagawa T et al (2009) Characterization of noncalcified coronary plaques and identification of culprit lesions in patients with acute coronary syndrome by 64-slice computed tomography. JACC Cardiovasc Imaging 2(2):153–160

Laudon DA et al (1999) Use of electron-beam computed tomography in the evaluation of chest pain patients in the emergency department. Ann Emerg Med 33(1): 15–21

Litt HI et al (2012) CT angiography for safe discharge of patients with possible acute coronary syndromes. N Engl J Med 366(15):1393–1403

Maurovich-Horvat P et al (2012) The napkin-ring sign indicates advanced atherosclerotic lesions in coronary CT angiography. JACC Cardiovasc Imaging 5(12): 1243–1252

Maurovich-Horvat P et al (2010) The napkin-ring sign: CT signature of high-risk coronary plaques? JACC Cardiovasc Imaging 3(4):440–444

McLaughlin VV, Balogh T, Rich S (1999) Utility of electron beam computed tomography to stratify patients presenting to the emergency room with chest pain. Am J Cardiol 84(3):327–328, A8

Miller CD et al (2012) Implications of 25% to 50% coronary stenosis with cardiac computed tomographic angiography in ED patients. Am J Emerg Med 30(4): 597–605

Puchner SB et al (2014) High-risk plaque detected on coronary CT angiography predicts acute coronary syndromes independent of significant stenosis in acute chest pain: results from the ROMICAT-II trial. J Am Coll Cardiol 64(7):684–692

Roe MT et al (2000) Clinical and therapeutic profile of patients presenting with acute coronary syndromes who do not have significant coronary artery disease. The Platelet Glycoprotein IIb/IIIa in Unstable Angina: Receptor Suppression Using Integrilin Therapy (PURSUIT) Trial. Circulation 102(10):1101–1106

Roffi M et al. (2015) 2015 ESC Guidelines for the management of acute coronary syndromes in patients presenting without persistent ST-segment elevation. Eur Heart J 37(3):ehv320

Rybicki FJ et al (2016) 2015 ACR/ACC/AHA/AATS/ACEP/ASNC/NASCI/SAEM/SCCT/SCMR/SCPC/SNMMI/STR/STS Appropriate Utilization of Cardiovascular Imaging in Emergency Department Patients With Chest Pain: A Joint Document of the American College of Radiology Appropriateness Criteria Comm. J Am Coll Cardiol 67(7):853–879

Schenker MP et al (2008) Interrelation of coronary calcification, myocardial ischemia, and outcomes in patients with intermediate likelihood of coronary artery disease: a combined positron emission tomography/computed tomography study. Circulation 117(13):1693–1700

Wells PS et al (2000) Derivation of a simple clinical model to categorize patients probability of pulmonary embolism: increasing the models utility with the SimpliRED D-dimer. Thromb Haemost 83(3): 416–420

Acute Aortic Syndromes: Aortic Dissection, Intramural Haematoma and Penetrating Aortic Ulcers

Elizabeth A. Dick, Maureen Dumba, Ali Alsafi, John M. Curtis, and Elika Kashef

Contents

E.A. Dick (✉) • M. Dumba • A. Alsafi • E. Kashef
Departments of Radiology, Imperial College London, London, UK
e-mail: Elizabeth.Dick@imperial.nhs.uk

J.M. Curtis
Aintree University Hospital, Liverpool, UK

Abstract

Acute Aortic Syndrome includes three non-traumatic potentially fatal pathologies of the thoracic aorta which commonly present with chest pain.

The three inter-related entities, Aortic Dissection, Intramural Haematoma (IMH) and Penetrating Atherosclerotic Ulcers (PAUs) share a common pathogenesis: disruption of the media layer. They can be difficult to distinguish from other causes of chest pain.

Differentiation between all three diseases cannot be achieved by history or clinical findings alone but requires imaging with multi-detector computed tomography (MDCT), the modality of choice.

In all three diseases, early diagnosis and treatment will improve outcome but treatment options vary between conservative managements, endovascular treatment and open surgery, based on the clinical and radiological features.

This chapter covers clinical presentation, imaging features, optimal imaging protocols and management of all three acute aortic syndromes.

1 Introduction

Acute aortic syndrome (AAS) includes three non-traumatic potentially fatal pathologies of the thoracic aorta which commonly present with

Med Radiol Diagn Imaging (2016)
DOI 10.1007/174_2016_31, © Springer International Publishing Switzerland

chest pain and affect 2.6–3.5 per 100,000 persons per annum (Abbas et al. 2014; Maddu et al. 2013).

The three interrelated entities, aortic dissection, intramural haematoma (IMH) and penetrating atherosclerotic ulcers (PAUs), share a common pathogenesis: disruption of the media layer (Maddu et al. 2013). They can be difficult to distinguish from each other and from other causes of chest pain including MI, oesophageal perforation and pulmonary emboli. Differentiation between all three diseases cannot be achieved by history or clinical findings alone but requires imaging (Maddu et al. 2013) with multi-detector computed tomography (MDCT), the modality of choice (Salvolini et al. 2008).

In all three diseases, early diagnosis and treatment will improve outcome (Hiratzka et al. 2010; Vilacosta et al. 2009), but treatment options vary between conservative managements, endovascular treatment and open surgery, based on the clinical and radiological features.

Since 1996, a group of over 30 international cardiothoracic research centres, the International Registry of Acute Aortic Dissections (IRAD), have collected data on patients with AAS (IRADonline org). The group publishes guidelines on clinical management in this rapidly changing field. IRAD's regular and frequent updates are an invaluable reference tool in the continuously evolving clinical management of patients with AAS.

2 Clinical Presentation

Patients with AAS present with excruciating pain (Maddu et al. 2013). This pain can be difficult to differentiate from other causes, but a sudden, persistent 'tearing' transthoracic sensation aids in differentiating it from other pathologies (Hiratzka et al. 2010; Lansman et al. 2010). The initial pain is thought to represent the initial disruption of the intima. In the case of dissection, this pain may change as the dissection progresses along the arterial tree. Other presenting symptoms include syncope, which may be due to cerebral ischaemia (McMahon and Squirrell 2010) or an indicator that cardiac tamponade has developed, which occurs in dissection of the ascending aorta as a primary presentation or a complication of a type B dissection and thus is a harbinger of high mortality (Abbas et al. 2014). Physical findings can be non-specific and variable particularly in elderly patients who may present without chest pain, instead with features of heart failure or a stroke (Maddu et al. 2013). One third of patients will have signs and symptoms of systemic involvement due to branch vessel involvement – a complication which should be considered in the clinical and imaging workup (Castaner et al. 2003).

Table 1 Risk factors for AAS

Hypertension
Genetic disorders such as Marfan and Turner syndrome, coarctation of the aorta
Inflammatory vasculitis, e.g. Behcet's disease, Takayasu arteritis
Infective arteritis
Iatrogenic factors (cardiac valve or aortic surgery)
Pregnancy
Phaeochromocytoma, corticosteroid treatment, cocaine use
Aortic root anomalies, e.g. valvular aortic stenosis, bicuspid aortic valves

There are multiple risk factors for the development of AAS (see Table 1) which act through a weakening of the media or by an increase in hydraulic pressure within the aorta. Hypertension is the most common association and may be uncontrolled (Hiratzka et al. 2010; Vilacosta et al. 2009). In patients under 40, those with a family history of connective tissue disorders, such as Marfan and Ehlers-Danlos syndromes, should be considered.

The outlook for patients depends on presentation. Patients with acute (less than 2 weeks duration of symptoms) AAS are at the greatest risk of morbidity and mortality (Abbas et al. 2014).

3 Imaging Protocol

MDCT is the gold standard imaging investigation for AAS with a sensitivity of 100 % and specificity of 98–99 % (Hiratzka et al. 2010). Although

Table 2 CT appearances in AAS (Maddu et al. 2013)

	Non-contrast CT	Post-contrast CT
Aortic dissection	May be normal in the acute setting OR inward displacement of intimal calcification	Intimal flap, >2 lumens (TL and FL) Flow through both true and false lumens +/– true lumen compression
Intramural haematoma	High attenuation crescentic thickening of aortic wall	Aortic wall thickening May have similar appearances to acute aortitis
Penetrating atherosclerotic ulcer	Difficult to diagnose on unenhanced CT	Focal ulceration penetrating through aortic intima to aortic wall

TL true lumen, *FL* false lumen

MRI and transoesophageal echo have similar sensitivity and specificity, MDCT is generally preferred in an acute setting because it is near-universally available and provides speedy acquisition and high accuracy (Salvolini et al. 2008). The ability to reconstruct in three planes and to assess aortic branches including aberrant anatomy makes CT invaluable for surgical and endovascular planning (Maddu et al. 2013; Agarwal et al. 2009). Both pre- and post-contrast CT should be obtained to differentiate between the three components of AAS (Maddu et al. 2013). Table 2 summarises the CT findings in all three entities of AAS (see later text for further explanations).

At least 64 detector rows are required to achieve multiplanar isotropic spatial resolution. ECG gating is required to reduce cardiac motion artefacts – this is particularly important in accurately diagnosing dissection at the aortic root and avoiding false positives due to cardiac motion artefact mimicking an acute dissection flap. ECG gating also improves coronary artery visualisation. The field of view for pre-contrast ECG-gated CT should extend from above the aortic arch to the inferior diaphragm. This should be acquired prospectively in mid diastole. Premedication with beta-blockers or other medications should be avoided (31 Chin in Abbas). On the non-contrast CT, high-density IMH can be identified, and local pleural or pericardial rupture can also be demonstrated (Abbas et al. 2014; Castaner et al. 2003). A bolus tracking CT angiogram achieving opacification of the aorta of >250 HU follows, covering from the thoracic inlet to the aortoiliac bifurcation or common femoral arteries, with precise timing of image acquisition and imaging parameters varying slightly with machines (Castaner et al. 2003). The usual volume of iodinated 370 mg/ml contrast medium of 120 ml is decreased in elderly patients to 80–100 ml in view of decreased cardiac output. The contrast should be injected via the right arm to avoid streak artefact from the left brachiocephalic vein near head and neck vessels. A saline flush of 20 ml further minimises streak artefact (Weininger et al. 2011). The patient is able to free breathe during abdominal aortic imaging, but chest imaging is acquired in breath-hold.

Multiplanar reformat assessment is advisable since it helps in the evaluation of the aortic root. Moreover, clinicians appreciate 2D and 3D reconstructions as they are useful for planning surgical or endovascular procedures (Agarwal et al. 2009). Maximum intensity projection reconstructions are valuable for visualisation of branch vessel involvement (Abbas et al. 2014).

Alternative techniques to MDCT in patients in whom iodinated contrast is contraindicated include transoesophageal echocardiography and MRI, but both of these techniques are time-consuming and not widely available in all hospital settings. Contrast-enhanced MR angiography has excellent spatial and contrast resolution and allows multiple vascular imaging phases and post-processing. Its limitations include the inability to demonstrate arterial wall or intimal calcification, lack of suitability for unstable patients or those with implanted electronic devices and the problem of artefacts due to stent placement

(McMahon and Squirrell 2010). Initial unenhanced CT followed by MRI (where feasible) or transoesophageal echocardiography may be a reasonable compromise in patients who cannot receive iodinated contrast or in whom repeated examinations are required, as CT will demonstrate IMH, intimal calcification displacement, rupture into pleural or pericardial space and aortic size (Abbas et al. 2014).

4 Classification in Acute Aortic Syndrome: The Stanford Classification

Classification of AAS is based on the location and extension of the dissection, with the Stanford system preferred over the DeBakey system in the emergency setting because it dictates immediate clinical management (broadly speaking, surgical= type A, medical=type B) (Maddu et al. 2013). Stanford type A affects the ascending aorta or aortic arch and accounts for 75 % of aortic dissection (Castaner et al. 2003). The dissection flap may extend to the descending aorta (McMahon and Squirrell 2010). Stanford type B begins distal to the left subclavian artery. For all three entities of AAS (dissection, IMH, PAU), the diagnosis of type A involvement requires immediate referral to a cardiothoracic surgical centre.

5 Acute Aortic Dissection

There are 2000 new cases of aortic dissection each year in the USA and 3000 in Europe (McMahon and Squirrell 2010). Dissection is the most common aortic emergency, being more prevalent than thoracoabdominal aortic aneurysm rupture (Castaner et al. 2003). Acute thoracic dissection is life-threatening and requires immediate diagnosis and treatment (Castaner et al. 2003): 75 % of deaths from aortic dissection occur within 2 weeks of clinical presentation.

The normal aortic wall has three layers (from external to internal: adventitia, media and intima) (Fig. 1). The pathophysiology of aortic dissection includes disruption of the aortic intima and inner layer of the media such that blood can track along the media (Macura et al. 2003) (Fig. 2). This propagation can be both retrograde and anterograde (Maddu et al. 2013) and results in formation of a true and a false lumen with the false lumen having pressures greater than or equal to the true lumen (Williams et al. 1997). Since the intervening 'intimal flap' between the two lumens consists of intima and media, it should more precisely be termed an 'intimomedial' flap. It is theorised that reduced elastic recoil of the dissection flap enables the false lumen to dilate. This resulting collapse of the true lumen is highly variable based on the number of fenestrations and tears between the true and false lumen, the chronicity of the flap and the degree of control of the patient's blood pressure. In our clinical experience, the patient's response to the compressed true lumen and their overall clinical status dictates further management (McMahon and Squirrell 2010; Williams et al. 1997). The overall degree of dilation of the false lumen depends on blood pressure, residual wall thickness and percentage of wall circumference involved in the dissection. The false lumen may subsequently compress or obstruct the true lumen. The dissection may remain patent as a false lumen, may thrombose or may recommunicate with the true lumen through fenestrations (Macura et al. 2003). Alternatively, it may rupture into a pericardial or pleural space (McMahon and Squirrell 2010). The greater the proportion of the media involved in the flap, the thinner the external wall of the false lumen, and therefore, the higher the risk of rupture (Roberts 1981). The initial intimal tear occurs at sites of greatest hydraulic pressure – usually the right lateral wall of the ascending aorta or the proximal segment of the descending aorta (Maddu et al. 2013).

5.1 Imaging Features

The presence of an intimomedial flap and the double-lumen aorta are both key features of aortic dissection. Further features include the origin and extent of dissection, which is the true and which is the false lumen, and whether branch vessels are affected (Hiratzka et al. 2010). A dissection flap is identified as a thin, uniform, low-

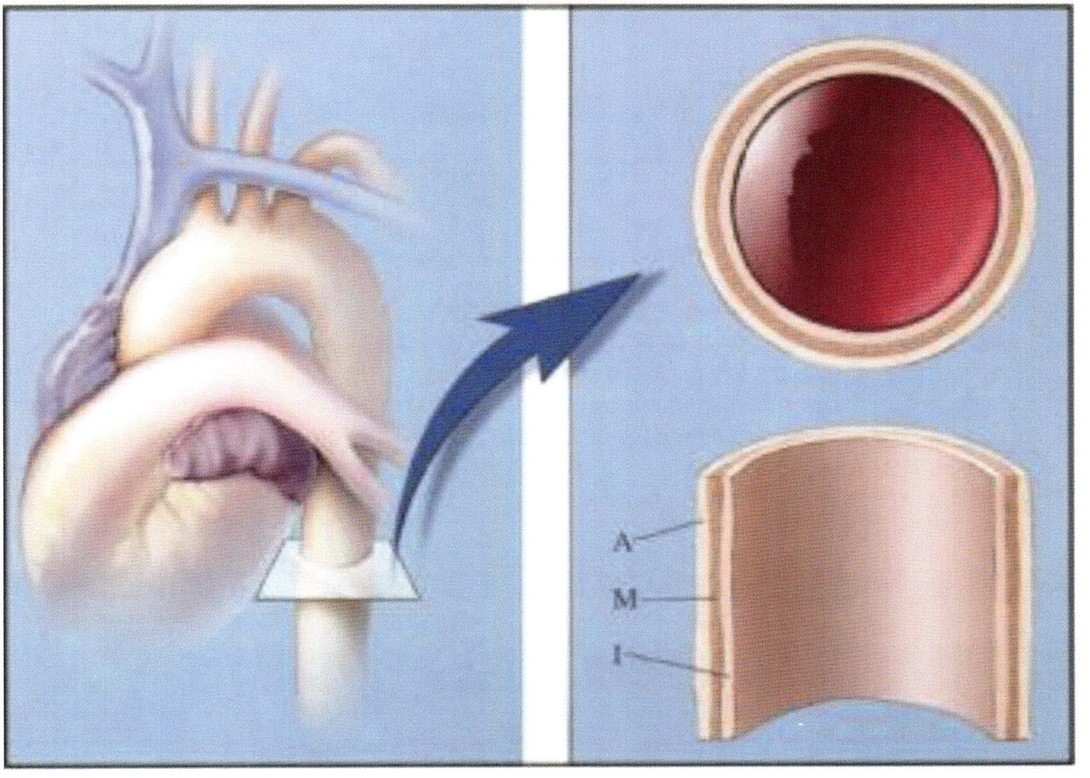

Fig. 1 Diagram shows three layers of normal aortic wall: from inner to outer, intima (*I*), media (*M*) and adventitia (*A*) (Reproduced from Macura et al. 2003, Pathogenesis in Acute Aortic Syndromes (Permission requested))

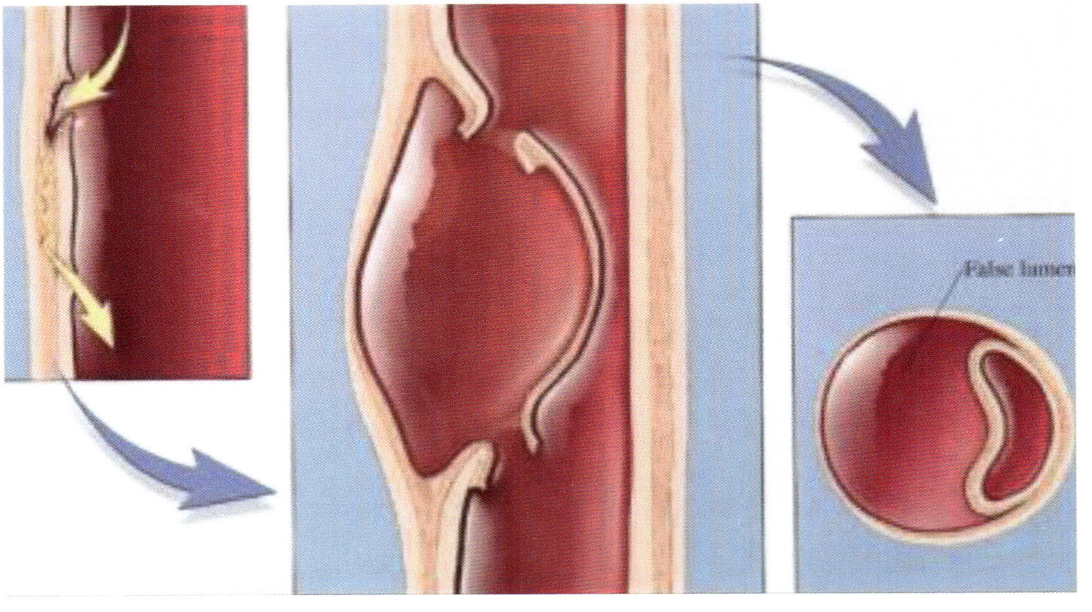

Fig. 2 The diagram illustrates events leading to aortic dissection from formation of entrance tear and exit tear of intima to splitting of aortic media and formation of intimomedial flap. Blood under pressure dissections medial longitudinally and double-channel aorta is formed with blood filling both true and false lumens (Reproduced from Macura et al. 2003, Pathogenesis in Acute Aortic Syndromes (Permission requested))

density flap on multiple contiguous slices, which is important in distinguishing it from artefactual flaps including streak artefact and cardiac motion. Streak artefacts have a variable width and orientation, radiate away from a high-density focus and may have high and low densities (Abbas et al. 2014). Cardiac motion artefact characteristically is seen in the right posterior and left anterior proximal aorta (Figs. 3 and 4).

It is particularly important to differentiate between the false and true lumen if endovascular treatment is planned (Castaner et al. 2003). The true lumen is continuous with the non-dissected portion of the aorta and can usually be identified (Maddu et al. 2013). Differentiating between the false and true lumen is more difficult when the aortic root is involved, for instance, in rare cases of intimointimal intussusception/circumferential dissection, which produce a circumferential flap with one lumen wrapped around the other lumen in the aortic arch. The inner lumen is usually the true lumen (Castaner et al. 2003).

The false lumen can be usually differentiated from the true lumen by the presence of slower flow (lower density opacification), wider channel and presence of thin 'cobweb' strands due to medial tissue within the false lumen (Litmanovich et al. 2009). The 'beak sign' occurs at the acute angle of the intimomedial flap and outer wall of the FL. Calcification may help to differentiate between the FL and TL – it has been described as only being seen in the wall of true lumen. The

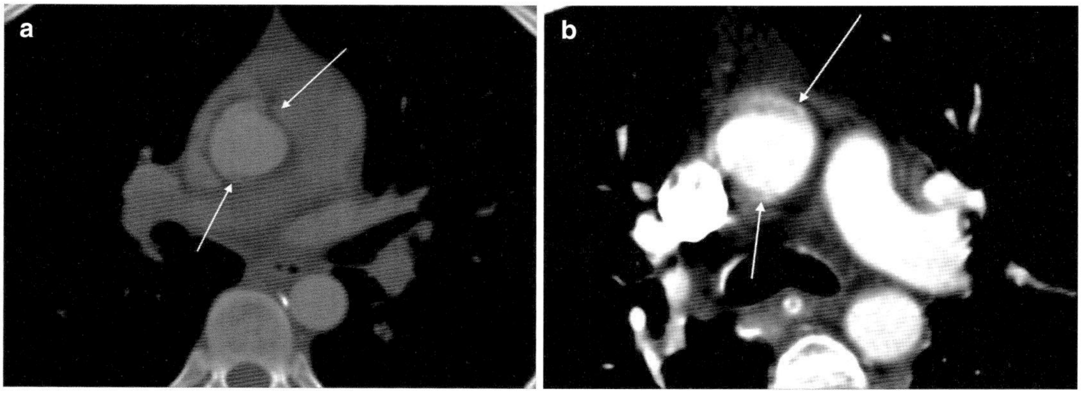

Fig. 3 Motion artefact. A cardiac motion artefact in the ascending aorta mimics a Stanford type A dissection in 2 different patients (**a** and **b**) (*arrowed*)

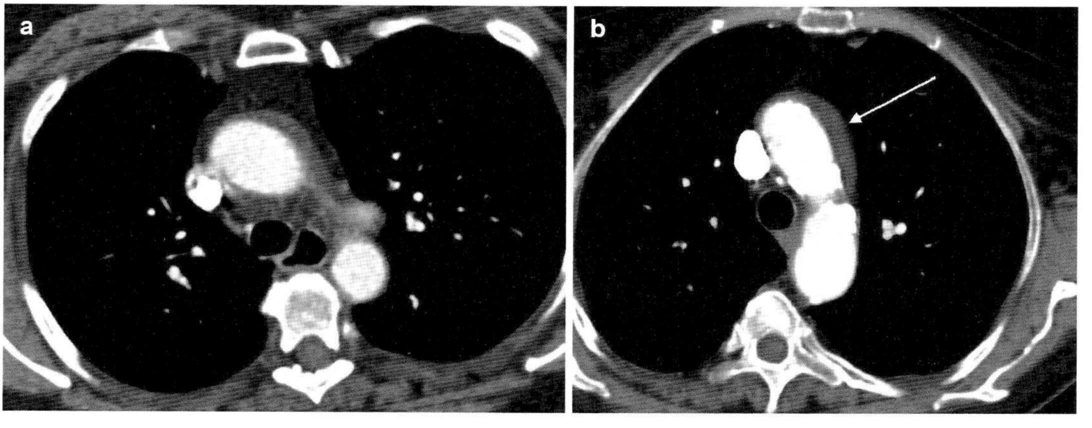

Fig. 4 Pseudodissection. A high superior pericardial recess mimics a Stanford type A dissection (*arrowed*)

Table 3 CT findings useful in differentiating between the TL and FL

CT finding	True lumen	False lumen
Communication with aorta	Directly communicates with aorta	Not connected to unaffected aorta
Intimomedial flap rupture		Communicates with false lumen
Calibre	Smaller than FL	Larger than TL
Intimal flap	Calcified	Surface of flap is convex
Enhancement	Enhances more than false lumen	Slower flow therefore hypodense to TL (in the arterial phase)
Other signs		Cobweb sign Beak sign 'Floating viscera' sign (true lumen is compressed but contrast is seen in visceral arteries)

Adapted from Maddu et al. (2013)

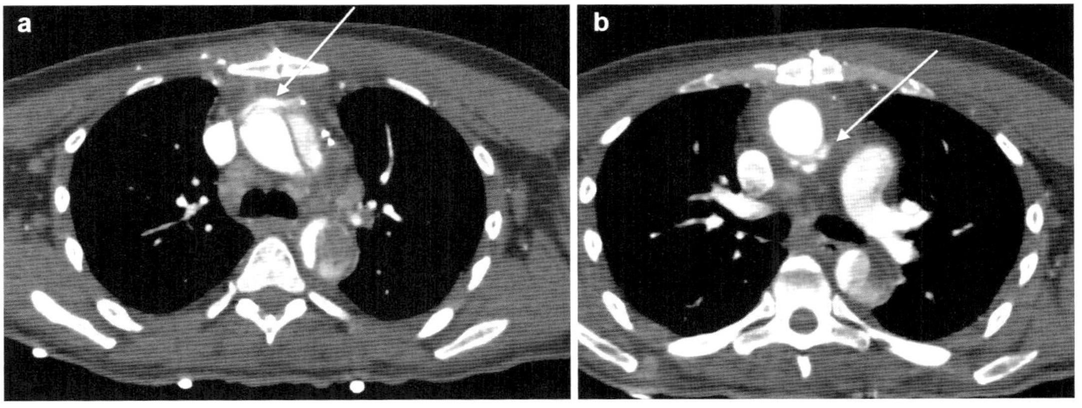

Fig. 5 Stanford type A dissection. Note extravasation of contrast from ascending aorta giving rise to mediastinal haematoma (*arrowed*)

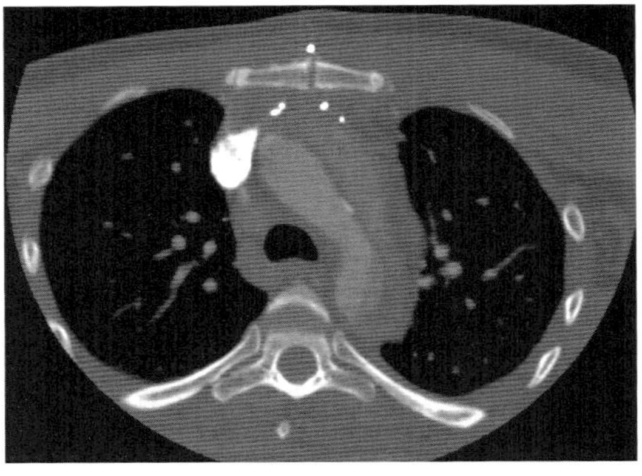

Fig. 6 Stanford type A aortic dissection. Note displacement of the intimal calcification by clot in the false lumen which lies lateral to the intimal flap

'floating viscera' sign occurs when the visceral arteries are opacified with contrast media, but the true lumen appears compressed (see Table 3) (Figs. 5, 6, 7 and 8).

Dissection with a thrombosed false lumen can be difficult to differentiate from aortic aneurysm with intraluminal thrombus, but the dissection will generally have a spiral shape, whereas the aneurysm and thrombus tend to maintain a constant circumferential relationship with the aortic wall. The mural thrombus usually has an irregular internal border, whereas dissection has a smooth internal border. Finally, intimal calcification is peripheral in an aortic aneurysm (Castaner et al. 2003).

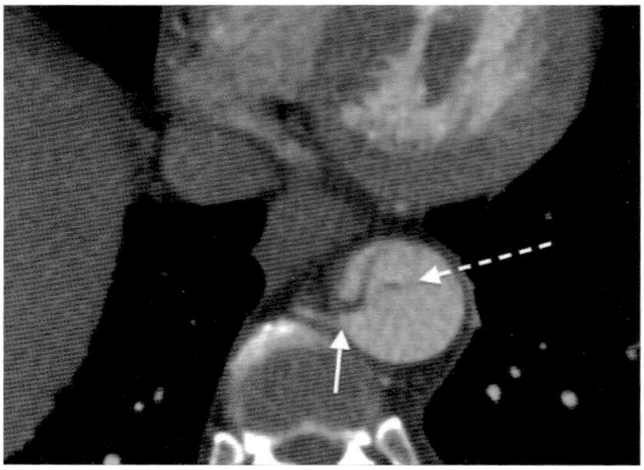

Fig. 7 Stanford type B dissection. Note the cobweb sign (*dotted arrow*) present which is caused by strands of fragmented media in the false lumen. Although not commonly seen, the cobweb sign is highly specific for the false lumen. Note the beak sign (*solid arrow*) caused by the false lumen as it contacts the junction of the intimal flap and aortic wall

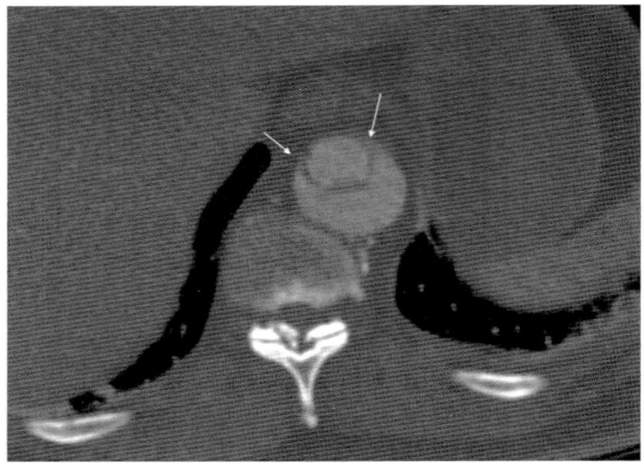

Fig. 8 The beak sign. The false lumen forms (*arrowed*) an acute angle with the aortic wall and the intimal flap. The true lumen is circular in cross-section; the false lumen is crescenteric

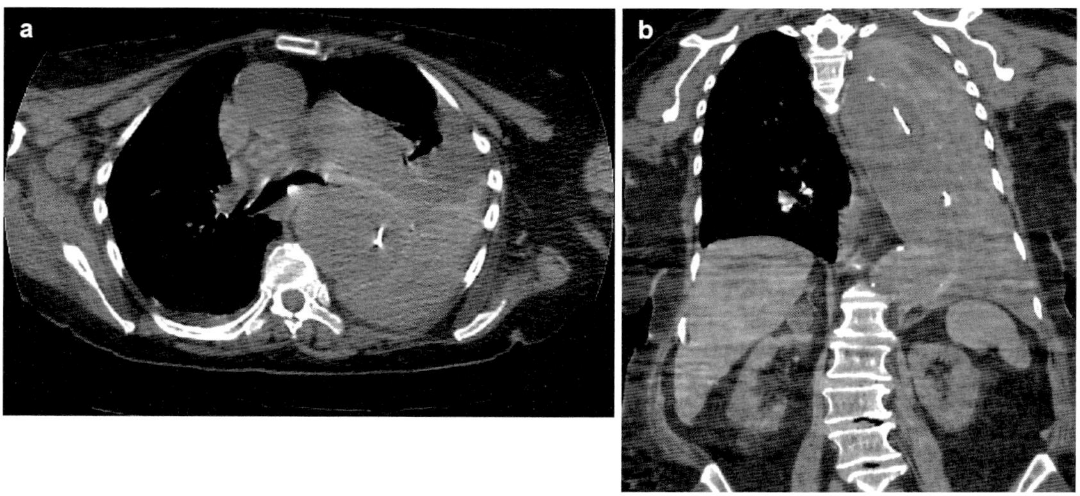

Fig. 9 Aortic dissection. Unenhanced CT thorax. Note inward displacement of intimal calcification by the false lumen

Complications of dissection include pericardial tamponade, acute aortic regurgitation, aortic rupture and major vessel occlusion (Hiratzka et al. 2010) (Fig. 9). Rupture is more common in ascending aortic dissection with rupture into the pericardium, left pleural cavity or mediastinum; hence, the treatment of ascending aorta dissection is always surgical (Abbas et al. 2014; Castaner et al. 2003). The radiologist can help the surgeon by assessing involvement of the coronary arteries in very proximal aortic dissection (Chiu et al. 2013). The risk of fatal aortic rupture in untreated proximal aortic dissection is 90 % with 75 % of ruptures taking place in the pericardium, left pleural cavity or mediastinum, where hyper-attenuating fluid will be demonstrated on unenhanced CT with extravasation on contrast-enhanced CT (Castaner et al. 2003). The presence of a pericardial effusion is a particularly ominous sign, suggesting a rupture or leak (Castaner et al. 2003) (Fig. 10). A rarer

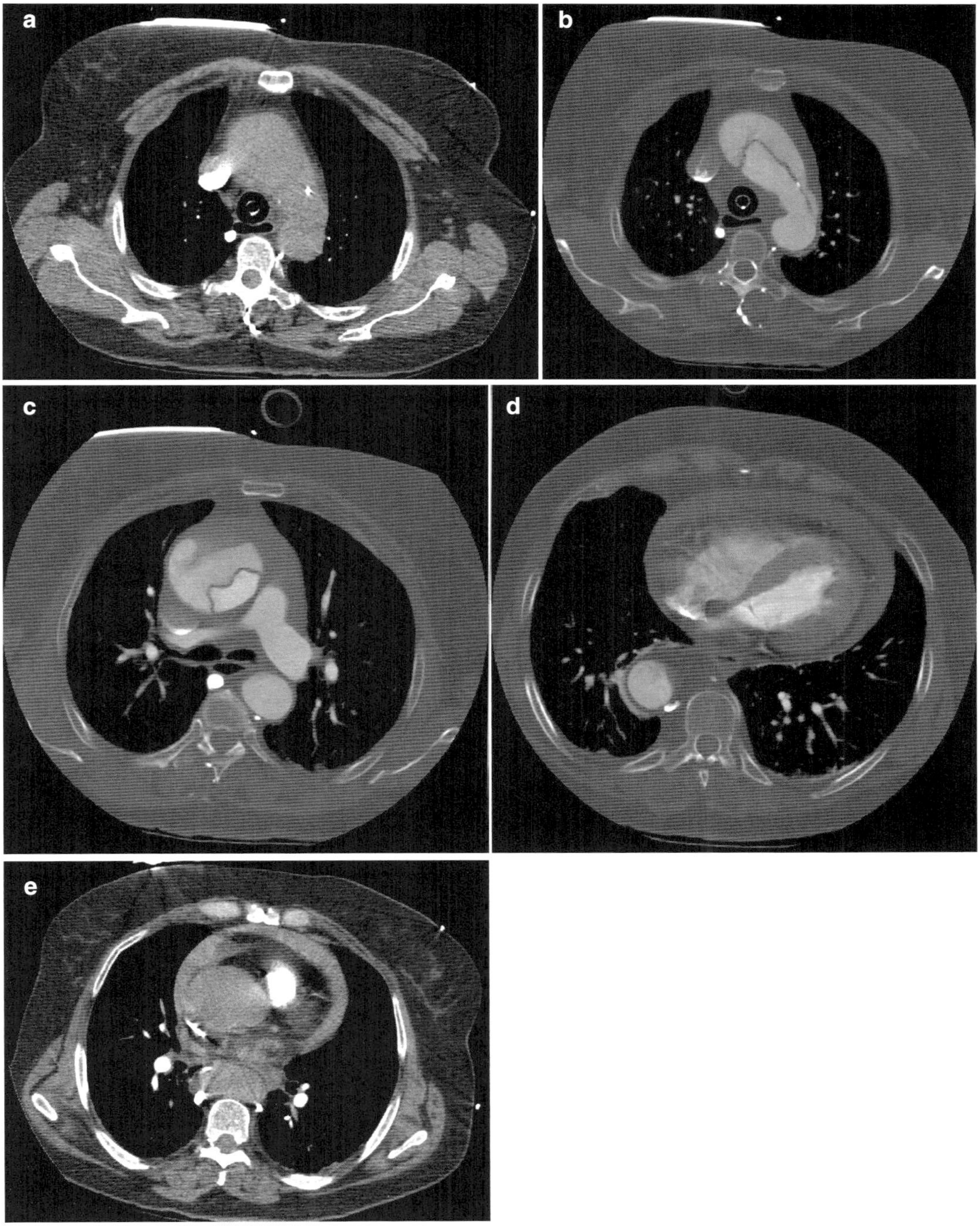

Fig. 10 Stanford type A aortic dissection on a CTPA study. (**a**) Note medial displacement of intimal calcification on the CTPA study. (**b** + **c**) Arterial phase showing calcified intimal flap. The false lumen lies lateral to the intimal flap. (**d** + **e**). Haemopericardium

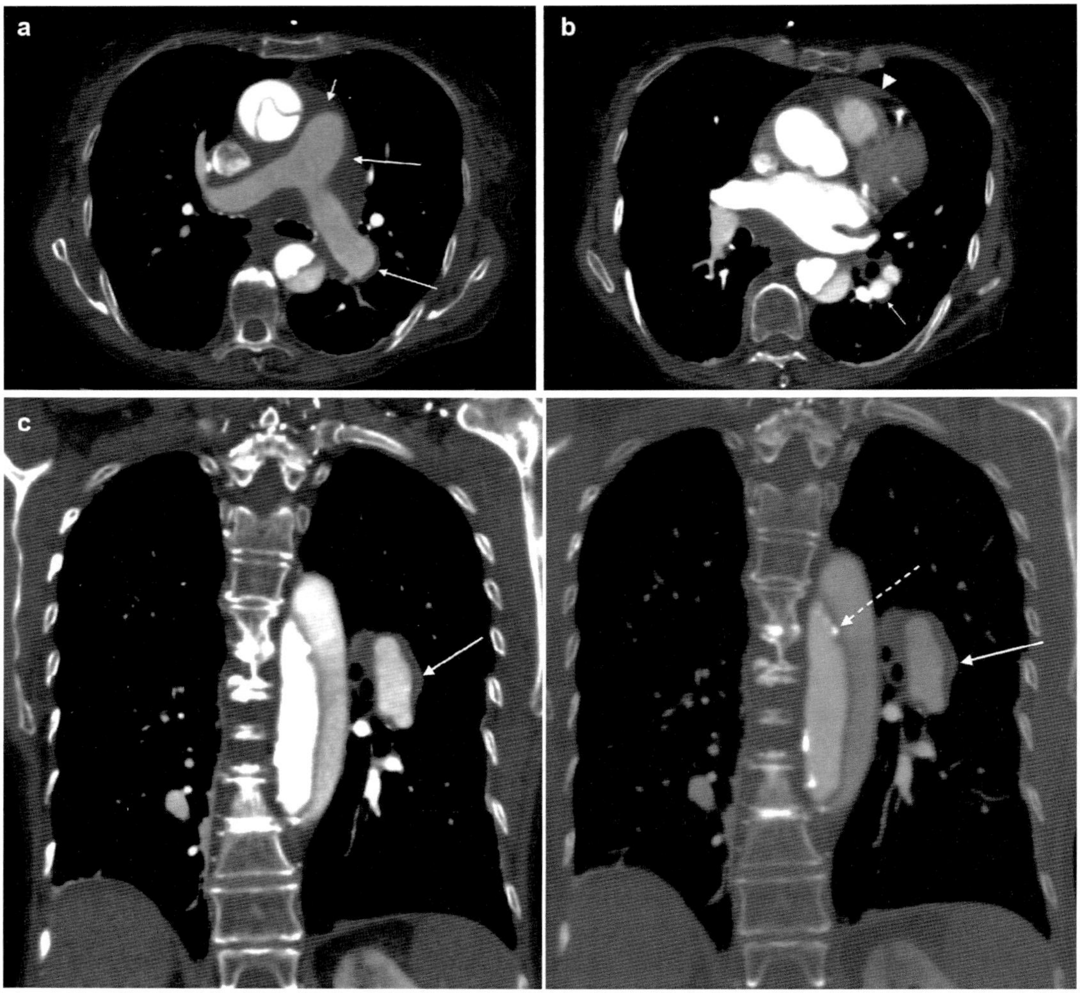

Fig. 11 (**a**) Type A aortic dissection with pulmonary artery sheath haematoma. Note the presence of haematoma (*arrows*) alongside the pulmonary artery caused by aortic dissection rupturing into the sheath of the pulmonary trunk. (**b**) Type A aortic dissection with pulmonary artery sheath haematoma. Note the presence of haematoma (*arrow*) alongside the pulmonary artery caused by aortic dissection rupturing into the sheath of the pulmonary trunk. Note haemopericardium (*arrowhead*). (**c**) Type A aortic dissection with pulmonary artery sheath haematoma. Note the presence of haematoma (*arrows*) alongside the pulmonary artery caused by aortic dissection rupturing into the sheath of the pulmonary trunk. Note displacement of the intimal calcification associated with acute aortic dissection (*dotted arrow*)

complication of type A dissection is mediastinal haematoma dissecting the sheath of the pulmonary arteries due to blood flow from the ascending aorta to the interstitial space around the pulmonary arteries (Castaner et al. 2003) (Fig. 11).

The presence of aberrant anatomy, such as an aberrant subclavian artery, and the involvement of all of the branches of the aorta should be addressed systematically with consideration of secondary ischaemia including whether the branch vessel is supplied by the true or false lumen. This is especially significant in coronary and head and neck vessel involvement (Litmanovich et al. 2009). Supra-aortic trunk involvement causing cerebral

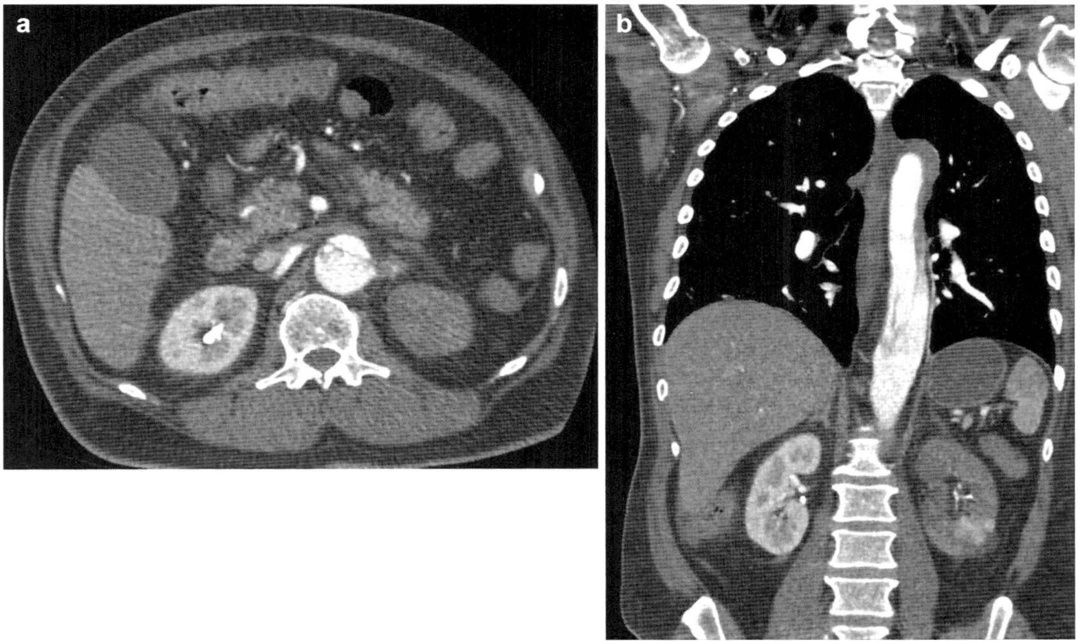

Fig. 12 Type B aortic dissection involving visceral arteries. The dissection flap has resulted in the false lumen being in continuity with the left renal artery. Note the large area of infarction in the left kidney

ischaemia is relatively rare (5–10 % (Castaner et al. 2003)), but involvement of these vessels carries a particularly poor prognosis (Litmanovich et al. 2009). Visceral branch vessel obstruction occurs in 1/3 of aortic dissection patients either due to the dissection flap extending across the lumen as a 'curtain' (dynamic occlusion) or into the wall of the branch vessel (static obstruction) (Abbas et al. 2014) (Fig. 12). It is key to remember that secondary ischaemia will not be visible on CT in the early stages, and therefore, a rising serum lactate level and true lumen compression together constitute the indication for intervention. Another theoretical mechanism of organ ischaemia is due to dissected aortic rupture causing blood to leak into structures surrounding an organ; however, this has not been our experience in clinical practice (Castaner et al. 2003). Finally, the presence or absence of dissection into the iliac and femoral vessels should be recorded and is particularly useful if endovascular treatment is contemplated.

6 IMH

IMH comprises 10–30 % of AAS patients and is defined as acute haemorrhage contained with the layers of the aortic wall (Lansman et al. 2010). IMH had been thought to be due to rupture of the vasa vasorum within the media without intimal interruption. However, there is increasing recognition based on autopsy findings that IMH may result from microscopic intimal tears (Maddu et al. 2013; Hiratzka et al. 2010; Chin and Fleischmann 2012), and with improved MDCT technology, intimal tears in IMH are becoming more easily visible (Kitai et al. 2011). Currently, there is a belief that IMH may be a variant or precursor of aortic dissection; in fact, it is likely that IMH is part of the acute aortic dissection spectrum. Essentially, the aortic wall layers are separated and filled with thrombus rather than free-flowing blood of a classic dissection (Maddu et al. 2013).

6.1 Imaging Features

IMH can only be confidently diagnosed on imaging: the most common finding being focal crescentic high attenuation (>45HU) within the thickened aortic wall on unenhanced CT that does not enhance and does not demonstrate a dissection flap. In our experience, IMH does not compress the aortic lumen. Intimal calcifications will be displaced by IMH (Castaner et al. 2003). IMH can be differentiated from a thrombosed false lumen of aortic dissection because IMH maintains a constant circumferential relationship with the aortic wall, whereas a dissection tends to spiral longitudinally (Maddu et al. 2013). IMH can however be difficult to differentiate from aortitis as both encase the aorta and both cause stranding.

Both IMH and PAU have an unpredictable evolution without treatment compared to dissection (Maddu et al. 2013). This is further complicated by different experiences in North America and Europe compared to Japan and Korea (Lansman et al. 2010). Clinically, IMH may resolve (reported to occur in 19 % of Western patients but more than 60 % of Korean patients (Lansman et al. 2010; Tittle et al. 2002)) or progress to dissection, aneurysm formation or rupture in approximately 45 % of patients (Abbas et al. 2014; Evangelista et al. 2005). Features that suggest risk of progression are listed below (Table 4). The 5-year mortality of IMH in the West is 50 %, and therefore, CT follow-up is required for conservatively treated patients (Abbas et al. 2014). However, mortality is lower in Korea and Japan: for example, in a recent series of 50 type A IMH patients from Japan, early and late progression was 30 and 10 % with an overall mortality of only 4 % (Kitai et al. 2009).

Table 4 Features suggesting risk of progression of IMH to aortic dissection

Ascending aorta involved
Aortic diameter >5 cm
Haematoma thickness >11 mm
Associated PAU (penetrating atherosclerotic ulcer) diameter >20 mm, depth > 10 mm
Temporal enlargement on serial imaging
Recurrent chest pain
Pleural or pericardial effusions, particularly if large or temporally progressive

7 PAU

PAUs comprise 2–8 % of AAS patients and develop from atherosclerotic aortic lesions which ulcerate into the internal elastic intima and media (Maddu et al. 2013; Vilacosta et al. 2009) (Fig. 13). PAUs usually occur in elderly patients with multiple atherosclerotic comorbidities such as coronary or peripheral arterial disease (Maddu et al. 2013). Younger patients with connective tissue disorders or a mycotic plaque are also at risk.

7.1 Imaging Features

PAUs can be differentiated from simple ulcerated atherosclerotic plaques because the intimal disruption leads to extension of blood into the media, visible on CT (Abbas et al. 2014; Litmanovich et al. 2009). In comparison, uncomplicated simple atherosclerotic ulcers remain within the intimal layer, and therefore, there is no extension of contrast beyond the intimal level. The presence of a focal contrast-filled outpouching of the aortic wall is diagnostic of a PAU. The outpouching has a jagged edge, and there is often extensive atheromatous disease and intimal calcification in keeping with the above-noted comorbidities (Maddu et al. 2013; Vilacosta et al. 2009). Wall thickening is also seen and this enhances (Kazerooni et al. 1992) (Fig. 14). PAUs are usually located in the middle or distal third of the descending aorta or less commonly within the aortic arch (Castaner et al. 2003). They rarely occur in the ascending aorta because rapid blood flow from the left ventricle provides protection against atherosclerosis (Welch et al. 1990). Deeper PAUs can be associated with an IMH (Abbas et al. 2014). The incidence of complications is high – up to 70 % (Maddu et al. 2013).

Complications of PAUs include false aneurysm formation, focal limited dissection and rup-

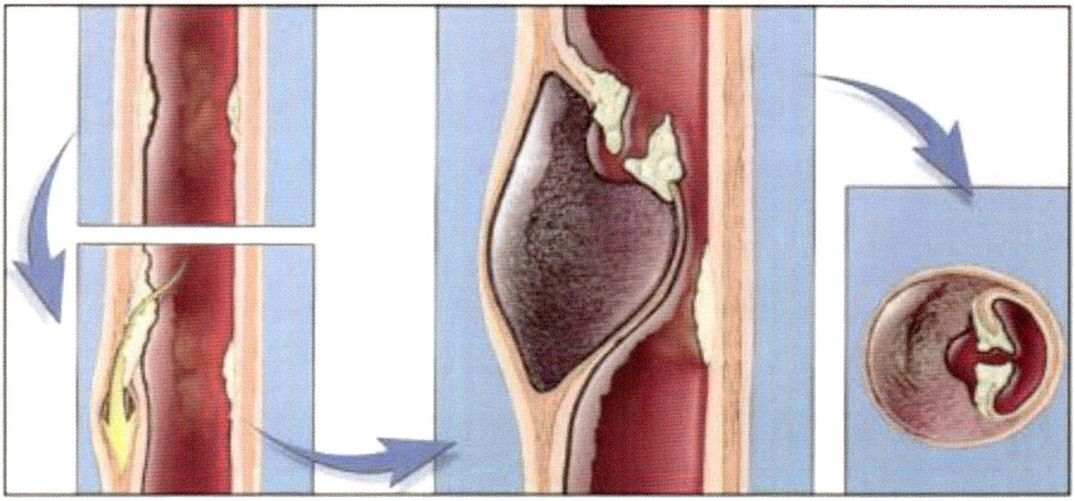

Fig. 13 Diagram shows events leading to penetrating aortic ulcer from formation of extensive aortic atheroma confined to the intimal layer through lesion progression to deep ulceration of plaque with penetration into media to entrance of blood from aortic lumen into media and splitting of media with intramural haematoma. Haematoma formation may extend along media resulting in long segment intramural haematoma (Reproduced from Macura et al. 2003, Pathogenesis in Acute Aortic Syndromes (Permission requested))

ture (Abbas et al. 2014; Vilacosta et al. 2009). In fact, some authors have theorised that most saccular aneurysms are caused by a PAU (Castaner et al. 2003).

8 Management of Aortic Dissection

Stanford A dissections have a mortality of 1–2% per hour after symptom onset if untreated (Abbas et al. 2014; DeSanctis et al. 1987). By 24 h mortality is 24% and by 14 days, 49% (Abbas et al. 2014). Some authorities suggest that a further subclassification of type A dissections should be created: type B*. This refers to dissections distal to the origin of the brachiocephalic artery, the significance of this being that some authors advocate nonoperative management (Lempel et al. 2014).

For uncomplicated type B dissection, medical management of hypertension alone is indicated since the 30-day mortality is 10% (van Bogerijen et al. 2014). However, patients with ischaemic complications such as renal failure or visceral ischaemia or who have signs of impending rupture should have immediate endovascular or surgical aortic repair (Maddu et al. 2013). Patients with partial thrombosis of the false lumen require intensive follow-up as they have a higher annual growth rate than dissections with patent or complete thrombosis of the false lumen (Maddu et al. 2013; Trimarchi et al. 2013). Risk factors for aortic dilation and adverse outcome are listed in Table 5.

If patients develop complications such as contained rupture or branch vessel ischaemia, invasive management may be needed, but this carries a risk of morbidity and mortality (31%) (Abbas et al. 2014; Piffaretti et al. 2006). Endovascular procedures such as stent grafting, branch vessel stenting and dissection flap fenestration may have a lower mortality and morbidity. However, requirement for reintervention is 7.2% over 12 months after a successful endovascular procedure, and the 12-month mortality is 11.4%; therefore, continued follow-up is indicated in these patients (Abbas et al. 2014).

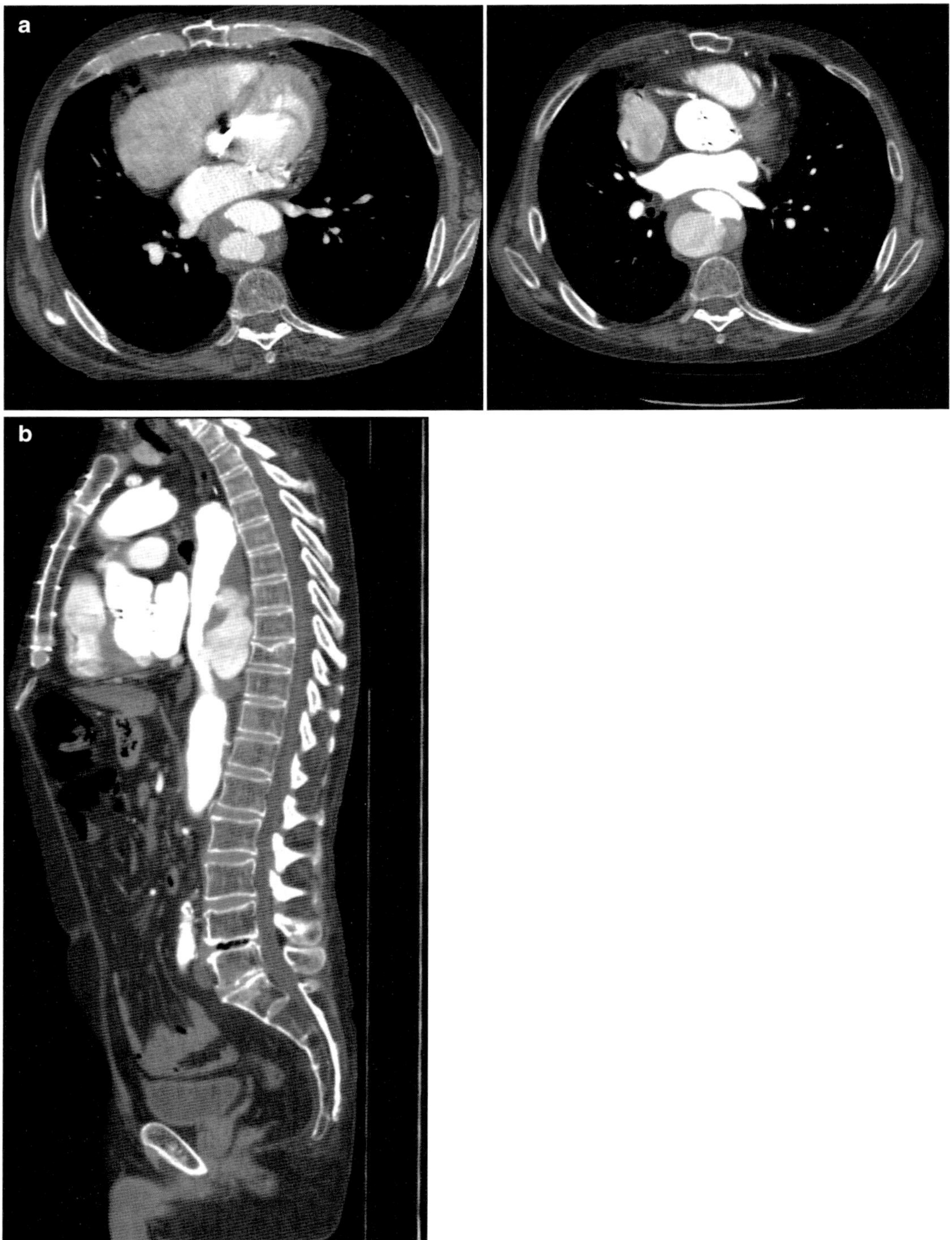

Fig. 14 (**a**) Penetrating atherosclerotic ulcer. There is a large intramural haematoma. Note the contrast-filled penetrating atherosclerotic ulcer. (**b**) Penetrating atherosclerotic ulcer. There is a large intramural haematoma. Note the contrast-filled penetrating atherosclerotic ulcer

Table 5 Risk factors for aortic dilation or adverse outcome in uncomplicated type B aortic dissection (van Bogerijen et al. 2014)

Male
Marfan syndrome
Aortic diameter >4 cm initial CT
Fusiform dilation of proximal descending aorta
Elliptical shape of true lumen
Saccular FL
Partial thrombosis FL
FL on inner curvature of aorta
Single entrance tear
Large entrance tear >10 mm within the proximal aspect of dissection

9 Management of IMH

The Stanford Classification is currently used for IMH in the West, and, as for dissection, early surgical repair has been advocated for type A IMH (Abbas et al. 2014). In the West, mortality rates with surgical repair of 8 % compare to 55 % with conservative measures (Abbas et al. 2014) and therefore, traditionally the diagnosis of IMH has merited urgent cardiothoracic surgical referral. However, reports from Eastern centres including meta-analyses have shown no difference in mortality between medical and surgical treatment (14 % versus 10 %) (Lansman et al. 2010). The divergence between Eastern and Western experience has not been explained, but it has led to a variety of approaches to the management of type A IMH, with a cautious adoption of the Eastern conservative strategy by some US and European centres (Lansman et al. 2010). Some Japanese and Korean centres use a 'time urgent' approach to patients with type A IMH, closely observing patients for 30 days after onset of symptoms before deciding on surgery based on certain criteria. Daily transthoracic echocardiography from days 0–5 followed by CT at day 5 and thereafter weekly CT and echocardiography is required for 30 days (Kitai et al. 2009) (see Table 6).

Patients with type B IMH without rupture can be treated conservatively (Coady et al. 2010). However, patients with type B IMH have a higher risk of mortality and rupture than a patient with type B dissection. Therefore, careful imaging and clinical follow-up are required. Endovascular treatment of type B IMH has so far been shown to have good outcomes (Coady et al. 2010).

Table 6 Criteria for timed surgery for type A IMH (Abbas et al. 2014)

Criteria for observation of type A IMH	Criteria for timed surgical intervention
Haemodynamically stable	Pain
Aortic diameter <5 cm	Increasing aortic diameter
Haematoma thickness <10 mm	Increasing thickness of IMH
No PAU	Increasing pericardial or pleural effusion
No large or progressive pericardial or pleural effusion	Progression to aortic dissection
No tamponade	Development of PAU
No end-organ malperfusion	Development of tamponade
	Development of end-organ malperfusion

10 Management of PAUs

There are conflicting reports about the natural history of PAUs (Lansman et al. 2010). Many consider PAUs to have an unfavourable prognosis, but others have reported successful conservative therapy including complete resolution of IMH within 1 year (Lansman et al. 2010). Therefore, decisions regarding conservative versus interventional management can be difficult. All authorities agree that pending or actual rupture requires urgent intervention (Lansman et al. 2010). The presence of extra-adventitial blood, grossly bulging IMH and temporally progressive haemothorax are further indicators for intervention (Coady et al. 2010). Surgical repair of a PAU is generally more complex and extensive than surgical repair of type B aortic dissection since much of the wall may have been damaged by ulceration and therefore require replacement (Castaner et al. 2003). Luminal irregularity requires extensive endografting and carries the risk of paraplegia (due to the occlusion of intercostal arteries (Lansman et al. 2010)). Endograft treatment has been reported to have a good outcome with a 12 % 30-day mortality (Lansman et al. 2010).

The management and outcomes in type B PAUs are similar to those for type B IMH (Coady et al. 2010). If a PAU is asymptomatic, it is more likely to warrant conservative management, but in all cases, patients with PAUs should be followed up with imaging (Maddu et al. 2013). The development of an aortic diameter >55 mm or >10 mm per annum and the presence of periaortic haematoma are in favour of subsequent intervention (Abbas et al. 2014).

11 Summary

- Acute aortic syndrome comprises three interrelated conditions with similar clinical presentations and distinct but related pathology: aortic dissection, intramural haematoma and penetrating atherosclerotic ulcer.
- All three conditions require prompt clinical and imaging assessment with early consideration of cardiothoracic surgery or intervention.
- In all three conditions, there is a significant mortality rate over time from presentation.
- There is controversy over the natural history of IMH in particular, but both IMH and PAU can be unstable.
- Stanford Classification, the extent of the disease and secondary complications determine conservative versus surgical/endovascular management.
- MDCT plays a pivotal role in early diagnosis and management.
- CT differentiation between aortic dissection, IMA and PAU are important as they influence management.
- In dissection, distinction between the true and false lumen is essential to guide endovascular treatment.
- The entire aorta must be evaluated and particular attention paid to possible branch vessel involvement.

References

Abbas A, Brown IW, Peebles CR, Harden SP, Shambrook JS (2014) The role of multidetector-row CT in the diagnosis, classification and management of acute aortic syndrome. Br J Radiol 87(1042):20140354

Agarwal PP, Chughtai A, Matzinger FR, Kazerooni EA (2009) Multidetector CT of thoracic aortic aneurysms. Radiographics 29(2):537–552

Castaner E, Andreu M, Gallardo X, Mata JM, Cabezuelo MA, Pallardo Y (2003) CT in nontraumatic acute thoracic aortic disease: typical and atypical features and complications. Radiographics 23 Spec No:S93–S110

Chin AS, Fleischmann D (2012) State-of-the-art computed tomography angiography of acute aortic syndrome. Semin Ultrasound CT MR 33(3):222–234

Chiu KW, Lakshminarayan R, Ettles DF (2013) Acute aortic syndrome: CT findings. Clin Radiol 68(7):741–748

Coady MA, Ikonomidis JS, Cheung AT, Matsumoto AH, Dake MD, Chaikof EL et al (2010) Surgical management of descending thoracic aortic disease: open and endovascular approaches: a scientific statement from the American Heart Association. Circulation 121(25):2780–2804

DeSanctis RW, Doroghazi RM, Austen WG, Buckley MJ (1987) Aortic dissection. N Engl J Med 317(17):1060–1067

Evangelista A, Mukherjee D, Mehta RH, O'Gara PT, Fattori R, Cooper JV et al (2005) Acute intramural hematoma of the aorta: a mystery in evolution. Circulation 111(8):1063–1070

Hiratzka LF, Bakris GL, Beckman JA, Bersin RM, Carr VF, Casey DE Jr et al (2010) 2010 ACCF/AHA/AATS/ACR/ASA/SCA/SCAI/SIR/STS/SVM guidelines for the diagnosis and management of patients with thoracic aortic disease: executive summary. A report of the American College of Cardiology Foundation/American Heart Association Task Force on Practice Guidelines, American Association for Thoracic Surgery, American College of Radiology, American Stroke Association, Society of Cardiovascular Anesthesiologists, Society for Cardiovascular Angiography and Interventions, Society of Interventional Radiology, Society of Thoracic Surgeons, and Society for Vascular Medicine. Catheter Cardiovasc Interv 76(2):E43–E86

IRADonline.org. http://www.iradonline.org/irad.html

Kazerooni EA, Bree RL, Williams DM (1992) Penetrating atherosclerotic ulcers of the descending thoracic aorta: evaluation with CT and distinction from aortic dissection. Radiology 183(3):759–765

Kitai T, Honda S, Okada Y, Tani T, Kim K, Kaji S et al (2009) Clinical outcomes in non-surgically managed patients with very severe versus severe aortic stenosis. Heart 97(24):2029–2032

Kitai T, Kaji S, Yamamuro A, Tani T, Kinoshita M, Ehara N et al (2011) Detection of intimal defect by 64-row multidetector computed tomography in patients with acute aortic intramural hematoma. Circulation 124(11 Suppl):S174–S178

Lansman SL, Saunders PC, Malekan R, Spielvogel D (2010) Acute aortic syndrome. J Thorac Cardiovasc Surg 140(6 Suppl):S92–S97; discussion S142–S146

Lempel JK, Frazier AA, Jeudy J, Kligerman SJ, Schultz R, Ninalowo HA et al (2014) Aortic arch dissection:

a controversy of classification. Radiology 271(3): 848–855

Litmanovich D, Bankier AA, Cantin L, Raptopoulos V, Boiselle PM (2009) CT and MRI in diseases of the aorta. AJR Am J Roentgenol 193(4):928–940

Macura KJ, Corl FM, Fishman EK, Bluemke DA (2003) Pathogenesis in acute aortic syndromes: aortic dissection, intramural hematoma, and penetrating atherosclerotic aortic ulcer. AJR Am J Roentgenol 181(2): 309–316

Maddu KK, Shuaib W, Telleria J, Johnson JO, Khosa F (2013) Nontraumatic acute aortic emergencies: part 1, acute aortic syndrome. AJR Am J Roentgenol 202(3):656–665

McMahon MA, Squirrell CA (2010) Multidetector CT of aortic dissection: a pictorial review. Radiographics 30(2):445–460

Piffaretti G, Tozzi M, Lomazzi C, Rivolta N, Caronno R, Castelli P (2006) Complications after endovascular stent-grafting of thoracic aortic diseases. J Cardiothorac Surg 1:26

Roberts WC (1981) Aortic dissection: anatomy, consequences, and causes. Am Heart J 101(2):195–214

Salvolini L, Renda P, Fiore D, Scaglione M, Piccoli G, Giovagnoni A (2008) Acute aortic syndromes: role of multi-detector row CT. Eur J Radiol 65(3):350–358

Tittle SL, Lynch RJ, Cole PE, Singh HS, Rizzo JA, Kopf GS et al (2002) Midterm follow-up of penetrating ulcer and intramural hematoma of the aorta. J Thorac Cardiovasc Surg 123(6):1051–1059

Trimarchi S, Tolenaar JL, Jonker FH, Murray B, Tsai TT, Eagle KA et al (2013) Importance of false lumen thrombosis in type B aortic dissection prognosis. J Thorac Cardiovasc Surg 145(3 Suppl):S208–S212

van Bogerijen GH, Tolenaar JL, Rampoldi V, Moll FL, van Herwaarden JA, Jonker FH et al (2014) Predictors of aortic growth in uncomplicated type B aortic dissection. J Vasc Surg 59(4):1134–1143

Vilacosta I, Aragoncillo P, Canadas V, San Roman JA, Ferreiros J, Rodriguez E (2009) Acute aortic syndrome: a new look at an old conundrum. Heart 95(14):1130–1139

Weininger M, Barraza JM, Kemper CA, Kalafut JF, Costello P, Schoepf UJ (2011) Cardiothoracic CT angiography: current contrast medium delivery strategies. AJR Am J Roentgenol 196(3):W260–W272

Welch TJ, Stanson AW, Sheedy PF 2nd, Johnson CM, McKusick MA (1990) Radiologic evaluation of penetrating aortic atherosclerotic ulcer. Radiographics 10(4):675–685

Williams DM, Lee DY, Hamilton BH, Marx MV, Narasimham DL, Kazanjian SN et al (1997) The dissected aorta: part III. Anatomy and radiologic diagnosis of branch-vessel compromise. Radiology 203(1):37–44

Thoracic Aortic Aneurysms, Fistula, and Thrombus

Maria Cristina Firetto, Marcello Petrini, Francesco Sala, Maurizio Domanin, Giovanni Terribile, and Pietro Raimondo Biondetti

Contents

M.C. Firetto, MD (✉) • M. Domanin, MD
G. Terribile • P.R. Biondetti, MD
Fondazione IRCCS Ca' Granda,
Ospedale Maggiore Policlinico, Milan, Italy
e-mail: firettomariacristina@gmail.com

M. Petrini, MD
Università degli Studi di Milano, Postgraduation School in Radiodiagnostics, Milan, Italy

F. Sala, MD
Department of Radiology, A.O. Papa Giovanni XXIII, Bergamo, Italy

Abstract

Thoracic aortic aneurysms (TAAs) are abnormal dilatation occurring in the thoracic aorta. They can be classified according to location, morphology, and etiology. TAAs can be divided into true aneurysms and false aneurysms (also called pseudoaneurysms). True aneurysms are usually associated with fusiform dilatation of the aorta and most commonly due to atherosclerosis. False aneurysms are typically saccular with a narrow neck and most commonly due to trauma, penetrating atherosclerotic ulcers, or infections (mycotic aneurysm). Atherosclerosis, genetic causes, aortitis, trauma, and dissection can be the causes of TAAs. MDCT allows the evaluation of TAAs in terms of morphologic features, extent, and signs of instability or impending rupture. Acute aortic thrombosis and aortic fistula with esophagus or bronchi are rare but life-threatening complications of aortic disease. Imaging findings may be subtle.

Med Radiol Diagn Imaging (2016)
DOI 10.1007/174_2016_44, © Springer International Publishing Switzerland

1 Thoracic Aortic Aneurysms

1.1 Definition

Aneurysm etymologically derives from the Greek "aneurysma," i.e., "dilation," and it is defined as a permanent dilatation of an artery having a ≥50 % increase in diameter compared with its expected normal diameter. Aneurysmal degenerations occurring in the thoracic aorta are defined as thoracic aortic aneurysms (TAAs). TAAs can be classified according to location, morphology, and etiology. While in the real aortic aneurysms all three layers (intima, media, and adventitia) of the aortic wall are present in the aneurysmal wall, in pseudoaneurysms one or more of these layers are absent due to the lesion that originates from them, for example, trauma or penetrating atherosclerotic aortic ulcers.

1.2 Location

The thoracic aorta consists of the aortic root, ascending aorta, aortic arch, and descending thoracic aorta (Agarwal et al. 2009). The aortic root consists of the annulus, sinuses of Valsalva, and sinotubular junction. The annulus, a fibrous band surrounding the aorta, is located at the aortoventricular junction. The Valsalva sinus is a dilatation of the aortic root just above the aortic valve. At its upper level, at sinotubular junction, the Valsalva sinus becomes the tubular ascending aorta. The ascending aorta extends from the root to the origin of the right brachiocephalic artery (also called innominate artery); the arch, from the right brachiocephalic artery to the attachment of the ligamentum arteriosum; and the descending aorta, from the ligamentum arteriosum to the aortic hiatus in the diaphragm (Lodi et al. 2004). The arch may be subdivided into proximal (right brachiocephalic artery to left subclavian artery) and distal (left subclavian artery to attachment of the ligamentum arteriosum) segments (Mukherjee and Rajagopalan 2007). The distal arch, also referred to as the isthmus, may be narrower than the proximal descending aorta (Mukherjee and Rajagopalan 2007).

A TAA is defined as a permanent abnormal dilatation of the thoracic aorta (Green and Klein 2007). Although the aortic diameter increases with age, the normal diameter of the midascending aorta should always be less than 4 cm, and that of the descending aorta no more than 3 cm (Aronberg et al. 1984).

TAAs may involve one or more aortic segments (Goldstein et al. 2015): 60 % of TAAs involve the aortic root and/or ascending tubular aorta, 40 % the descending aorta, 10 % the arch, and 10 % the thoracoabdominal aorta (Isselbacher 2005).

1.3 Morphology and Pathophysiology

1.3.1 Morphology

An arterial blood vessel has the following three layers: intima (a thin inner layer made of endothelial cells, easily traumatized), media (a thick middle layer, composed of smooth muscle cells and multiple layers of elastic laminae that provide tensile strength, distensibility, and elasticity), and adventitia (a rather thin outer layer, made of collagen and vasa vasorum). The wall of a *true aneurysm* (Fig. 1a, b) involves all three layers, and the aneurysm is contained inside the endothelium. It is usually associated with fusiform dilatation of the aorta and is most commonly due to atherosclerosis (Posniak et al. 1990). The wall of a *false or pseudoaneurysm* involves only the outer layer, and it is contained by the adventitia or periadventitial tissues. It is typically saccular (Fig. 2a–e) with a narrow neck, and it is most commonly due to trauma, penetrating atherosclerotic ulcers, or infections (mycotic aneurysm) (Lesko et al. 1997). There are also various morphologic shapes of the aortic root and ascending aorta, some of which suggest specific etiologies. For example, *annuloaortic ectasia*, a condition characterized by dilated sinuses of Valsalva with effacement of the sinotubular junction producing a pear-shaped aorta that tapers to a normal aortic arch, is most commonly associated with Marfan syndrome (Fig. 3a, b).

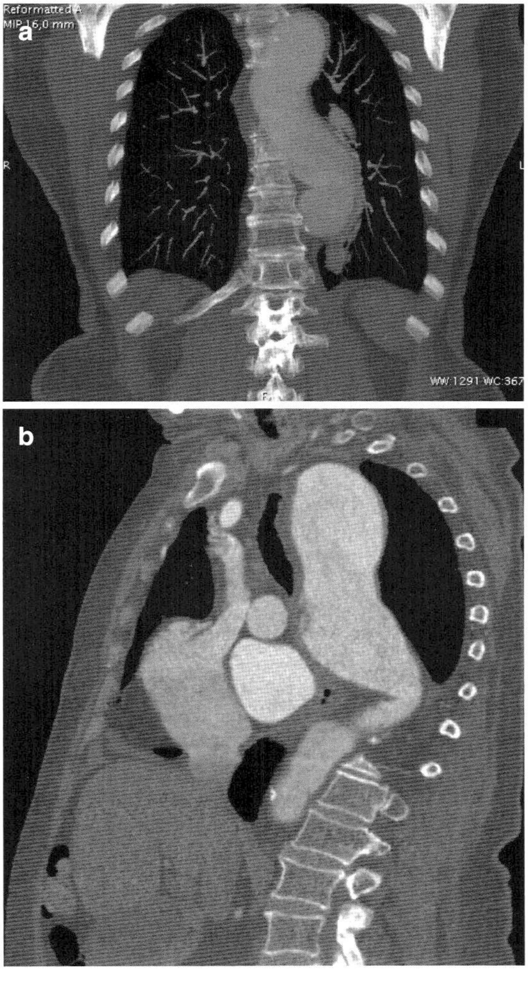

Fig. 1 Thoracic aortic aneurysm in a 59-year-old man. Contrast-enhanced coronal MIP image (**a**) and sagittal MPR image (**b**) show a true aneurysm, with fusiform dilatation of the descending aorta

1.3.2 Pathophysiology

The pathogenesis of aneurysm is extremely complex and not completely understood; most likely, aneurysms result from the interaction of multiple factors, systemic and local hemodynamic features (Michel et al. 2011). The elastic properties of the aorta are important for its normal function. The elasticity of the wall allows the aorta to accept the pulsatile output of the left ventricle in systole and to modulate continued forward flow during diastole. With aging, the medial elastic fibers become thinned and fragmented, with the increase in collagen and ground substance. Elasticity and compliance of the aortic wall are progressively lost, with the increase in pulse pressure and with progressive dilatation of the aorta (Goldstein et al. 2015). Many authors suggest that a group of enzymes called matrix metalloproteinases (MMPs) plays a significant role in the destruction of extracellular matrix in the aortic wall. MMPs lead to the degradation of these structural proteins with elastic fiber fragmentation and loss and degeneration of the tunica media with loss of elasticity and weakening of the aortic wall and consequent dilation (Sakalihasan et al. 2005). Hemodynamic factors probably play a fundamental role in the formation of aortic aneurysms. The human aorta is a relatively low-resistance circuit for circulating blood while the lower extremities have higher arterial resistance (Hoshina et al. 2003). Repeated hydrostatic trauma may injure a diseased aortic wall and contribute to aneurysmal development. In case of concomitant systemic hypertension, it can accelerate the expansion of known aneurysms and may contribute to their initial formation (Piccinelli et al. 2013). Wall rupture follows the basic principles of material failure, i.e., an aneurysm breaks open when mural stress or deformation meets an appropriate failure criterion. The law of Laplace states that wall tension is proportional to the pressure and to the radius of the arterial conduit ($T = P \times R$). As diameter increases, wall tension increases, which contributes to increasing diameter and risk of rupture. Also increased pressure and aneurysm size aggravate wall tension and therefore increase the risk of rupture. The use of the law of Laplace to predict AAA rupture potential is erroneous, because the AAA wall geometry is not a simple cylinder or sphere with a single radius of curvature, and wall stress alone is not sufficient to predict AAA rupture. So AAA diameter cannot be considered as the only determinant factor of either wall strength or wall stress (Piccinelli et al. 2013). Various indices have been proposed to create a more reliable and patient-specific criteria for clinical practice. Despite many progresses, the majority of the proposed criteria for risk stratification and decision making still rely on

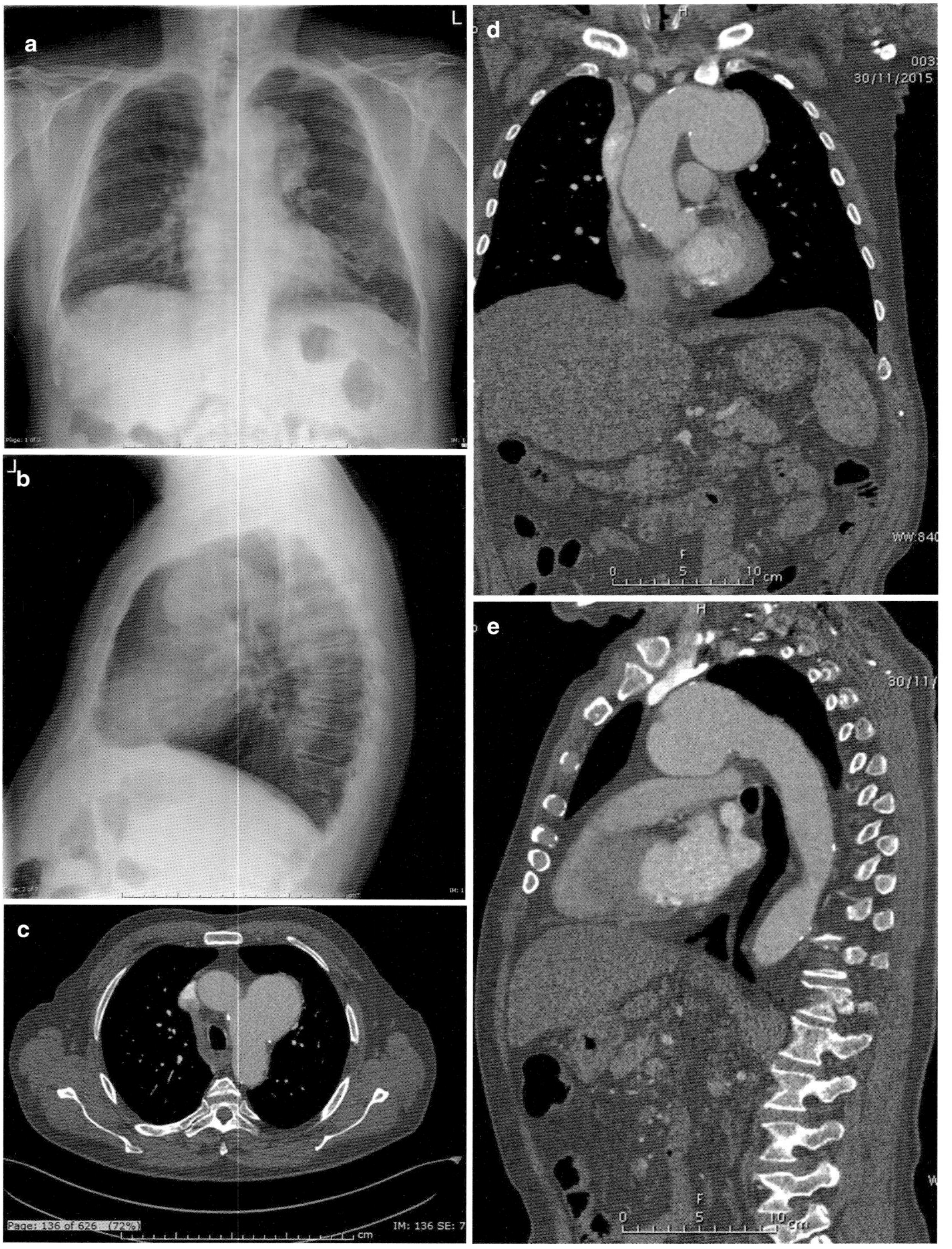

Fig. 2 PA and lateral X-rays (**a**, **b**) show widened mediastinum, opacification of the aortopulmonary window, and rightward deviation of the trachea. Axial (**c**), coronal (**d**), and sagittal (**e**) MPR CT images show saccular dilatation of the proximal descending aorta

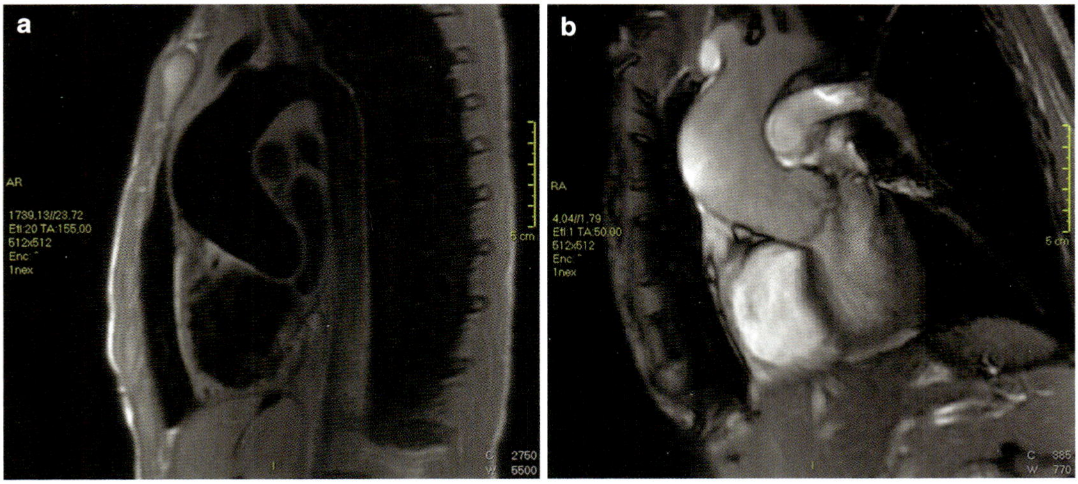

Fig. 3 Marfan syndrome and annuloaortic ectasia in a 42-year-old woman. (**a**) T1-weighted and (**b**) gradient echo sagittal oblique MRI show a pear-shaped aorta that tapers to a normal aortic arch, a characteristic finding in Marfan syndrome

empirical measurements rather than on the analysis of biomechanical properties (Creasy et al. 1997); among these are maximum AAA diameter (Greenhalgh 2004), currently the prevalent index for the evaluation of risk of rupture; AAA expansion rate (Hirose and Takamiya 1998); wall stiffness (Fillinger et al. 2003); intraluminal thrombus thickness (Speelman et al. 2010); and AAA wall peak stress (Raghavan et al. 2000; McGloughlin and Doyle 2010). The presence of anisotropic displacement of the AAA lumen boundary and their link to hemodynamic forces have been assessed, highlighting a new possible role for hemodynamics in the study of AAA progression (Piccinelli et al. 2013).

1.4 Etiology

Atherosclerosis is the cause of approximately 70 % of all TAAs (Lesko et al. 1997) and contributes to the formation of aortic aneurysms secondary to the degeneration of the components of the aortic wall. Atherosclerotic aneurysms are the most common type; usually they are seen in the elderly and typically characterized by intimal calcification and fibrous plaques along the aorta. The majority of them are fusiform, up to 20 % may be saccular (Posniak et al. 1990), and they occur in the descending thoracic aorta and rarely involve only the ascending aorta (Lesko et al. 1997) (Fig. 4a, b).

Because an abdominal aortic aneurysm occurs in 28 % of patients with TAA, initial CT evaluation may include the entire thoracoabdominal aorta (Bickerstaff et al. 1982).

Many authors consider *genetic causes* as a leading factors in the formation and development of aortic aneurysms. Inherited disorders of connective tissue contribute to the formation of aortic aneurysms. *Marfan syndrome* is a multisystemic connective tissue, autosomal dominant inherited disorder (Goldstein et al. 2015). One of the hallmark features is dilatation or dissection of the aortic root (Daimon et al. 2008). Aortic aneurysms without annuloaortic ectasia are also common. Annuloaortic ectasia, especially with dilatation of the aortic root, is found in 60–80 % of adults with Marfan syndrome. It usually begins with dilatation of the aortic sinuses, which progresses first into the sinotubular junction, than into the aortic annulus. Dilatation of the aortic root causes aortic valve insufficiency that may progress to aortic root dissection or rupture (Vasan et al. 1995). The aortic aneurysms rarely show intimal calcification or atherosclerotic thrombosis; they occur

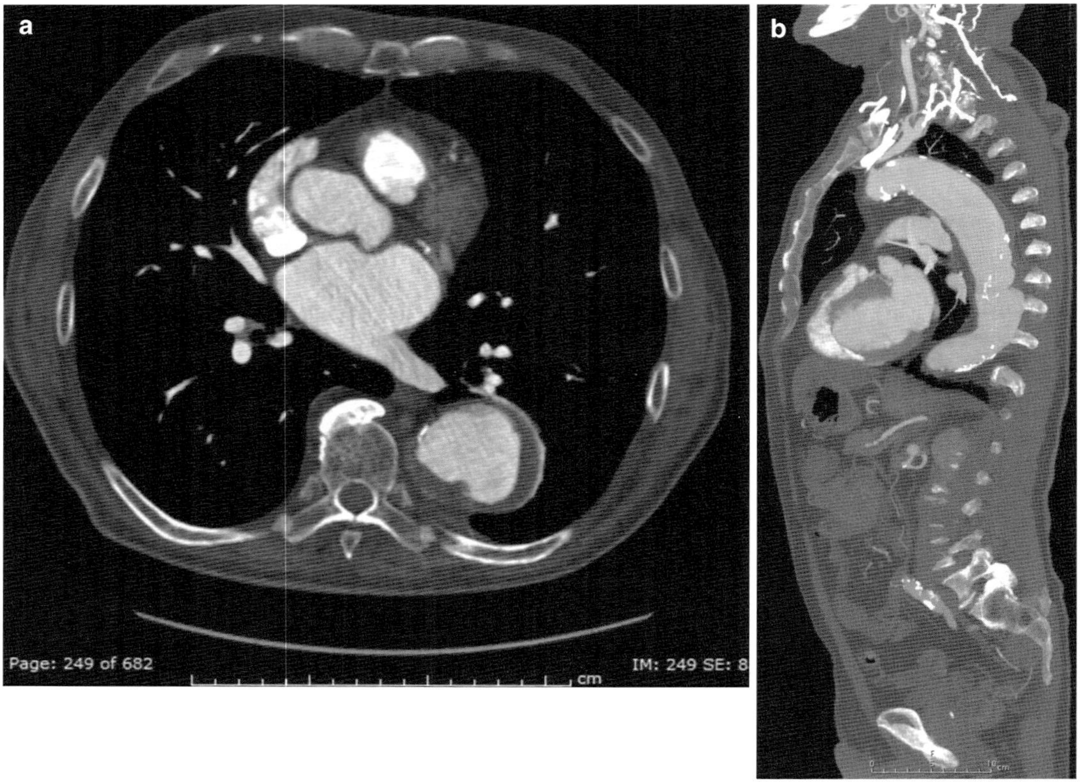

Fig. 4 Descending TAA in an 82-year-old man. Contrast-enhanced (**a**) axial CT image shows an atherosclerotic aorta, with fusiform aneurysm. (**b**) Sagittal MIP image shows the overall extent of the aneurysm in the descending aorta

commonly and develop more rapidly in younger patients. After the initial diagnosis of aortopathy by TTE, CT or MRI is recommended to confirm the size of the aorta and to document the diameters of the distal ascending aorta, aortic arch, and descending aortic segments. Repeated CT or MRI, about every 3 years, is recommended to reassess the aortic arch and the descending aorta. Prophylactic surgery for annuloaortic ectasia is recommended when the diameter of the Valsalva sinus exceeds 5.5 cm in an adult and 5.0 cm in a child, when the diameter of the Valsalva sinus is less than 5.0 cm but in a rapid rate of aortic aneurysm expansion (increase in dilatation by more than 1 cm per year), or when there is a family history of aortic dissection (Wolak et al. 2008; Kälsch et al. 2013; De Backer et al. 2006). Composite surgical replacement of the aortic root and valve is commonly performed with or without coronary reimplantation (Fig. 5a, b).

Other genetic conditions associated with aortic dilatation are bicuspid valve-related aortopathy (BAV), Loeys–Dietz syndrome, Turner syndrome, familial TAA, and Ehlers–Danlos syndrome. *Ehlers–Danlos syndrome* (EDS) is an autosomal dominant disorder with vascular involvement (arterial dilatation and rupture). The imaging characteristics of aortic aneurysms in Ehlers–Danlos syndrome resemble those in Marfan syndrome.

Aortitis is a general term that refers to a broad category of infectious or noninfectious conditions, in which there is abnormal inflammation of the aortic wall. These inflammatory conditions have different clinical and morphologic features and variable prognoses (Restrepo et al. 2011). The differentiation between infectious (mycotic) and noninfectious aneurysms is important because, as mycotic aneurysms are treated with antibiotic therapy and surgical debridement with

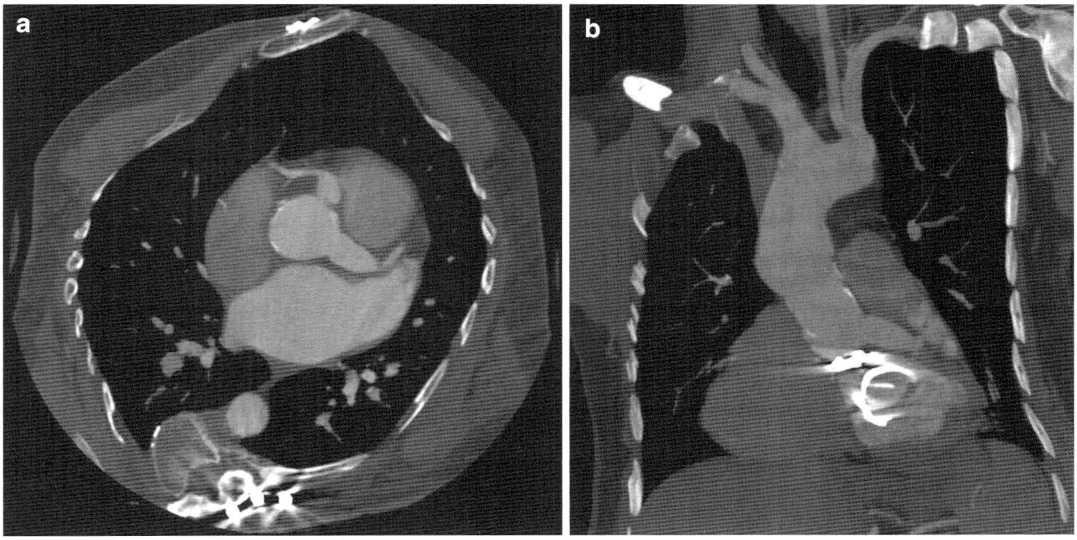

Fig. 5 Axial–oblique (**a**) and coronal–oblique MIP (**b**) CT sections at the level of the coronary artery origin, after ascending aorta replacement with graft. Note the persistent dilation of both proximal left and right coronary arteries

or without surgical revascularization, noninfectious aneurysms are managed by steroids and immunosuppressive drugs (Nagpal et al. 2015).

Noninfectious aortitis may be part of a systemic disorder (Gornik and Creager 2008). The association between rheumatic diseases and aortic involvement is well known, but the prevalence of aortic involvement in the different rheumatic diseases is quite variable. Rheumatic diseases (Slobodin et al. 2006) with a high prevalence (>10 %) of aortic involvement include Takayasu arteritis (Fig. 6a–c), giant cell arteritis (GCA), long-standing ankylosing spondylitis, Cogan syndrome (interstitial keratitis, iritis, conjunctival or subconjunctival hemorrhage, fever, aortic insufficiency) (Fig. 7a, b), and relapsing polychondritis. Rheumatic diseases in which aortic involvement is an uncommon well-documented complication include rheumatoid arthritis, seronegative spondyloarthropathies, Behçet disease, and systemic lupus erythematosus (SLE). Aortitis most commonly affects the ascending aorta in rheumatoid arthritis (Fig. 8a, b), ankylosing spondylitis, giant cell arteritis, and relapsing polychondritis (Posniak et al. 1990). These conditions may also be associated with aortic valve insufficiency. Aortitis in rheumatic fever can be segmental, limited to the ascending aorta, or it can involve the abdominal aorta or the entire aorta (Lande and Berkmen 1976; Posniak et al. 1990). Takayasu arteritis commonly affects the aortic arch and its major branches, with variable involvement of the abdominal aorta and pulmonary arteries; although Takayasu arteritis typically causes arterial stenosis and occlusion, aneurysms may also occur. Inflammatory aneurysms differ from atherosclerotic aneurysms because of the presence of dense perianeurysmal fibrosis and thickened aortic wall (Restrepo et al. 2011). The prevalence is 5–25 % of all abdominal aortic aneurysms. Inflammatory aneurysms of the ascending aorta and aortic arch are much less frequent, usually associated with concomitant inflammatory aneurysms in the abdominal aorta (Girardi and Coselli 1997). CT shows a hypoattenuating mass with periaortic wall thickening that spares the posterior wall. After intravenous administration of contrast material, rapid luminal opacification is followed by delayed enhancement of the soft-tissue component.

Infected (mycotic) aneurysms. Infectious aortitis is secondary to gram-positive bacteria such as the *Staphylococcal* species, *Enterococcus* species, and *Streptococcus pneumonia*, responsible

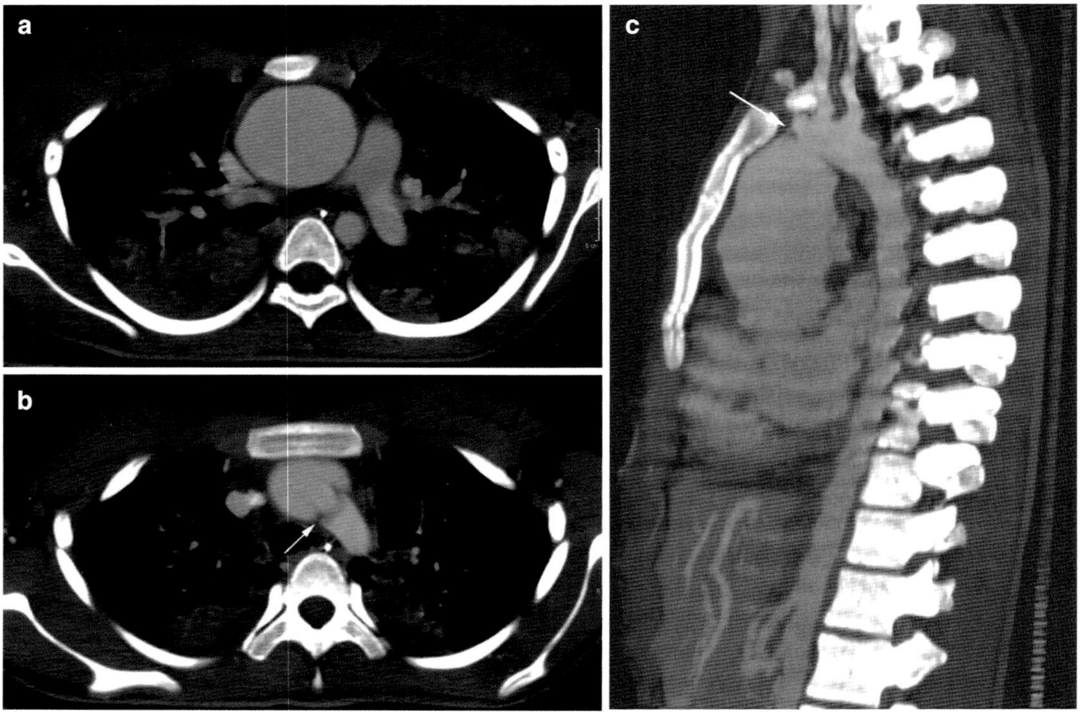

Fig. 6 Axial (**a**, **b**) and sagittal (**c**) CT MIP images in a patient with Takayasu arteritis. Fusiform aneurysm of the ascending aorta (**a**, **c**) and atypical coarctation at the level of the aortic arch (*arrows* in **b**, **c**) are well demonstrated

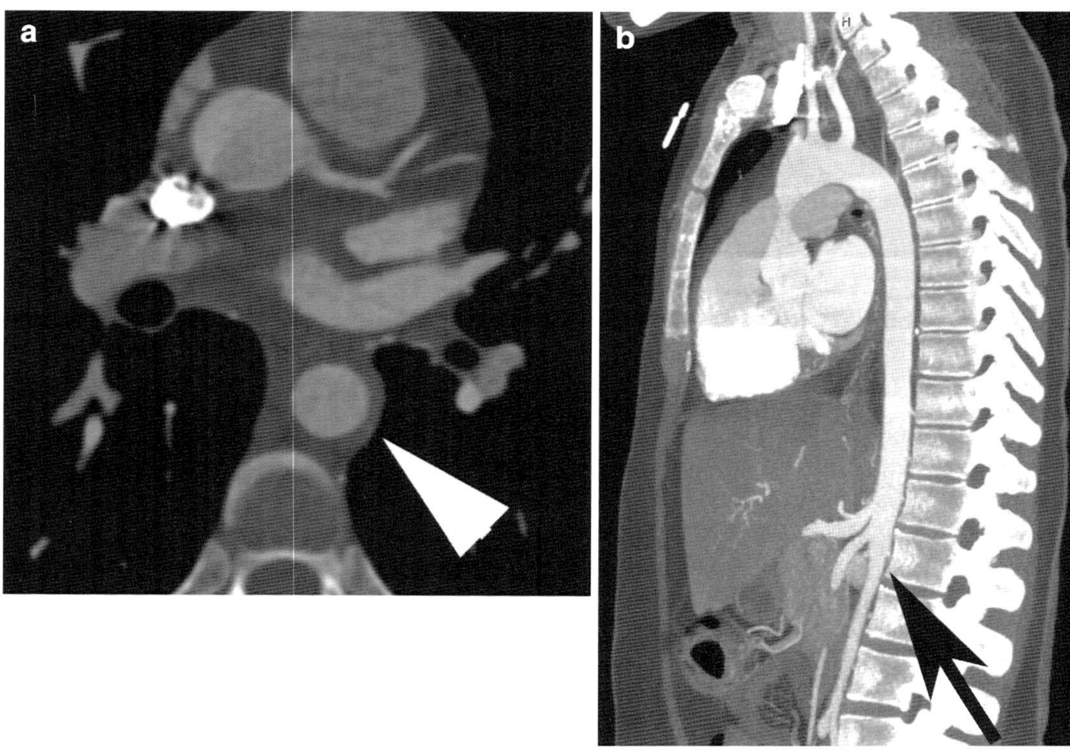

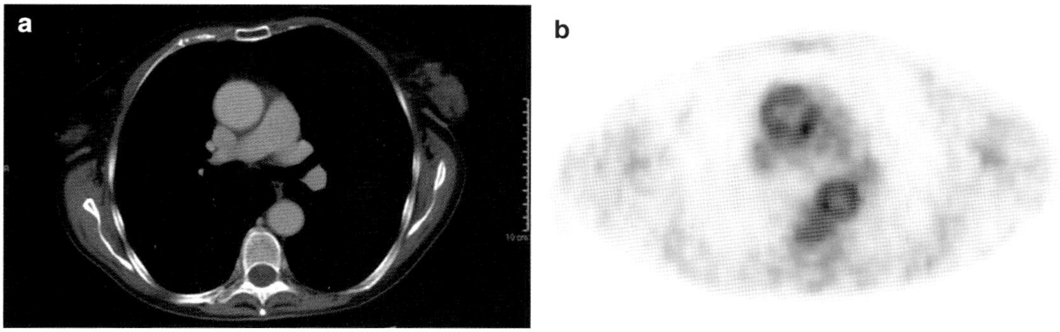

Fig. 8 Axial CT (**a**) and PET (**b**) images of a patient with rheumatoid arteritis. There is questionable wall thickening of the normal caliber thoracic aorta at CT (**a**). PET shows abnormal uptake of the aortic wall due to the inflammatory changes

of 60 % of the infections. Gram-negative bacilli (*Salmonella* species in the majority of cases) are also a frequent cause of aortic infection; however, they are more prevalent in infectious abdominal aortitis (Revest et al. 2007). Aortic infection by *Mycobacterium tuberculosis*, an uncommon problem in developed countries, may occur as a result of the extension to the aortic wall of a contiguous infective focus such as infected mediastinal lymph nodes or lung lesions. *Treponema pallidum* is a rare etiology today, with a historical importance. Aortic infection by unusual bacteria and nonbacterial (fungi) microorganisms is extremely rare; however, this possibility must be considered in immunocompromised patients (Gornik and Creager 2008). Infected (mycotic) aneurysms are uncommon, and they usually involve segments not commonly involved by atherosclerosis (Lee et al. 2008). Although the infraabdominal aorta is the most frequently involved segment of the aorta, there is also a combined involvement of the descending thoracic, thoracoabdominal, and suprarenal aorta (Oderich et al. 2001). Early changes of aortitis preceding aneurysm formation include an irregular arterial wall, periaortic edema as fat stranding or a hypoattenuating concentric rim at CT, a periaortic soft-tissue mass, and periaortic gas. Concentric or eccentric periaortic inflammatory soft tissue can develop, as a homogeneous contrast-enhancing mass at CT (Ting and Cheng 1997; Tsao et al. 2002; Azizi et al. 2004). The inflammatory mass can develop necrosis with a heterogeneous attenuation at CT, with rim enhancement or poor enhancement after administration of contrast material (Gomes and Choyke 1992). Periaortic mass and fat stranding are the most common imaging findings of infected aortic aneurysms, and they are found in 48 % of cases (Macedo et al. 2004). Periaortic gas is an uncommon feature (Vogelzang and Sohaey 1988; Macedo et al. 2004). At CT, an infected aortic aneurysm appears as a focal, contrast-enhancing dilatation, usually saccular. The lumen can be central or eccentric and it can be a single compartment or multiloculated. Disrupted arterial wall calcifications can occur adjacent to the infected aneurysm (Sueyoshi et al. 1998; Azizi et al. 2004). Calcification within the aneurysmal wall and thrombus within an infected aneurysm are uncommon (Gomes and Choyke 1992). An infected aneurysm can rapidly develop and enlarge (Sueyoshi et al. 1998; Macedo et al. 2004), and subsequently it can rupture due to high systemic arterial pressure.

Fig. 7 Axial (**a**) and sagittal MIP (**b**) CT images of a patient with Cogan syndrome, showing circumferential wall thickening of the normal caliber descending aorta (*arrow head* in **a**) and abrupt narrowing of the abdominal aorta distal to the mesenteric artery origin (*arrow* in **b**)

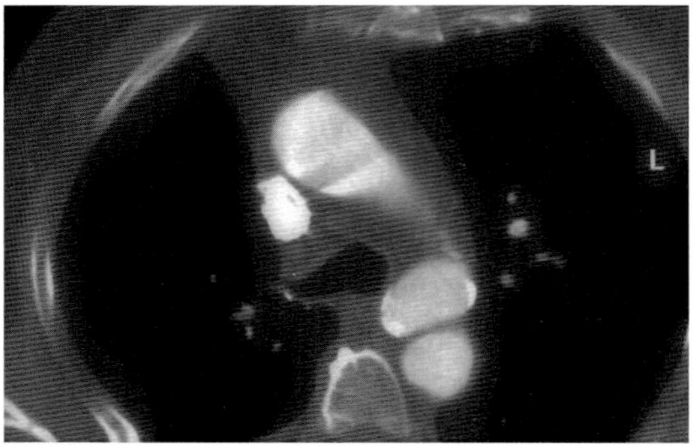

Fig. 9 Axial CT in a patient with chronic posttraumatic pseudoaneurysm of the aortic isthmus. There is no mediastinal hematoma and there are some calcifications along the aneurysmal wall

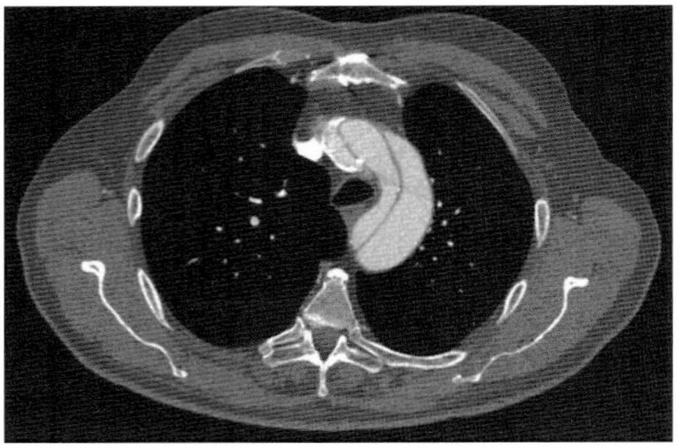

Fig. 10 Axial CT image at the aortic arch level in a patient with chronic dissection. The dilated aortic arch with intimal flap, false and true lumens are well demonstrated

Posttraumatic aneurysms or, better, pseudoaneurysms, following blunt trauma may result from rapid deceleration, which is the most accepted mechanism of injury (Agarwal et al. 2009), with shearing and bending stress on the aortic wall. According to this theory, during the sudden deceleration, the distal transverse arch moves forward while the proximal descending thoracic aorta remains stationary, held back by the ligamentum arteriosum and the intercostal vessels (Javadpour et al. 2002). Another proposed mechanism is the "osseous pinch," where an anteroposterior compression force results in posteroinferior displacement of the manubrium, first rib, and medial clavicle, which impinge on the aorta and compress it against the thoracic spine posteriorly (Crass et al. 1990). A third possible mechanism of aortic injury is represented by the sudden increase of intraluminal blood pressure due to trauma with the so-called water hammer effect (Creasy et al. 1997). The most common site of injury, seen in survived trauma victims, is the aortic isthmus (90 % of cases), followed by the ascending aorta and the descending aorta near the diaphragmatic hiatus (Mukherjee and Rajagopalan 2007). Chronic pseudoaneurysms develop in 2.5 % of patients who survive the initial trauma. These often calcify (Fig. 9), may contain thrombus (Heystraten et al. 1986), and have the potential to enlarge progressively, rupturing even years after the initial trauma (Posniak et al. 1990).

Aortic dissection is an abnormal passage of blood, through an intimal tear, into the media, producing a false lumen separated from the true lumen by an intimal flap. A previous aortic dissection, with a persistent false channel, may produce aneurysmal dilatation of the false lumen. These are false aneurysms, contained only by the outer media and adventitia, enlarging over time (Fig. 10).

1.5 Pitfalls

Normal aortic variants can mimic an aortic aneurysm. Three of these are ductus diverticulum, Kommerell's diverticulum, and aortic spindle.

1.5.1 Ductus Diverticulum

Ductus diverticulum consists of a convex focal bulge along the anterior undersurface of the isthmic region of the aortic arch (Gotway and Dawn 2003). Although ductus diverticulum is commonly believed to be a remnant of the closed ductus arteriosus, it has been suggested that this entity may actually represent a remnant of the right dorsal aortic root (Grollman 1989). It is particularly important to differentiate ductus diverticulum from a posttraumatic aortic pseudoaneurysm, which most commonly occurs at the aortic isthmus. In contrast to a pseudoaneurysm, ductus diverticulum has smooth margins with gently sloping symmetric shoulders and forms obtuse angles with the aortic wall (Gotway and Dawn 2003).

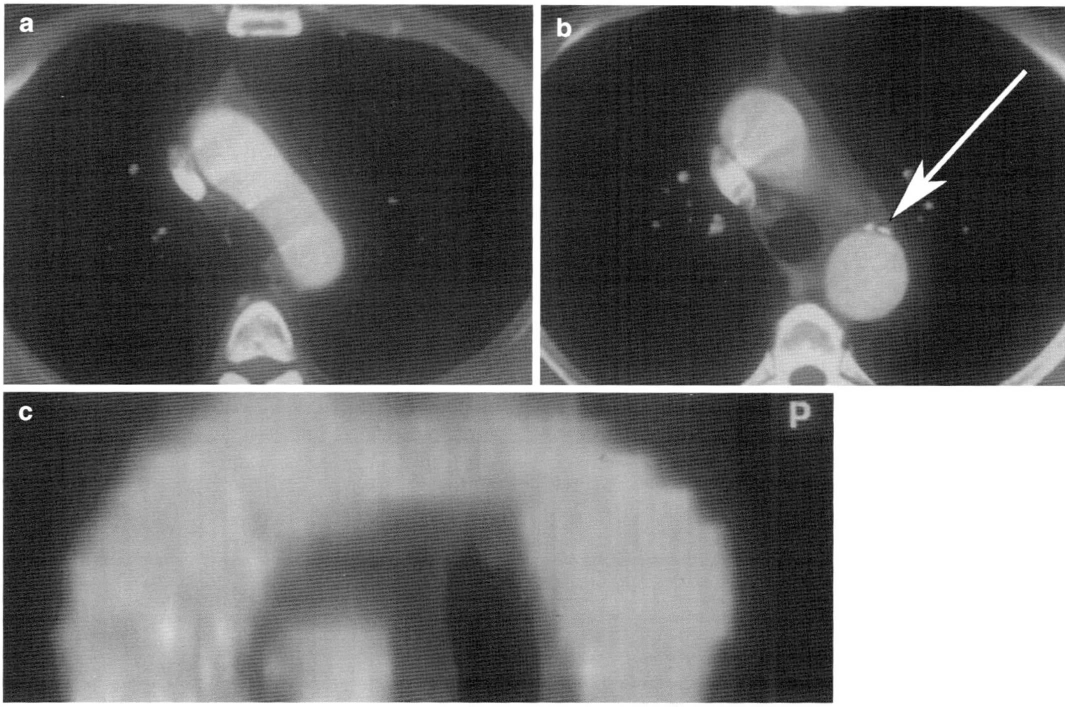

Fig. 11 Axial CT images (**a**, **b**) and sagittal–oblique MPR image (**c**) of aortic spindle, which is a normal mild dilation of the most proximal descending thoracic aorta. Note the calcific densities at the level of ductus arteriosus insertion (*arrow*)

1.5.2 Aortic Spindle

Aortic spindle is a smooth, circumferential bulge located below the isthmus, in the first portion of the descending aorta. It should not be confused with an aneurysm (Agarwal et al. 2009) (Fig. 11a–c).

1.5.3 Kommerell's Diverticulum

Right aortic arch (RAA) is an uncommon anatomical variant, occurring in about 0.1 % of the population (Shuford et al. 1986). Two main types are commonly seen: mirror-image branching (type I), commonly associated with congenital cyanotic heart disease, and aberrant left subclavian artery (LSA) (type II) (Yeo et al. 2015). Type II RAA is often accompanied by a Kommerell's diverticulum, an aneurismal diverticulum that develops at the origin of the LSA and the proximal aspect of descending aorta (Edwards 1948). Because of the atherosclerotic changes occurring in the arterial wall during life, in adults it is generally not possible to distinguish a true diverticulum (Kommerell's diverticulum, an embryonic remnant) from an acquired aneurysm of the origin of the aberrant LSA. Patients with type II RAA are often asymptomatic; they are diagnosed incidentally in adulthood or when complications arise from compression of the mediastinal structures, caused by a growing Kommerell's diverticulum (Hastreiter et al. 1966). However, it was originally described as a diverticular outpouching at the origin of an aberrant right subclavian artery with a left-sided aortic arch (Fig. 12a, b).

1.6 Complications

1.6.1 Rupture

The risk of rupture of TAAs increases with the size of the aneurysm (Gotway and Dawn 2003).

Indications for surgical treatment are summarized in the Guidelines of the American Heart Association (Hiratzka et al. 2010):

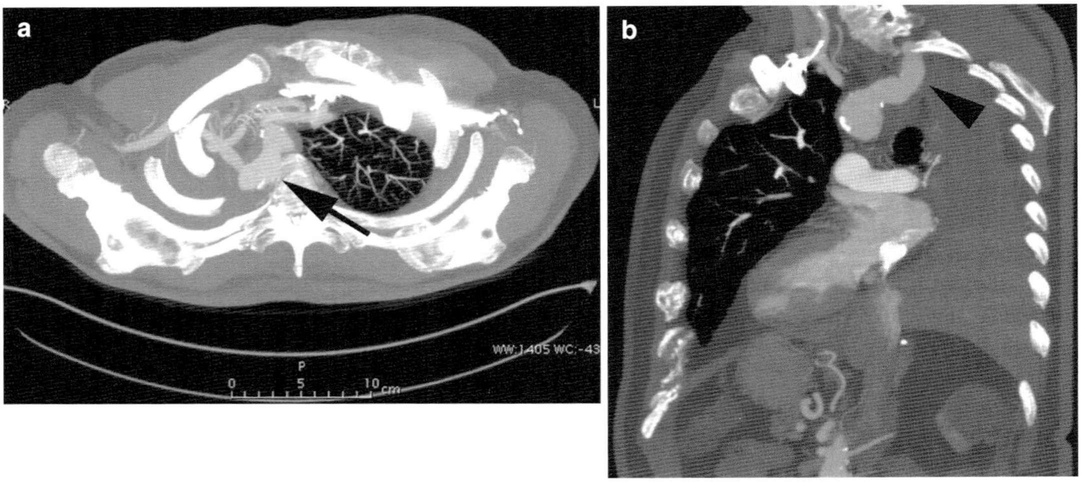

Fig. 12 Axial (**a**) and sagittal oblique (**b**) CT MIP images in a patient post-right pneumonectomy, with retroesophageal right aberrant subclavian artery with proximal aneurysmal dilation: Kommerell's diverticulum (*arrow* in **a**, *arrowhead* in **b**)

- Aortic size – ascending aortic diameter ≥5.5 cm or twice the diameter of the normal contiguous aorta; descending aortic diameter ≥6.5 cm; subtract 0.5 cm from the cutoff measurements if the following are present: Marfan syndrome, family history of aneurysm or connective tissue disorder, bicuspid aortic valve, aortic stenosis, dissection, and patient undergoing another cardiac operation; growth rate ≥1 cm/year
- Symptomatic aneurysm
- Traumatic aortic rupture
- Acute type B aortic dissection with associated rupture, leak, distal ischemia
- Pseudoaneurysm
- Large saccular aneurysm
- Mycotic aneurysm
- Aortic coarctation
- Bronchial compression by aneurysm
- Aortobronchial or aortoesophageal fistula

Contraindications are always individualized on patient's ability to undergo a major surgery. High-risk patients and elderly persons must be always considered for less invasive procedures. Patients with end-stage renal disease, respiratory insufficiency, cirrhosis, or other major comorbid conditions are the most critical.

CT is the modality of choice for identifying aneurysmal rupture. *CT findings of aneurysm rupture.* Thoracic aortic aneurysms can rupture into the mediastinum (Fig. 13a, b), pleural cavity, pericardium, or adjacent luminal structures such as the airways or the esophagus. CT findings are a high-attenuation hematoma on nonenhanced scans and an active contrast material extravasation from the aortic lumen on contrast-enhanced scans (Agarwal et al. 2009). An important imaging feature, in a contained rupture of TAA, is the "draped aorta sign": it occurs when the posterior wall of the aorta is not identifiable as distinct from adjacent structures or when it closely follows the contour of adjacent vertebral bodies (Halliday and al-Kutoubi 1996). *Imaging features suggestive of instability or impending rupture* include increased aneurysmal size, a low thrombus-to-lumen ratio, and hemorrhage into a mural thrombus (Rakita et al. 2007). Nonruptured aneurysms generally contain more thrombus than ruptured aneurysms and thrombus-to-lumen ratio decreases with the increase of the aneurysmal size (Pillari et al. 1988). It is intuitive that a thick circumferential thrombus is protective against rupture and an enlargement of the patent lumen is indicative of partial lysis of the thrombus, which predisposes an aneurysm to rupture (Pillari et al. 1988; Mower

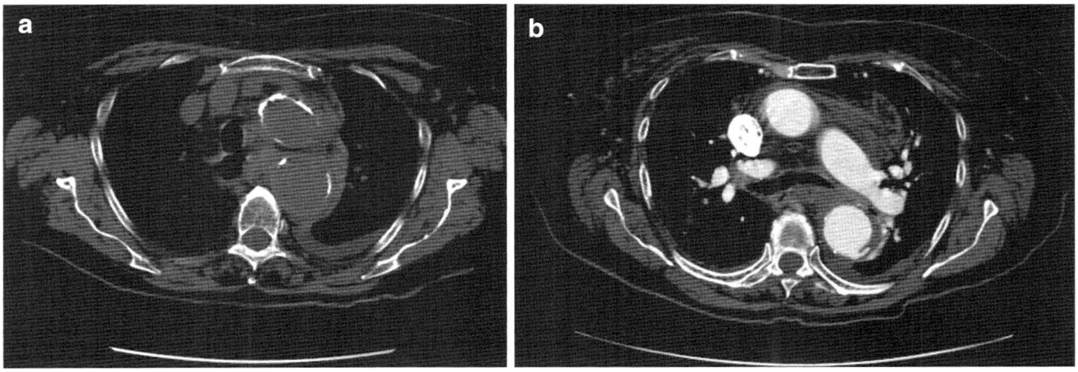

Fig. 13 Unenhanced (**a**) and enhanced (**b**) axial CT scan of a patient with ruptured aortic aneurysm. Unenhanced image (**a**) shows discontinuity in wall calcifications, high-attenuation hematoma, and draping of the posterior aortic wall. Enhanced image (**b**) shows active extravasation of contrast material into the thrombus. Both images demonstrate blood into mediastinum and left pleural cavity

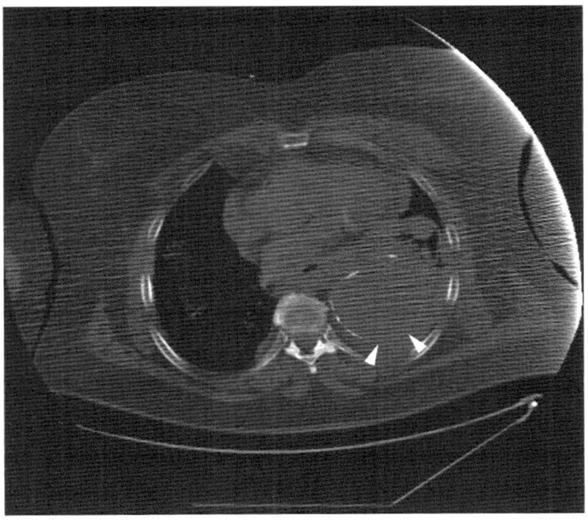

Fig. 14 Unenhanced axial CT sections of a patient with contained rupture of aneurysmal descending aorta. The discontinuity of wall calcifications is clearly shown on the posterior and lateral side of aorta (*arrow heads*)

et al. 1997). A focal discontinuity in the circumferential wall calcifications (Fig. 14) is more commonly observed in unstable or ruptured aneurysms (Siegel et al. 1994); this finding is really important when, in comparison with a previous CT, the area of discontinuity in mural calcifications is new. A well-defined peripheral crescent of increased attenuation (Fig. 15a, b) within the thrombus of a large TAA is a CT sign of acute or impending rupture (Mehard et al. 1994; Gonsalves 1999). This finding is best appreciated on unenhanced CT images. It represents an internal dissection of blood into the peripheral thrombus or into the aneurysm wall, when the ability of the thrombus to protect the aneurysm from rupture is shrinking (Arita et al. 1997). It is one of the earliest and most specific CT signs of the rupture process (Mehard et al. 1994; Siegel et al. 1994; Arita et al. 1997; Gonsalves 1999). A TAA can develop fistulous communication with the tracheobronchial tree and the esophagus. The aortobronchial fistula manifests clinically as hemoptysis (Lesko et al. 1997) and at CT as consolidation in the adjacent lung due to hemorrhage; the fistulous communication cannot be easily seen at CT (Coblentz and Sallee 1988). Most aortobronchial fistulas (90 %) occur between the descending aorta and the left lung (MacIntosh et al. 1991). Aortoesophageal fistula is less common. It manifests clinically as hematemesis and dysphagia (Cho et al. 2004) and at CT as mediastinal hematoma, as an intimate relationship of the aneurysm to the esophagus, and, rarely, as contrast material extravasation into the esophagus (Green and Klein 2007).

1.6.2 Compression of Adjacent Structures

TAAs can produce symptoms by compressing adjacent structures, such as superior vena cava syndrome due to compression of the superior vena cava, stridor or dyspnea due to airway

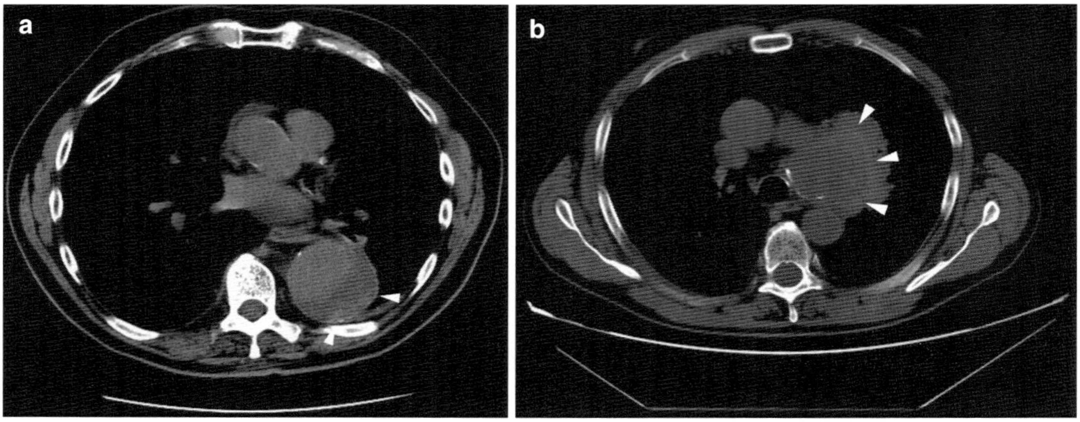

Fig. 15 Unenhanced axial CT scan of two different patients with hemorrhage into a mural thrombus. A peripheral crescent-shaped area of hyperattenuation (*arrow heads* in **a**, **b**), corresponding to the hematoma into the mural thrombus, is displayed in (**a**) a patient with impending rupture of an aneurysmal descending aorta with thrombus and (**b**) in a patient with contained rupture of aortic arch aneurysm into the mediastinum (**b**)

compression, hoarseness due to compression of the recurrent laryngeal nerve, and dysphagia due to esophageal compression (Posniak et al. 1990).

1.7 Clinical Presentation

Thoracic aortic aneurysms often grow slowly and usually without symptoms, making them difficult to detect. TAAs are usually found incidentally after chest radiographs or during other imaging studies. Most patients are hypertensive or can have a history of vascular disease in different districts, such as coronary or carotid arteries, but, in general, they remain relatively asymptomatic until the aneurysm expands.

The most common symptom is pain. Chest or back pain in presence of TAA is predictive of aortic rupture. Ascending aortic aneurysms tend to cause anterior chest pain, whereas arch aneurysms more likely cause pain radiating to the neck. Descending thoracic aneurysms more likely cause back pain localized between the scapulae. When located at the level of the diaphragmatic hiatus, the pain occurs in the mid-back and epigastric region; however, identifying the area of aortic involvement on the basis of the specific location of pain is not always reliable and can be misleading. Large ascending aortic aneurysms can cause superior vena cava obstruction with distended neck veins. Ascending aortic aneurysms also may develop aortic insufficiency and heart failure. Arch aneurysms, where stretching of the recurrent laryngeal nerves is present, may cause hoarseness. Descending thoracic aneurysms and thoracoabdominal aneurysms may compress the trachea and/or bronchi and cause dyspnea, stridor, wheezing, or cough. Compression of the esophagus results in dysphagia. They can also erode the surrounding structures and result in aortobronchial or aortoesophageal fistulas with, respectively, hemoptysis, hematemesis, or gastrointestinal bleeding. Erosion into the spine causes back pain or instability. Spinal cord compression or thrombosis of spinal arteries may result in paraparesis or paraplegia. Descending thoracic aneurysms may thrombose or embolize clot and atheromatous debris distally to visceral, renal, or lower extremity arteries.

The most common complications of TAAs are acute rupture and dissection with rupture into the pericardium, causing tamponade, or dissection into the aortic valve, causing acute aortic insufficiency, or into the coronary arteries, causing myocardial infarction (Safi et al. 2012; Upchurch 2014).

1.8 CT Technique and CT Data Manipulation

In the clinical setting of acute nontraumatic chest pain, case history, physical examination, ECG, and laboratory risk markers should be immediately obtained. Chest X-ray is useful to rule out many nonvascular causes of acute chest pain such as pleural effusions, pneumothorax, etc. In the field of nontraumatic vascular emergencies, CT has a primary role with a sensitivity and a specificity near 100 % for acute aortic pathologies, while MRI is indicated mainly for follow-up of aortic pathologies due to longer scan time, limited availability, and increased cost (Nagpal et al. 2015).

The CT protocol starts with unenhanced scan to visualize intramural hematoma that can be misdiagnosed as atherosclerotic thrombus in the arterial phase CT scan (Chiu et al. 2013). The scan should be extended above the aortic arch (for aortic branches) and caudally to the femoral heads to cover aorta entirely. Then contrast-enhanced CT with high infusion rate (4–5 mL/s) is performed to achieve a target opacification of the aorta >250 HU, obtained in the arterial phase with a test bolus or a bolus-tracking technique. The contrast should be injected through the right upper extremity to avoid artifacts from left innominate vein in the area of the aortic arch. A saline flush of 30–40 mL should be injected following contrast medium to minimize streak artifact from superior vena cava (Weininger et al. 2011). Delayed images are recommended after stent–graft repair of aortic aneurysm to detect endoleaks (Task et al. 2014). ECG gating when available is very useful to avoid cardiac motion artifacts impairing the evaluation of thoracic aorta and coronary origin. ECG-gated imaging both in precontrast and in postcontrast CT, from above aortic arch to diaphragmatic hiatus, should be included in the standard protocols for thoracic vascular emergency. Prospective ECG gating is performed at mid-diastole if heart rate is <70 beats per minute, while it is acquired in end-systole in patients with heart rate >70 beats per minute (Abbas et al. 2014). High-quality images of aortic root and proximal coronary tracts can be obtained without ECG gating using newer CT scanners (128 slice CT) with fast gantry rotation time and iterative reconstruction algorithm to reduce both X-ray dose and contrast media volume (Russo et al. 2015).

MDCT images are initially evaluated in axial sections, but two-dimensional and three-dimensional reformatting techniques such as multiplanar reformation (MPR), maximum intensity projection (MIP), and virtual rendering (VR) allow better diagnosis of aortic pathology. In particular to obtain correct measurement of the aortic diameters, it is necessary to use MPR images perpendicular to the centerline of the aortic lumen to avoid overestimation (Fig. 16a). Measurements of the aortic lumen on the transaxial CT images are incorrect when the central axis of the aorta is not perpendicular but oblique to the transaxial CT image (Fig. 16b).

MIP is a useful tool to display vascular map (Fig. 17) but doesn't demonstrate the 3D relationship with nonvascular structures, while volume rendering (VR) allows to display vascular anatomy and provides, at the same time, definition of the surrounding structures (Fishman et al. 2006) (Fig. 18). It is the only way to transfer to the referring clinician the 3D perspective of the aortic aneurysm.

A standard report describing thoracic aorta should include the following measurements (Agarwal et al. 2009):

- Sinus
- Sinoaortic junction
- Midascending aorta
- Proximal aortic arch
- Midaortic arch
- Proximal descending aorta
- Aorta at diaphragm

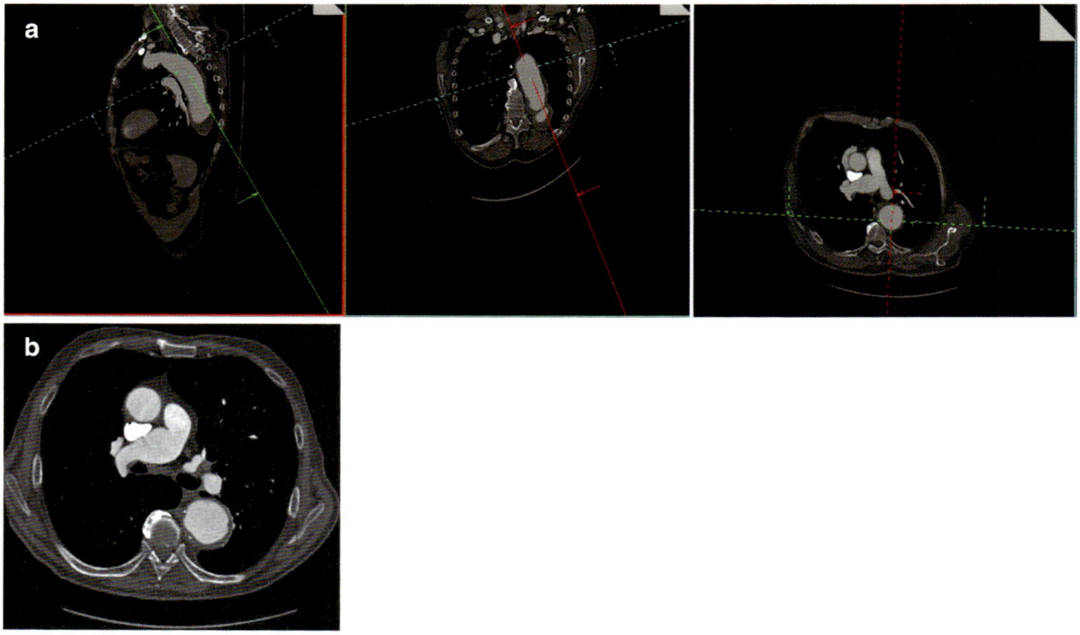

Fig. 16 A 77-year-old woman with descending aortic aneurysm. Multiplanar postcontrast CT images show the correct (**a**) technique of wall-to-wall measurement of the descending aortic aneurysm perpendicular to its center line. Pure axial postcontrast CT image of the same patient shows the incorrect (**b**) measurement technique of the aneurysm due to overestimation

Every report of an aneurysmal thoracic aorta must include the relationships between the aneurysm and the aortic branches, to assess the possibility of endovascular repair. Minimum length of 15 mm from aortic lesion and left subclavian artery/celiac trunk and maximum aortic landing zone diameter of 40 mm without circumferential thrombus within the landing zone are essential to perform endovascular procedure (Garzón et al. 2005).

2 Thoracic Aortic Thrombosis

2.1 Introduction

With the advent of recently developed imaging techniques and the routine exploration using TEE after any embolic events, the presence of thrombi in the aorta has been increasingly identified. The primary source of peripheral arterial embolism (PAE) is cardiac in more than 85 % of cases (Reber et al. 1999). Among noncardiac sources, the aorta has been reported in up to 5 % of cases to be the origin of PAE (Gagliardi et al. 1988).

Thrombus formation can be found both in atheromatous and in apparently normal aorta.

2.2 Definition, Etiology, and Clinical Presentation

Aortic mural thrombi usually arise as a consequence of preexisting aortic pathology. Thrombogenic lesions such as aneurysm, complex atherosclerotic plaque with protruding atheromas, and/or dissection are found to underlie the vast majority of aortic thrombi (Rossi et al. 2002).

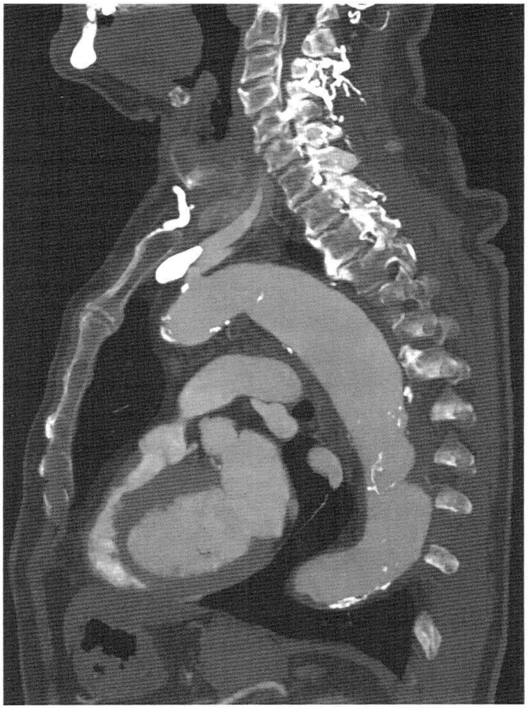

Fig. 17 MPR sagittal view with MIP CT image of thoracic aorta aneurysm

Common well-recognized embolic sources of aortic thrombosis include intracardiac thrombus or myxoma.

Thrombi in the thoracic aorta are even much less common, particularly in apparently normal aorta. It has been initially associated to premature atherosclerosis, as a result of prior trauma, but some authors suggested as a separate clinical entity.

Primary aortic mural thrombus (PAMT) is defined as a thrombus formation in a morphologically normal aorta without any evidence of cardiac source.

In 1958, H. Gaylis described the first case of PAMT: the thrombus was located in the abdominal aorta (Gaylis 1958). Later, Machleder et al. confirmed this clinical entity: in 10,671 consecutive autopsies, he found 95 cases of mural thrombus of the thoracoabdominal aorta and reported an incidence of 0.45 % (48 cases) of nonaneurysmal aortic mural thrombus, with 17 % of these patients having evidence of distal embolization (Machleder et al. 1986).

Because the disease is mostly asymptomatic, the true incidence of PAMT remains unknown. In two large series that evaluated patient with PAE, the incidence reported was higher and varies from 5 to 20 % (Verma et al. 2014).

Verma et al. identified 19 PAMT in a retrospective study of 88 patients who underwent extensive evaluation of acute occlusion of extremities or visceral arteries. Mural thrombus was located in the thoracic aorta in ten patients (52 %) and in the abdominal aorta in nine (48 %) (Verma et al. 2014).

The most frequent thoracic location of PAMT is the region of the aortic isthmus and the portion distal to the aortic arch, at the side opposite to the origin of the subclavian artery (Choukroun et al. 2002). Also, localization of aortic thrombus in the ascending aorta has been described (Pousios et al. 2009).

PAMT is more frequent in young women, and it has been associated in patients with essential thrombocytosis (Fang et al. 2001) and Crohn's disease (Lehmann et al. 2001). Smoking, steroid therapy, elevated fibrinogen levels and/or hypercoagulability, and numerous underlying pathologies have been reported.

Underlying pathologies described in morphologically normal thoracic aortic thrombosis
Predisposing factor[a]
Essential thrombocythemia
Protein C or S deficiency
Antiphospholipid syndrome
Heparin-induced thrombocytopenia
Hyperhomocysteinemia
Iatrogenic (e.g., intra-aortic balloon pumping)
Aortic wall tumor
Cancer
Chemotherapy
Homozygous plasminogen activator inhibitor type 1 (PAI-1)
Factor V Leiden
Familiar dysfibrinogenemia
Antithrombin III deficiency
Blunt aortic trauma
Drug abuse
Elevated factor VIII
Aspergilloma
Rheumatic disease
Crohn's disease (Lehmann et al. 2001)
Pancreatitis (Verbeeck et al. 2014)

[a]Modified from Tsilimparis et al. (2011)

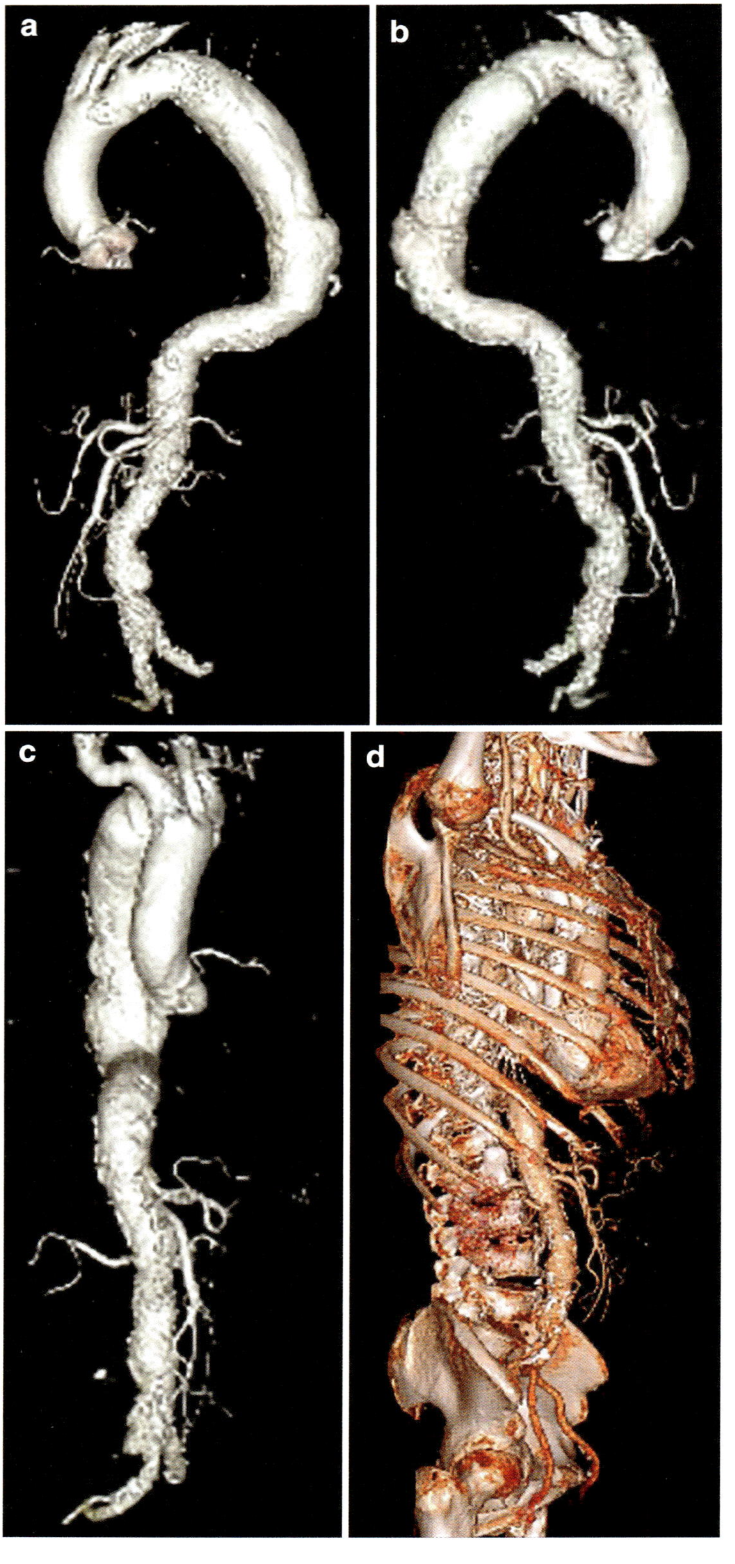

Fig. 18 3D volume-rendered CT images of thoracic aorta aneurysm in lateral (**a**, **b**) and frontal view (**c**). In (**d**) 3D volume-rendered CT image of the same patient without bone elimination

In all patients who underwent surgery, histopathological examination revealed microscopic features of atherosclerosis limited to the insertion site (Laperche et al. 1997).

Clinical presentation is variable and mainly characterized by peripheral or mesenteric embolization arising from detachment of large thrombi within the visceral aortic segment. In some cases, cerebral transient ischemic attack, acute pancreatitis, and exacerbation of Crohn's disease symptoms are associated.

2.3 Diagnostic Workup

The diagnostic workup for aortic thrombosis includes TEE and cardiologic evaluation combined with imaging modalities (CT and/or MRI) and laboratory screening test for hypercoagulable disorders.

The differential diagnosis of PAMT must be established with primary aortic tumors (Thalheimer et al. 2004) and certainly with aortic dissection because of the urgent therapeutic implications.

A diagnosis can be achieved by TEE, CT, MRI, and digital subtraction angiography (DSA). Currently, because of the rarity of the disease, there are no robust studies comparing the various imaging techniques; consequently, there is a lack of consensus on the relative role (comparative effectiveness) of these imaging modalities and on the ideal way of managing PAMT.

Review of published data on aortic mural thrombus until 2014 revealed fewer than 250 cases, the majority of which were single case reports (Fayad et al. 2013).

Several authors have earlier reported TEE to be an adequate method for detecting PAMT (Lau et al. 1997) with some suggesting TEE to be comparatively more sensitive than CT or MRI (Tunick et al. 1991).

However, these studies were published before recent advancements in CT and MRI imaging with high- spatial resolution images. Currently, the recommended approach for a complete diagnostic workup requires the synergistic use of at least two modalities, TEE (mainly for exploration of cardiac cavities) and CT or MRI for the detection of thrombi and the evaluation of thrombus and of the entire aorta (Tsilimparis et al. 2011; Verma et al. 2014; Abissegue et al. 2015).

TEE allows a thorough examination of both the heart and the thoracic aorta. It plays a key role because it is the gold standard (sensitivity>95 %) in identifying a cardiac source (thrombi in atrial fibrillation, valvulopathy, myocardial infarction) of embolism (85 % of all arterial thrombosis). Cardiac CT and of course cardiac MR have been proposed as an alternative method (Romero et al. 2013; Shapiro et al. 2007; Goldstein et al. 2015). On the other hand, echocardiography is less consistently able to image the distal ascending aorta, aortic arch, and descending thoracic aorta. To image these segments, CT and MR are preferred (Goldstein et al. 2015).

CT is the imaging modality of choice for diagnosis of most aortic pathologies, preoperative planning, and follow-up after invasive or medical treatment. This status reflects its widespread availability, accuracy, and applicability.

PAMT is recognized on CT as a hypodense endoluminal filling defect in a non-aneurysmatic and non-atherosclerotic aorta (Fig. 19a).

Multiplanar reconstructions obtained are very effective at distinguishing a subtle and pedunculated thrombus from intimal flaps, tears, or dissection (Fig. 19a–e).

The morphologic feature of the thrombus (sessile vs. pedunculated), the location, and the length of the aortic segment involved (Fig. 20a–c) could be predictors of embolic potential of such a lesion (Verma et al. 2014; Karalis et al. 1991).

Furthermore, CT allows simultaneous imaging of vascular structures, including the vessel wall and of viscera, and can assess severe complications due to distal vessel embolism detecting visceral malperfusion, splenic, hepatic, renal, or intestinal infarction or peripheral arterial occlusion (Vernhet et al. 2004).

Noteworthy, CT is able to demonstrate both aortic source of embolism (atherosclerotic plaque or rare aortic tumors) and extra-aortic diseases associated with PAMT (Crohn's disease, pancreatitis, or malignancies) (Verbeeck et al. 2014).

MRI is a second-line imaging modality in assessing aortic disease because of some

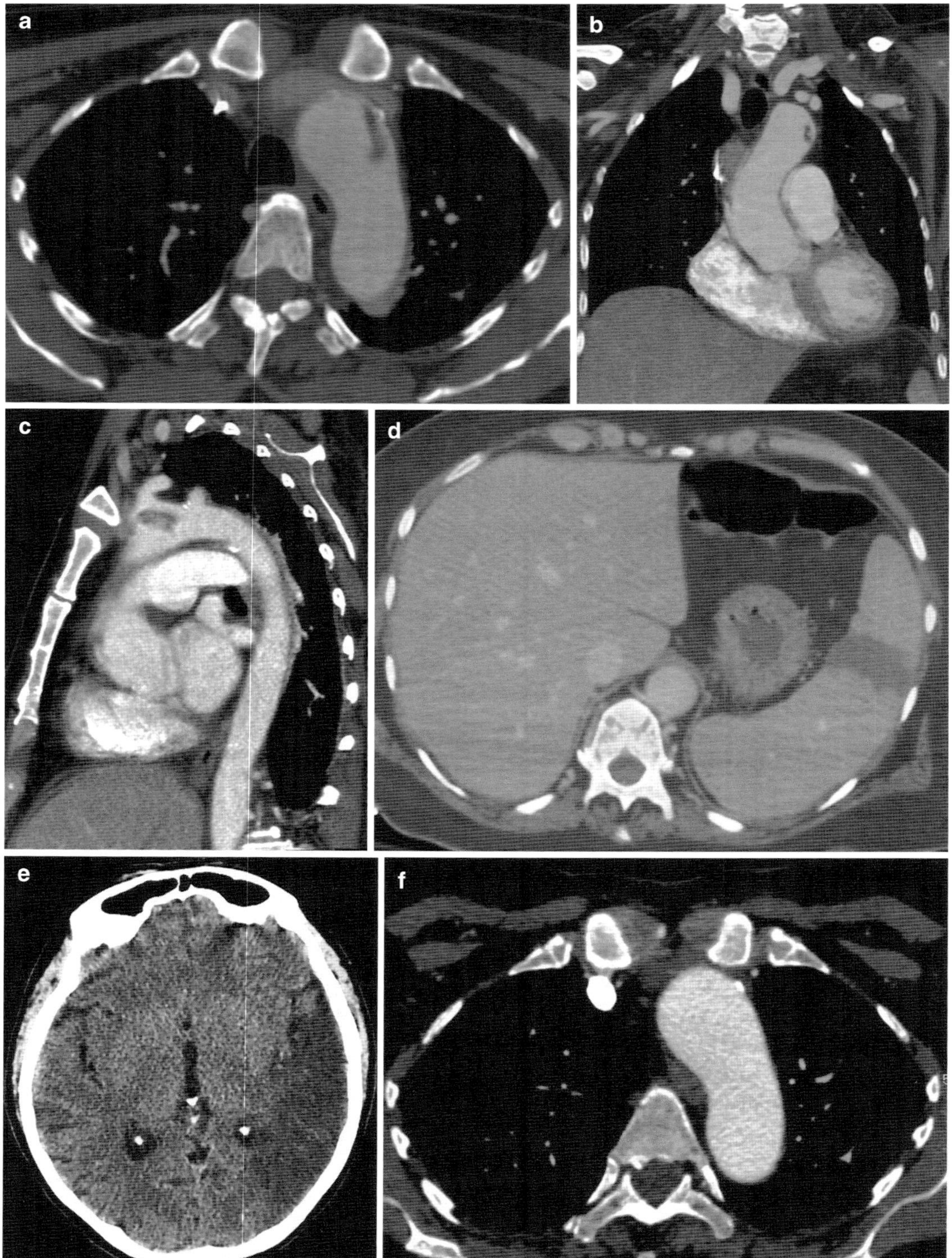

Fig. 19 A 50-year-old woman presented to ED with abdominal pain. After a negative abdominal US, she developed aphasia and underwent head CT and TEE investigation. On the basis of TEE, thoracic aortic dissection was suspected. CT demonstrates a filling defect in a non-aneurysmatic aortic arch adjacent to a small calcified plaque (**a**) and a splenic infarction (**d**). Reformatted images (**b**, **c**) help in differentiating floating thrombus from intimal flap. Head CT demonstrated a left temporal lobe ischemia (**e**). After anticoagulant therapy, the thrombus disappeared (**f**)

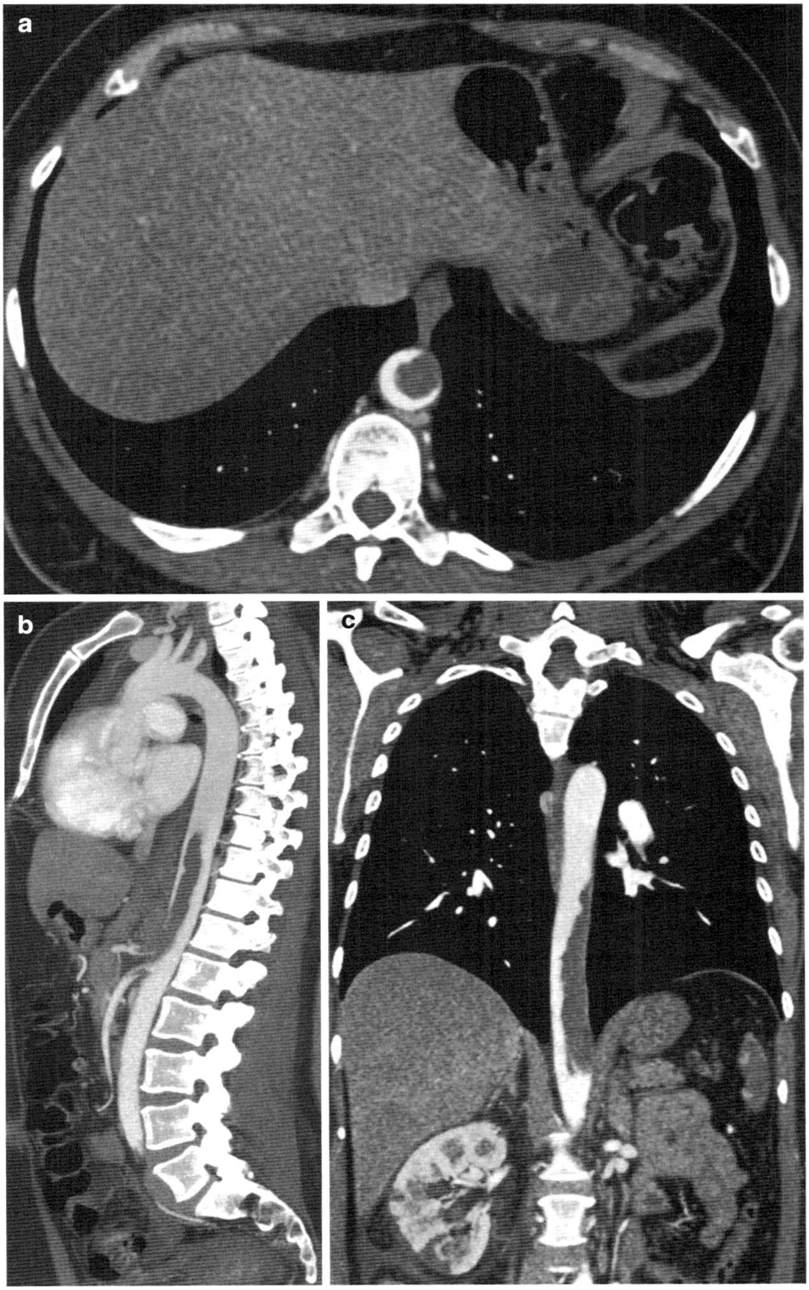

Fig. 20 Axial CT image (**a**) demonstrates an endoluminal filling defect in the non-aneurysmatic descending aorta of a young woman. Sagittal (**b**) and coronal (**c**) reformatted images demonstrate the features of the sessile thrombus located in the descending thoracic aorta and extended to celiac and superior mesenteric arteries and causing right kidney infarctions

disadvantages: the examination time is longer than CT; it benefits from patient cooperation (breath hold), in the turbulent flow that accompanies many cardiovascular diseases may suffer from artifacts that generate false-positive images and is limited in emergency situations. On the other hand, MRI is excellent for differentiating primary intramural hematoma from atherosclerotic plaque and intraluminal thrombus. MRI can noninvasively distinguish various components of the plaque, such as fibrous cap, lipid core, and thrombus, thereby assessing plaque stability (Oppenheim et al. 2009). Furthermore, MRI offers the possibility of diagnosing primary aortic or cardiac neoplasm in the differential diagnosis with thrombi.

Myxomas are the most common type of primary cardiac tumor (25–50 %), and in 75 % of cases, they originate from the left atrium. In MRI, these benign lesions are hypointense or isointense in T1-weighted sequences and hyperintense in T2-weighted sequences, with inhomogeneous contrast enhancement pattern. This is useful in the differential diagnosis with thrombi that should not enhance (Motwani et al. 2013).

Aortic sarcoma and cardiac angiosarcoma are very rare and aggressive malignant neoplasms that often are already metastatic at the diagnosis. Aortic sarcomas are broadly categorized as either primarily luminal or primarily mural. The luminal type often forms intraluminal polyps or extends along the intima causing peripheral emboli or aortic obstruction. The mural type originates from the media or adventitia and usually extends beyond the aorta (Bendel et al. 2011).

MRI shows inhomogeneous signal intensity in T1-weighted and T2-weighted sequences (sometimes can appear hyperintense in T1-weighted sequences with fat suppression due to its methemoglobin content in case of subacute hemorrhage), with inhomogeneous enhancement in postcontrast images.

Von Falck et al. observed in three patients with sarcomas of the aorta a pedunculated appearance ($n = 2/3$), an atypical location for a thrombus ($n = 2$), an expansion beyond the vessel wall ($n = 1/3$), contrast enhancement in MRI ($n = 2/2$, MRI was available in two patients) or MDCT ($n = 1/1$, MDCT was available in one patient), and metabolic activity as demonstrated by F-18 FDG PET/CT ($n = 1/1$; SUVmax = 3.6–5.5, PET was available in one patient) (von Falck et al. 2013).

2.4 Treatment

How to treat this potentially devastating aortic thrombus is a management dilemma.

Embolism from large vessel thrombi is potentially lethal, and it has been managed surgically in a few reported cases (Lehmann et al. 2001; Rossi et al. 2002; Mohammadi et al. 2007). Also, thrombolysis, thromboaspiration, and endovascular stent grafting have been utilized (Hausmann et al. 1992; Fueglistaler et al. 2005). Therefore, no guidelines for its management have been established.

In recent years, medical management of large intra-aortic thrombosis with systemic long-term anticoagulation with warfarin has been proposed with good results. Failure to continue warfarin therapy resulted in problems. Surgical treatment should be reserved only for selected cases of recurrent embolism or persistent symptomatology related to thrombus despite proper anticoagulation.

3 Aortobronchial Fistula

3.1 Definition, Etiology, and Clinical Presentation

Aortobronchial fistula (ABF) is a direct communication which occurs between the aorta and the bronchial tree. ABF was first described by Keefer in 1934 (Demeter and Cordasco 1980; Keefer 1934).

Primary ABF occurred rarely in patients who have no history of surgical intervention although the true incidence could be underestimated because more than 30 % are diagnosed at autopsy (Léobon et al. 2002). ABF is almost always associated to an underlying TAA. Compression of the tracheobronchial tree by enlargement of the TAA or low-grade inflammatory process associated may induce pressure necrosis, which can lead to erosion of both the aortic and bronchial walls.

The left bronchial tree is more frequently involved in ABF with the communication usually localized between the aneurysm and the membranous wall of the bronchus.

Secondary ABF is relatively more frequent and occurs postoperatively, after the implantation of a prosthetic vascular graft in the thoracic aorta (Favre et al. 1994; MacIntosh et al. 1991; Dorweiler 2001).

ABF can also occur in case of pseudoaneurysm as complication of aortic coarctation repair by means of patch aortoplasty (Milano et al. 1999) or after deployment of self-expanding bronchial stent to relieve extrinsic compression of a left main bronchus by a dissected descending aorta (Katayama et al. 2000).

When fistula between the aorta and bronchial lumina is created, patient presents hemoptysis that is usually massive, but occasionally is minor and intermittent. Hemoptysis is defined as the expectoration of blood that originates from the tracheobronchial tree or pulmonary parenchyma. Although hemoptysis is not specific to ABF, it is the most common presenting symptom and occurs in over 95% of cases (Demeter and Cordasco 1980). Common causes of hemoptysis include chronic bronchitis, bronchiectasis, pneumonia, fungal infections, tuberculosis, malignancy, and rarely pulmonary vasculitis (Ketai et al. 2014). The differential diagnosis is broad; the severity and the prognosis of the underlying disease are very variable. Most cases are benign and hemoptysis is a self-limiting event.

ABF must be strongly suspected when hemoptysis occurs in a patient who has had a TAA or has undergone to thoracic aortic surgery. Even the first of hemoptysis can be fatal, and a very high mortality rate accompanies recurrence, which can be a consequence of lysis or displacement of the temporary clot.

3.2 Diagnostic Workup

Diagnostic modalities for studying hemoptysis include chest radiography (CXR), bronchoscopy, CT, and DSA (Larici et al. 2014).

Life-threatening hemoptysis is rare and requires urgent investigations and appropriate treatment. The diagnosis of the vascular source of hemoptysis should be clarified in order to decide the treatment (surgical or endovascular).

In 95% of cases of hemoptysis, systemic arterial supply to the lungs (mainly bronchial arteries) is the origin of the bleeding (Bruzzi et al. 2006). Exceptionally, hemoptysis is related to the aorta. Unfortunately, the ability to diagnose ABF is further confounded by the lack of a diagnostic test that can definitely demonstrate the fistula (Riesenman et al. 2009). Chest radiograph (CXR) is the initial imaging modality. The sensitivity of CXR in this clinical context is not high. Radiography can help to lateralize the bleeding and can often help to detect underlying parenchymal and pleural abnormalities (Hsiao et al. 2001). Lung consolidation, resulting from hemorrhage into lung, is the most common radiographic finding in aortobronchopulmonary fistula (Coblentz and Sallee 1988). A more specific finding is the demonstration of a thoracic aortic aneurysm, which can be seen on the chest radiograph in 46% of cases.

If CXR demonstrates an aortic dilatation combined with an opacification of the airspace that obscures the adjacent outline of the arch or the descending aorta, a diagnosis of ABF should be suspected even in case of no previous history of aortic surgery.

With minor and intermittent hemoptysis, the diagnosis may go unrecognized. This may end in death as in some reports when the minor and intermittent hemoptysis lead to the mistaken diagnosis of bronchitis (Demeter and Cordasco 1980; Oldham et al. 1983; Garrett et al. 1965; Graeber et al. 1980). CT evaluation is mandatory.

CT can identify the site of bleeding as accurately as bronchoscopy and detect underlying disease with high sensitivity (Revel et al. 2002). The site of hemorrhage is usually localized on the basis of the presence of liquified material in segmental and lobar bronchi and of hazy consolidation or ground-glass infiltrates in the lung parenchyma, findings that represent intra-alveolar hemorrhage (Bruzzi et al. 2006).

When these findings are mainly adjacent to the aorta, radiological features of TAA must be accurately evaluated (Fig. 21a, b, d). Although CT will rarely show the communication between the lung and the aorta because the fistula is

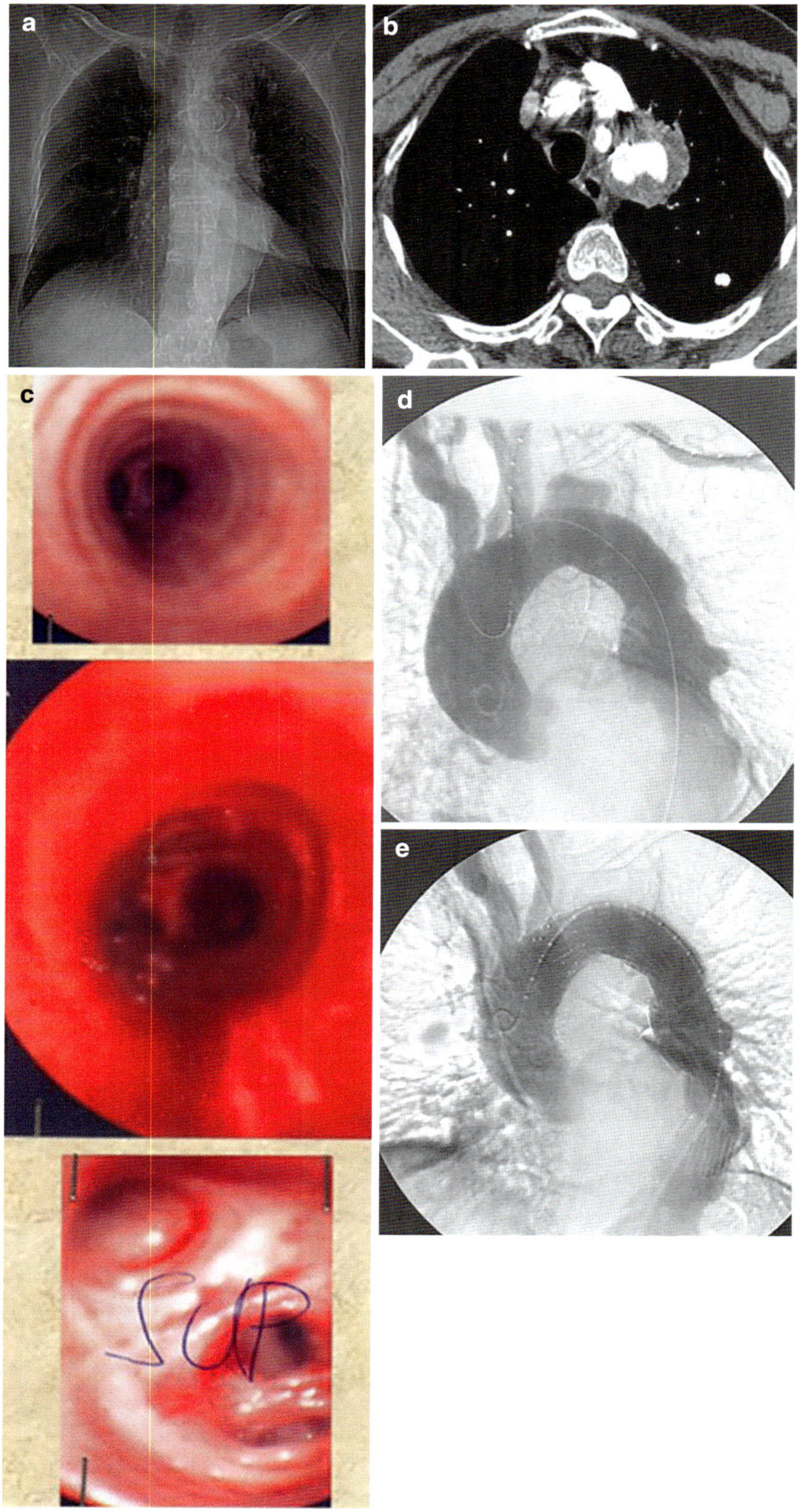
a
b
c
d
e
SUP

usually filled with clot (Graeber et al. 1980), the diagnosis of ABF is highly suggestive in this clinical setting (Pinilla et al. 2006).

Bronchoscopy (Fig. 21c) and DSA are often part of the evaluation of hemoptysis, and bronchoscopy could be directly visualize the fistula; however, both of these modalities often can fail to demonstrate the ABF (Liu et al. 2004) and may potentially induce massive hemorrhage dislodging clots overlying the fistula tract (Picichè et al. 2003).

4 Aortoesophageal Fistula

4.1 Definition, Etiology, and Clinical Presentation

Aortoesophageal fistula (AEF) is an uncommon cause of massive gastrointestinal hemorrhage that is associated with high morbidity and mortality and consists in direct communication between aorta and esophagus.

AEFs are classified as either primary or secondary. The main causes of primary AEFs are the erosion of a thoracic aortic aneurysm, foreign body ingestion such as bone from animal foods or sharp metal objects, and advanced esophageal malignancy (Lee et al. 2010; Hollander and Quick 1991; da Silva et al. 1999; Nandi and Ong 1978).

Cases of esophageal diverticulum associated with a secondary infective TAA complicated by AEF development have also been reported (Yasuda et al. 2002).

Secondary AEF occurs as complications of aortic reconstructive surgery with or without the placement of an aortic stent graft.

The exact pathophysiological mechanism of AEF remains unknown. Investigators suggested that the pathogenesis is related to esophageal ischemia secondary to elevated pressure in the posterior mediastinum, inflammation of the resorbed hematoma, mechanical compression by a large aneurysm and secondary erosion, or the geometric change in the aortic arch and the descending aorta after TEVAR. The radial force of the graft against the native aortic wall can be a causative factor (Okita et al. 2014; Hollander and Quick 1991; Czerny et al. 2014; von Segesser 1997). Primary infection or inflammation of the aneurysmal wall is also a potential cause of AEF (Hollander and Quick 1991).

The number of primary AEF resulting from aneurysm rupture is in apparent decline for the emerging use of open surgical and endovascular treatment of TAA at early stages. However, with the growing number of surgical repair of thoracic aneurysms and interventional procedures, postoperative AEF has become increasingly evident over time. The incidence of AEF as complication of open repair of the thoracic and thoracoabdominal aorta ranges from 0.5 to 1.7 % (Kieffer et al. 2003; Lawrie et al. 1994; Svensson et al. 1993). Diagnosis of AEF is rarely characterized by massive hematemesis. Patients usually present with the classic manifestations of midthoracic pain, sentinel arterial hemorrhage, and exsanguination after a symptom-free interval (Chiari's triad). In a few cases, AEF can be suspected on the basis of isolated sepsis or septic embolism in a lower extremity (Seymour 1978).

Other suggestive findings include dysphagia and/or chest pain and previous surgery involving the thoracic aorta (Kieffer et al. 2003).

4.2 Diagnostic Workup

Most diagnostic tests have significant individual limitations. The identification of massive upper

Fig. 21 A 70-year-old woman with intermittent hemoptysis. Chest radiography (scout view) demonstrated ill-defined aortic arch outline with calcified plaque (**a**). CT axial image detected multiple ulcerated atheromatous plaque (**b**) and an aneurysmatic aortic arch. Bronchoscopy (**c**) found a blood clot in the upper left lobe bronchus close to the aortic arch. TEVAR treatment was indicated: DSA demonstrated multiple aortic parietal bulging (**d**), the bigger in the aortic arch before the placement of the graft (**e**). After TEVAR, hemoptysis stopped gastrointestinal hemorrhage that is bright red and arterial in nature is characteristic. Endoscopy of the upper gastrointestinal tract might aid in the detection of fistula. Endoscopic findings may be directly due to visualization of pulsatile blood into the esophagus or a pulsatile adherent blood clot. More subtle findings during endoscopy might point in direction of a fistula, such as submucosal hematoma shown as a blue-gray discoloration of the esophageal wall. However, the sensitivity of detection of fistulae via endoscopy is a mere 38 % (Perdue et al. 1980).

Although no single imaging modality demonstrates AEF with sufficient sensitivity and specificity, computed tomography (CT) is the imaging modality of choice for evaluations in the emergency setting (Figs. 22a–c and 23a–c). The clinical manifestations are often crucial to the diagnosis of aortoenteric fistula (Vu et al. 2009).

The most specific but quite rare sign of AEF is the identification on CT of direct extravasation of contrast from the aorta into the esophagus (Fig. 22d, e) (Vu et al. 2009; Raman et al. 2013), but during the symptom-free interval, radiological evidence of AEF may be absent due to the transient clot formation (Khawaja and Varindani 1987).

Similarly, the leakage of enteric contrast directly into the periaortic space is a highly specific sign, but extremely rare (Fig. 22f).

Other important signs to assess are esophageal wall thickening, effacement of the periaortic fat plane, and periaortic soft tissue/fluid.

Identification of an aortic aneurysm or a penetrating atherosclerotic ulcer adjacent to a mediastinal soft-tissue mass or to a mediastinal hematoma is helpful for ascertaining the precise location of a primary aortoenteric fistula (Hughes et al. 2007).

The diagnosis of secondary AEF is dependent on a number of other nonspecific, but suggestive, findings, including effacement of the periaortic fat plane (Fig. 22b), focal thickening and tethering of the esophageal wall immediately adjacent to the aorta (Fig. 22d, e), periaortic free fluid and soft-tissue thickening, and disruption of a graft (Fig. 22d, e) or significant graft migration (Low et al. 1990).

However, CT normal findings in the immediate postoperative period should not be misinterpreted as a fistula. Perigraft soft-tissue edema, fluid, and ectopic gas may be normal immediately after surgery. After 3–4 weeks, any ectopic gas is abnormal and should be considered a sign of perigraft infection and possibly fistulization (Hughes et al. 2007; Vu et al. 2009). The perigraft soft-tissue thickening, fluid, or hematoma should resolve within 2–3 months after surgery (Vu et al. 2009).

Because of their overlapping CT features, aortoenteric fistula and perigraft infection may be difficult or impossible to differentiate. However, the specific CT findings that correlate strongly with the presence of aortoenteric fistula include ectopic gas (Fig. 22b), focal esophageal wall thickening, breach of the aortic wall, and extravasation of contrast material into the esophageal lumen (Fig. 22d, e) (Low et al. 1990; Hughes et al. 2007; Hagspiel et al. 2007; Vu et al. 2009).

Esophageal ingested foreign body such as bones is easily detectable (sensitivity 100 %) by CT (Fig. 22c) even if they migrated in the mediastinum and both radiography and endoscopy are negative (Marco De Lucas et al. 2004).

Foreign bodies in the thoracic esophagus tend to be lodged at the level of the left primary bronchus, where the aortic arch presses against

Fig. 22 Primary AEF fistula in a 65-year-old woman with hematemesis and a history of ingested bone. A pseudoaneurysm of the descending thoracic aorta is visible in the arterial phase (axial image **a**). Ectopic gas is detectable in the mediastinal hematoma that surrounds the pseudoaneurysm (**b**, venous phase) and occupies the fat plane between the esophagus and the aorta. Parasagittal MPR (**c**) demonstrates both the small foreign body (*arrow*) close to the left main bronchus and the pseudoaneurysm. Patient developed also a severe mediastinitis and three months post-TEVAR she had hematemesis. Axial (**d**) and coronal reformatted (**e**) images demonstrate contrast leakage in the esophagus and AOF localized where the esophageal wall is tethered to the aorta. Although the infected graft was removed and with the placement of esophageal stent, the fistula was fatal. Radiograph (**f**) demonstrates oral contrast leakage in the mediastinum

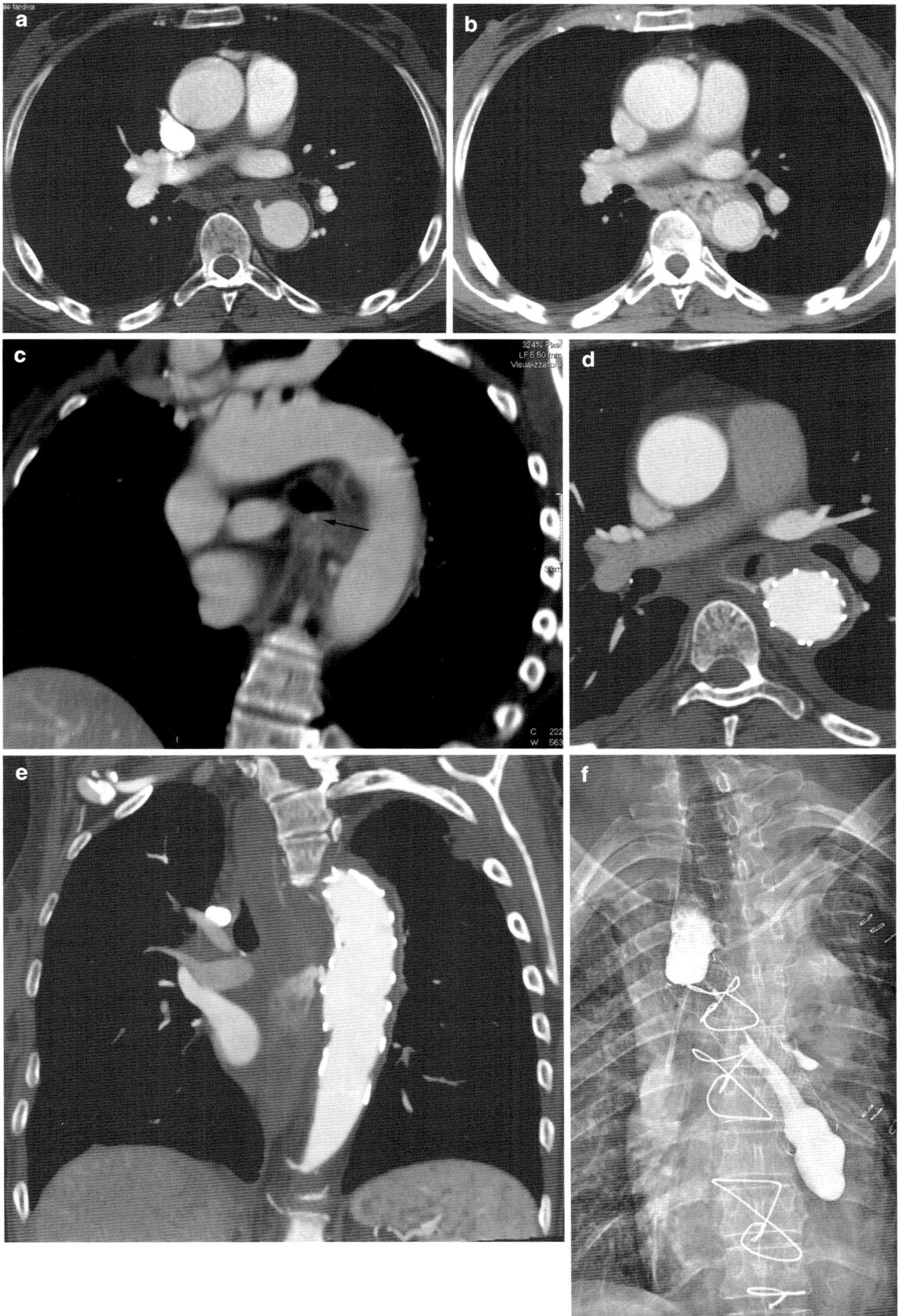
a
b
c
d
e
f

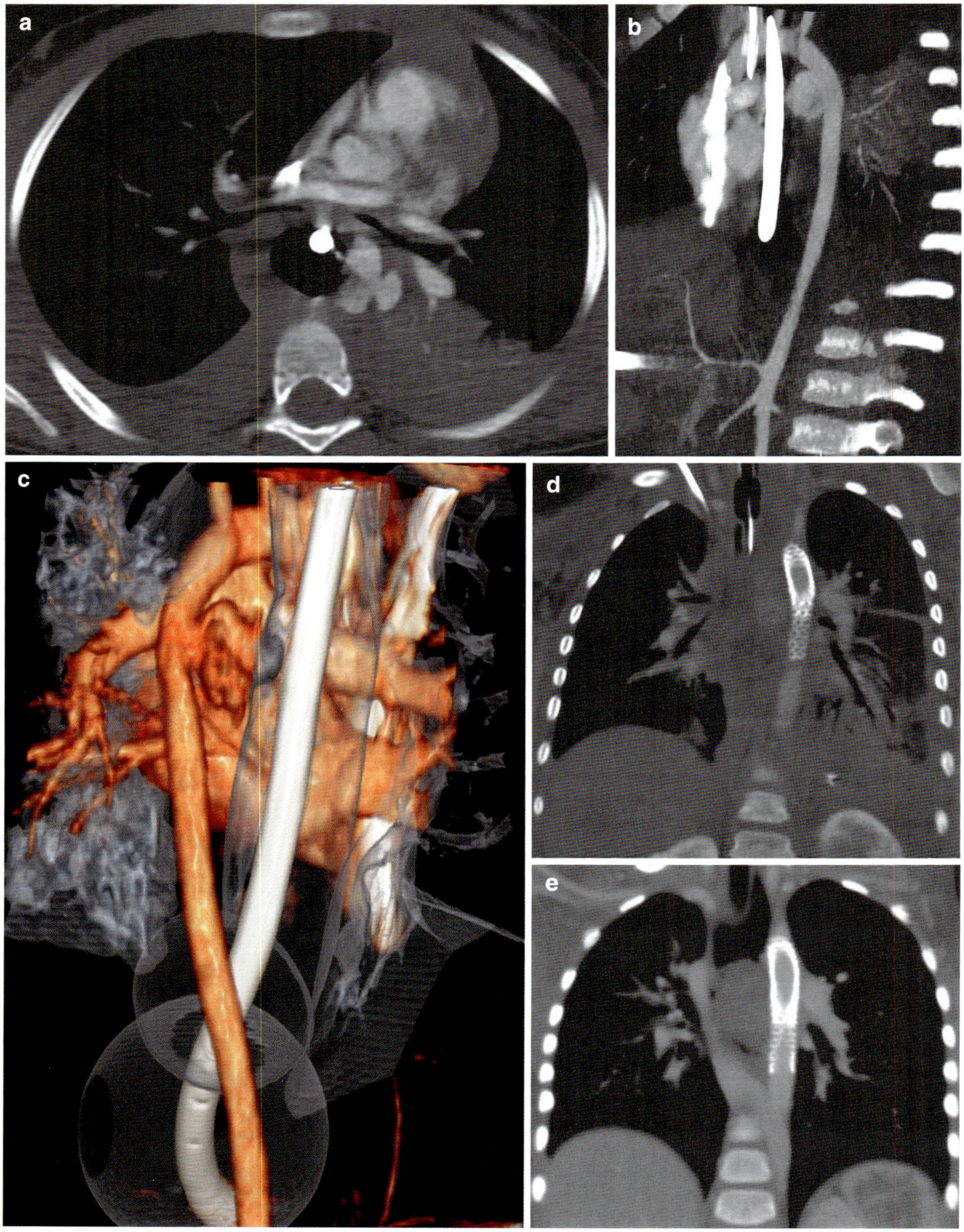

Fig. 23 Primary AEF in a 4-year-old patient presenting with massive hematemesis. Axial CT image (**a**), sagittal MIP (**b**), and VR posterior view (**c**) demonstrate a large pseudoaneurysm. Esophagus is distended by an insufflated Sengstaken–Blakemore balloon (**c**). Immediately after TEVAR, CT coronal image (**d**) demonstrated the excluded pseudoaneurysm, filled with residual contrast, which in the following CT evolved in a large hypodense hematoma (**e**) with narrowing the adjacent esophageal lumen (**f**)

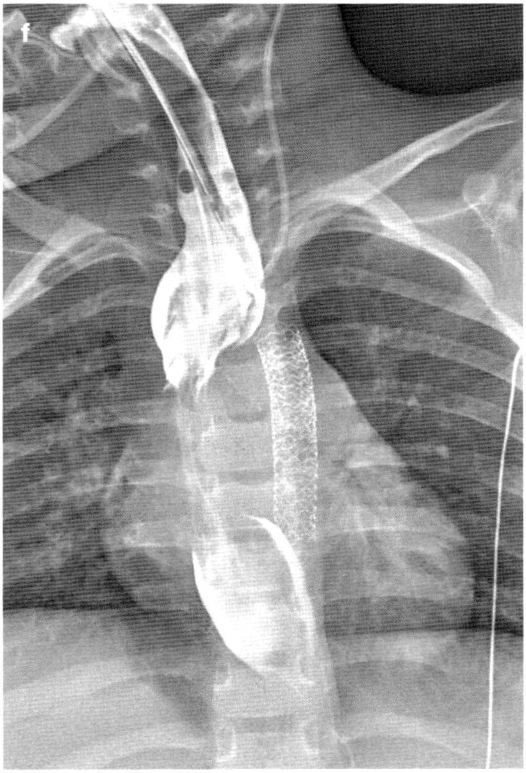

Fig. 23 (continued)

the esophagus and creates a relatively narrow lumen (Wei et al. 2015).

Interestingly, Wei Y. et al. analyzed the clinical data of 22 patients with ingested foreign bodies retrospectively and developed a classification system based on CT findings for esophageal injuries and used this system and the clinical presentation to guide treatment. Depending on the CT findings, the esophageal injuries were divided into four grades: Grade I, non-penetrating injury; Grade II, penetrating injury with minimal infection; Grade III, potential AEF; and Grade IV, definite AEF (Wei et al. 2015). CT findings in Grade III were suggestive of esophageal perforation and severe intrathoracic infections such as mediastinitis, chest empyema, and abscess with foreign body close to the aorta (<2 mm). In Grade IV, CT findings were aortic wall perforation, pseudoaneurysm, and mediastinal abscess.

4.3 AEF and ABF Treatment

Surgical treatment of AEF and ABF requires replacement of the thoracic aorta associated with adjunctive procedures to repair the esophageal or tracheobronchial lesion with a high rate of perioperative mortality and morbidity. Recently, the use of TEVAR (Figs. 21e and 23d, e) has been proposed as mini-invasive treatment. Although the excellent technical result in the immediate postoperative period, there are several limitations due to the high risk of contamination of the graft. For this reason, TEVAR should be considered as a "bridge" intervention to the open treatment.

References

Abbas A, Brown IW, Peebles CR et al (2014) The role of multidetector-row CT in the diagnosis, classification and management of acute aortic syndrome. Br J Radiol 87:20140354. doi:10.1259/bjr.20140354

Abissegue YG, Lyazidi Y, Chtata H et al (2015) Acute systemic embolism due to an idiopathic floating thrombus of the thoracic aorta: success of medical management: a case report. BMC Res Notes 8:181

Agarwal PP, Chughtai A, Matzinger FRK, Kazerooni EA (2009) Multidetector CT of thoracic aortic aneurysms. Radiographics 29:537–552. doi:10.1148/rg.292075080

Arita T, Matsunaga N, Takano K et al (1997) Abdominal aortic aneurysm: rupture associated with the high-attenuating crescent sign. Radiology 204:765–768

Aronberg DJ, Glazer HS, Madsen K, Sagel SS (1984) Normal thoracic aortic diameters by computed tomography. J Comput Assist Tomogr 8:247–250

Azizi L, Henon A, Belkacem A et al (2004) Infected aortic aneurysms: CT features. Abdom Imaging 29:716–720

Bendel EC, Maleszewski JJ, Araoz PA (2011) Imaging sarcomas of the great vessels and heart. Semin Ultrasound CT MR 32:377–404

Bickerstaff LK, Pairolero PC, Hollier LH et al (1982) Thoracic aortic aneurysms: a population-based study. Surgery 92:1103–1108

Bruzzi JF, Remy-Jardin M, Delhaye D et al (2006) Multidetector row CT of hemoptysis. Radiographics 26:3–22. doi:10.1148/rg.261045726

Chiu KWH, Lakshminarayan R, Ettles DF (2013) Acute aortic syndrome: CT findings. Clin Radiol 68:741–748. doi:10.1016/j.crad.2013.03.001

Cho Y, Suzuki S, Katogi T, Ueda T (2004) Esophageal perforation of aortic arch aneurysm treated free of mediastinitis without manipulating esophagus. Japanese J Thorac Cardiovasc Surg Off Publ Japanese Assoc Thorac Surg Nihon Kyōbu Geka Gakkai zasshi 52:314–317

Choukroun EM, Labrousse LM, Madonna FP, Deville C (2002) Mobile thrombus of the thoracic aorta: diagnosis and treatment in 9 cases. Ann Vasc Surg 16:714–722
Coblentz L, Sallee DS (1988) Aortobronchopulmonary complicating aortic diagnosis in four cases fistula aneurysm. Ann Surg 150:535–538
Crass JR, Cohen AM, Motta AO et al (1990) A proposed new mechanism of traumatic aortic rupture: the osseous pinch. Radiology 176:645–649
Creasy JD, Chiles C, Routh WD, Dyer RB (1997) Overview of traumatic injury of the thoracic aorta. Radiographics 17:27–45. doi:10.1148/radiographics.17.1.9017797
Czerny M, Eggebrecht H, Sodeck G et al (2014) New insights regarding the incidence, presentation and treatment options of aorto-oesophageal fistulation after thoracic endovascular aortic repair: the European Registry of Endovascular Aortic Repair Complications. Eur J Cardiothorac Surg 45:452–457
da Silva ES, Tozzi FL, Otochi JP et al (1999) Aortoesophageal fistula caused by aneurysm of the thoracic aorta: successful surgical treatment, case report, and literature review. J Vasc Surg 30: 1150–1157
Daimon M, Watanabe H, Abe Y et al (2008) Normal values of echocardiographic parameters in relation to age in a healthy Japanese population: the JAMP study. Circ J 72:1859–1866
De Backer J, Loeys B, Devos D et al (2006) A critical analysis of minor cardiovascular criteria in the diagnostic evaluation of patients with Marfan syndrome. Genet Med 8:401–408
Demeter SL, Cordasco EM (1980) Aortobronchial fistula: keys to successful management. Angiology 31:431–435
Dorweiler B (2001) Endovascular treatment of acute bleeding complications in traumatic aortic rupture and aortobronchial fistula. Eur J Cardiothorac Surg 19:739–745
Edwards JE (1948) Anomalies of the derivatives of the aortic arch system. Med Clin North Am 32:925–949
Fang M, Agha S, Lockridge L et al (2001) Medical management of a large aortic thrombus in a young woman with essential thrombocythemia. Mayo Clin Proc 76:427–431
Favre JP, Gournier JP, Adham M et al (1994) Aortobronchial fistula: report of three cases and review of the literature. Surgery 115:264–270
Fayad ZY, Semaan E, Fahoum B et al (2013) Aortic mural thrombus in the normal or minimally atherosclerotic aorta. Ann Vasc Surg 27:282–290
Fillinger MF, Marra SP, Raghavan ML, Kennedy FE (2003) Prediction of rupture risk in abdominal aortic aneurysm during observation: wall stress versus diameter. J Vasc Surg 37:724–732
Fishman EK, Ney DR, Heath DG et al (2006) Volume rendering versus maximum intensity projection in CT angiography: what works best, when, and why. Radiographics 26:905–922. doi:10.1148/rg.263055186
Fueglistaler P, Wolff T, Guerke L et al (2005) Endovascular stent graft for symptomatic mobile thrombus of the thoracic aorta. J Vasc Surg 42:781–783
Gagliardi JM, Batt M, Khodja RH, Le bas P (1988) Mural thrombus of the aorta. Ann Vasc Surg 2:201–204
Garrett HE, Ricks RK, Lewis JM et al (1965) Hemoptysis secondary to aortopulmonary fistula; a report of two cases of successful treatment by operation. J Thorac Cardiovasc Surg 49:588–593
Garzón G, Fernández-Velilla M, Martí M et al (2005) Endovascular stent-graft treatment of thoracic aortic disease. Radiographics 25(Suppl 1):S229–S244. doi:10.1148/rg.25si055513
Gaylis H (1958) Aortic thrombosis. Circulation XVII:941
Girardi LN, Coselli JS (1997) Inflammatory aneurysm of the ascending aorta and aortic arch. Ann Thorac Surg 64:251–253
Goldstein SA, Evangelista A, Abbara S et al (2015) Multimodality imaging of diseases of the thoracic aorta in adults: from the American Society of Echocardiography and the European Association of Cardiovascular Imaging. J Am Soc Echocardiogr 28:119–182. doi:10.1016/j.echo.2014.11.015
Gomes MN, Choyke PL (1992) Infected aortic aneurysms: CT diagnosis. J Cardiovasc Surg (Torino) 33:684–689
Gonsalves CF (1999) The hyperattenuating crescent sign. Radiology 211:37–38
Gornik HL, Creager MA (2008) Aortitis. Circulation 117:3039–3051
Gotway MB, Dawn SK (2003) Thoracic aorta imaging with multislice CT. Radiol Clin North Am 41: 521–543
Graeber GM, Farrell BG, Neville JF, Parker FB (1980) Successful diagnosis and management of fistulas between the aorta and the tracheobronchial tree. Ann Thorac Surg 29:555–561
Green E, Klein S (2007). Multidetector row CT angiography of thoracic aorta. In P. Boiselle and C. White (Eds.), New techniques in cardiothoracic imaging. New York, NY: Informa Healthcare pp 105–126
Greenhalgh R (2004) Comparison of endovascular aneurysm repair with open repair in patients with abdominal aortic aneurysm (EVAR trial 1), 30-day operative mortality results: randomised controlled trial. Lancet 364:843–848
Grollman JH (1989) The aortic diverticulum: a remnant of the partially involuted dorsal aortic root. Cardiovasc Intervent Radiol 12:14–17
Hagspiel KD, Turba UC, Bozlar U et al (2007) Diagnosis of aortoenteric fistulas with CT angiography. J Vasc Interv Radiol 18:497–504
Halliday KE, al-Kutoubi A (1996) Draped aorta: CT sign of contained leak of aortic aneurysms. Radiology 199:41–43. doi:10.1148/radiology.199.1.8633170
Hastreiter AR, D'Cruz IA, Cantez T et al (1966) Right-sided aorta. I. Occurrence of right aortic arch in various types of congenital heart disease. II. Right aortic arch, right descending aorta, and associated anomalies. Br Heart J 28:722–739
Hausmann D, Gulba D, Bargheer K et al (1992) Successful thrombolysis of an aortic-arch thrombus in a patient after mesenteric embolism. N Engl J Med 327:500–501

Heckstall RL, Hollander JE (1998) Aortoesophageal fistula: recognition and diagnosis in the emergency department. Ann Emerg Med 32:502–505

Heystraten FM, Rosenbusch G, Kingma LM, Lacquet LK (1986) Chronic posttraumatic aneurysm of the thoracic aorta: surgically correctable occult threat. AJR Am J Roentgenol 146:303–308

Hiratzka LF, Bakris GL, Beckman JA et al (2010) ACCF/AHA/AATS/ACR/ASA/SCA/SCAI/SIR/STS/SVM guidelines for the diagnosis and management of patients with thoracic aortic disease: executive summary a report of the American College of Cardiology Foundation/American Heart Association Task Force on Practice Guidelines, American Association for Thoracic Surgery, American College of Radiology, American Stroke Association, Society of Cardiovascular Anesthesiologists, Society for Cardiovascular Angiography and Interventions, Society of Interventional Radiology, Society of Thoracic Surgeons, and Society for Vascular Medicine. J Am Coll Cardiol 55:e27–e129

Hirose Y, Takamiya M (1998) Growth curve of ruptured aortic aneurysm. J Cardiovasc Surg (Torino) 39:9–13

Hollander JE, Quick G (1991) Aortoesophageal fistula: a comprehensive review of the literature. Am J Med 91:279–287

Hoshina K, Sho E, Sho M et al (2003) Wall shear stress and strain modulate experimental aneurysm cellularity. J Vasc Surg 37:1067–1074

Hsiao EI, Kirsch CM, Kagawa FT et al (2001) Utility of fiberoptic bronchoscopy before bronchial artery embolization for massive hemoptysis. AJR Am J Roentgenol 177:861–867

Hughes FM, Kavanagh D, Barry M et al (2007) Aortoenteric fistula: a diagnostic dilemma. Abdom Imaging 32:398–402

Isselbacher EM (2005) Thoracic and abdominal aortic aneurysms. Circulation 111:816–828

Javadpour H, O'Toole JJ, McEniff JN et al (2002) Traumatic aortic transection: evidence for the osseous pinch mechanism. Ann Thorac Surg 73:951–953

Kälsch H, Lehmann N, Möhlenkamp S et al (2013) Body-surface adjusted aortic reference diameters for improved identification of patients with thoracic aortic aneurysms: results from the population-based Heinz Nixdorf Recall study. Int J Cardiol 163:72–78

Karalis DG, Chandrasekaran K, Victor MF et al (1991) Recognition and embolic potential of intraaortic atherosclerotic debris. J Am Coll Cardiol 17:73–78

Katayama Y, Suzuki H, Mizutani T (2000) Aorto-bronchial fistula after implantation of a self-expanding bronchial stent in a patient with aortic dissection. Japanese J Thorac Cardiovasc Surg Off Publ Japanese Assoc Thorac Surg Nihon Kyōbu Geka Gakkai zasshi 48:73–75

Keefer CSMK (1934) The pulmonary and pleural complications of aortic aneurysms. Am Heart J 10:208

Ketai LH, Mohammed T-LH, Kirsch J et al (2014) ACR appropriateness criteria® hemoptysis. J Thorac Imaging 29:W19–W22. doi:10.1097/RTI.0000000000000084

Khawaja FI, Varindani MK (1987) Aortoesophageal fistula. Review of clinical, radiographic, and endoscopic features. J Clin Gastroenterol 9:342–344

Kieffer E, Chiche L, Gomes D (2003) Aortoesophageal fistula: value of in situ aortic allograft replacement. Ann Surg 238:283–290

Lande A, Berkmen YM (1976) Aortitis: pathologic, clinical and arteriographic review. Radiol Clin North Am 14:219–240

Laperche T, Laurian C, Roudaut R, Steg PG (1997) Mobile thromboses of the aortic arch without aortic debris : a transesophageal echocardiographic finding associated with unexplained arterial embolism. Circulation 96:288–294

Larici AR, Franchi P, Occhipinti M et al (2014) Diagnosis and management of hemoptysis. Diagnos Interv Radiol 20:299–309. doi:10.5152/dir.2014.13426

Lau LS, Blanchard DG, Hye RJ (1997) Diagnosis and management of patients with peripheral macroemboli from thoracic aortic pathology. Ann Vasc Surg 11:348–353

Lawrie GM, Earle N, De Bakey ME (1994) Evolution of surgical techniques for aneurysms of the descending thoracic aorta: twenty-nine years experience with 659 patients. J Card Surg 9:648–661

Lee W-K, Mossop PJ, Little AF et al (2008) Infected (mycotic) aneurysms: spectrum of imaging appearances and management. Radiographics 28:1853–1868. doi:10.1148/rg.287085054

Lee RY, Flaherty L, Khushalani NI et al (2010) Aorto-esophageal fistula: a rare fatal case caused by esophageal malignancy. J Gastrointest Oncol 1:64–65

Lehmann JM, Shnaker A, Silverberg D et al (2001) Arterial thromboembolism from a distal aortic thrombus in a patient with Crohn's disease. Isr Med Assoc J 3:226–227

Léobon B, Roux D, Mugniot A et al (2002) Endovascular treatment of thoracic aortic fistulas. Ann Thorac Surg 74:247–249

Lesko N, Link K, Grainger R (1997) The thoracic aorta, 3rd edn. Churchill Livingstone, Edinburgh, pp 854–857

Liu S-F, Chen Y-C, Lin M-C, Kao C-L (2004) Thoracic aortic aneurysm with aortobronchial fistula: a thirteen-year experience. Heart Lung 33:119–123. doi:10.1016/j.hrtlng.2003.12.008

Lodi R, Rajagopalan B, Blamire AM et al (2004) Abnormal cardiac energetics in patients carrying the A3243G mtDNA mutation measured in vivo using phosphorus MR spectroscopy. Biochim Biophys Acta 1657:146–150. doi:10.1016/j.bbabio.2004.05.003

Low RN, Wall SD, Jeffrey RB et al (1990) Aortoenteric fistula and perigraft infection: evaluation with CT. Radiology 175:157–162

Macedo TA, Stanson AW, Oderich GS et al (2004) Infected aortic aneurysms: imaging findings. Radiology 231:250–257

Machleder HI, Takiff H, Lois JF, Holburt E (1986) Aortic mural thrombus: an occult source of arterial thromboembolism. J Vasc Surg 4:473–478
MacIntosh EL, Parrott JC, Unruh HW (1991) Fistulas between the aorta and tracheobronchial tree. Ann Thorac Surg 51:515–519
Marco De Lucas E, Sádaba P, Lastra García-Barón P et al (2004) Value of helical computed tomography in the management of upper esophageal foreign bodies. Acta Radiol 45:369–374
McGloughlin TM, Doyle BJ (2010) New approaches to abdominal aortic aneurysm rupture risk assessment: engineering insights with clinical gain. Arterioscler Thromb Vasc Biol 30:1687–1694
Mehard WB, Heiken JP, Sicard GA (1994) High-attenuating crescent in abdominal aortic aneurysm wall at CT: a sign of acute or impending rupture. Radiology 192:359–362
Michel J-B, Martin-Ventura J-L, Egido J et al (2011) Novel aspects of the pathogenesis of aneurysms of the abdominal aorta in humans. Cardiovasc Res 90:18–27
Milano A, De Carlo M, Mussi A et al (1999) Aortobronchial fistula after coarctation repair and blunt chest trauma. Ann Thorac Surg 67:539–541
Mohammadi S, Trahan S, Miro S, Dagenais F (2007) Images in cardiovascular medicine. Large free-floating intra-aortic thrombus. Circulation 116:e142–e143
Motwani M, Kidambi A, Herzog BA et al (2013) MR imaging of cardiac tumors and masses: a review of methods and clinical applications. Radiology 268:26–43
Mower WR, Quiñones WJ, Gambhir SS (1997) Effect of intraluminal thrombus on abdominal aortic aneurysm wall stress. J Vasc Surg 26:602–608
Nagpal P, Khandelwal A, Saboo SS et al (2015) Modern imaging techniques: applications in the management of acute aortic pathologies. Postgrad Med J 91:449–462. doi:10.1136/postgradmedj-2014-133178
Nandi P, Ong GB (1978) Foreign body in the oesophagus: review of 2394 cases. Br J Surg 65:5–9
Oderich GS, Panneton JM, Bower TC et al (2001) Infected aortic aneurysms: aggressive presentation, complicated early outcome, but durable results. J Vasc Surg 34:900–908
Okita Y, Yamanaka K, Okada K et al (2014) Strategies for the treatment of aorto-oesophageal fistula. Eur J Cardiothorac Surg 46:894–900
Oldham KT, Johansen K, Winterscheid L, Larson EB (1983) Remembrance of things past: aortobronchial fistula 15 years after thoracic aortic homograft. West J Med 139:225–228
Oppenheim C, Naggara O, Touzé E et al (2009) High-resolution MR imaging of the cervical arterial wall: what the radiologist needs to know. Radiographics 29:1413–1431
Perdue GD, Smith RB, Ansley JD, Costantino MJ (1980) Impending aortoenteric hemorrhage: the effect of early recognition on improved outcome. Ann Surg 192:237–243
Piccinelli M, Vergara C, Antiga L et al (2013) Impact of hemodynamics on lumen boundary displacements in abdominal aortic aneurysms by means of dynamic computed tomography and computational fluid dynamics. Biomech Model Mechanobiol 12:1263–1276
Picichè M, De Paulis R, Fabbri A, Chiariello L (2003) Postoperative aortic fistulas into the airways: etiology, pathogenesis, presentation, diagnosis, and management. Ann Thorac Surg 75:1998–2006
Pillari G, Chang JB, Zito J et al (1988) Computed tomography of abdominal aortic aneurysm. An in vivo pathological report with a note on dynamic predictors. Arch Surg 123:727–732
Pinilla I, Bret M, Cuesta E et al (2006) Role of computed tomography and magnetic resonance imaging in aortobronchial fistula diagnosis following aortic coarctation reparative surgery. Report of two cases. J Cardiovasc Surg (Torino) 47:221–227
Posniak HV, Olson MC, Demos TC et al (1990) CT of thoracic aortic aneurysms. Radiographics 10:839–855
Pousios D, Velissaris T, Duggan S, Tsang G (2009) Floating intra-aortic thrombus presenting as distal arterial embolism. Interact Cardiovasc Thorac Surg 9:532–534
Raghavan ML, Vorp DA, Federle MP et al (2000) Wall stress distribution on three-dimensionally reconstructed models of human abdominal aortic aneurysm. J Vasc Surg 31:760–769
Rajagopalan S, Sanz J, Ribeiro VG, Dellegrottaglie S (2007) CT angiography of the thoracic aorta with protocols. In D. Mukherjee and S. Rajagopalan (Eds.), CT and MR angiography of the peripheral circulation: practical approach with clinical protocols, London, England: Informa Healthcare pp 91–110
Rakita D, Newatia A, Hines JJ et al (2007) Spectrum of CT findings in rupture and impending rupture of abdominal aortic aneurysms. Radiographics 27:497–507. doi:10.1148/rg.272065026
Raman SP, Kamaya A, Federle M, Fishman EK (2013) Aortoenteric fistulas: spectrum of CT findings. Abdom Imaging 38:367–375. doi:10.1007/s00261-012-9873-7
Reber PU, Patel AG, Stauffer E et al (1999) Mural aortic thrombi: an important cause of peripheral embolization. J Vasc Surg 30:1084–1089
Restrepo CS, Ocazionez D, Suri R, Vargas D (2011) Aortitis: imaging spectrum of the infectious and inflammatory conditions of the aorta. Radiographics 31:435–451. doi:10.1148/rg.312105069
Revel MP, Fournier LS, Hennebicque AS et al (2002) Can CT replace bronchoscopy in the detection of the site and cause of bleeding in patients with large or massive hemoptysis? AJR Am J Roentgenol 179:1217–1224. doi:10.2214/ajr.179.5.1791217
Revest M, Decaux O, Cazalets C et al (2007) Thoracic infectious aortitis: microbiology, pathophysiology and treatment. La Rev médecine interne/fondée par la Société Natl Fr médecine interne 28:108–115

Riesenman PJ, Brooks JD, Farber MA (2009) Thoracic endovascular aortic repair of aortobronchial fistulas. J Vasc Surg 50:992–998. doi:10.1016/j.jvs.2009.03.001
Romero J, Husain SA, Kelesidis I et al (2013) Detection of left atrial appendage thrombus by cardiac computed tomography in patients with atrial fibrillation: a meta-analysis. Circ Cardiovasc Imaging 6:185–194
Rossi PJ, Desai TR, Skelly CL et al (2002) Paravisceral aortic thrombus as a source of peripheral embolization – report of three cases and review of the literature. J Vasc Surg 36:839–843
Russo V, Garattoni M, Buia F et al (2015) 128-slice CT angiography of the aorta without ECG-gating: efficacy of faster gantry rotation time and iterative reconstruction in terms of image quality and radiation dose. Eur Radiol. doi:10.1007/s00330-015-3848-3
Safi H, Estrera A, Sheinbaum R, Miller C (2012) Indications, techniques and results of open repair of ascending and transverse aortic arch aneurysms, 6th edn. Wiley-Blackwell, Oxford, UK
Sakalihasan N, Limet R, Defawe OD (2005) Abdominal aortic aneurysm. Lancet (London, England) 365:1577–1589
Seymour EQ (1978) Aortoesophageal fistula as a complication of aortic prosthetic graft. AJR Am J Roentgenol 131:160–161
Shapiro MD, Neilan TG, Jassal DS et al (2007) Multidetector computed tomography for the detection of left atrial appendage thrombus: a comparative study with transesophageal echocardiography. J Comput Assist Tomogr 31:905–909
Shuford WH, Sybers RG, Gordon IJ et al (1986) Circumflex retroesophageal right aortic arch simulating mediastinal tumor or dissecting aneurysm. AJR Am J Roentgenol 146:491–496
Siegel CL, Cohan RH, Korobkin M et al (1994) Abdominal aortic aneurysm morphology: CT features in patients with ruptured and nonruptured aneurysms. AJR Am J Roentgenol 163:1123–1129
Slobodin G, Naschitz JE, Zuckerman E et al (2006) Aortic involvement in rheumatic diseases. Clin Exp Rheumatol 24:S41–S47
Speelman L, Schurink GWH, Bosboom EMH et al (2010) The mechanical role of thrombus on the growth rate of an abdominal aortic aneurysm. J Vasc Surg 51:19–26
Sueyoshi E, Sakamoto I, Kawahara Y et al (1998) Infected abdominal aortic aneurysm: early CT findings. Abdom Imaging 23:645–648
Svensson LG, Crawford ES, Hess KR et al (1993) Experience with 1509 patients undergoing thoracoabdominal aortic operations. J Vasc Surg 17:357–368; discussion 368–370
Task A, Erbel R, Germany C et al (2014) 2014 ESC Guidelines on the diagnosis and treatment of aortic diseases. Eur Heart J 35:2873–2926. doi:10.1093/eurheartj/ehu281
Thalheimer A, Fein M, Geissinger E, Franke S (2004) Intimal angiosarcoma of the aorta: report of a case and review of the literature. J Vasc Surg 40:548–553
Ting AC, Cheng SW (1997) Femoral pseudoaneurysms in drug addicts. World J Surg 21:783–786; discussion 786–787
Tsao JW, Marder SR, Goldstone J, Bloom AI (2002) Presentation, diagnosis, and management of arterial mycotic pseudoaneurysms in injection drug users. Ann Vasc Surg 16:652–662
Tsilimparis N, Hanack U, Pisimisis G et al (2011) Thrombus in the non-aneurysmal, non-atherosclerotic descending thoracic aorta – an unusual source of arterial embolism. Eur J Vasc Endovasc Surg 41:450–457
Tunick PA, Culliford AT, Lamparello PJ, Kronzon I (1991) Atheromatosis of the aortic arch as an occult source of multiple systemic emboli. Ann Intern Med 114:391–392
Uittenbogaart M, Sosef MN, van Bastelaar J (2014) Sentinel bleeding as a sign of gastroaortic fistula formation after oesophageal surgery. Case Rep Surg 2014:614312
Upchurch G (2014) Thoracic and Thoracoabdominal Aortic Aneurysms. In J. Cronenwett and K. Johnston (Eds.). Rutherford's vascular surgery. Philadelfia, Pennsylvania, USA: Elsevier. 8th ed., pp 2084–2101
Vasan RS, Larson MG, Levy D (1995) Determinants of echocardiographic aortic root size. The Framingham Heart Study. Circulation 91:734–740
Verbeeck N, Cavez N, Plawny L et al (2014) Primary aortic thrombosis : role of enhanced multislice CT demonstrated in three exceptional cases. JBR-BTR J Belge Radiol 97:76–80
Verma H, Meda N, Vora S et al (2014) Contemporary management of symptomatic primary aortic mural thrombus. J Vasc Surg 60:1524–1534. doi:10.1016/j.jvs.2014.08.057
Vernhet H, Serfaty JM, Serhal M et al (2004) Abdominal CT angiography before surgery as a predictor of postoperative death in acute aortic dissection. AJR Am J Roentgenol 182:875–879
Vogelzang RL, Sohaey R (1988) Infected aortic aneurysms: CT appearance. J Comput Assist Tomogr 12:109–112
von Falck C, Meyer B, Fegbeutel C et al (2013) Imaging features of primary Sarcomas of the great vessels in CT, MRI and PET/CT: a single-center experience. BMC Med Imaging 13:25. doi:10.1186/1471-2342-13-25
von Segesser L (1997) Aortobronchial and aortoesophageal fistulae as risk factors in surgery of descending thoracic aortic aneurysms. Eur J Cardiothorac Surg 12:195–201
Vu QDM, Menias CO, Bhalla S et al (2009) Aortoenteric fistulas: CT features and potential mimics. Radiographics 29:197–209
Wei Y, Chen L, Wang Y et al (2015) Proposed management protocol for ingested esophageal foreign body and aortoesophageal fistula: a single-center experience. Int J Clin Exp Med 8:607–615
Weininger M, Barraza JM, Kemper CA et al (2011) Cardiothoracic CT angiography: current contrast medium delivery strategies. Am J Roentgenol 196:W260–W272. doi:10.2214/AJR.10.5814

Wolak A, Gransar H, Thomson LEJ et al (2008) Aortic size assessment by noncontrast cardiac computed tomography: normal limits by age, gender, and body surface area. JACC Cardiovasc Imaging 1:200–209

Yasuda F, Shimono T, Tonouchi H et al (2002) Successful repair of an aortoesophageal fistula with aneurysm from esophageal diverticulum. Ann Thorac Surg 73:637–639

Yeo DL, Haider S, Alexandra C, Zhen C (2015) Blunt traumatic aortic injury of right aortic arch in a patient with an aberrant left subclavian artery. Yale J Biol Med 88:93–97

Pulmonary Embolism

Raffaella Basilico, Manuela Mereu,
Rosa Lucia Patea, Francesco D'Alessandro,
Paola Franchi, Anna Rita Larici,
and Antonio R. Cotroneo

Contents

Abstract

Pulmonary embolism is a common clinical problem that is associated with considerable morbidity and mortality. Although early diagnosis of pulmonary embolism is one of the critical factors affecting outcomes, clinical presentation is often nonspecific and can mimic that of several other conditions. Therefore, clinicians often have to rely on a combination of physical examination and laboratory resultsd and imaging tests to determine the correct diagnosis. Currently, imaging offers a variety of fast and accurate tests that can provide anatomic and functional information, thus allowing early diagnosis. Nowadays, CT angiography represents the cornerstone of diagnostic evaluation of pulmonary embolism and new technological improvements, such as Dual Source CT, have increased the accuracy of CT in this clinical setting. Nevertheless, concerns about radiation exposure and side effects of contrast medium administration with CT angiography indicate that a role for ventilation/perfusion scintigraphy in the evaluation of patients with suspected pulmonary

R. Basilico (✉) • M. Mereu • R.L. Patea
F. D'Alessandro • A.R. Cotroneo
Department of Imaging, University of Chieti, Via dei Vestini, Chieti 66 100, Italy
e-mail: raffaellabasilico@gmail.com

P. Franchi • A.R. Larici
Department of Radiological Sciences, Fondazione Policlinico A. Gemelli, Catholic University, Largo A. Gemelli 8, 00168 Roma, Italy

Med Radiol Diagn Imaging (2016)
DOI 10.1007/174_2016_65, © Springer International Publishing Switzerland

embolism is still to consider. In this chapter we will review the CT pulmonary angiography protocols, the CT findings of acute pulmonary embolism, we will describe some pitfalls that can led to pulmonary embolism misdiagnosis. Furthermore, we will compare the diagnostic performance of ventilation-perfusion scintigraphy vs CT angiography and present some cases of non-thrombotic causes of pulmonary embolism.

1 Introduction

Managing pulmonary embolism (PE) is a common clinical practice issue, and it represents a significant component of any acute medical workload.

An incidence of 0.6–1.2 per 1000 persons per year has been reported (Mos et al. 2012).

Mortality rate reaches 30 % for untreated PE (Dalen and Alpert 1975), even though with treatment, the mortality rate decreases to 2.5–10 % (Carson et al. 1992; Barritt and Jordan 1960).

The clinical presentation of PE is varied and may include pleuritic chest pain, haemoptysis, dyspnoea and tachypnoea, nonspecific symptoms that are present in many chest diseases.

Because clinical presentations tend to be nonspecific, the diagnosis of PE still represents a challenge, and the diagnostic testing has a crucial role in this context, specifically imaging. The aim of imaging is to accurately confirm or rule out the diagnosis of PE, and upon imaging results, if indicated, an anticoagulant treatment can be safely initiated (Phillips et al. 2015).

2 Acute Pulmonary Embolism

Pulmonary embolism (PE) and deep vein thrombosis (DVT) are the target and the aetiology of venous thromboembolism (VTE) which represents the third most frequent cardiovascular disease after ischaemic heart disease and cerebrovascular disease, with an overall annual incidence of 100–200 per 100,000 inhabitants (Kuriakose and Patel 2010). VTE results from the interaction between patient-related (usually permanent) risk factors and setting-related (usually temporary) risk factors (Heit 2008). The latter are represented by surgery, trauma immobilization, pregnancy, oral contraceptive use, hormone replacement therapy and cancer, which is a well-recognized predisposing factor of VTE (Konstantinides et al. 2014).

Acute PE is the most serious clinical presentation of VTE. The wide spectrum of clinical presentations, ranging from lack of symptoms to sudden death, and the complications such as embolization and recurrent pulmonary arterial hypertension with heart failure justify the high rates of mortality, morbidity and hospitalization (Cohen et al. 2007).

A prompt diagnosis of PE can be difficult since the clinical signs and symptoms are not specific. Blood pressure decrease and shock are rare but important clinical presentations, as they are indicative of massive pulmonary embolism and/or severely reduced pulmonary haemodynamic reserve. In this scenario, the 2014 ESC Guidelines on the diagnosis and management of acute pulmonary embolism stratify patients with PE as high-risk patient in the presence of shock or persistent arterial hypotension and not high-risk patient in the absence of these conditions. This classification has relevant implications for both diagnosis and therapeutic strategies (Konstantinides et al. 2014).

High-risk patients should undergo CT angiography examination if it is immediately available. When CT angiography is not available, bedside transthoracic echocardiography is the most useful initial test for the evaluation of acute pulmonary hypertension and right ventricular (RV) dysfunction. In patients with suspected PE without shock or hypotension, clinical assessment probability through Geneva and Wells score is the logical first step and allows PE to be ruled out in around 30 % of patients. The sum of the scores assigned with these scores underlines the likelihood of pulmonary embolism, which can be low, intermediate or high. Even for patients who have a high probability of PE, as for those in shock, a CT angiography should be promptly

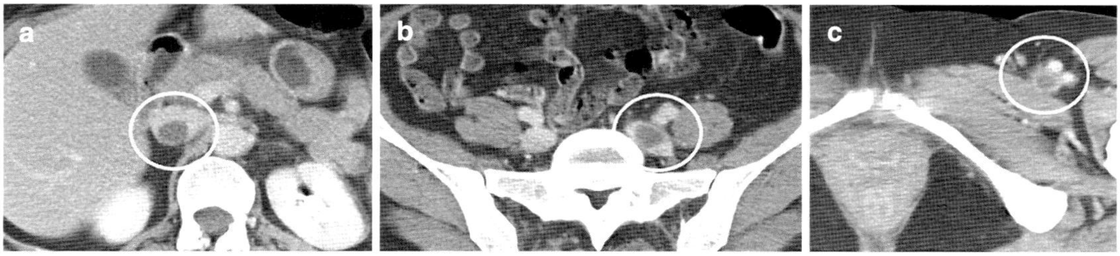

Fig. 1 CT venography scans show the presence of intraluminal filling defects in the inferior vena cava (*circle* in **a**), the left common iliac vein (*circle* in **b**) and the left femoral vein (*circle* in **c**)

performed. For patients with a low or intermediate risk, the d-dimer plasma dosage is the first diagnostic test recommended by the guidelines: its positivity identifies only patients who must undergo CT angiography, while for those in which the d-dimer is negative, no further workup is required (Konstantinides et al. 2014).

Nowadays CT angiography has become the modality of choice for imaging patients with suspected PE (Ghaye and Dondelinger 2007; Perrier et al. 2001). It allows adequate visualization of the pulmonary arteries down to at least the segmental level (Ghaye et al. 2001), and it is possible to obtain perfusion images.

2.1 CT Pulmonary Angiography Technique (CTPA)

The rapid advances of MDCT technology determined a continued evolution of techniques and protocols which vary between the different generation scanners and different vendors (Patel and Kazerooni 2005). The key concepts for CT pulmonary angiography are acquisition of the entire lung in a single short breath hold in full-suspended respiration with thinner collimation (1.25 mm or less) using power injectors for rapid contrast delivery to obtain an adequate enhancement of the pulmonary arteries. An 18–20 gauge intravenous cannula is placed in the antecubital vein, with arms in upright position. The degree and quality of pulmonary arterial enhancement depend on the amount of concentration of contrast, injection rate and the scan delay. In our institution with a 128-slice scanner, we use about 70 mL of contrast medium at a flow rate of 3–4 mL/s for CTPA imaging of the chest alone and for a combined CTPA and CT venography (CTV) 110–120 mL of contrast. The timing of contrast bolus is of crucial importance. A fixed scan delay (20–25 s) is not recommended especially in patients with cardiac dysfunction. The best approach is to use the timing bolus or bolus tracking. We routinely use the bolus tracking method in which a cursor, placed in the main pulmonary artery, triggers scanning at a preset threshold (100–120 UH). Because most PE originates from thrombi in the lower extremity veins, Loud and colleagues (Loud et al. 2001) first demonstrated the potential role of CT venography in combination with CTPA. CT venography is performed after a 2.5–4 min delay following start of injection bolus for CTPA. Scans acquired with an incremental or helical technique are obtained from the tibial plateaus to the iliac crests. Deep vein thrombosis is seen as a low-attenuation filling defect partially or totally occluding the vein (Fig. 1a–c). The use and the role of CT venography remain contradictory, making evidence-based consensus difficult. Combined CTPA with CTV provides "one-stop shopping", which has proved popular with referring physicians, patients and radiologists. It is also superior to ultrasound (US) for evaluating the inferior vena cava and iliac veins especially in obese patients and those with anomalous and complicated venous anatomy. On the other side, the main disadvantage is the additional radiation dose.

Clearly, compression ultrasound (CUS) is well accepted, has low cost and does not expose the patient to radiation. Numerous comparative studies have shown that there is approximately 97 % agreement between CT venography and CUS (Cham et al. 2005; Katz et al. 2002). CT venography and CUS have also been shown to be equivalent in patients in the intensive care unit (Taffoni et al. 2005). The PIOPED II study of 711 CT venograms showed 95 % concordance between CUS and helical CT venography (Stein et al. 2006).

In general, Fleischner Society (Remy-Jardin et al. 2007) recommend the use of CT venography when emphasis must be placed on a complete vascular examination that can be accomplished expeditiously; when there are concerns about radiation exposure, they recommend substituting lower extremity US. When evaluation of the lower extremity veins is not clinically important, CT venography can be omitted (Remy-Jardin et al. 2007; Pena and Dennie 2012).

2.2 CT Findings of Acute Pulmonary Embolism

CT angiography allows the direct visualization of emboli as arterial filling defect that partially or totally occludes the enhanced artery (Ghaye et al. 2002). A partial arterial defect surrounded by contrast material produces the so-called "polo mint" sign on images acquired perpendicular to the long axis of the vessel (Fig. 2) and the "railway track" images sign on longitudinal images of the vessel (Fig. 3). A partial filling defect can place peripherally forming acute angles with the arterial wall (Fig. 4). When the embolus totally occludes the artery, the involved vessel may be enlarged (Fig. 5) compared with the corresponding patent vessel of the opposite site (Han et al. 2003). A vessel "cut-off" sign is seen when the distal artery is not opacified owing to the presence of occlusive disease. Central filling defects can sometimes already be highlighted on CT scans without contrast medium as hyperdense images at the level of the main pulmonary arteries (Fig. 6a, b). The visualization of the thrombus on chest CT without contrast medium is related to the "age" of the clot and the haematocrit of the patient at the time of the survey. The gradual retraction of the thrombus is associated to the reduction of its water content resulting in an increase of density values up to 50–80 UH (Kanne et al. 2003).

In the presence of PE, parenchymal CT findings can be seen as areas of ground glass opacity or consolidation representing pulmonary haemorrhage that usually resolve within a week.

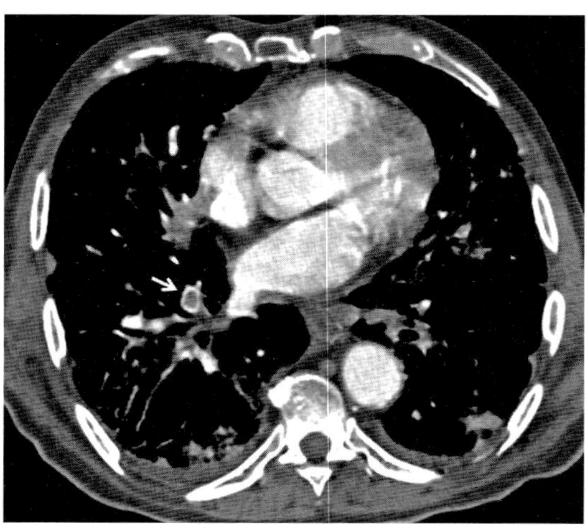

Fig. 2 CT scan demonstrates a pulmonary embolus that affects the segmental artery of the anterior basal segment of the right lower lobe; the embolus (*arrow*) is surrounded by contrast material reproducing the so-called "polo mint" sign

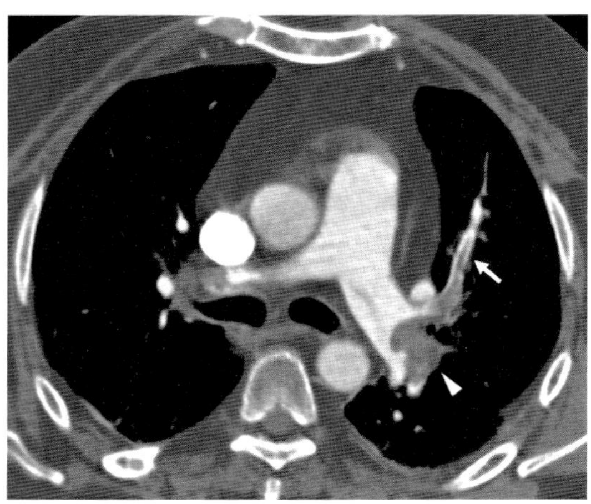

Fig. 3 Enhanced CT scan shows an acute pulmonary embolus that causes a partial filling defect surrounded by contrast material "railway track" sign (*arrow*). One more acute pulmonary embolus affects the left main pulmonary artery (*arrowhead*)

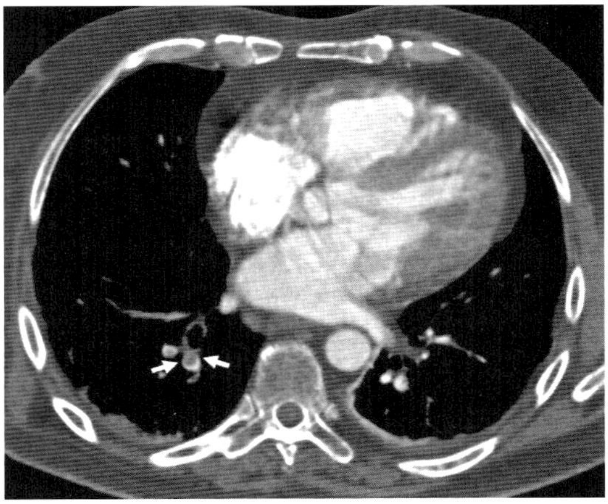

Fig. 4 CT angiography shows a pulmonary embolus that affects the segmental artery of the posterior basal segment of the right lower lobe; the embolus is peripherally located forming acute angle with the vessel wall (*arrows*)

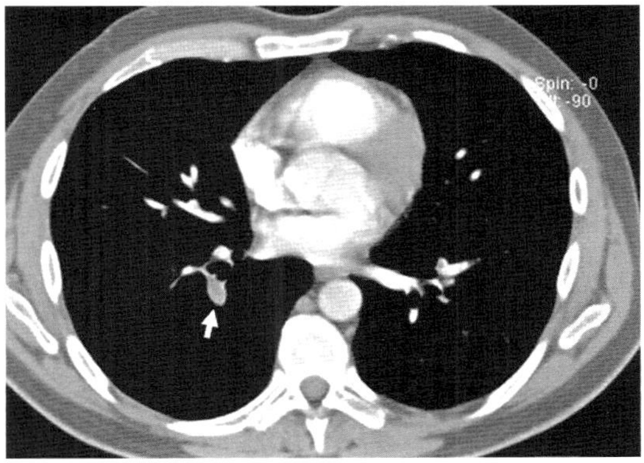

Fig. 5 CT scan shows a complete occlusion of a segmental artery of the right lower lobe with a prominent enlargement of the vessel (*arrow*)

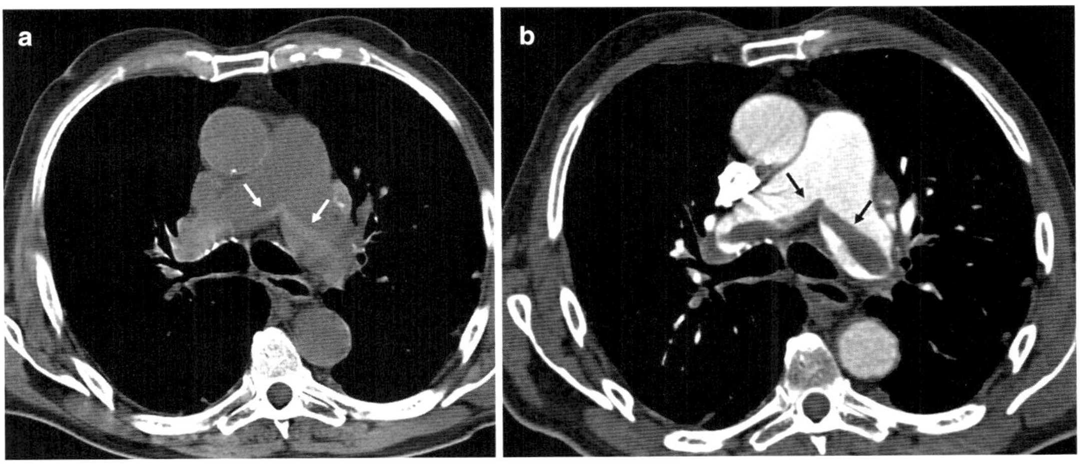

Fig. 6 CT scans at the level of the pulmonary trunk. Unenhanced multidetector CT scan (**a**) shows bilateral central high-attenuation emboli (*arrows*); enhanced CT scan (**b**) confirms the presence of the central emboli (*black arrows*)

Pulmonary infarction is more frequently seen in lower lobes as a wedge-shaped area of consolidation with the apex towards the hilum and with central hypodense areas representing secondary pulmonary lobules spared from the disease process (Fig. 7a). It is often possible to highlight the presence of an intraluminal filling defect in the arterial branching afferent to the pulmonary infarction (Fig. 7b).

Pulmonary infarction is seen in about 10% of patient with PE, and it gradually reduces in size in 3–5 weeks retaining its triangular morphology. The excavation of pulmonary infarction is rare; it can also be found in the absence of infectious processes especially if the pulmonary infarction has a transverse diameter >4 cm and generally occurs after 2 weeks of onset of the infarct (Fig. 7d). Linear parenchymal bands, atelectasis, focal oligaemia and small pleural effusion are less frequent features.

CT can also highlight findings suggestive of right ventricular failure as dilation of the right

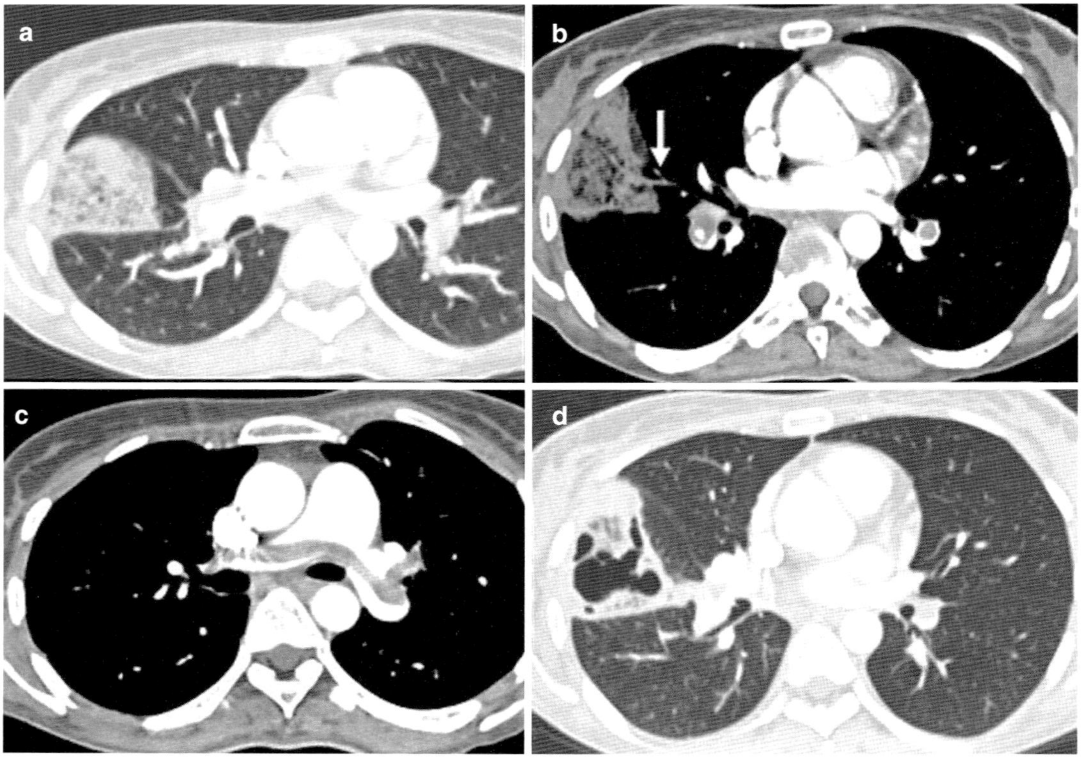

Fig. 7 Chest CT scan (**a**) shows a wedge-shaped, subpleural consolidation in the middle lobe with central hypodense areas due to lung infarction; there is a vessel totally occluded (*arrow* in **b**) and coursed towards the apex of the consolidation. A central bilateral emboli are also demonstrated (**c**). One-month chest CT follow-up showing excavation of the lung infarction (**d**)

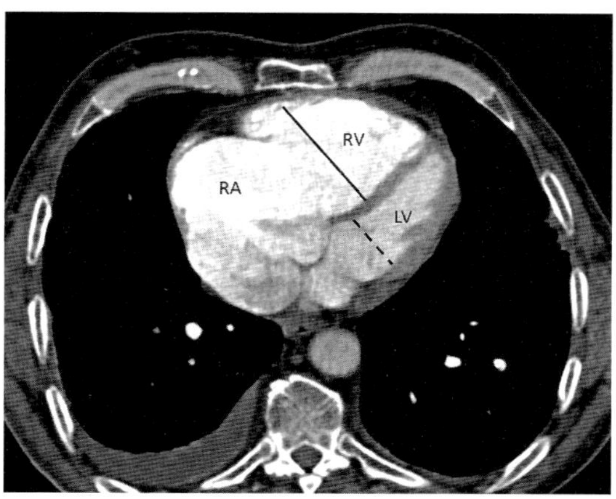

Fig. 8 Right ventricular strain: CT scans show dilation of the right atrium (*RA*) and the right ventricle (*RV*). The short-axis diameter of the RV (*continuous line*) is greater than that of the left ventricle (*LV*, *dotted line*). The interventricular septum is bowed towards the LV

ventricle, with right ventricular cavity transverse diameter greater than the left, with or without the presence of reflux of contrast medium in the hepatic veins and deviation of the interventricular septum towards the left ventricle (Fig. 8).

2.3 Acute Pulmonary Embolism Misdiagnosis

Several conditions can be responsible of acute PE misdiagnosis (Wittram et al. 2004). Respiratory motion artefacts are the most common cause of indeterminate CT pulmonary angiography. These artefacts are best seen with lung window settings and can create the "seagull" sign. Images obtained in large patients have more quantum noise making the evaluation of segmental and

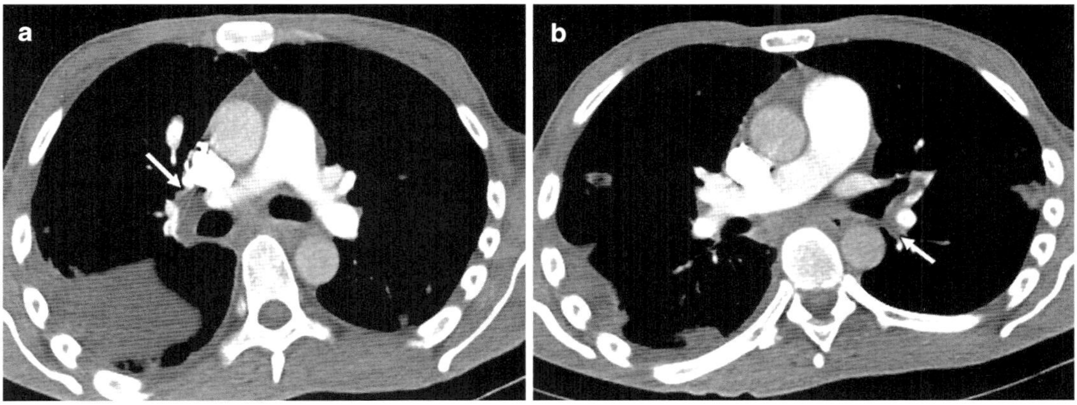

Fig. 9 (**a**, **b**) Chest CT scans show hilar and bronchial lymph nodes (*arrows*) that can mimic pulmonary emboli

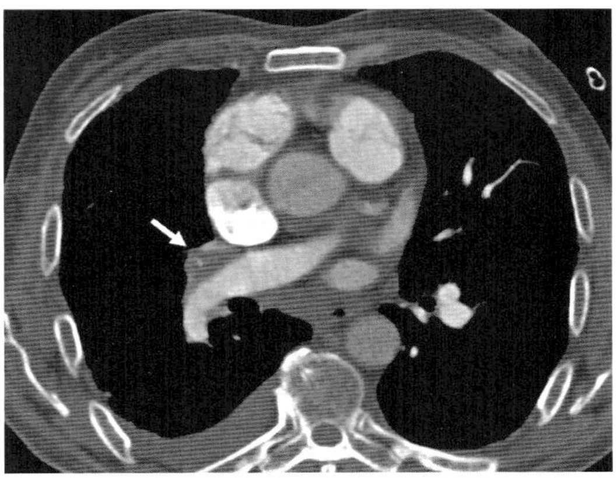

Fig. 10 Chest scan demonstrates a peripheral filling defect in the interlobar artery (*arrow*) with obtuse angle with vessel wall

subsegmental vessel very difficult. A soft tissue reconstruction algorithm should be used to avoid high attenuation around vessels. We recommend using pulmonary embolism-specific settings with a window width and level of 800 and 100 HU, respectively. Streak artefacts from dense contrast material within the superior vena cava or from a central venous catheter can obscure emboli or can mimic PE. These artefacts can be distinguished from pulmonary emboli for their radiating nature and the nonanatomic morphology (Pena and Dennie 2012). These artefacts can be reduced by flushing the superior vena cava with saline solution using dual chamber injectors. A poor contrast opacification of pulmonary arteries can be also a cause of misdiagnosis of PE. Hilar lymph nodes can be confused with emboli even if, nowadays, thanks to the use of thinner collimations, lymph nodes are easily differentiated from emboli (Fig. 9a, b). Low-density mucus-filled bronchi and pulmonary veins can also mimic pulmonary filling defect. The review of sagittal and coronal reformatted images can be helpful in difficult cases.

3 Chronic Pulmonary Embolism

Most cases of pulmonary emboli resolve without sequelae. In a small percentage of patients with PE, especially when large emboli are present, these can undergo organization, retraction and recanalization, with the possibility of determining frameworks of pulmonary hypertension and cor pulmonale (Hoeper et al. 2006). The most frequent CT findings are complete occlusion of a vessel that is smaller than adjacent patent vessel, a peripheral filling defect with obtuse angles with the vessel wall (Fig. 10), web or flap within a contrast material-filled artery, presence of calcifications in the context of the parietal thrombus or calcification of the pulmonary arteries (Fig. 11a, b) and contrast material flowing through thickened often smaller arteries due to recanalization (Fig. 12b). The main pulmonary artery is typically enlarged (diameter, >29 mm) for the onset

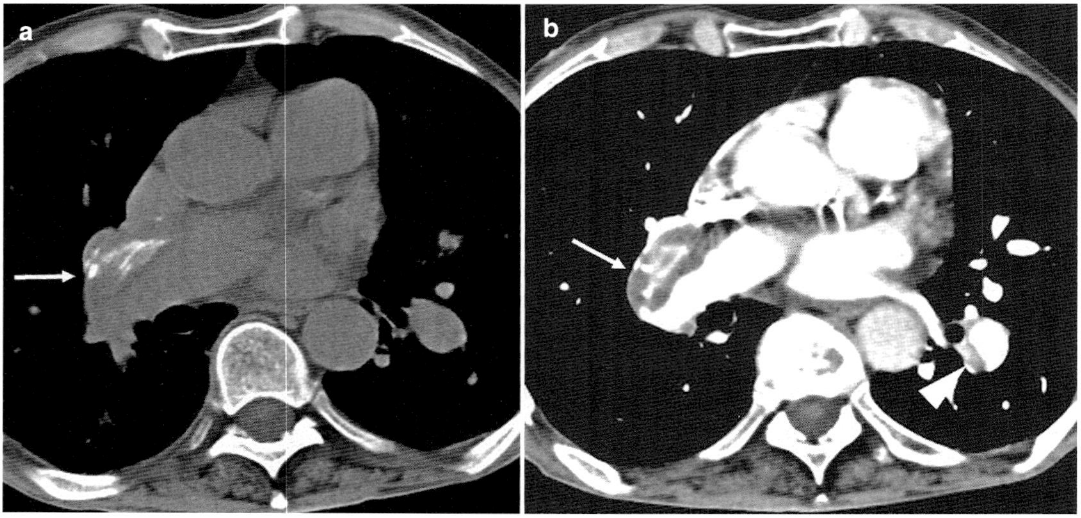

Fig. 11 CT scans at the level of the right pulmonary artery in a patient with chronic pulmonary embolism show a peripherally located thrombus in the right pulmonary artery (*arrows* in **a** and **b**) with calcification within (**a, b**). There is also a peripheral thrombus in the left lower lobe artery (*arrowhead* in **b**)

of pulmonary arterial hypertension, and bronchial artery dilation is also present (Fig. 12a). Pulmonary parenchymal CT findings in chronic PE consist of "mosaic pattern": lung areas with a different density in a patchy distribution resulting from irregular perfusion of lung parenchyma (Fig. 13) (Pena and Dennie 2012).

Chronic pulmonary embolism in the appropriate clinical setting should be differentiated from pulmonary artery sarcoma (PAS). It is a rare tumour with poor prognosis, and it should be considered as a possible diagnosis in the absence of thromboembolic risk factors and when there is no evidence of cancer elsewhere. Patients are generally in their 50s and do not show any response to anticoagulation.

Pulmonary artery sarcoma is an uncommon cause of intraluminal filling defect causing often a unilateral hilar enlargement (Cox et al. 1997; Hu et al. 2009). CT angiography of the chest shows tissue which tends to occupy the full diameter of the vessel with vascular involvement of the common trunk (85 % of cases) and the main branches (left pulmonary artery, 65 %; right pulmonary artery, 71 %); inhomogeneous enhancement of the intraluminal pulmonary tissue due to haemorrhage, necrosis and calcification (Fig. 14); increase in vessel calibre; and extra-luminal extension of the tissue. Pulmonary nodules can also be an expression of metastases (Long et al. 2010).

4 Ventilation-Perfusion Scintigraphy Versus Computed Tomography

Over the last decade, different imaging modalities have been established as useful tools in the diagnosis of PE, with various ranges of diagnostic performance being reported. Choice of the imaging modality varies by site, with usage of a particular modality influenced by a combination of site history, availability of equipment, physician personal preference and patient suitability (Phillips et al. 2015).

For 30 years ventilation/perfusion (V/Q) lung scanning has been the preferred non-invasive imaging procedure in patients with suspected PE. However, a complex probability scoring system and a relative high number of non-diagnostic scans have dampened enthusiasm about this procedure.

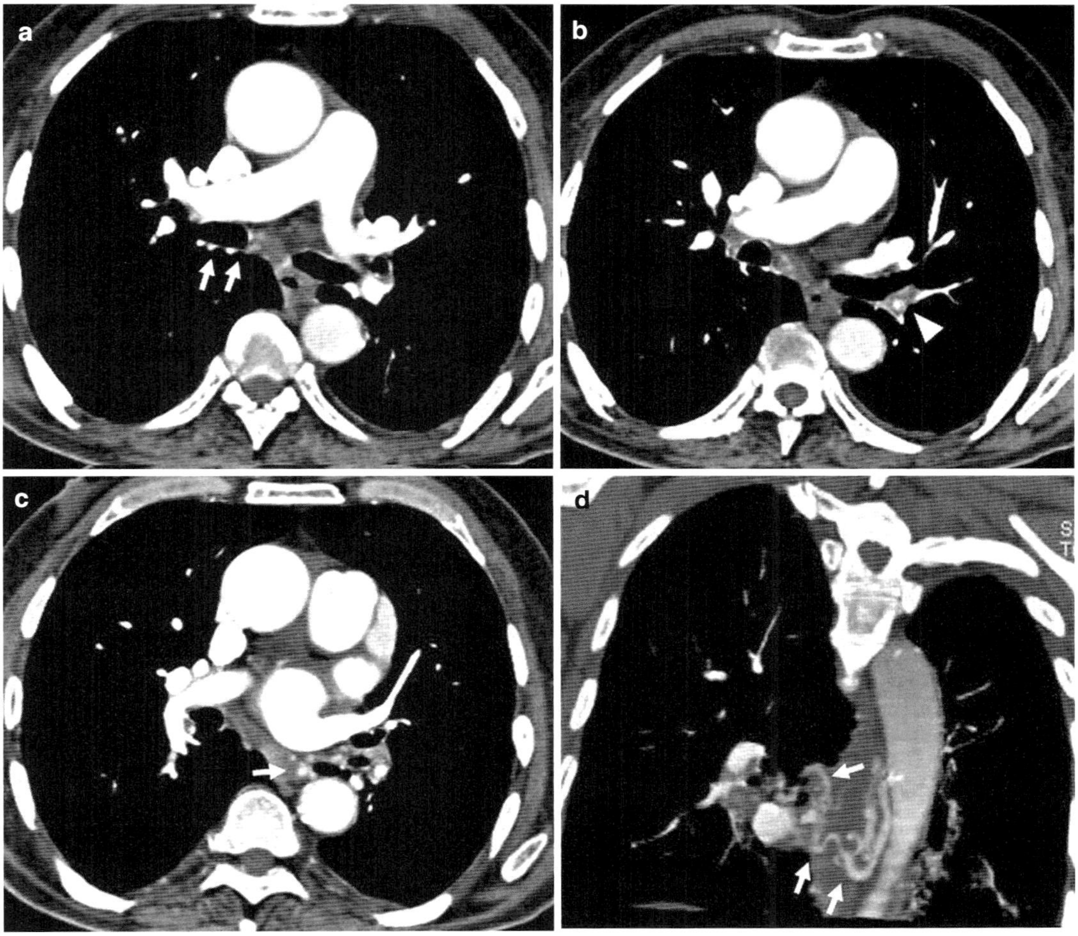

Fig. 12 CT scans in patient with chronic pulmonary embolism showing a small recanalized left pulmonary artery with contrast material in the central lumen (*arrowhead* in **b**). Dilated bronchial and collateral vessels are also evident (*arrows* in **a**, **c**, **d**)

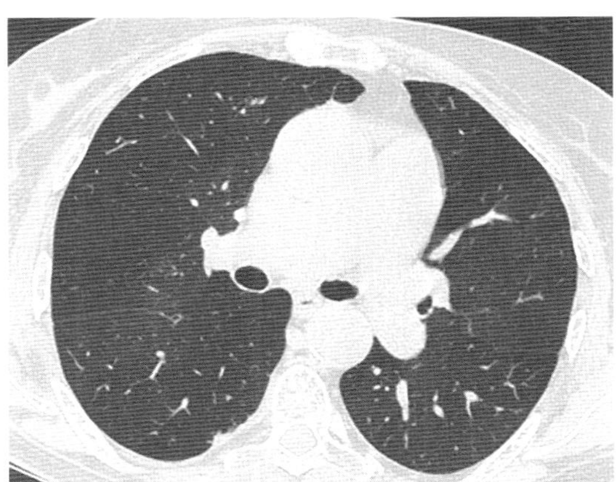

Fig. 13 CT scan at the level of the pulmonary trunk in a patient with chronic pulmonary embolism showing a mosaic perfusion pattern. The dark regions are underperfused, and vessels are smaller than the adjacent patent vessel in the normally perfused lung

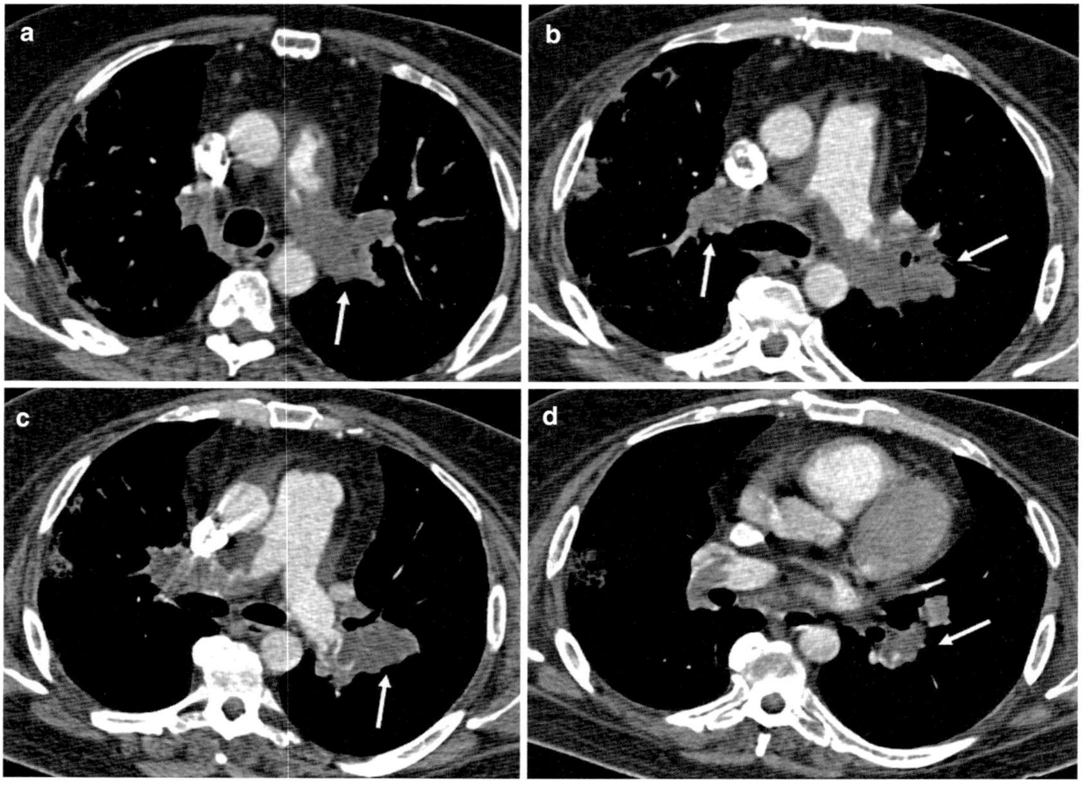

Fig. 14 Contrast-enhanced CT scans show a heterogeneous enhancing lobulated tissue (*arrows*) in the main pulmonary artery and in the left and right branches with involvement of lobar and segmental arteries bilaterally. The enlargement of the involved vessels is also evident

In the past decade, CTPA has proven to be a more accurate test with relatively few inadequate studies and has been welcomed by clinicians (Stein et al. 2006). Nevertheless, concerns about radiation exposure and side effects of contrast medium administration with CTPA indicate that a role for V/Q scintigraphy in the evaluation of patients with suspected PE is still to consider (Freeman 2008).

4.1 Scintigraphy: Technical Considerations, Diagnostic Accuracy and Novel Imaging

Diagnostic ventilation/perfusion (V/Q) scintigraphy involves simultaneous imaging of the distribution of pulmonary blood flow and alveolar ventilation.

The main clinical indication for this technique is the evaluation of PE. The principle underlying the "scintigraphic diagnosis" of PE is that, whereas pulmonary perfusion is abnormal, the pulmonary parenchyma usually remains intact and ventilation remains normal. This gives rise to the so-called mismatched perfusion defect, the hallmark of pulmonary embolic disease.

As regards technical aspects, perfusion and ventilation scanning are two different processes of the same resulting examination.

Perfusion scanning (*Q*) is performed by the intravenous injection of a radiotracer, which is trapped in the lung on first pass. The tracer used in the clinical practice, nowadays, is macroaggregated human serum albumin (MAA) labelled with technetium-99m (Tc-99m). These particles have a size range of 10–100 μm and cause microembolization of pulmonary capillaries and precapillary arterioles, reflecting regional perfusion. Routinely, about 400,000 particles are injected. As there are over 280 billion pulmonary capillaries and 300 million precapillary arterioles, only a small fraction of the pulmonary bed will be obstructed; thus, even in patients with pulmonary vascular disease (pulmonary hypertension), it can be used safely. Provided the particles mix completely in the blood prior to microembolization, the distribution of radioactivity is proportional to the distribution of pulmonary blood flow (Heck and Duley 1974). A Tc-99m lung perfusion scan provides an effective radiation dose equivalent of 1 mSv/100 MBq.

Ventilation scanning (*V*) is currently performed using radiolabelled aerosols, unlike in the past when radioactive inert gases were the most widely used agents for ventilation imaging. Aerosol ventilation imaging has become popular largely because of technical improvements in the delivery systems and the small size of particles. Aerosols are generally made of Tc-99m diethylenetriaminepentaacetic acid (DTPA). The aerosol administration requires cooperation of the patient, who is asked to breathe through a mouthpiece, with a nose clip in place, for several minutes. Tc-99m DTPA diffuses through the alveolo-capillary membrane to the blood (Mason et al. 2001). Another type of aerosol available is "Technegas", made of extremely small carbon particles (0.005–0.2 μm), generated in a high-temperature furnace (Senden et al. 1997). The small particle size implies that they are distributed in the lungs almost like a gas and are deposited in alveoli by diffusion.

V/Q lung scanning in the presence of PE has the typical diagnostic feature of a perfusion defect in a region of normally ventilated lung, the mismatched perfusion defect. The size of defect may range from appreciably smaller than a segment (subsegmental) to about the size of a segment (segmental) or, very rarely, of a lobe or whole lung. A non-segmental defect is one that does not correspond to segmental anatomy. A minimum of four views (anterior, posterior and both posterior obliques) is recommended for the accurate evaluation of V/Q lung scanning, and occasionally, lateral and anterior obliques may be useful.

The pathologic basis of the mismatched perfusion defect is that in an uncomplicated pulmonary embolism, in otherwise healthy individuals, the pulmonary architecture remains intact, and ventilation is therefore normal. However, when embolism is followed by lung infarction, a ventilation defect appears, although it is usually smaller than the perfusion defect because the lung around the periphery of the perfusion defect continues to ventilate. The diagnostic feature of a pulmonary infarct, therefore, is an incompletely matched perfusion defect. In many patients, however, V/Q scan is non-diagnostic, and further investigation is required (Macdonald et al. 2005). V/Q scan provides a higher effective radiation dose with respect to the Q scan alone. Phillips JJ et al. in a recent review of medical literature reported that the effective dose for correct diagnosis with V/Q scan was 3.46 mSv (Phillips et al. 2015).

The V/Q scan has been widely used as the first-line radiologic examination in the diagnosis of suspected PE. In the mid-1980s, the multicentre Prospective Investigation of Pulmonary Embolism Diagnosis (PIOPED) study evaluated the diagnostic utility of the V/Q scan for 731 patients with conclusive pulmonary angiogram results for PE (PIOPED Investigators 1990). The study demonstrated that all patients with pulmonary embolism had abnormal V/Q scans of high, intermediate or low probability, but so did most without pulmonary embolism (sensitivity, 98 %; specificity, 10 %) and indicated the diagnostic utility of the V/Q scan to be limited to the small proportion of patients with high-probability results or to those with normal/near-normal or low-probability scans in conjunction with low clinical likelihood of the disease. The PIOPED study showed that the combination of pretest clinical assessment and V/Q scintigraphy could diagnose or exclude PE accurately, but such readings were possible in only 28 % of patients. Unfortunately, this leaves a large group of patients with non-diagnostic results that were insufficiently conclusive to guide definitive clinical management.

The risk of missed PE may result in death. Alternatively, treating patients unnecessarily for PE exposes them to the risk of life-threatening complications from anticoagulation, which has been reported being of 5 % at 1 year (Petty et al. 1988).

For all these reasons, the PIOPED criteria were reviewed in order to increase accuracy of V/Q scan (Sostman et al. 1994). More recently, in the retrospective analysis of the PIOPED II trial data retrieved from patients who had undergone both V/Q scintigraphy and CTPA, the V/Q scan diagnostic criteria for PE have been recategorized into "PE present", "PE absent" and "non-diagnostic test". Results showed a definitive V/Q scan reading in 73.5 % of patients and a non-diagnostic scan rate reduced to 26.5 %, with a sensitivity and specificity of 77 % and 98 %, respectively (Sostman et al. 2008a). Authors concluded that V/Q scan scintigraphy can be considered an appropriate imaging procedure in patients with suspected PE for whom CTPA may be disadvantageous, as in those with iodinated contrast medium allergy or impaired renal function, particularly if outpatients.

The investigators of Prospective Investigative Study of Acute Pulmonary Embolism Diagnosis (PISAPED) suggested a new set of diagnostic criteria, intended to diagnose or exclude PE using incorporation of clinical prediction rules, the Q scan alone and chest radiograph. They used the archived PIOPED II data and images to test their hypothesis and found a sensitivity of 80 %, a specificity of 97 %, with 0 % of non-diagnostic results (Sostman et al. 2008b). These results indicate that Q scintigraphy combined with chest radiography can provide diagnostic accuracy similar to that of V/Q with the additional benefits of lower cost and lower radiation dose.

Single-photon emission computed tomography (SPECT) is a technique that provides three-dimensional volumetric images and has the potential to improve the diagnostic accuracy of the nuclear medicine imaging for PE. SPECT improves the performance of V/Q imaging thanks to better spatial resolution, in particular regarding detection of peripherally located perfusion defects, and limited overlapping of the perfusion defects by other structures.

Recent V/Q SPECT studies conducted in over 3000 cases showed a sensitivity of 96–99 % and a specificity of 91–98 % for PE (Bajc et al. 2009a). The rate of non-diagnostic findings has been reported between 1 and 3 %.

V/Q SPECT is non-invasive, is well-tolerated and can be performed in all patients. With efficient technique and effective organization, V/Q SPECT takes only 20 min of acquisition time, and the radiation exposure is low (effective dose of 2.12 mSv) with respect to the planar V/Q scan (Phillips et al. 2015). Furthermore, it allows quantification of PE, and that option has a relevant impact on choice of treatment in some centres and frequently provides alternative diagnosis of comorbid conditions as COPD, left heart failure and pneumonia (Bajc and Jonson 2011).

However, V/Q SPECT is uniquely useful for follow-up and research and not employed in the emergency setting, where CTPA is the host, even if, according to some authors (Bajc and Jonson 2011), its outstanding qualities merit consideration of its use as the primary diagnostic method for PE in all hospitals in which nuclear medicine is practiced.

4.2 Computed Tomography Pulmonary Angiography (CTPA): Diagnostic Accuracy and Novel Imaging

CTPA has emerged as an alternative modality for imaging of PE. Since the introduction of multidetector CT, CTPA has become the method of choice for imaging the pulmonary vasculature when PE is suspected in routine clinical practice.

The diagnostic accuracy of multidetector CT is directly linked to the dramatic improvement in image quality made possible by advances in CT technology over the past decade. The improvements in spatial and temporal resolution, as well as the overall increased quality of pulmonary arterial opacification, have allowed the routine analysis of pulmonary arteries down to the subsegmental level (Patel et al. 2003). These technical advances have improved image quality both in outpatients (Revel et al. 2005) and in dyspnoeic inpatients of the intensive care units or with underlying respiratory disease (Kelly et al. 2006; Tillie-Leblond et al. 2006).

Sensitivity and specificity of multidetector CTPA vary between 83 % and 100 % and 89 % and 97 %, respectively (Qanadli et al. 2000; Winer-Muram et al. 2004; Stein et al. 2006). Moreover, the negative predictive value of a CTPA (99.4 %) in ruling out pulmonary embolism was demonstrated to be comparable to that of pulmonary angiography (Quiroz et al. 2005), and in 2007, multidetector CT angiography has fulfilled the conditions to replace pulmonary angiography as the reference standard for diagnosis of acute PE (Remy-Jardin et al. 2007). Additional attractive features of CTPA include that it provides direct visualization of the thrombus within the pulmonary arteries and a simple positive or negative result in most of the cases (Wittram 2007; Hoang et al. 2008). The test may be able to determine an alternative explanation for symptoms if pulmonary embolism is excluded, and it may also offer clues to the aetiology of PE, such as the presence of previously undetected malignancy (Bierry et al. 2008).

Furthermore, it has proven technically feasible to assess the proximal venous system of the legs with CT venography performed during the same procedure as CTPA (Stein et al. 2006) and to provide prognostic information by demonstrating signs of right ventricular dysfunction (Ocak and Fuhrman 2008), which has been shown to be independently predictive of 30-day mortality.

For all these reasons, CTPA has been enthusiastically embraced by the medical community as an excellent minimally invasive examination for the evaluation of PE, widely used in all categories of adult patients (inpatients, outpatients, emergency room patients). On the other hand, as a result of this wide application, serious concerns regarding high-radiation exposure associated with CT have arose. However, it is worth noting that the risk of death from undiagnosed PE far exceeds the risk of radiation-induced malignancy (Remy-Jardin et al. 2007) and there is strong scientific evidence that in pregnant women, the foetal dose from V/Q scintigraphy (640–800 μGy) is considerably higher than that from CTPA (3–131 μGy) (Winer-Muram et al. 2002; Russell et al. 1997).

Since spiral CT offers a diagnosis of PE within a matter of seconds along with a lot of additional information on the lung parenchyma, heart and great vessels, pulmonary scintigraphy has widely been replaced with CT for this indication. However, the information gained with both modalities is not quite the same. CT displays clots in vessels irrespective of their effect on perfusion, and scintigraphy displays perfusion defects irrespective of their cause. Thus, CT is able to answer the question for PE more precisely, while scintigraphy may provide a more accurate estimation of the perfusion, which should be pathophysiologically more relevant.

Dual-source CT (DSCT) can nowadays provide both anatomical and functional information of the whole lungs, by combining pulmonary CTPA with an assessment of pulmonary iodine map in a single spiral contrast-enhanced CT acquisition.

DSCT uses two orthogonally mounted X-ray tubes and detectors. As each tube can be set at a different tube potential (80 kVp for one tube and 140 kVp for the other), DSCT allows simultaneous dual-energy CT (DECT) image. Iodine attenuates X-ray spectra very differently at 80 and 140 kVp settings. The obtained DECT data can be readily post-processed to determine the amount of iodinated contrast material in any voxel. A mathematic algorithm is used to create an iodine map by means of known attenuation range values for iodine at 80 and at 140 kVp to calculate its relative contribution to each voxel. In particular, the calculation of iodine distribution in the lung parenchyma, which is related to the microvascular circulation in the lung, can generate colour-coded pulmonary blood volume (PBV) maps that can be considered a surrogate indicator of pulmonary perfusion (Ameli-Renani et al. 2014). On the other hand, diagnostic evaluation of morphology and anatomy is achieved combining image data from both energy levels to create a hybrid image that is equivalent to a standard scan acquired at 120 kVp.

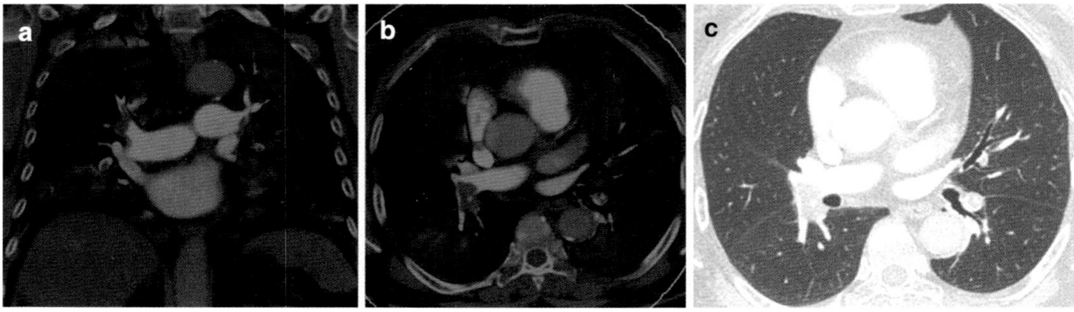

Fig. 15 (**a–c**) Bilateral pulmonary embolism in a 69-year-old woman. Fused DECT angiographic image/iodine perfusion maps (**a**, **b**) simultaneously showing bilateral arterial filling defects, larger on the right with proximal extension in the lobar arteries and interlobar artery, and concordant wedge-shaped perfusion defects in the right upper lobe (**a**, **b**). Axial CT image at lung window setting (**c**), selected at the same anatomic level as (**b**), does not show any abnormality in the corresponding lung parenchyma

In the context of PE diagnosis, DECT technology has the capacity to improve the diagnostic accuracy through a comprehensive analysis of lung "perfusion" and pulmonary vessel opacification obtained during a single chest contrast-enhanced CT scan performed with dual-energy mode.

PBV images can be used to search the defect resulting from emboli. Normal PBV images were defined as showing homogeneous contrast enhancement in the normal colour-code range with dependent symmetric lung iodine distribution. PBV defects, which can be considered "perfusion" defects consistent with PE, include those that are peripherally located, wedge shaped and in a segmental or lobar distribution (Fink et al. 2008) (Fig. 15a–c).

PBV imaging from DECT could assist in the detection of pulmonary emboli that are not evident by conventional CTPA. Thieme et al. (2008) found that corresponding perfusion defects were observed in DECT and scintigraphy in two patients in whom there was no evidence of intravascular clots in angiographic CT images. Lu et al. (2010) reported a case of a patient in whom the initial conventional CTPA did not visualize abnormal findings, while the magnified view of the targeted pulmonary arteries corresponding to an area of hypoperfusion in PBV images showed a subtle subsegmental filling defect. These findings indicate that DECT has the potential to improve the detection of small pulmonary emboli, which may be of clinical importance because even small emboli require treatment to prevent chronic PE and pulmonary artery hypertension in several clinical scenarios, specifically in patients with poor cardiopulmonary reserve.

Aside from visualizing PBV defects to diagnose PE, DECT can be used for monitoring PE treatment (Zhang et al. 2009). Following anticoagulant therapy or thrombolysis therapy, complete resolution of pulmonary arterial and corresponding perfusion defects indicate that pulmonary emboli have been dissolved. Thieme et al. (2008) suggested that contrast enhancement defects visualized in PBV images might be a better prognostic marker for therapy monitoring, as it is easier and more intuitively relevant to quantify the extent of perfusion defects than to quantify the clot burden. This study showed the potential of DECT as "one-stop shop" for the diagnostic workup of lung disease by offering a simultaneous assessment of vasculature, perfusion and high-resolution morphology in a single breath-hold exam, with radiation exposure not higher than that of single-source CTPA (Pontana et al. 2008). The ability to assess perfusion in CT may make an additional scintigraphy dispensable and help to avoid the corresponding radiation exposure.

To date, there have been limited studies assessing the correlation between pulmonary embolism-related perfusion defects seen at DECT and those seen at V/Q scintigraphy (Thieme et al. 2008)

and SPECT (Thieme et al. 2012). Thieme et al. (2008) reported limited diagnostic accuracy for PBV maps, with 75 % sensitivity and 80 % specificity for pulmonary embolism in a per-patient analysis, but these increased to 83 % and 99 %, respectively, in a per-segment analysis. DECT PBV perfusion defects related to SPECT imaging had a sensitivity of 77 % and a specificity of 98 % in a follow-up study by the same group (Thieme et al. 2012). A complete concordance between defects seen at DECT PBV imaging and scintigraphy is unlikely. Not only are these measures not precisely physiologically equivalent, but V/Q scintigraphy is performed during shallow respiration, whereas DECT PBV maps reflect full inspiration. Nevertheless, the degree of agreement between DECT PBV and scintigraphic images is encouraging, particularly on a clinically significant per-segment basis. Nowadays, DECT PBV is not usually used in the clinical context of emergency for assessing PE, even if future developments will surely induce a more wide employment of this CT technique.

4.3 Comparison of Modalities

In the diagnosis of PE, nuclear medicine methods used to serve as first-line imaging modalities for a long time. V/Q SPECT could show a higher diagnostic accuracy when compared to planar V/Q scintigraphy. However, in the last years, nuclear medicine imaging methods have lost clinical impact in the diagnosis of PE due to the technical improvements in the field of CTPA, which offers high spatial and temporal resolution as well as additional morphological information when compared to nuclear medicine techniques. Moreover, CTPA has undeniable advantages in the setting of emergency.

Guidance on which modality to use varies. Currently in the UK, the National Institute of Health & Clinical Excellence (NICE) (Howard and Hughes 2013) recommends immediate CTPA or immediate interim anticoagulant therapy followed by a CTPA, if a CTPA cannot be performed immediately. Similarly, the European Society of Cardiology (Konstantinides et al. 2014) describes CTPA as the method of choice for the investigation of PE. Conversely, the European Association of Nuclear Medicine broadly recommends V/Q SPECT over CTPA, where available (Bajc et al. 2009b), on the basis of the advantages of V/Q SPECT, including absence of contrast agent injection, lower radiation burden and better estimation of PE extent based upon the functional impact.

A recent elegant work by Phillips JJ et al. aimed to comparing different imaging techniques for PE detection (planar V/Q, V/Q SPECT and CTPA), by performing a systematic literature review and aggregating available data using a summary ROC analysis (Phillips et al. 2015). In addition, this study has quantified the diagnostic costs per correct result and the radiation burden per correct diagnosis for each technique. Authors found that CTPA and V/Q SPECT show equivalent diagnostic performance and both clearly outperform planar V/Q. The cost per correct diagnosis indicated that CTPA was least expensive and V/Q SPECT was shown to be the most effective per unit of radiation dose received. This would suggest that V/Q SPECT should be favoured over CTPA when radiation dose is a concern, for example, in radiosensitive patients (young, pregnant, etc.). Nevertheless, the modern effective dose-reduction strategies of which the last generation CT scanners are equipped and which would further reduce radiation burden have not been taken into consideration in the available studies in medical literature. Also in patients with contrast medium allergy or renal failure, V/Q SPECT may be a valid diagnostic alternative for PE.

A clear advantage that CTPA has over SPECT in the evaluation of patients with suspected PE is the chance of finding alternative diagnoses to explain symptoms, the speed of exam execution and the ready availability within 24 h.

4.4 Conclusions

In an emergency clinical background of suspected PE, CTPA is the modality of choice to detect or exclude PE because of its very high accuracy, availability, rapidity and low cost compared to the other imaging modalities. However, in patients for whom CTPA may be disadvantageous, V/Q scintigraphy or Q scintigraphy alone often yields diagnostically definitive results and can be considered appropriate pulmonary imaging procedures. V/Q SPECT has a better performance when compared to planar scintigraphic imaging and yields lower radiation burden; however, it is not routinely used as a primary diagnostic method for PE. Nowadays, DECT has the capacity to improve further the diagnostic accuracy of PE through comprehensive analysis of lung "perfusion" and CTPA obtained during a single contrast-enhanced chest CT, without adding radiation dose.

5 Non-thrombotic Pulmonary Embolism

Non-thrombotic pulmonary embolism is an uncommon condition caused by embolization of different materials, and it is often associated with specific imaging findings (Rossi et al. 2000).

5.1 Fat Embolism

Fat (or lipid) embolism is the most common among non-thrombotic pulmonary embolism. It occurs after multiple fractures of long bones and pelvis, mostly in patients with fractures of the middle-proximal femoral shaft. The percentages of this complication range from 2 to 20 % in different studies and mortality close to 10 %. Although these emboli can virtually reach any organ, the consequences of this "embolic rain" are more clearly visible in the lungs, brain and skin (Han et al. 2003). The pathogenic mechanisms of fat embolism are not completely understood but presumably are twofold. The first mechanism is the production of free fatty acids, which determine a toxic reaction in the endothelium, amplified by inflammatory mediators. The second theory is represented by mechanical obstruction of the pulmonary artery branches by fat emboli. Clinical manifestations occur 1–3 days after the trauma due to the involvement of the lungs, brain and skin (Malagari et al. 2003).

Three to four percent of patients develop the fat embolism syndrome (FES, fat embolism syndrome) characterized by respiratory distress, brain abnormalities and cutaneous petechiae. The diagnosis of fat embolism syndrome requires the presence of a major criterion and at least four minor criteria. Based on Gurd's and Wilson's criteria, the major criteria are petechial rash, respiratory insufficiency and cerebral involvement. Minor criteria are tachycardia, fever, retinal changes, jaundice, renal signs, thrombocytopenia, anaemia, high erythrocyte sedimentation rate (ESR), fat macroglobinaemia (Gurd and Wilson 1974).

Chest X-ray (Fig. 16a, b) and chest CT (Fig. 16c, d) findings resemble those of acute respiratory distress syndrome from any cause and consist of widespread homogenous and heterogeneous areas of increased opacity. CT angiography does not show the presence of vascular filling defects because the fat embolus involves capillaries.

Differential diagnosis should be made with pulmonary oedema and pulmonary contusion. In the first case, CT scans demonstrate smooth septal interlobular thickening, pleural effusion and ground glass opacities, while in the pulmonary contusion, CT alterations occur immediately after the trauma, whereas alterations due to fat embolism occur after 24–48 h from injury.

5.2 Cement Embolism

This condition is a complication of percutaneous vertebroplasty, and it is caused by migration of polymethyl methacrylate's particles in the pulmonary vessels via external vertebral venous plexus. A symptomatic onset is rare. The percentage of embolization to the lungs is unknown, as patients are not submitted to radiographic examination of the chest before and after the procedure (Choe et al. 2004). Both chest X-ray and CT may demonstrate linear

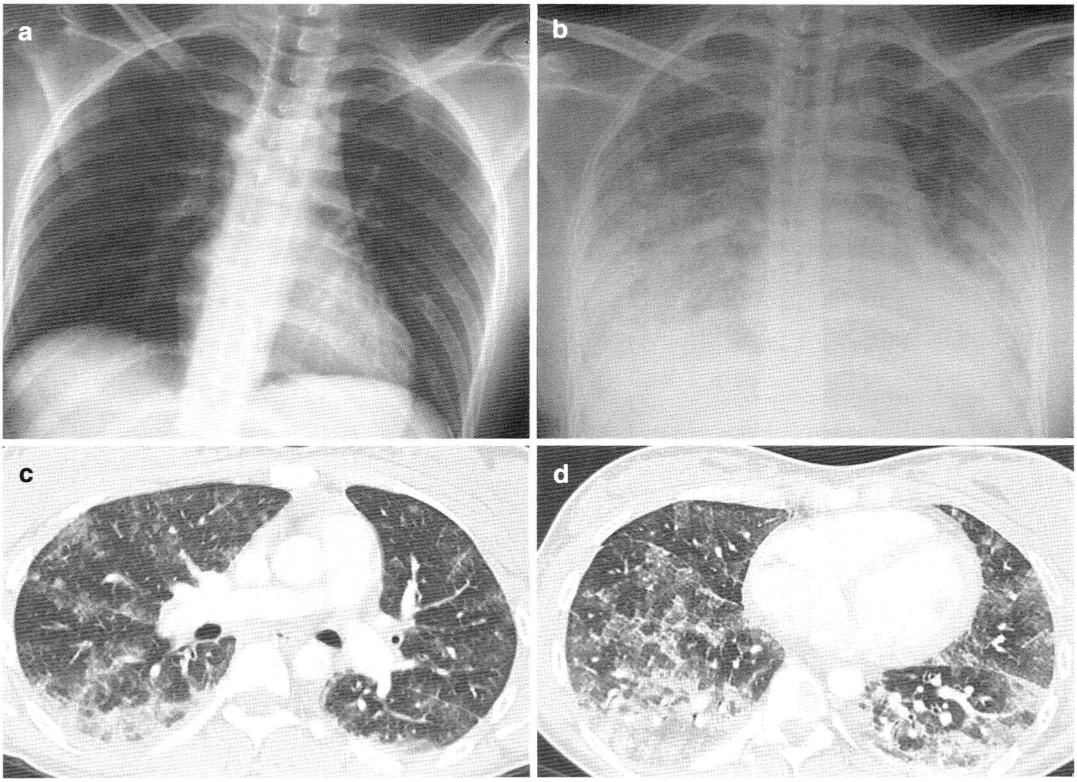

Fig. 16 Twenty-five-year-old woman with a tibial fracture treated with osteosynthesis. Chest X-ray immediately after trauma doesn't show any abnormality (**a**). After 2 days, the patient had a rapid onset of dyspnoea, and a chest X-ray was performed showing multiple bilateral alveolar opacities engaging especially the lower lobes (**b**). CT scans (**c**, **d**) confirm areas of ground glass opacities, consolidation and minimal smooth septal thickening. No pulmonary filling defects were seen on enhanced CT scans (not shown)

images of increased opacity or attenuation outlining the pulmonary arteries (Fig. 17a–d).

5.3 Septic Embolism

Septic embolism occurs after embolization of fragments of infected emboli, usually by bacteria and less frequently fungi or parasites. The predisposing factors include tricuspid valve endocarditis, alcoholism, infections of the skin and immunodeficiency's condition (particularly lymphoma). The septic emboli can also be found in patients with central venous catheters or permanent pacemaker (Han et al. 2003). Chest CT shows peripheral nodules of different sizes, with blurred margins, sometimes with excavation or subpleural, triangular areas of consolidation (Fig. 18a–c). Sometimes an arterial branch directly related to the hump of the consolidation, "feeding vessel sign", can also be seen.

CT angiography can show increased calibre of pulmonary arteries and pseudoaneurysms.

5.4 Air Embolism

Air embolism is a pathological condition that arises when one or more air bubbles can block blood flow within a vessel. Iatrogenic causes of air embolism include transthoracic biopsy, baro-

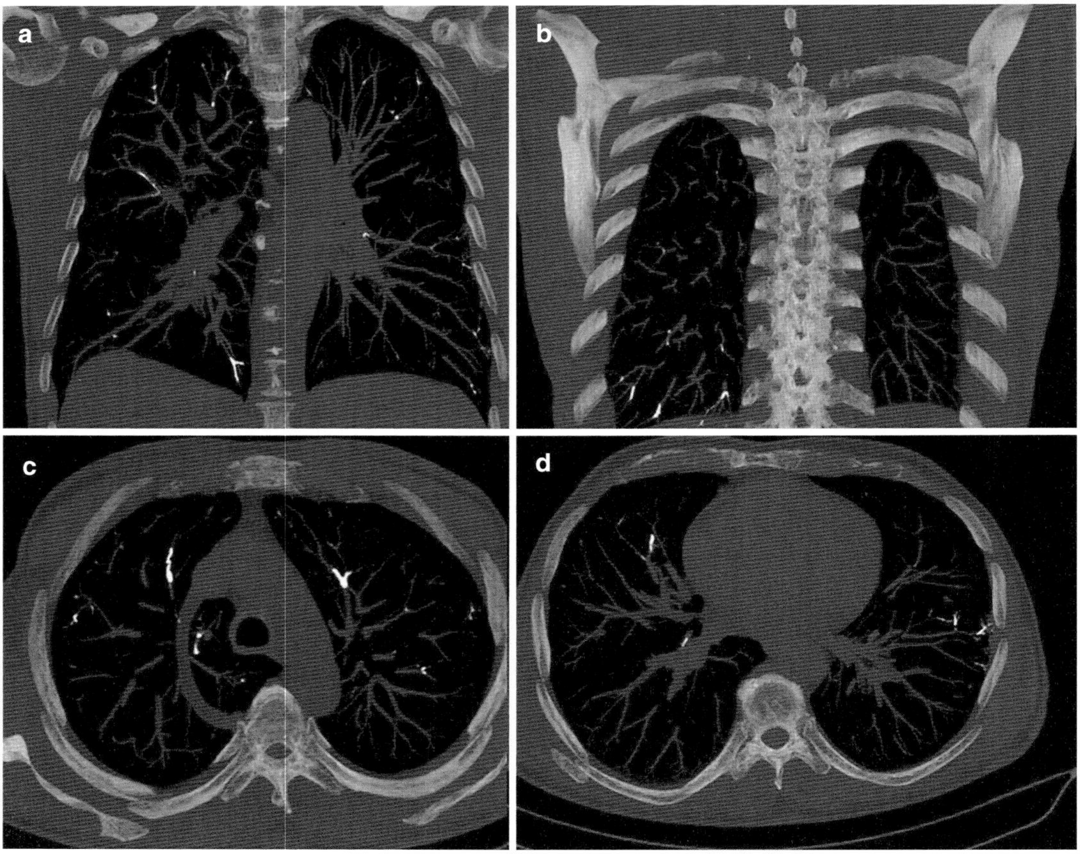

Fig. 17 MIP-reformatted CT images in coronal (**a**, **b**) and axial (**c**, **d**) planes showing multiple polymethyl methacrylate emboli in segmental and subsegmental levels. Patient had undergone lumbar percutaneous vertebroplasty 2 months before

trauma caused by positive-pressure ventilation, haemodialysis and the placement of central venous catheters (Han et al. 2003).

The risk of death depends on the amount of air introduced and the speed of introduction: 300–500 mL and 100 mL/s, respectively, represent the minimum amount of air and the speed of lethal injections to humans. Chest X-ray can be completely normal or sometimes can show areas of hyperlucency projecting to the heart or pulmonary vessels. On chest CT, it is possible to point out air bubbles within the pulmonary arteries and veins (Fig. 19a, b).

5.5 Hydatid Embolism

The hydatid embolism is a rare complication of heart and liver echinococcosis. Embolization of hydatid material can occur by (a) breaking of the cysts, especially if localized at cardiac level; (b) "jump" of the embryo through the porta-caval anastomosis, with the spread of hydatid material in the right cardiac chambers and from here in the pulmonary arteries; or (c) direct transfer of hydatid material (daughter cysts and scolices) in the pulmonary vascular bed through the "vasa vasorum" (Mereu et al. 2001). The slow growth of hydatid cysts in pulmonary arterial branches

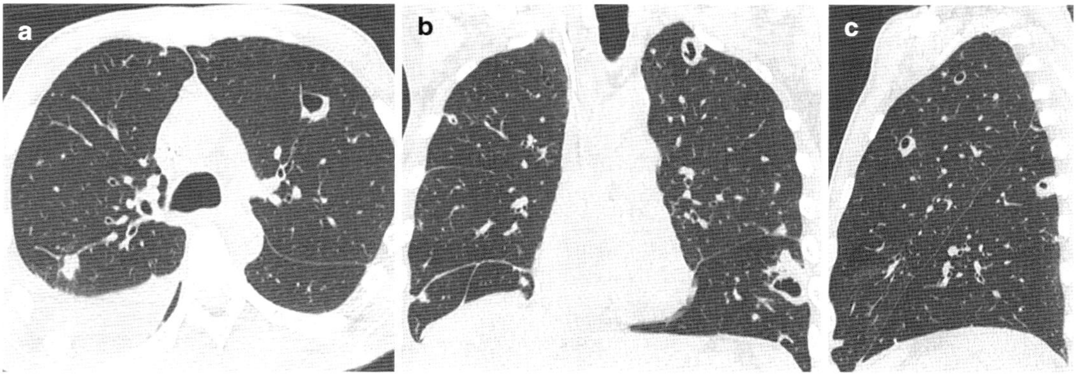

Fig. 18 CT scan above the carina (**a**) and coronal (**b**) and sagittal (**c**) reformatted images showing multiple cavitary nodules and consolidations bilaterally. This was consistent with septic embolism in a 34-year-old intravenous drug abuser with *human immunodeficiency virus*

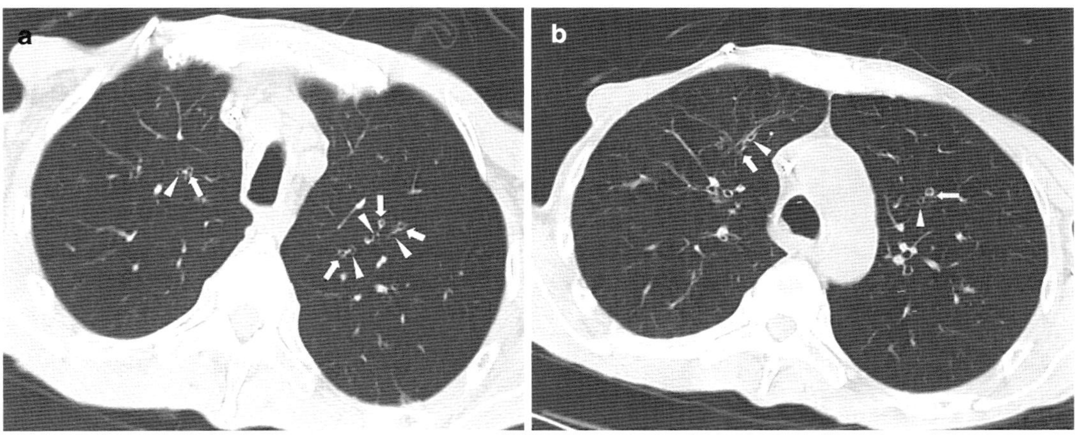

Fig. 19 CT examination in a patient with cancer of the larynx and recent placement of central venous catheter. CT scans show air in the segmental arteries of the upper lobes (*arrows* in **a**, **b**); normal bronchi are pointed out by *arrowheads*

explains the absence of symptoms in the early phase because of adequate compensation through the arteries (Han et al. 2003). The symptoms may be caused by compression of the hydatid cysts of vital structures as well as the reduction or interruption of blood flow and are represented by coughing, chest pain, dyspnoea and haemoptysis. Other clinical manifestations may be sudden death for massive pulmonary embolism, pulmonary hypertension with subacute and right ventricular failure or chronic pulmonary hypertension (Pena and Dennie 2012). Chest CT demonstrates occlusion of pulmonary arterial branches by hypodense material, direct visualization of the cystic lesions and increasing the calibre of the vessel concerned (inconstant finding) (Fig. 20a–c).

5.6 Tumour Embolism

It may be observed in patients with hepatocellular carcinoma, breast, renal, gastric and prostate cancer or choriocarcinoma. Tumour intravascular embolization can be observed up

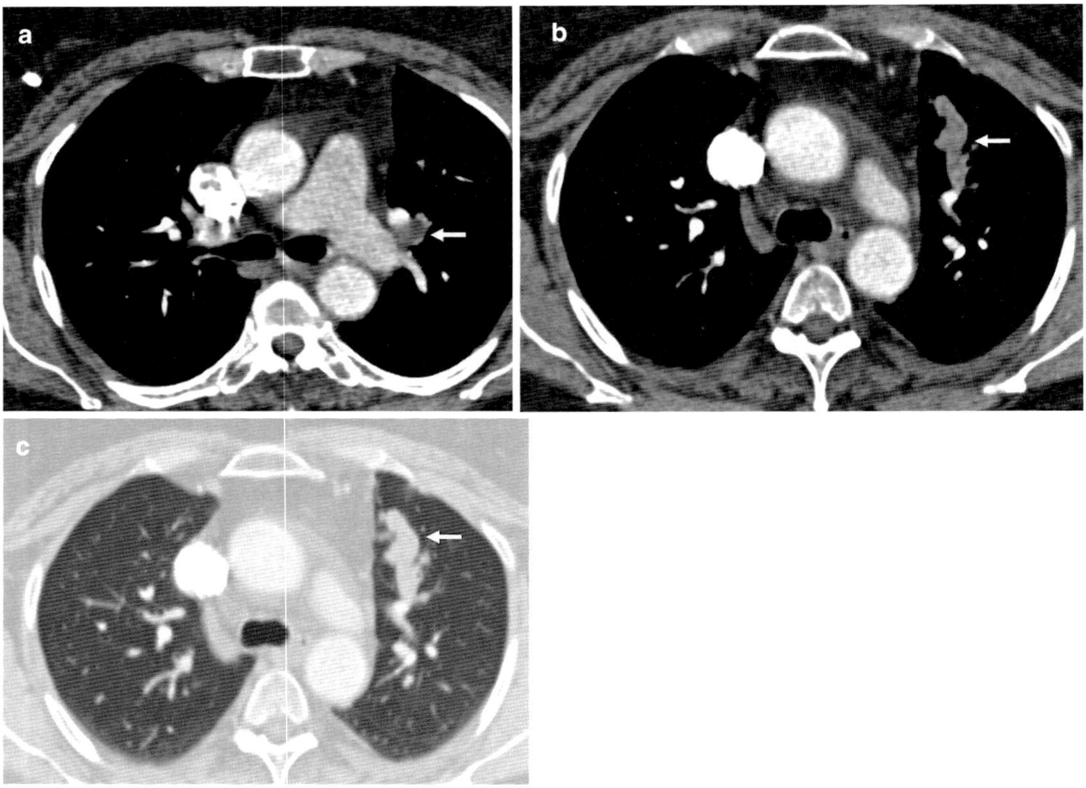

Fig. 20 CT examination in patient with previous history of anaphylactic shock for a ruptured hepatic hydatid cyst. Enhanced chest CT scans with mediastinal (**a**, **b**) and lung (**c**) window setting show endoluminal defects with low density in the left upper lobe artery (*arrows*), with prominent enlargement of the vessel

to 26 % of autopsy. Clinical symptoms may be represented by wheezing, coughing and signs of hypoxia and pulmonary hypertension. The radiographic findings are often minimal or nonspecific, making the radiological diagnosis difficult (Tack et al. 2001). CT findings are areas of focal or diffuse consolidation representing areas of pulmonary infarction, increase in the calibre of pulmonary arteries (pulmonary hypertension) and prominence of small peripheral arterial branches with "tree-in-bud" pattern supported by filled centrilobular arteries by tumour microemboli (Fig. 21) associated with a thrombotic microangiopathy in which the tumour emboli are responsible of wide fibrocellular intimal proliferation that causes thrombosis and obliteration of the lumen.

5.7 Miscellaneous Foreign Body Embolism

Central venous catheters are routinely used in oncology; spontaneous rupture and embolization of a catheter are rare complications (Han et al. 2003). The most common sites of embolization are the basilic vein and pulmonary arteries (Fig. 22a, b).

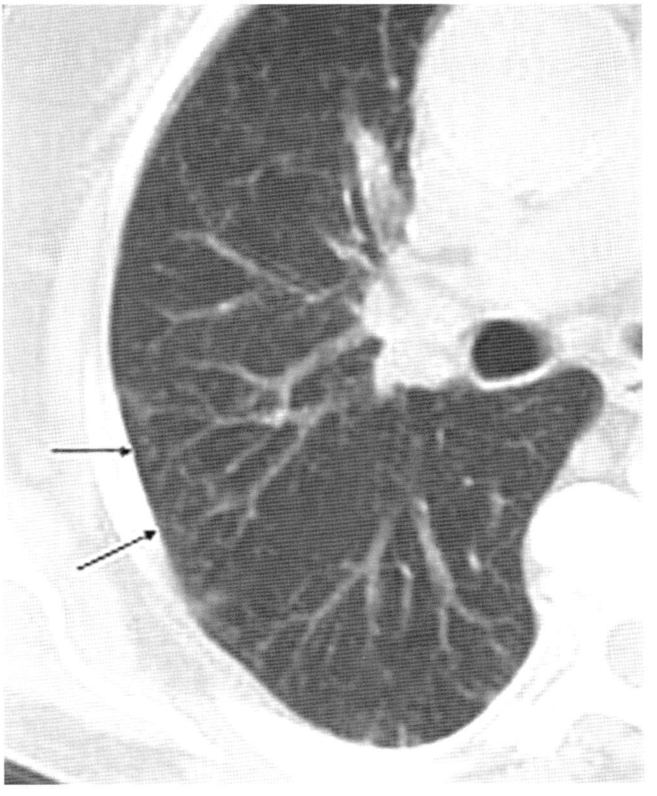

Fig. 21 CT scan shows multifocal tree-in-bud appearance (*arrows*) caused by tumour emboli

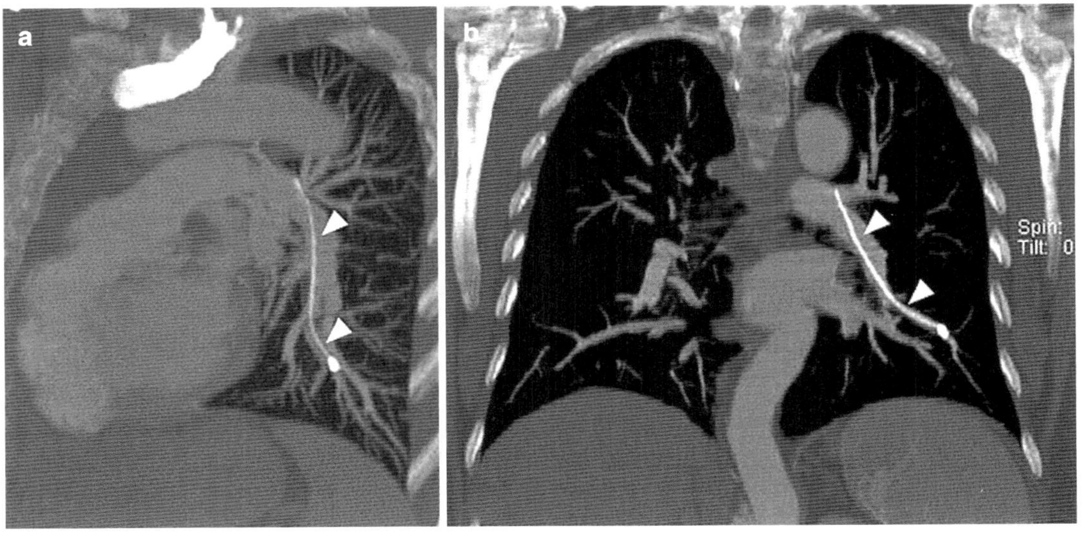

Fig. 22 MIP Sagittal (**a**) and coronal (**b**) reformatted CT images show the presence of a fragment of central venous catheter (*arrowheads*) migrated in the left main pulmonary artery and left lower lobe artery

References

Ameli-Renani S, Rahman F, Nair A et al (2014) Dual-energy CT for imaging of pulmonary hypertension: challenges and opportunities. Radiographics 34(7):1769–1790

Bajc M, Jonson B (2011) Ventilation/perfusion SPECT for diagnosis of pulmonary embolism and other diseases. Int J Mol Imaging 2011:682949

Bajc M, Neilly J, Miniati M et al (2009a) EANM guidelines for ventilation/perfusion scintigraphy. Eur J Nucl Med Mol Imaging 36:1528–1538

Bajc M, Neilly JB, Miniati M et al (2009b) EANM guidelines for ventilation/perfusion scintigraphy: part 1. Pulmonary imaging with ventilation/perfusion single photon emission tomography. Eur J Nucl Med Mol Imaging 36(8):1356–1370

Barritt DW, Jordan SC (1960) Anticoagulant drugs in the treatment of pulmonary embolism: a controlled trial. Lancet 1:1309–1312

Bierry G, Holl N, Kellner F et al (2008) Venous thromboembolism and occult malignancy: simultaneous detection during pulmonary CT angiography with CT venography. AJR Am J Roentgenol 191:885–889

Carson JL, Kelley MA, Duff A et al (1992) The clinical course of pulmonary embolism. N Engl J Med 326: 1240–1245

Cham MD, Yankelevitz DF, Henschke CI (2005) Thromboembolic disease detection at indirect CT venography versus CT pulmonary angiography. Radiology 234:591–594

Choe DH, Marom EM, Ahrar K et al (2004) Pulmonary embolism of polymethyl methacrylate during percutaneous vertebroplasty and kyphoplasty. AJR Am J Roentgenol 183:1097–1102

Cohen AT, Agnelli G, Anderson FA et al (2007) Venous thromboembolism (VTE) in Europe. The number of VTE events and associated morbidity and mortality. Thromb Haemost 98(4):756–764

Cox JE, Chiles C, Aquino SL et al (1997) Pulmonary artery sarcomas: a review of clinical and radiologic features. J Comput Assist Tomogr 21:750–755

Dalen J, Alpert JS (1975) Natural history of pulmonary embolism. Prog Cardiovasc Dis 14:257–270

Fink C, Johnson TR, Michaely HJ et al (2008) Dual-energy CT angiography of the lung in patients with suspected pulmonary embolism: initial results. Rofo 180:879–883

Freeman LM (2008) Don't bury the V/Q scan: it's as good as multidetector CT angiograms with a lot less radiation exposure. J Nucl Med 49:5–8

Ghaye B, Dondelinger RF (2007) When to perform CTA in patients suspected of PE? Eur Radiol 18:500–509

Ghaye B, Szapiro D, Mastora I et al (2001) Peripheral pulmonary arteries: how far in the lung does multi-detector row spiral CT allow analysis. Radiology 219(3):629–636

Ghaye B, Remy J, Remy-Jardin M (2002) Non-traumatic thoracic emergencies: CT diagnosis of acute pulmonary embolism: the first 10 years. Eur Radiol 12:1886–1905

Gurd AR, Wilson RE (1974) The fat embolism syndrome. J Bone Joint Surg Br 56:408–416

Han D, Lee KS, Franquet T et al (2003) Thrombotic and nonthrombotic pulmonary arterial embolism: spectrum of imaging findings. Radiographics 23:1521–1539

Heck LL, Duley JW (1974) Statistical considerations in lung imaging with 99mTc albumin particles. Radiology 113(3):675–679

Heit JA (2008) The epidemiology of venous thromboembolism in the community. Arterioscler Thromb Vasc Biol 28(3):370–372

Hoang JK, Lee WK, Hennessy OF (2008) Multidetector CT pulmonary angiography features of pulmonary embolus. J Med Imaging Radiat Oncol 52:307–317

Hoeper MM, Mayer E, Simonneau G et al (2006) Chronic thromboembolic pulmonary hypertension. Circulation 113:2011–2020

Howard LS, Hughes RJ (2013) NICE guideline: management of venous thromboembolic diseases and role of thrombophilia testing. Thorax 68(4):391–393

Hu XP, Xu JP, Liu NN (2009) Primary pulmonary artery sarcoma: surgical management and differential diagnosis with pulmonary embolism and pulmonary valve stenosis. J Card Surg 24:613–616

Kanne JP, Gotway MB, Thoongsuwan N et al (2003) Six cases of acute central pulmonary embolism revealed on unenhanced multidetector CT of the chest. AJR Am J Roentgenol 180:1661–1664

Katz DS, Loud PA, Bruce D et al (2002) Combined CT venography and pulmonary angiography: a comprehensive review. Radiographics 22(Spec Issue):S3–S19

Kelly AM, Patel S, Carlos RC et al (2006) Multidetector-row CT pulmonary angiography and indirect venography for the diagnosis of venous thromboembolic disease in intensive care unit patients. Acad Radiol 13:486–495

Konstantinides S, Agnelli A, Danchin G et al (2014) 2014 ESC guidelines on the diagnosis and management of acute pulmonary embolism. Eur Heart J 14:3033–3073

Kuriakose J, Patel S (2010) Acute pulmonary embolism. Radiol Clin North Am 48:31–50

Long SS, Johnson P, Hruban RH et al (2010) CT features of pulmonary artery sarcoma: critical aid to a challenging diagnosis. Emerg Radiol 17:153–155

Loud PA, Katz DS, Bruce D et al (2001) Deep venous thrombosis with suspected pulmonary embolism: detection with combined CT venography and pulmonary angiography. Radiology 219:498–501

Lu GM, Wu SY, Yeh BM, Zhang LJ (2010) Dual-energy computed tomography in pulmonary embolism. Br J Radiol 83(992):707–718

Macdonald WB, Patrikeos AP, Thompson RI et al (2005) Diagnosis of pulmonary embolism: ventilation perfusion scintigraphy versus helical computed tomography pulmonary angiography. Australas Radiol 49(1):32–38

Malagari K, Economopoulos N, Stoupis C et al (2003) High resolution CT findings in mild pulmonary fat embolism. Chest 123:1196–1201

Mason GR, Peters AM, Bagdades E et al (2001) Evaluation of pulmonary alveolar epithelial integrity by the detection of restriction to diffusion of hydrophilic solutes of different molecular sizes. Clin Sci 100(3):231–236

Mereu M, Guidotti A, Marano R et al (2001) Embolia polmonare multipla idatidea: descrizione di un caso. Radiol Med 102:397–399

Mos I, Klok F, Kroft L et al (2012) Imaging tests in the diagnosis of pulmonary embolism. Semin Respir Crit Care Med 33:138–143

Ocak I, Fuhrman C (2008) CT angiography findings of the left atrium and right ventricle in patients with massive pulmonary embolism. AJR Am J Roentgenol 191: 1072–1076

Patel S, Kazerooni EA (2005) Helical CT for the evaluation of acute pulmonary embolism. AJR Am J Roentgenol 185:135–149

Patel S, Kazerooni EA, Cascade PN (2003) Pulmonary embolism: optimization of small pulmonary artery visualization at multi–detector row CT. Radiology 227:455–460

Pena E, Dennie C (2012) Acute and chronic pulmonary embolism: an in-depth review for radiologists through the use of frequently asked questions. Semin Ultrasound CT MR 33:500–521

Perrier A, Howarth N, Didier D et al (2001) Performance of helical computed tomography in unselected outpatient with suspected pulmonary embolism. Ann Intern Med 135:88–97

Petty GW, Lennihan L, Mohr JP et al (1988) Complications of long term anticoagulation. Ann Neurol 23:570–574

Phillips JJ, Straiton J, Staff RT (2015) Planar and SPECT ventilation/perfusion imaging and computed tomography for the diagnosis of pulmonary embolism: a systematic review and meta-analysis of the literature, and cost and dose comparison. Eur J Radiol 84(7):1392–1400

PIOPED Investigators (1990) Value of the ventilation/perfusion scan in acute pulmonary embolism. Results of the prospective investigation of pulmonary embolism diagnosis (PIOPED). JAMA 263(20):2753–2759

Pontana F, Faivre JB, Remy-Jardin M et al (2008) Lung perfusion with dual-energy multidetector- row CT (MDCT) feasibility for the evaluation of acute pulmonary embolism in 117 consecutive patients. Acad Radiol 15:1494–1504

Qanadli SD, Hajjam ME, Mesurolle B et al (2000) Pulmonary embolism detection: prospective evaluation of dual-section helical CT versus selective pulmonary arteriography in 157 patients. Radiology 217:447–455

Quiroz R, Kucher N, Zou KH et al (2005) Clinical validity of a negative computed tomography scan in patients with suspected pulmonary embolism: a systematic review. JAMA 293:2012–2017

Remy-Jardin M, Pistolesi M, Goodman LR et al (2007) Management of suspected acute pulmonary embolism in the era of CT angiography: a Statement from the Fleischner Society. Radiology 245(2):315–329

Revel MP, Petrover D, Hernigou A et al (2005) Diagnosing pulmonary embolism with four–detector row helical CT: prospective evaluation of 216 outpatients and inpatients. Radiology 234:265–273

Rossi SE, Goodman PC, Franquet T. Nonthrombotic pulmonary emboli. Am J Roentgenol. 2000 Jun;174(6):1499–508.

Russell JR, Stabin MG, Sparks RB, Watson E (1997) Radiation absorbed dose to the embryo/fetus from radiopharmaceuticals. Health Phys 73:756–769

Senden TJ, Moock KH, Gerald JF et al (1997) The physical and chemical nature of technegas. J Nucl Med 38(8):1327–1333

Sostman HD, Coleman RE, DeLong DM et al (1994) Evaluation of revised criteria for ventilation-perfusion scintigraphy in patients with suspected pulmonary embolism. Radiology 193(1):103–107

Sostman HD, Stein PD, Gottschalk A et al (2008a) Acute pulmonary embolism: sensitivity and specificity of ventilation-perfusion scintigraphy in PIOPED II study. Radiology 246:941–946

Sostman HD, Miniati M, Gottschalk A et al (2008b) Sensitivity and specificity of perfusion scintigraphy combined with chest radiography for acute pulmonary embolism in PIOPED II. J Nucl Med 49(11):1741–1748

Stein PD, Fowler SE, Goodman LR et al (2006) Multidetector computed tomography for acute pulmonary embolism. N Engl J Med 354:2317–2327

Tack D, Nollevaux MC, Gevenois PA (2001) Tree-in-bud pattern in neoplastic pulmonary emboli. AJR Am J Roentgenol 176:1421–1422

Taffoni MJ, Ravenel JG, Ackerman SJ (2005) Prospective comparison of indirect CT venography versus venous sonography in ICU patients. AJR Am J Roentgenol 185:457–462

Thieme SF, Becker CR, Hacker M et al (2008) Dual energy CT for the assessment of lung perfusion — correlation to scintigraphy. Eur J Radiol 68:369–374

Thieme SF, Graute V, Nikolaou K et al (2012) Dual energy CT lung perfusion imaging: correlation with SPECT/CT. Eur J Radiol 81(2):360–365

Tillie-Leblond I, Marquette CH, Perez T et al (2006) Pulmonary embolism in patients with unexplained exacerbation of chronic obstructive pulmonary disease: prevalence and risk factors. Ann Intern Med 144:390–396

Winer-Muram HT, Boone JM, Brown HL et al (2002) Pulmonary embolism in pregnant patients: fetal radiation dose with helical CT. Radiology 224:487–492

Winer-Muram HT, Rydberg J, Johnson MS et al (2004) Suspected acute pulmonary embolism: evaluation with multi-detector row CT versus digital subtraction pulmonary arteriography. Radiology 233:806–815

Wittram C (2007) How I do it: CT pulmonary angiography. AJR Am J Roentgenol 188:1255–1261

Wittram C, Maher M, Yoo A et al (2004) CT angiography of pulmonary embolism: diagnostic criteria and causes of misdiagnosis. Radiographics 24:1219–1238

Zhang LJ, Yang GF, Zhao YE et al (2009) Detection of pulmonary embolism using dual-energy computed tomography and correlation with cardiovascular measurements: a preliminary study. Acta Radiol 50: 892–901

Index

DOI 10.1007/174_2016, © Springer International Publishing Switzerland

B

D

E

Printed by Printforce, the Netherlands